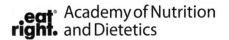
Academy of Nutrition and Dietetics

SECOND EDITION

Health Professional's Guide *to* Gastrointestinal Nutrition

EDITORS

Laura E. Matarese, PhD, RDN, LDN, FADA, FASPEN, FAND

Gerard E. Mullin, MD, AGAF, FACG, FACN

Kelly A. Tappenden, PhD, RDN, FASPEN

eat right. Academy of Nutrition and Dietetics

Academy of Nutrition and Dietetics
120 S. Riverside Plaza, Suite 2190
Chicago, IL 60606

Health Professional's Guide to Gastrointestinal Nutrition, Second Edition

ISBN 978-0-88091-216-7 (print)
ISBN 978-0-88091-217-4 (eBook)
Catalog Number 450523 (print)
Catalog Number 450523e (eBook)

10 9 8 7 6 5 4 3 2 1

For more information on the Academy of Nutrition and Dietetics, visit
www.eatright.org.

Library of Congress Cataloging-in-Publication Data
Library of Congress Cataloging-in-Publication Data

Names: Matarese, Laura E., editor. | Mullin, Gerard E., editor. |
  Tappenden, Kelly A., editor.
Title: Health professional's guide to gastrointestinal nutrition / Laura E.
  Matarese, PhD, RDN, LDN, FADA, FASPEN, FAND, Gerard E. Mullin, MD, AGAF,
  FACG, Kelly A. Tappenden, PhD, RDN, FASPEN.
Description: Second edition. | Chicago, IL : Academy of Nutrition and
  Dietetics, [2022] | Includes bibliographical references and index.
Identifiers: LCCN 2022038257 (print) | LCCN 2022038258 (ebook) | ISBN
  9780880912167 (print) | ISBN 9780880912174 (eBook)
Subjects: LCSH: Gastrointestinal system--Diseases--Nutritional aspects.
Classification: LCC RC802 .H43 2022 (print) | LCC RC802 (ebook) | DDC
  616.3/30654--dc23/eng/20220829
LC record available at https://lccn.loc.gov/2022038257
LC ebook record available at https://lccn.loc.gov/2022038258

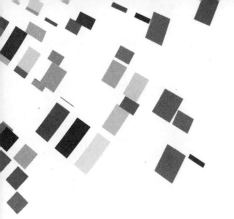

Contents

SECTION 1

Gastrointestinal Nutrition Assessment and Diagnostics

SECTION 2

Nutrition and Gastrointestinal-Related Disorders

List of Boxes, Tables, and Figures

BOXES

TABLES

FIGURES

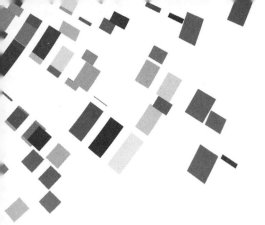

Frequently Used Terms and Abbreviations

AAD	antibiotic-associated diarrhea
AANH	artificially administered nutrition and hydration
AGB	adjustable gastric banding
AN	anorexia nervosa
ARFID	avoidant/restrictive food intake disorder
BCAA	branched-chain amino acid
BCFA	branched-chain fatty acid
BED	binge eating disorder
BEE	basal energy expenditure
BN	bulimia nervosa
BPD/DS	biliopancreatic diversion with duodenal switch
BTF	blenderized tube feeding
CACS	cancer anorexia-cachexia syndrome
CAM	complementary and alternative medicine
CBT	cognitive behavioral therapy
CDI	*Clostridioides difficile* infection
CF	cystic fibrosis
CRP	C-reactive protein
CVC	central venous catheters
DASH	Dietary Approaches to Stop Hypertension
DHA	docosahexaenoic acid
DRI	Dietary Reference Intake
DXA	dual-energy x-ray absorptiometry
EFA	essential fatty acid
EN	enteral nutrition
EoE	eosinophilic esophagitis
EPA	eicosapentaenoic acid
ERAS	enhanced recovery after surgery
FFQ	food frequency questionnaire
FODMAP	fermentable oligosaccharides, disaccharides, monosaccharides, and polyols
FOS	fructo-oligosaccharide
FPIAP	food protein–induced allergic proctocolitis
FPIES	food protein–induced enterocolitis syndrome
GERD	gastroesophageal reflux disease
G-tube	gastrostomy tube
GOS	galacto-oligosaccharide
GRV	gastric rehydration volume
HEN	home enteral nutrition

HPEN	home parenteral and enteral nutrition
HPN	home parenteral nutrition
IBD	inflammatory bowel disease
IBS	irritable bowel syndrome
IgE	Immunoglobulin E
IL-6	Interleukin-6
ILE	intravenous lipid emulsion
IV	intravenous
LCT	long-chain triglycerides
LGG	*Lacticaseibacillus rhamnosus* GG
MCT	medium-chain triglycerides
MST	Malnutrition Screening Tool
NAFLD	nonalcoholic fatty liver disease
NUTRIC	Nutrition Risk in the Critically Ill
OIT	oral immunotherapy
ORS	oral rehydration solution
OSFED	other specified feeding or eating disorder
PEG	percutaneous endoscopic gastrostomy
PEI	pancreatic exocrine insufficiency
PEJ	percutaneous endoscopic jejunostomy
PERT	pancreatic enzyme replacement therapy
PG-SGA	patient-generated subjective global assessment
PICC	peripherally inserted central catheter
PN	parenteral nutrition
PNAC	parenteral nutrition–associated cholestasis
QOL	quality of life
RMR	resting metabolic rate
RYGB	Roux-en-Y gastric bypass
SBS	short bowel syndrome
SCFA	short-chain fatty acid
SDM	surrogate decision maker
SG	sleeve gastrectomy
SGA	subjective global assessment
SIBO	small intestine bacterial overgrowth
SMA	superior mesenteric artery
SOFA	sequential organ failure assessment
STEP	serial transverse enteroplasty
T1DM	type 1 diabetes mellitus
T2DM	type 2 diabetes mellitus
TNF	tumor necrosis factor
UBW	usual body weight
UFED	unspecified feeding or eating disorder
VLCD	very low-calorie diet

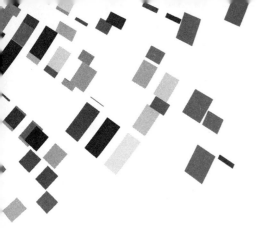

About the Editors

Laura E. Matarese, PhD, RDN, LDN, FADA, FASPEN, FAND is a professor of Medicine in the Division of Gastroenterology, Hepatology, and Nutrition, Department of Internal Medicine and Adjunct Professor of Surgery at the Brody School of Medicine at East Carolina University in Greenville, NC. She has over 40 years of experience in nutrition support and gastrointestinal nutrition. She is the author of numerous manuscripts, bookzs, chapters, abstracts, and videos and currently serves on the editorial boards of several journals. She has lectured extensively, both nationally and internationally and has held numerous positions within the Academy of Nutrition and Dietetics, the Commission on Dietetic Registration, and the American Society for Parenteral and Enteral Nutrition. Dr Matarese is the past president of the National Board of Nutrition Support Certification and currently serves as a councillor for the Obesity, Metabolism and Nutrition section of the American Gastroenterological Association and on the Board of Advisors of The Oley Foundation. She is the recipient of numerous honors and awards. Prior to matriculation to East Carolina University, Dr Matarese held positions at the University of Cincinnati Medical Center, the Cleveland Clinic, and the Starzl Transplant Institute at the University of Pittsburgh.

Gerard E. Mullin, MD, AGAF, FACG, FACN, is an associate professor of medicine at the Johns Hopkins University School of Medicine. He is board-certified in internal medicine and gastroenterology. Nationally and internationally renowned for his work in nutrition, Dr Mullin has more than 30 years of clinical experience in the field of gastroenterology. In 2009, he was selected by the American Dietetic Association as honorary member of the year. At this time, Dr Mullin was the youngest person to receive an Honorary membership from the American Dietetic Association. He also received the Grace A. Goldsmith award presented by the American College of Nutrition in November 2011. This special award acknowledges a scientist who is under the age of 50 years for significant achievements in the field of nutrition. Dr Mullin is a reviewer and also serves on the editorial board of numerous gastroenterology journals.

Kelly A. Tappenden, PhD, RDN, FASPEN received her PhD in nutrition and metabolism at the University of Alberta, underwent post-doctoral training at the University of Texas Medical School in Houston, and joined the faculty at the University of Illinois at Urbana in 1997 as an Assistant Professor. She was promoted to Associate Professor in 2003 and Professor in 2008. In 2011, she was named a University of Illinois Distinguished Teacher-Scholar—the premier campus award recognizing excellence in teaching and learning—and in 2012, the Kraft Foods Human Nutrition Endowed Professor. Dr Tappenden's current position is Professor and Head of the Department of Kinesiology and Nutrition at the University of Illinois at Chicago. Dr Tappenden's research program focuses on intestinal failure, mechanisms regulating epithelial function, and patient malnutrition. For these contributions, she has received multiple awards, published over 100 peer-reviewed papers, and delivered over 500 invited lectures. Dr Tappenden served as the 33rd President of the American Society for Parenteral and Enteral Nutrition from 2008 to 2009, Chair of the Nutrition, Metabolism and Obesity section of the American Gastroenterology Association Institute from 2009 to 2013, and presently represents the American Society for Nutrition on the Federation of American Societies for Experimental Biology Board of Directors. Dr Tappenden has been the Editor-in-Chief of the *Journal for Parenteral and Enteral Nutrition* since 2010.

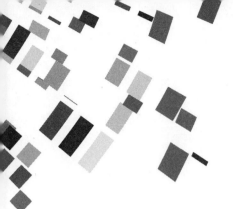

Contributors

Maria S. Altieri, MD, MS
Assistant Professor, Bariatric and Minimally Invasive Surgery
Associate Program Director, General Surgery Residency
Brody School of Medicine at East Carolina University
Greenville, NC

Sumeet K. Asrani, MD, MSc
Doctor, Liver Consultants of Texas
Dallas, TX

Stephanie Merlino Barr, MS, RDN, LD
Neonatal Nutritionist, MetroHealth Medical Center
Cleveland, OH

Albert Barrocas, MD, FACS, FASPEN
Adjunct Professor of Surgery,
Tulane University School of Medicine
Atlanta, GA

Therese Berry, MS, RDN, LD, CNSC
Infusion Nutrition Support Dietitian,
Coram CVS Specialty Infusion Services
Cleveland, OH

Justin Brandler, MD
Gastroenterology and Hepatology Fellow, University of Michigan
Ann Arbor, MI

Jennifer R. Bridenbaugh, MS, RD, CNSC
Assistant Professor, School of Health Professions,
Rutgers University
New Brunswick, NJ

Lawrence J. Cheskin, MD, FACP, FTOS
Professor and Chair, Nutrition and Food Studies,
George Mason University
Fairfax, VA

William D. Chey, MD
Nostrant Collegiate Professor of Gastroenterology and Nutrition
Sciences; Chief, Division of Gastroenterology & Hepatology,
Michigan Medicine
Ann Arbor, MI

Kelly Green Corkins, MS, RD-AP, CSP, LDN, FAND, FASPEN
Clinical Pediatric Dietitian III, Le Bonheur Children's Hospital
Memphis, TN

Mark R. Corkins, MD, CNSC, FASPEN, AGAF, FAAP
St Jude Chair of Excellence in Pediatric Gastroenterology,
Division Chief of Pediatric Gastroenterology, Hepatology and
Nutrition, The University of Tennessee Health Science Center
Memphis, TN

Melissa Corson, MD
Gastroenterology Fellow, University of California
Los Angeles School of Medicine
Los Angeles, CA

Gail A. Cresci, PhD, RD, LD
Associate Professor of Pediatrics, Cleveland Clinic Lerner
College of Medicine and Staff in Departments of Pediatric
Gastroenterology and Inflammation & Immunity
Cleveland, OH

Sheila Crowe, MD, FRCPC, FACP, FACG, AGAF
Professor of Medicine, Director of Research, Division of
Gastroenterology, University of California, San Diego
La Jolla, CA

Wendy J. Dahl, PhD
Associate Professor, University of Florida
Gainesville, FL

Mark DeLegge, MD
Partner, DeLegge Medical
Awendaw, SC

Eric J. DeMaria, MD, FACS, FASMBS
Professor and Chief, General and Bariatric Surgery,
East Carolina University
Greenville, NC

Anoushka Dua, MD
Resident Physician, University of California, Los Angeles, David
Geffen School of Medicine
Los Angeles, CA

Jacqueline P. Dziuba, MS, RDN, LDN
Registered Dietitian Nutritionist, Department of Bariatric
Surgery, East Carolina University
Greenville, NC

Amy K. Fischer, MS, RD, CDN
Dietitian, Montefiore Medical Center
New York, NY

Mallory Foster, RD, CNSC, CCTD
Clinical Dietitian, University of Virginia Health System
Charlottesville, VA

Jane Gervasio, PharmD, BCNSP
Professor and Chair of Pharmacy Practice, Butler University
Indianapolis, IN

Jennifer Leah Goetz, MD
Instructor, Child, Adolescent & General Psychiatrist,
McLean Hospital, Harvard Medical School
Belmont, MA

James H. Grendell, MD
Professor of Medicine, New York University Long
Island School of Medicine; Chief, Division of
Gastroenterology, Hepatology & Nutrition,
New York University Langone Hospital—Long Island
Mineola, NY

Angela S. Guarda, MD
Associate Professor of Psychiatry and Behavioral Sciences,
Johns Hopkins School of Medicine
Baltimore, MD

M.Linley Harvie, MD
Pediatric Gastroenterologist, GI for Kids, PLLC
Knoxville, TN

Glenn Harvin, MD
Associate Professor, Division Chief of Gastroenterology,
Hepatology and Nutrition, Brody School of Medicine at East
Carolina University
Greenville, NC

**Jeanette M. Hasse, PhD, RD, LD, CNSC, CCTC,
FASPEN, FADA**
Transplant Nutrition Manager, Baylor Simmons Transplant
Institute; Baylor University Medical Center
Dallas, TX

Tiffani L. Hays, MS, RD, LDN
Director, Pediatric Clinical Nutrition Education and Practice,
Johns Hopkins Health System
Baltimore, MD

Hannah D. Holscher, PhD, RD
Associate Professor, University of Illinois
Urbana, IL

Riley L. Hughes, PhD
Postdoctoral Research Associate, University of Illinois
Urbana, IL

Eden Koo, MD
Research Fellow, University of Michigan
Ann Arbor, MI

Vanessa J. Kumpf, PharmD, BCNSP, FASPEN
Clinical Pharmacist Specialist,
Vanderbilt University Medical Center
Nashville, TN

Dennis Kumral, MD
Assistant Professor of Medicine, Division of
Gastroenterology and Hepatology, University of Virginia
Charlottesville, VA

Jennifer Lefton, MS, RD-AP, CNSC, FAND
Nutrition Consultant
Arlington, VA

Berkeley Limketkai, MD, PhD
Associate Clinical Professor, University of
California Los Angeles School of Medicine
Los Angeles, CA

John Leung, MD
Board Certified Gastroenterologist and Allergist;
Founder and CEO of Boston Specialists
Boston, MA

Amanda Lynett, MS, RDN
Registered Dietitian Nutritionist, Michigan Medicine
Ann Arbor, MI

Angela A. MacDonald, DCN, RD
Clinical Dietitian, Nutritional Management Services
London, Canada

Natalie Manitius, MPH, RDN
Registered Dietitian, University of California Los Angeles
Division of Digestive Diseases
Los Angeles, CA

Mary J. Marian, DCN, RDN, CSO, FAND, FASPEN
Professor of Practice/Director, Didactic Program in Dietetics,
University of Arizona
Tucson, AZ

Robert Martindale, MD, PhD
Professor of Surgery, Division of Gastrointestinal and General Surgery, School of Medicine; Medical Director for Hospital Nutrition Services, Oregon Health and Science University
Portland, OR

Laura E. Matarese, PhD, RDN, LDN, FADA, FASPEN, FAND
Professor, Division of Gastroenterology, Hepatology and Nutrition, Brody School of Medicine at East Carolina University
Greenville, NC

Kris M. Mogensen, MS, RD-AP, LDN, CNSC
Team Leader Dietitian Specialist, Brigham and Women's Hospital
Boston, MA

Gerard E. Mullin, MD, AGAF, FACG, FACN
Co-Chair John Hopkins Hospital Nutrition Advisor Committee, Associate Professor of Medicine, Johns Hopkins Hospital
Baltimore, MD

Alyssa M. Parian, MD
Assistant Professor of Medicine, Johns Hopkins University
Baltimore, MD

Walter J. Pories, MD, FACS
Professor of Surgery, Biochemisty, and Kinesiology, East Carolina University
Greenville, NC

Jaclyn Quinlan, MPH, RD, LDN
Clinical Dietitian, Boston Specialists
Boston, MA

Denise Baird Schwartz, MS, RD, FADA, FAND, FASPEN
Bioethics Committee Community Member, Providence Saint Joseph Medical Center
Burbank, CA

Ezra Steiger, MD, FACS, FASPEN, AGAF
Consultant Digestive Disease and Surgery Institute, Cleveland Clinic
Cleveland, OH

Arlene Stein, MS, RD, CDN, CNSC
Nutrition Support Dietitian, New York University Langone Hospital—Long Island
Mineola, NY

Kelly A. Tappenden, PhD, RDN, FASPEN
Professor, Department Head, Kinesiology and Nutrition, University of Illinois at Chicago
Chicago, IL

Jenifer L. Thompson, MS, RD, CSP
Advanced Practice Dietitian, Johns Hopkins Hospital
Baltimore, MD

Anna Tuttle, MS, RD, LDN, CNSC
Clinical Dietitian III, Le Bonheur Children's Hospital
Memphis, TN

Tammy L. Wagner, PhD, RDN
Program Director, George Mason University
Middletown, VA

Malissa Warren, RDN, LDN, CNSC
Advanced Practice Nutrition Support Dietitian, Nutrition and Food Services, VA Portland Health Care System/Department of Surgery, Oregon Health and Science University
Portland, OR

Maeson L. Zietowski
Clinical Assistant, Boston Food Allergy Center
Chicago, IL

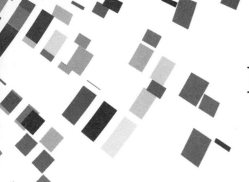

Reviewers

Stephanie Merlino Barr, MS, RDN, LD
Neonatal Nutritionist, MetroHealth Medical Center
Cleveland, OH

Britta Brown, MS, RD, LD, CNSC
Clinical Dietitian, Hennepin Healthcare
Minneapolis, MN

Patsy Catsos, MS, RDN
President, Patsy Catsos Advanced Nutrition
New London, NH

Marlee Coldwell, RD
Registered Dietitian, Ignite Nutrition Inc
Calgary, Canada

Pamela Cureton, RDN, LDN
Clinical and Research Dietitian, University of Maryland
Baltimore, MD

Melinda Dennis, MS, RDN, LD
Nutrition Coordinator, Celiac Center, Beth Israel
Deaconess Medical Center
Boston, MA

Holly Estes Doetsch, MS, RD, LD
Clinical Instructor, The Ohio State University,
Medical Dietetics Division
Columbus, OH

Kelsey Gabel, PhD, RD
Clinical Assistant Professor, University of Illinois at Chicago
Chicago, IL

Nana Gletsu-Miller, PhD
Associate Professor, Indiana University Bloomington,
School of Public Health
Bloomington, IN

Natasha Haskey, RD, PhD
Clinician Researcher/Independent Nutrition Consultant
Kelowna, Canada

Bob Hutkins, PhD
Professor, Department of Food Science and Technology,
University of Nebraska
Lincoln, NE

Kellene A. Isom, PhD, MS, RD, CAGS
Assistant Professor, Nutrition, California State
Polytechnic University, Pomona
Pomona, CA

Nancee Jaffe, MS, RDN
Dietitian Senior Supervisor, UCLA Vatche and
Tamar Manoukian Division of Digestive Diseases
Los Angeles, CA

Maria Karimbakas, RD, CNSC
Program Manager, Optum Intestinal Rehab Program
Cincinnati, OH

Elieke Demmer Kearns, PhD, RD
Scientific Affairs Lead, Bobbie Baby Inc
Chicago, IL

Tiffany A. Leon, MS, RD
Senior Manager Training and Professional Programs, Food
Allergy Research and Education (FARE)
McLean, VA

Diana Mager, PhD, MSc, RD
Professor, Clinical Nutrition, Department of Pediatrics,
Department of Agriculture, Food & Nutritional Sciences,
University of Alberta
Edmonton, Canada

Yvonne McKenzie, MSc, MBDA
Specialist Dietitian in Gastrointestinal Nutrition
and Irritable Bowel Syndrome
Oxford, United Kingdom

Mayumi Nakamura, MPH, RD, CSP
Clinical Dietitian, Children's Hospital Los Angeles
Los Angeles, CA

Tracy L. Oliver, PhD, RDN, LDN
Associate Professor, Villanova University
Villanova, PA

Maria Petzel, RD, CSO, LD, CNSC, FAND
Senior Clinical Dietitian, The University of Texas
MD Anderson Cancer Center
Houston, TX

Alyssa Price, MS, RDN, LD, CNSC
Clinical Dietitian, Dayton Children's Hospital
Cincinnati, OH

Kristen M. Roberts, PhD, RDN, LD, CNSC, FAND, FASPEN
Associate Professor-Clinical, The Ohio State University
Columbus, OH

Carol J. Rollins, MS, RD, PharmD, CNSC, BCNSP, FASHP, FASPEN
Clinical Professor, University of Arizona, College of Pharmacy
Tucson, AZ

Mary Ellen Sanders, PhD
Executive Science Officer, International Scientific
Association for Probiotics and Prebiotics
Centennial, CO

Amber Smith, MBA, RD, TMP, PMP
Director, Nutrition Services, University of California
San Francisco Medical Center
San Francisco, CA

Beth Taylor, DCN, RD-AP, FCCM
Research Scientist/Nutrition Support Specialist,
Barnes-Jewish Hospital
St Louis, MO

Carina Venter, PhD, RD
Associate Professor of Pediatrics, Section of Allergy &
Immunology, University of Colorado Denver School of Medicine,
Children's Hospital Colorado
Denver, CO

Taylor C. Wallace, PhD, CFS, FACN
Principal and CEO, Think Healthy Group, LLC; Adjunct
Professor, Department of Nutrition and Food Studies,
George Mason University;
Editor-in-Chief, *Journal of Dietary Supplements*
Washington, DC

Melissa Wallinga, MS, RD, CSPCC, LD
Pediatric ICU Dietitian, St Luke's Children's Hospital
Boise, ID

Marion F. Winkler, PhD, RD, LDN, CNSC
Professor of Surgery (Teaching Scholar), Alpert Medical
School of Brown University; Surgical Nutrition
Specialist, Rhode Island Hospital
Providence, RI

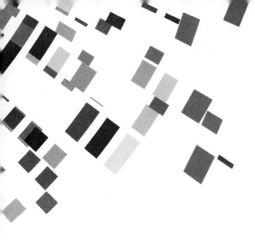

Foreword

THIS SECOND EDITION OF THE *Health Professional's Guide to Gastrointestinal Nutrition* is a comprehensive review of the assessment and management of hospitalized and home-based patients with gastrointestinal-related conditions. The 25 chapters are unique in their involvement of physician and dietitian authors to broaden the book's use for medical and dietetics students as well as practitioners. The editors, Laura Matarese, Gerry Mullin, and Kelly Tappenden, are all recognized experts and thought leaders in the field of gastrointestinal nutrition and nutrition support. This has enabled them to attract expert authors to evaluate and present state-of-the-art evidence on nutrition science and contribute practical solutions to difficult and complex clinical problems in their designated chapters on a variety of common gastrointestinal conditions and feeding techniques.

One point that comes through strongly in the key chapters on enteral and parenteral feeding is the need to perform a full nutritional status evaluation, together with an assessment of short- and long-term survival, before starting nutritional support. This is important as the developments in interventional feeding, well summarized in this book, have allowed anybody, even the sickest ICU patient, to be fed. This must be balanced against the recognition that all forms of nutrition support, parenteral or enteral, have potential complications, which might actually worsen outcome if not indicated. This book provides up-to-date guidelines on the indications, treatments, and potential complications of nutrition interventions and provides strategies on how to avoid complications while optimizing patient care and outcome.

Chapters of note cover contemporary gastronintestinal-related issues, including nutraceuticals and obesity, as well as adding a new and expanded section covering the importance of the human microbiome in influencing health and disease and the ability of food, including prebiotics and probiotics, and addressing specific diets to possibly prevent dysbiosis-associated diseases. Among the many gastronintestinal conditions covered, there are an increasing array of investigations and interventions available based on current literature and experience-based knowledge that offer cutting-edge gastrointestinal nutrition care. This includes the practical management of patients with short bowel intestinal failure, irritable bowel syndrome, as well as other complex and chronic conditions before and after discharge, with an emphasis on regular, long-term follow up to help support the patient and their family with ongoing and life-saving nutrition therapy.

Stephen J. D. O'Keefe, MBBS, MSc, MD, FRCP
Professor of Medicine
Division of Gastroenterology
University of Pittsburgh
Director African Microbiome Institute
University of Stellenbosch
South Africa

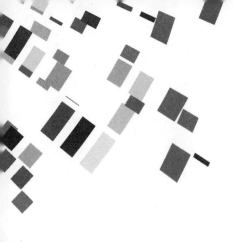

Preface

THE GASTROINTESTINAL (GI) SYSTEM IS OFTEN UNDERAPPRECIATED DESPITE ITS VAST COMPLEXITY, which includes the mouth, pharynx, esophagus, stomach, biliary system, pancreas, liver, small intestine, large intestine, rectum, and anus. Functionally, the GI system is essential for the digestion and absorption of nutrients that sustain us, the immunity that protects us, and the metabolism that fuels us. Further, the GI system orchestrates function among distant organs and communicates with our central nervous system. An additional ecosystem is now known to exist within the GI system that provides and impacts many physiological processes. Despite all these critical, ongoing actions, we often take the GI system for granted until there is a problem.

With the success of the first edition of the *Health Professional's Guide to Gastrointestinal Nutrition*, we were asked to lead the development of a second edition. The book's purpose is to help registered dietitian nutritionists (RDNs) and other health care providers understand both the complexities of the GI system and the changes that occur in various disease states, with the goal of providing the best nutrition care for their patients. As a practice-oriented guide, this book is intended to help RDNs, physicians, interns, and students identify and alleviate or resolve the nutritional problems related to the GI tract that affect the health and quality of life of our patients.

For ease of use, the book is divided into five sections. **Section 1: Gastrointestinal Nutrition Assessment and Diagnostics** begins with a comprehensive chapter on nutrition assessment of the patient with GI disorders, which is the first step in the Nutrition Care Process. These patients frequently experience nutrition-related problems, including nutrient deficiencies due to the inability to digest and absorb nutrients. An overview of tests and procedures commonly performed for patients with GI disorders is provided in a separate chapter to identify the indications, preparation, and risks involved in diagnosing various disease states.

Section 2: Nutrition and Gastrointestinal-Related Disorders includes 10 chapters that examine specific GI tract diseases. There is a wealth of information on disease etiologies, symptoms, diagnostic techniques, and nutritional implications. These chapters also offer practical suggestions about selecting nutrition interventions that are appropriate for specific patients. The specific topics in this section include inflammatory bowel disease (Chapter 3), short bowel syndrome (Chapter 4), irritable bowel syndrome (Chapter 5), celiac disease (Chapter 6), liver disease (Chapter 7), pancreatic disease (Chapter 8), pediatric-originating gastrointestinal disorders (Chapter 9), and gastrointestinal oncology (Chapter 10).

Section 3: Nutrition and Gastrointestinal Related Systemic Disorders focuses on nutrition intervention for common systemic conditions with gastrointestinal implications. This section covers medical treatment of obesity (Chapter 11), eating disorders (Chapter 12), and food allergies and intolerances (Chapter 13).

With the emergence of evidence on the critical role of the gut microbiome in health and disease, a new **Section 4: Overview of the Intestinal Microbiome** addresses this area of critical knowledge for health care professionals. Physiological functions of the intestinal microbiome, diagnoses related to altered microbial communities, and nutritional strategies for optimizing the microbial community are included in chapters on the intestinal microbiome (Chapter 16), prebiotics (Chapter 17), and probiotics (Chapter 18).

Section 5: Surgical and Therapeutic Interventions for Gastrointestinal Disorders includes ten chapters. Chapters 17 and 18 focus on GI surgeries (bariatric and other GI surgeries), which explore how surgical interventions are used to address serious health problems and how these might alter digestion and absorption. Chapters 19 to 22 focus on nutrition support, including the uses of enteral and parenteral nutrition in adult and pediatric patients, as well as the special challenges of administering nutrition support in the home care setting. The information in these chapters complements and expands upon the coverage of nutrition support interventions for specific GI disorders found in many of the earlier chapters of this book. Chapter 23 is a guide to drug-nutrient interactions that may occur with the medications used to treat GI disorders. Chapter 24 address the use of nutraceutical supplements. Although further rigorous, scientific investigation of the use of nutraceuticals is needed, this chapter can help readers separate the more promising options from those that have not demonstrated efficacy. Chapter 25 frames the ethical and legal issues that health care professionals may face when providing GI nutrition interventions, particularly when a patient or authorized caregiver chooses to refuse artificial nutrition and hydration.

There are many ways to use this book. You may wish to start at the beginning and read from cover to cover. Alternatively, we encourage you to turn to the chapters that are most relevant to the types of care you provide or begin with the topics that are least familiar to you. Whatever your strategy, our goal is that you find this *Health Professional's Guide to Gastrointestinal Nutrition* to be an essential evidence-based professional resource in your clinical practice.

Laura E. Matarese, PhD, RDN, LDN, FADA, FASPEN, FAND
Gerard E. Mullin, MD, AGAF, FACG, FACN
Kelly A. Tappenden, PhD, RDN, FASPEN

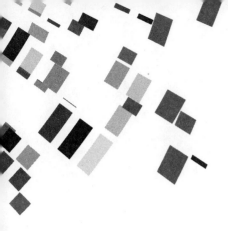

Acknowledgments

No achievement, great or small, is effectively accomplished in isolation. This book was truly a team effort of the editors and authors who graciously shared their expertise. Equally important to making this volume a success was the exceptional editorial assistance received from Betsy Hornick, MS, RDN, at the Academy of Nutrition and Dietetics. She kept us focused, on track, and provided us with superb publishing guidance. We would be remiss if we did not acknowledge the expert input from our reviewers. Their objectivity and directed comments helped to shape the book.

Many people have supported us throughout this endeavor. To our family and friends who tolerated our many absences while we finished this book, we thank you. We are grateful to our colleagues who over the years have become dear friends, many of whom contributed chapters. Finally, a very special and heartfelt thanks goes to the patients who have allowed us to care for them. We learned from them. They kept us grounded and reminded us of what is truly important in life. They were and remain an inspiration to us, professionally and personally.

Laura E. Matarese, PhD, RDN, LDN, FADA, FASPEN, FAND
Gerard E. Mullin, MD, AGAF, FACG, FACN
Kelly A. Tappenden, PhD, RDN, FASPEN

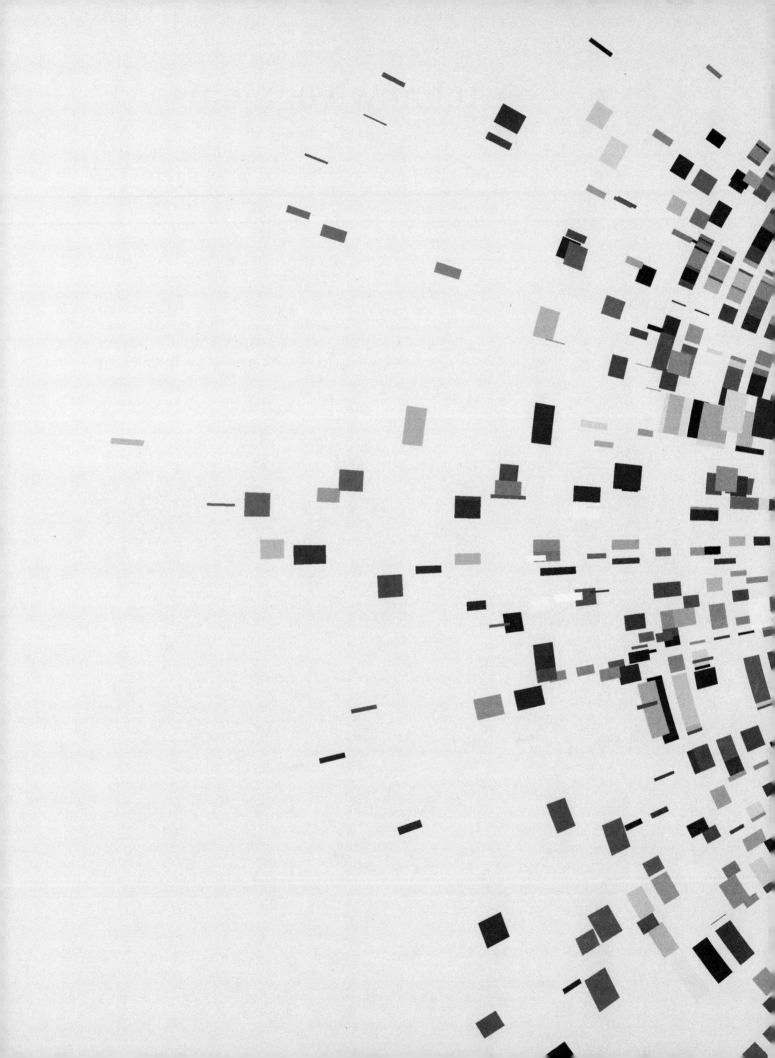

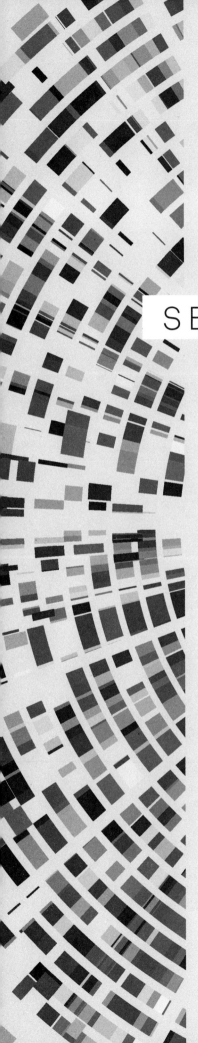

Gastrointestinal Nutrition Assessment and Diagnostics

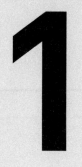

Nutrition Assessment for Patients With Gastrointestinal Disorders

Kris M. Mogensen, MS, RD-AP, LDN, CNSC

KEY POINTS

- Disorders of the gastrointestinal system can have a significant adverse impact on nutritional status by impairing ingestion, digestion, and absorption of food and nutrients, increasing nutritional losses and nutrient requirements, and ultimately influencing morbidity and mortality.
- The nutrition assessment is a comprehensive evaluation of the nutritional status of an individual. Nutrition screening occurs before the comprehensive nutrition assessment to identify patients who are malnourished or at risk for developing malnutrition.
- A complete nutrition assessment includes evaluating dietary data, biochemical test and procedure results; anthropometric measures; nutrition focused physical findings; and a personal, medical, and social history with the ultimate goal of improving clinical outcomes in patients with gastrointestinal disorders.

Introduction

Disorders of the gastrointestinal (GI) system can have an adverse impact on nutritional status by impairing ingestion, digestion, and absorption of food and nutrients and increasing nutritional losses and nutrient requirements.[1] Nutritional status has a profound influence on morbidity and mortality from illness in the acute care setting in both patients who are non-critically ill and critically ill.[2-6] In the clinical setting, nutrition assessment is a comprehensive evaluation of the nutritional status of an individual patient. Nutrition screening occurs before the comprehensive nutrition assessment to help identify patients who are malnourished or at risk for developing malnutrition to assure timely and appropriate nutrition assessment.[7] Once a patient is identified as at risk, the patient should then undergo nutrition assessment.

As the first step of the Nutrition Care Process, nutrition assessment is defined as "a systematic method for obtaining, verifying, and interpreting data needed to identify nutrition-related problems, their causes, and significance."[8] Nutrition assessment involves an initial evaluation of the patient, and ongoing monitoring and periodic reassessment is important to refine the individualized nutrition care plan to help maintain or improve the assessed status. The types of data collected during the assessment vary on a case-by-case basis but are organized into five general categories (see Box 1.1).[8] No single method is ideal for nutrition assessment; the use of a combination of methods is needed to effectively characterize nutritional status. All nutrition assessment methods provide indirect estimates of the process measured. Thus, the data obtained are usually compared to reference data to determine indicators of nutritional status.

BOX 1.1

Components of a Nutrition Assessment[8]

Food/nutrition-related history

Food and nutrient intake

Medication and dietary supplement intake, including herbs and other botanicals

Knowledge, beliefs, and attitudes

Food availability

Physical activity

Nutrition-related quality of life

Biochemical data, medical tests, and procedures

Laboratory data (eg, electrolytes, glucose, renal, liver, gastrointestinal profiles)

Tests (eg, gastric emptying time, resting metabolic rate)

Anthropometric measurements

Height

Weight

Body mass index

Weight history

Weight change

Nutrition focused physical findings

Physical appearance

Skin, hair, and nail assessment

Muscle and fat wasting

Edema assessment

Swallow function

Abdominal exam

Evaluation of enteral access devices (eg, gastrostomy or jejunostomy), if present

Stool frequency and consistency

Ileostomy or colostomy output, including volume and consistency

Appetite

Affect

Client history

Personal history (eg, age, gender, race, language, education)

Medical, health, and family history

Treatments and use of complementary and alternative medicine

Social history (eg, socioeconomic status, housing situation)

Nutrition Screening

Nutrition screening is a vital first step in determining which patients should be referred to the registered dietitian nutritionist (RDN) for nutrition assessment and care plan development. The American Society for Parenteral and Enteral Nutrition (ASPEN) defines nutrition screening as "a process to identify an individual who may be malnourished or at risk for malnutrition to determine if a comprehensive nutrition assessment and appropriate intervention are indicated."[9] The Academy of Nutrition and Dietetics expands this definition to include nutrition concerns beyond malnutrition, defining nutrition screening as "the process of identifying and referring those individuals and populations who are at risk for nutrition-related problems, are appropriate for nutrition care services, and would benefit from the Nutrition Care Process."[10]

Nutrition screening may be done by many health care professionals, including medical assistants, nurses, and nutrition and dietetics technicians, registered.[11] Physicians may also do nutrition screenings, particularly in the critical care setting.[12] Screening tools should be quick and easy for the clinician to use. More importantly, the tool should be valid and reliable for the population or care setting. In 2020, the Academy of Nutrition and Dietetics published a position paper on nutrition screening tools and recommended that the Malnutrition Screening Tool (MST) be used in all care settings to screen adults for malnutrition.[11,13] Although the MST was initially developed for the acute care setting, it has been validated in acute care, long-term care, and outpatient settings.[11] It has a moderate degree of validity, a moderate degree of agreement, and a moderate degree of inter-rater reliability in identifying malnutrition risk in adults, supported by Grade 1 evidence with good generalizability. Other screening tools performed well in some areas of validity but did not have Grade 1 evidence.[11] An MST score of 2 or greater means that the patient is at nutritional risk and should be promptly referred to an RDN for a full nutrition assessment.[13]

In the critical care setting, a more in-depth screening process is recommended to capture the risk of malnutrition and severity of illness, recognizing the impact of inflammation and the hypermetabolic and hypercatabolic state on nutritional status.[12] In the Society of Critical Care Medicine (SCCM)/ASPEN critical care guidelines, two screening tools are recommended: the Nutrition Risk Screening 2002 (NRS-2002) and the Nutrition Risk in the Critically Ill (NUTRIC) score, both of which are acceptable for use in the intensive care unit (ICU).[12] The NRS-2002 has two parts: The initial screening is used to identify the presence of malnutrition or risk of nutritional compromise. If the patient has a positive indicator for one of four initial screening questions, the final screening is done, which includes an assessment of nutritional risk and severity of illness to generate a risk score.[14] A score of 3 or higher indicates that the patient requires a full nutrition assessment and development of a nutrition care plan; a score of 5 or higher suggests that the patient is at high risk.[12,14] Those with high nutritional risk benefit from the initiation of early nutrition support therapy.[12] The NUTRIC score does not include specific nutritional measures, but it is a scoring system that includes age, Acute Physiology and Chronic Health Evaluation II (APACHE II) score, sequential organ failure assessment (SOFA) score, number of comorbidities, days from hospital admission, and interleukin-6 (IL-6) level.[15] A score is generated from these parameters. Because IL-6 is not available at all institutions, a modified NUTRIC score has been validated for use without IL-6 to allow institutions without the means to measure this inflammatory marker to use the scoring system.[16] A NUTRIC score of 6 to 10, or a modified NUTRIC score of 5 to 9, suggests that the patient is at high risk for worse clinical outcomes and would benefit from aggressive nutrition support intervention.[15,16] The NRS-2002, NUTRIC score, and modified NUTRIC score have been validated in the ICU population, demonstrating that those at high nutritional risk benefit from early nutrition intervention with improved clinical outcomes including reduced complications (including infectious complications) and mortality.[15-20] Box 1.2 summarizes key elements and populations of the screening tools discussed in this section.

Malnutrition Screening Tool (MST)

Screening elements

Weight loss, including amount lost

Change in appetite

Recommended populations

Adults in all care settings

Nutrition Risk Screening 2002 (NRS-2002)

Screening elements

Initial screening:

- BMI less than 20.5
- unintentional weight loss in the past 3 months
- reduced intake in the past week
- severe illness (in the intensive care unit [ICU])

If any element of the initial screen is positive, final screening is conducted to evaluate:

- degree of impaired nutritional status, based on degree and time frame of unintentional weight loss, BMI, and reduced intake
- severity of illness

Recommended populations

European Society for Clinical Nutrition and Metabolism (ESPEN) recommends for hospitalized patients; American Society for Parenteral and Enteral Nutrition (ASPEN) recommends for patients who are critically ill

Nutrition Risk in the Critically Ill (NUTRIC)

Screening elements

Age

Acute Physiology and Chronic Health Evaluation II (APACHE II) score

Sequential organ failure assessment (SOFA) score

Number of comorbidities

Days from hospital admission to ICU admission

Interleukin-6 (IL-6) level

Recommended populations

Patients who are critically ill; validated with and without IL-6 level

Food/Nutrition-Related History

The food/nutrition-related history can include data related to dietary intake as well as such diet-related information as knowledge and beliefs about food and nutrition, medication and supplement use, and physical activity. Evaluation of usual dietary intake (ie, diet history) is an important part of the nutrition assessment. Commonly used methods for assessing food/nutrition-related history include the following:

- diet history
- 24-hour recall

- food record or diary
- food frequency questionnaire (FFQ)
- mobile health tracking applications

Each method has its advantages and disadvantages. In addition, the accuracy of these methods for predicting actual dietary intake is a matter of debate.[21-23]

Diet recall methods, such as the diet history and 24-hour recall, are commonly used in the clinical setting. The diet history helps the clinician assess a patient's usual dietary intake over an extended period of time, such as the past month or the past year. The 24-hour recall method estimates the patient's usual intake based on reported dietary intake in the past 24 hours. Multiple 24-hour recalls are sometimes necessary because 1 day of intake is not typically representative of usual intake.[24]

With food records, the patient records the types and amounts of food and beverages consumed for a predefined period of time, usually 1 to 7 days, and the clinician estimates the usual intake based on this information. Unlike the diet history and 24-hour recall methods, food records do not rely on memory.

The FFQ asks patients how many times a day, week, or year they consume certain foods (depending on the dietary component of interest). The clinician can use a patient's responses to the questionnaire to estimate intake of the dietary parameter of interest. The FFQ is often used in the research setting.

Mobile health tracking devices, including apps that can be installed on smartphones, are gaining in popularity.[25] A review noted that in 2017 there were 325,000 mobile health apps available in major app stores for download.[26] The available apps cover a wide range of monitoring tools including fitness, sleep, and food intake. Apps for tracking food intake can be much more convenient than a pen-and-paper food record or diary. Some apps offer nutrient analysis of food items by allowing the consumer to take a digital picture of the food item to be consumed, but these are still in development, and research is ongoing in this area. The apps vary in accuracy, so clinicians should be careful when using food tracking apps in a research setting.[25] Clinicians should also consider the patient's resources (eg, type of device and memory available for the app) and comfort level with technology before recommending a specific app for monitoring intake.[27,28] Knowledge of a variety of apps with different levels of complexity will allow RDNs to make app recommendations tailored to their patients' needs.

All these data-gathering methods can provide valuable information about a patient's dietary intake, which can then be compared to the patient's nutritional requirements to estimate adequacy of the diet. For patients who cannot participate in an interview (eg, patients who are critically ill requiring mechanical ventilation or patients with neurologic disorders), clinicians may need to rely on family members or caretakers to provide information about a patient's food/nutrition-related history. For patients receiving home nutrition support therapy—home enteral nutrition (EN) or parenteral nutrition (PN), or both—the home-infusion clinician may provide valuable insight into the patient's home-infusion history, including tolerance to the EN or PN regimen and ability to adhere to the infusion prescription.

In the acute care setting, calorie counts may be used to quantify oral intake. The patient may keep a food record or food diary during the hospital stay, but for patients who are ill and unable to keep these records, a family member, bedside nurse, patient care assistant, or other professional (eg, a trained food service professional) may do the monitoring. Extensive training or other innovations, such as taking pictures of food trays after a meal, may improve accuracy.[29] The RDN or designee then calculates energy and protein intake of the food consumed. The reliability of intake data depends on accuracy of the recorded food intake. For hospitalized patients receiving EN, monitoring of intake and output records can help identify interruptions in infusion and the need to adjust the infusion time to ensure consistent and adequate feeding.

Biochemical Data, Medical Tests, and Procedures

Biochemical tests using blood and urine provide quantitative data about nutritional status. They can supply useful information about recent nutrient intakes and nutrient deficiencies. However, because the results of biochemical tests can be influenced by non-nutrition-related factors, such as medications, fluid status, and other metabolic processes (eg, inflammation[30]), these findings should be evaluated in conjunction with other nutrition assessment methods. Biochemical assessment can include the following tests[8]:

- protein profile (eg, albumin, prealbumin, transferrin, C-reactive protein)
- vitamin and mineral profiles
- acid-base balance
- electrolyte and renal profile
- essential fatty acid profile
- nutritional anemia profile (eg, hemoglobin, hematocrit, mean corpuscular volume, vitamin B12, folate, and iron panel)
- lipid profile
- GI profile (eg, total bilirubin, direct bilirubin, alanine aminotransferase, aspartate aminotransferase, amylase, lipase)

Malabsorptive disorders are common with GI diseases. Malabsorption can involve defective digestion and absorption of carbohydrate, protein, fat, vitamins, and minerals, either in combination or independently. Biochemical tests and other procedures used in the diagnosis of malabsorptive disorders in patients with GI diseases are described in Chapter 2. Patients with malabsorptive disorders are at increased risk for vitamin and trace element deficiencies and, therefore, often require supplementation with a multivitamin, multivitamin with minerals, or individual micronutrients, depending on the location of the disorder (eg, vitamin B12 supplementation is usually required for patients with disorders that affect the terminal ileum). See Table 1.1 for laboratory tests used to assess vitamin and trace element status.[31-34]

Medical tests and procedures are an important part of the nutrition assessment process. For example, a computed tomography (CT) scan of the abdomen may help to identify GI complications, such as ileus or obstruction, which will help determine the patient's ability to start an oral diet or EN or the need to consider PN. A video swallow examination in a recently extubated patient can provide valuable information about the patient's ability to take an oral diet, need for a texture-modified diet, or need to continue taking nothing by mouth. The RDN should monitor for results of tests and procedures that will help develop and refine the nutrition care plan.

TABLE 1.1 Assessment of Vitamin and Trace Element Status[31-34]

Nutrient	Laboratory assay	Normal values[a]	Signs of deficiency	Toxicity symptoms
Water-soluble vitamins				
Thiamin (B1)	Whole blood	>3.0-7.7 mcg/dL	Beriberi, mental confusion, Wernicke encephalopathy, congestive heart failure	Rare: irritability, headache, insomnia
Riboflavin (B2)	Erythrocyte glutathione reductase activity coefficient	<1.2	Mucositis, dermatitis, photophobia, cheilosis, normocytic anemia	Unknown
Niacin (B3)	Urinary niacin metabolites	>2 mg per g creatinine	Headaches, diarrhea, dermatitis, pellagra, memory loss	Flushing, rash, irritation, vasodilation

Table continues

Nutrient	Laboratory assay	Normal values[a]	Signs of deficiency	Toxicity symptoms
Pantothenic acid (B5)	Urinary pantothenic acid	>1 mg/dL	Fatigue, malaise, headache, insomnia	Diarrhea
Pyridoxine (B6)	Plasma pyridoxal 5'-phosphate (PLP)	39-98 nmol/L	Dermatitis, neuritis, microcytic anemia	Peripheral neuropathy
	Urinary excretion of B6 metabolite	>3 mcmol/d		
Biotin (B7)	Whole blood or serum biotin	>200 pg/mL	Dermatitis, lethargy, anorexia, alopecia, paresthesia, conjunctivitis	Unknown
Folate (B9)	Serum folate	>3 ng/mL	Megaloblastic anemia, diarrhea, lethargy	Pernicious anemia, convulsive seizures
Cyanocobalamin (B12)	Serum B12[b]	170-250 pg/mL	Megaloblastic anemia, neuropathy, stomatitis, glossitis, pernicious anemia	Unknown
Ascorbic acid (C)	Plasma ascorbic acid	>0.4 mg/dL	Hemorrhaging skin, nose, gastrointestinal tract; weakness; bleeding gums; impaired wound healing	Osmotic diarrhea, oxalate kidney stones, interferes with anticoagulation therapy
Choline[c]	Plasma choline	≥10 mcmol/L	Fatty liver, liver damage, elevated aminotransferase	Fishy body odor, sweating, salivation, hypotension
Fat-soluble vitamins				
A	Serum retinol	30-100 mcg/dL	Night blindness, dermatitis, xerophthalmia, keratomalacia	Acute: nausea, vomiting, headache, dizziness, chronic peeling skin, gingivitis, alopecia
D	Serum 25-hydroxyvitamin D	≥20 ng/mL	Osteomalacia, rickets, muscle weakness	Excess bone and soft tissue calcification, kidney stones, hypercalcemia
E	Plasma or serum α-tocopherol	0.5-2.0 mg/dL	Increased platelet aggregation hemolytic anemia, neuronal axonopathy, myopathy	Impaired neutrophil function, thrombocytopenia
K	Plasma phylloquinone	0.15-1.0 mcg/L	Bleeding, purpura, bruising	Bruising, bleeding, jaundice
Trace elements				
Chromium	Serum value	0.05-5.0 mcg/L	Glucose intolerance, peripheral neuropathy, increased serum cholesterol, hyperlipidemia, insulin resistance	Unknown

Table continues

TABLE 1.1 Assessment of Vitamin and Trace Element Status[31-34] (continued)

Nutrient	Laboratory assay	Normal values[a]	Signs of deficiency	Toxicity symptoms
Copper	Serum value Ceruloplasmin level	70-140 mcg/dL 20-35 mg/dL	Neutropenia, microcytic anemia, osteoporosis, decreased hair and skin pigmentation, dermatitis	Uncommon: nausea, vomiting, epigastric pain, diarrhea
Iodine[d]	Urine	100-199 mcg/L	Hyperplasia of thyroid, goiter, reduced metabolic rate, hypercholesterolemia	Rhinorrhea, headache, parotitis, acne
Iron	Serum ferritin	M: 40-300 mcg/L F: 20-200 mcg/L	Microcytic hypochromic anemia, pallor, koilonychia, glossitis, impaired behavioral and intellectual performance, fatigue	Cirrhosis, cardiomegaly, pancreatic damage
Manganese	Serum value	5-15 mcg/L	Nausea, vomiting, dermatitis, changes in hair color, hypocholesterolemia	Extrapyramidal symptoms, encephalitis-like symptoms, hyperirritability
Molybdenum	Neutron	0.58-0.8 mcg/L	Tachycardia, tachypnea, altered mental status, vision changes, headache, nausea, vomiting	Increased copper excretion
Selenium	Plasma or serum value	63-160 mcg/L	Muscle weakness and pain, cardiomyopathy	Hair loss, dermatitis, brittle nails, tooth decay, fatigue
Zinc	Serum value[e]	80-120 mcg/dL	Dermatitis, hypogeusia, diarrhea, apathy, depression, impaired wound healing	Nausea, vomiting, headache

[a] Reference ranges for adult patients. Reference values may vary by laboratory.
[b] Metabolites that result from vitamin B12 deficiency (ie, methylmalonic acid and homocysteine) may be sensitive indicators of B12 deficiency. Normal serum methylmalonic acid levels are 0.08 to 0.56 mcmol/L, and normal homocysteine levels are 5 to 15 mcmol/L.
[c] Although not a vitamin, choline is an essential nutrient and is, therefore, included in this table.
[d] Serum thyroid-stimulating hormone and free thyroxine can be used as initial screening. These surrogate markers for iodine deficiency can be used initially in place of a 24-hour urine iodine study.
[e] During systematic inflammatory response syndrome, serum zinc will decrease to about half of normal and remain depressed until the syndrome resolves.

Anthropometric Measurements

Anthropometry includes measurements of body size, weight, and proportions. Anthropometric measurements used for nutrition assessment can include the following parameters[8]:

- height or length
- weight
- frame size
- weight change
- BMI
- growth pattern indexes or percentile ranks
- body compartment estimates (eg, fat mass, fat-free mass)

Anthropometric measures can be used, in conjunction with other assessment methods, as indicators of overall nutritional status. However, these measures are not useful for identifying specific nutrient deficiencies. Anthropometric assessments are particularly important in patients with GI disorders because wasting syndrome is a common adverse effect of the disease process.[1]

Body Weight

Body weight provides a gross evaluation of overall fat and muscle stores. Ideal body weight (IBW) is often calculated using the Hamwi method[35]:*

- Males: 106 lb for the first 5 ft in height, 6 lb for each inch taller than 5 ft
- Females: 100 lb for the first 5 ft in height, 5 lb for each inch taller than 5 ft

Usual body weight (UBW) may be a more applicable parameter to use when evaluating patients with GI dysfunction. A report of weight change may be subject to the patient's memory but can be confirmed with measured weights if a clinician has access to outpatient records. The UBW provides a useful tool for assessing changes in weight status over time. IBW and UBW may be used to evaluate the degree of overnutrition or undernutrition. Recent unintentional weight loss is a strong indicator of declining nutritional status.[36] Weight loss of more than 10% of UBW within a 6-month period is considered clinically significant.[37] Weight gain could indicate repletion of lean and fat tissue, overnutrition, or presence of edema. Percentages of IBW, UBW, and recent weight can all be used to evaluate weight status.[38] Assessment of weight status can be difficult in patients who are critically ill because of changes in fluid status and the challenges of correlating weight changes to fluid balance.[39,40] Patients who are critically ill requiring mechanical ventilation may not be able to communicate a weight history. Careful review of outpatient records, if such records are available, is essential to obtaining a weight history and determining the optimal weight to use for the nutrition assessment. For patients who are critically ill who were not weighed before volume resuscitation (eg, in severe pancreatitis), an outpatient weight that was measured closest to the ICU admission date may be a more appropriate weight to use for assessment.

Percentage of Ideal Body Weight

To calculate a patient's percentage of IBW, divide the current weight by the IBW and multiply the result by 100. The results are interpreted as follows[38]:

- mild malnutrition: 80% to 90% of IBW
- moderate malnutrition: 70% to 79.9% of IBW
- severe malnutrition: less than 70% of IBW

Percentage of Usual Body Weight

To calculate a patient's percentage of UBW, divide the current weight by the UBW and multiply the result by 100. The results are interpreted as follows[38]:

- mild malnutrition: 85% to 95% of UBW
- moderate malnutrition: 75% to 84.9% of UBW
- severe malnutrition: less than 75% of UBW

---

* Specific recommendations for transgender people were not provided.

Time Frame of Weight Change

The time frame of weight loss is an important part of the assessment of percentage of UBW. The clinician should obtain the time frame of the weight change either from the patient interview or from documented weight records. After calculating the percentage of UBW, the time frame of weight change should be interpreted as follows:

$$\% \text{ Weight Change} = \frac{(\text{Usual body weight} - \text{Current body weight})}{\text{Usual body weight}} \times 100$$

The results are interpreted as follows[38]:

- *Significant weight loss* is defined as 1% to 2% in 1 week; 5% in 1 month; 7.5% in 3 months; or 10% in 6 months.
- *Severe weight loss* is defined as weight loss that exceeds the preceding amounts.

BMI

BMI is commonly used to classify weight status and assess healthy weight, malnutrition, and obesity. It is calculated using relative weight for height (as shown in the following equations) and is significantly correlated with total body fat content.[41]

$$\text{BMI} = \frac{\text{Weight in kg}}{(\text{Height in m})^2}$$

or

$$\text{BMI} = \frac{\text{Weight in lb}}{(\text{Height in inches})^2} \times 703$$

Guidelines for interpretation of BMI in adults are presented in Table 1.2.[41,42] For children and adolescents aged 19 years and younger, assessment of BMI is age- and gender-specific. Refer to the appropriate reference tables available from the Centers for Disease Control and Prevention (www.cdc.gov/growthcharts).

TABLE 1.2 Interpretation of Body Mass Index in Adults[41,42]

BMI	Classification
≤15.9	Severe thinness
16.0-16.9	Moderate thinness
17.0-18.4	Mild thinness
18.5-24.9	Normal weight
25.0-29.9	Overweight
30.0-34.9	Obesity class I
35.0-39.9	Obesity class II
≥40	Obesity class III

Body Composition

Historically, body composition (ie, fat mass and fat-free mass) has been estimated using skinfold measurements, such as midarm circumference, midarm muscle circumference, and skinfold thickness. Although not frequently used in the clinical setting, skinfold measurements (serial measures) can be used to evaluate changes in lean and fat mass over time in individual patients. Other methods for clinical evaluation of body composition include dual-energy x-ray absorptiometry (DXA), ultrasound (US), and bioelectrical impedance analysis (BIA). Recent clinical guidelines published by ASPEN recommend DXA for the evaluation of fat mass only, because validity of use for the evaluation of lean body mass is still unknown. Guidelines for the use of US and BIA could not be provided.[43] CT has been used in the research setting and may also be used in the clinical setting, by appropriately trained practitioners, to evaluate fat and muscle mass.[44]

Waist Circumference

Waist circumference is an assessment of abdominal fat. It is measured (in inches or centimeters) by placing a standard measuring tape around the bare abdomen just above the hip bone. Independent of BMI, a high waist circumference is a risk factor for several diseases, including diabetes, hyperlipidemia, hypertension, and cardiovascular disease. A waist circumference of more than 40 inches (102 cm) in men and more than 35 inches (88 cm) in women is associated with increased disease risk.[45]

Nutrition Focused Physical Findings

Nutrition focused physical findings are described as "nutrition-related physical characteristics associated with pathophysiological states derived from a nutrition focused physical examination, interview, or the medical record." These findings are examined to assess overall physical appearance, muscle and subcutaneous fat wasting, swallow function, appetite, and affect. Signs and symptoms of micronutrient deficiencies as well as essential fatty acid deficiency, which may be of significant concern in patients with GI disorders, may be identified during the nutrition focused physical examination. See Box 1.3 for clinical findings from the physical examination associated with nutrient deficiencies. Both subjective and objective physical findings are assessed during the nutrition focused physical examination, which includes evaluations of the following factors and systems[8]:

- overall appearance
- body language
- cardiovascular-pulmonary system (eg, edema, shortness of breath)
- extremities, muscles, and bones
- GI system (mouth to rectum)
- head and eyes
- nerves and cognition
- skin
- vital signs (eg, blood pressure, heart rate, temperature)

The nutrition focused physical examination may be limited in patients who are critically ill, particularly the evaluation of extremities, muscles, and bones. The presence of an endotracheal tube, tracheostomy, central venous catheters, orogastric or nasogastric tubes, or compression boots may make it difficult for the RDN to conduct a comprehensive evaluation. Coordination with the patient's bedside nurse to assist with the examination or to plan the examination for times when the patient is being turned to evaluate for pressure injuries or while being washed may allow for a more comprehensive examination.

BOX 1.3

Clinical Findings From Physical Examination Associated With Nutrient Deficiencies

Hair

Clinical findings	Possible deficiency
Alopecia	Protein
Dry, dull, lackluster, brittle, sparse	Protein, iron, zinc, essential fatty acids
Dyspigmentation	Biotin, protein
Flag sign (alternating bands of light and dark hair)	Protein

Skin and nails

Clinical findings	Possible deficiency
Xerosis	Vitamin A, essential fatty acids
Follicular hyperkeratosis	Vitamin A, essential fatty acids
Perifollicular petechiae	Vitamin C, vitamin K
Dermatitis	Essential fatty acids, niacin, riboflavin, zinc
Pallor	Iron, folate, vitamin B12
Nasolabial seborrhea	Niacin, riboflavin, vitamin B6
Koilonychia	Iron

Eyes

Clinical findings	Possible deficiency
Xerophthalmia	Vitamin A
Bitot spots	Vitamin A
Night blindness	Vitamin A
Angular palpebritis	Riboflavin

Mouth

Clinical findings	Possible deficiency
Cheilosis	Vitamin B6, riboflavin, niacin
Angular stomatitis	Riboflavin, vitamin B6, iron
Bleeding or spongy gums	Vitamin C
Magenta tongue	Riboflavin
Atrophic papillae	Iron, niacin, folate, vitamin B12
Glossitis	Niacin, folate, iron, vitamin B6, vitamin B12
Dysgeusia	Zinc

Box continues

BOX 1.3 (CONTINUED)

Cardiovascular

Clinical findings	*Possible deficiency*
Irregular or abnormal rhythm or rate	Potassium excess or deficiency, calcium or phosphorus deficiency, magnesium deficiency or excess

Musculoskeletal

Clinical findings	*Possible deficiency*
Muscle wasting	Protein-energy malnutrition
Bowlegs	Vitamin D, calcium
Beading of ribs	Vitamin D, protein-energy malnutrition

Neurologic

Clinical findings	*Possible deficiency*
Mental confusion	Thiamin, vitamin B12, vitamin B6
Dementia	Niacin, vitamin B12

Client History

The client history includes information related to personal, medical, family, and social history with the potential to affect nutritional status. Box 1.4 outlines the data to be included in the client history.[8]

Assessment of Energy Requirements

Patients Who Are Critically Ill

Patients who are critically ill have unique metabolic alterations compared to patients who are noncritically ill and ambulatory. These changes are summarized in Box 1.5. Patients who are critically ill have higher protein losses and increased metabolic demand for protein. Protein losses can be minimized but not completely abolished with nutrition support therapy alone.[46] The goals of nutrition support therapy for the patient who is critically ill are to minimize protein loss, maintain immune function, avoid metabolic complications, and attenuate the metabolic response to stress.[12] An accurate assessment of energy requirements is an important step in meeting these goals.

Underfeeding or overfeeding patients who are critically ill can lead to significant complications. Underfeeding calories can lead to impaired immune response, muscle catabolism, poor wound healing (particularly for surgical patients), and development of pressure injuries. Overfeeding can lead to hyperglycemia, hyperinsulinemia, hypokalemia, hypophosphatemia, excess carbon dioxide production, difficulty weaning from the ventilator, hepatic steatosis, and azotemia.[47,48] Indirect calorimetry is used to calculate energy expenditure by measurement of respiration gas exchange (oxygen consumption and carbon dioxide production) and is considered the gold standard for assessing energy requirements, particularly in patients who are critically ill.[49] Measuring energy expenditure can help to avoid the complications associated with underfeeding or overfeeding. Because the equipment used to conduct indirect calorimetry is expensive and requires technical expertise, its use in the clinical setting is limited. For clinicians without access to indirect calorimetry, predictive equations are necessary to determine energy requirements for the patient who is critically ill.

BOX 1.4

Data to Include in a Client History[8]

Personal history

Age, gender, sex, race

Ethnicity

Language

Literacy factors

Education

Role in family

Tobacco use

Physical disability

Mobility

Medical history

Chief nutrition complaint

Cardiovascular

Endocrine, metabolic

Excretory

Gastrointestinal

Gynecologic

Hematologic, oncologic

Immunologic

Musculoskeletal

Neurologic

Psychological

Treatments and therapy

Medical treatment, medical therapy

Surgical treatment

Palliative care, end-of-life care

Family and social history

Socioeconomic status

Living and housing situation

Domestic issues

Social and medical support

Geographic location of home

Occupation

Religion

History of recent crisis

Daily stress level

BOX 1.5

Metabolic Changes During Critical Illness

Shock or resuscitation phase

Low cardiac output

Hypotension

Poor tissue perfusion

Reduced oxygen consumption

Acute catabolic phase

Glycogenolysis

Gluconeogenesis

Proteolysis

Increased oxygen consumption

Increased carbon dioxide production

Hypermetabolism

Hyperglycemia

Overall catabolism

Anabolic phase

Energy expenditure returns to normal

Normoglycemia

Anabolism

According to the Academy of Nutrition and Dietetics 2012 Critical Illness Evidence-Based Nutrition Practice Guideline,[50] the Penn State University (PSU) 2003b equation for resting metabolic rate (RMR) has the highest prediction accuracy and should be used in nonobese, critically ill, mechanically ventilated adults. See Box 1.6 for this equation.[51]

BOX 1.6

Estimating Energy Requirements for Adults Who Are Mechanically Ventilated and Without Obesity[51]

Penn State University 2003b Equation

$$RMR = Mifflin\ (0.96) + V_E\ (31) + T_{max}\ (167) - 6,212$$

Where RMR is resting metabolic rate, Mifflin is Mifflin-St. Jeor RMR equation (see Box 1.9), V_E is minute ventilation in L/min, and T_{max} is maximum temperature over previous 24 hours in degrees Celsius.

According to the Academy of Nutrition and Dietetics 2012 Critical Illness Evidence-Based Nutrition Practice Guideline, the PSU 2003b equation has the highest prediction accuracy in critically ill, mechanically ventilated adults with obesity who are aged 60 years or less. However, for patients who are obese aged 60 years or older, the PSU 2010 equation has the highest prediction accuracy.[50] See Box 1.7 for the PSU 2010 equation.[52]

BOX 1.7

Estimating Energy Requirements for Adults With Obesity Who Are Mechanically Ventilated[52]

Penn State University 2010 Equation

$$RMR = Mifflin\ (0.71) + V_E\ (64) + T_{max}\ (85) - 3,085$$

Where RMR is resting metabolic rate, Mifflin is Mifflin-St. Jeor RMR equation (see Box 1.9), V_E is minute ventilation in L/min, and T_{max} is maximum temperature over previous 24 hours in degrees Celsius.

The SCCM and ASPEN have published guidelines for estimating energy requirements in patients who are critically ill as well. Both societies advocate the use of indirect calorimetry, but many institutions do not have access to this technology. The societies recommend a simplified, weight-based method for determining energy requirements. For nonobese adults, 25 to 30 kcal/kg is recommended. Hypocaloric, high-protein feeding is recommended for critically ill obese patients to help avoid specific complications, such as hyperglycemia and excessive carbon dioxide production while preserving lean body mass.[12] For patients with a BMI of 30 to 50, energy requirements should be calculated using 11 to 14 kcal/kg of actual weight, and for patients with a BMI of greater than

50, energy requirements should be calculated using 22 to 25 kcal/kg of IBW.[12,53] Interestingly, a secondary data analysis found no significant difference in mortality or time to discharge alive in a large cohort (n=5,672) of patients who are critically ill whose energy requirements were calculated using complex equations vs weight-based equations.[54]

Patients Who Are Noncritically Ill

In patients who are noncritically ill, basal energy expenditure (BEE) can be estimated using predictive equations, as an alternative to indirect calorimetry. The Harris-Benedict equation[55] is one of the oldest and most widely used predictive equations for calculating BEE. See Box 1.8.

BOX 1.8

Harris-Benedict Equation

$$\text{Male: BEE} = 66 + (13.7 \times W) + (5 \times H) - (6.8 \times A)$$

$$\text{Female: BEE} = 655 + (9.6 \times W) + (1.7 \times H) - (4.7 \times A)$$

Where BEE is basal energy expenditure, W is body weight in kg, H is height in cm, and A is age in years.

In addition, estimated energy needs may be based on RMR, as calculated by the Mifflin-St. Jeor equation.[6] See Box 1.9.

BOX 1.9

Mifflin-St. Jeor Equation

$$\text{Male: RMR} = (9.99 \times W) + (6.25 \times H) - (4.92 \times A) + 5$$

$$\text{Female: RMR} = (9.99 \times W) + (6.25 \times H) - (4.92 \times A) - 161$$

Where W is body weight in kg, H is height in cm, and A is age in years.

This equation seems to be the most accurate for estimation of energy needs among individuals who are obese and nonobese who are not critically ill.[57]

Assessment of Protein Requirements

Protein Requirements

In healthy individuals, the Recommended Dietary Allowance for protein in men and women* is 0.8 g/kg/d.[58] Estimated protein requirements may be based on specific disease states or metabolic stress states and may increase to levels of up to 2 g/kg/d depending on level of

---

* Specific recommendations for transgender people were not provided.

hypermetabolism, stress, and exogenous losses.[59] The body of a 70-kg male includes approximately 11 kg protein, with about 43% of it in the form of skeletal muscle.[60]

The rate of endogenous protein breakdown (catabolism) decreases during energy deprivation. An unstressed individual loses approximately 12 to 18 g protein per day after about 10 days of starvation, which equates to approximately 2 oz (57 g) of muscle tissue (2 to 3 g nitrogen). During metabolic stress, protein breakdown increases exponentially to approximately 30 to 60 g/d after surgery, 60 to 90 g/d with infection, 100 to 130 g/d with severe sepsis, and more than 175 g/d with burns or head injuries.[61] In chronic illness, skeletal muscle becomes the largest single contributor to protein loss.[62] The SCCM and ASPEN recommend a protein intake of 1.2 to 2 g/kg for patients who are critically ill. For patients who are critically ill who are obese, the societies recommend using IBW for calculations and providing at least 2 g/kg IBW for patients with class I and II obesity and at least 2.5 g/kg IBW for patients with class III obesity.[12]

Nitrogen Balance

Nitrogen balance studies are sometimes used to evaluate the adequacy of protein intake. Nitrogen balance studies indicate the relationship between protein intake and nitrogen removal from the renal system. Positive nitrogen balance cannot confirm anabolism because it lacks the specificity of stable isotopic amino acid studies.[63,64] The conversion factor commonly used for dietary protein is 6.25 g nitrogen per 1 g protein. Accurate 24-hour urine collection is difficult to obtain, and significant error may consequently be introduced into nitrogen balance calculations. See Box 1.10.

BOX 1.10

Nitrogen Balance Calculation

Nitrogen balance (g/d) = nitrogen intake (g/d) − nitrogen loss (g/d)

$$= \frac{(\text{Protein Intake})}{6.25} - \left[\frac{\text{UUN (g/d)}}{0.8} + 2.5\text{ g}\right]$$

Where UUN = urine urea nitrogen, UUN/0.8 represents UUN + urinary nonurea nitrogen, and 2.5 is the sum of fecal and integumental nitrogen.

Hepatic Transport Proteins

Historically, hepatic transport proteins have been used as markers of malnutrition. Low levels of these acute-phase proteins are correlated with morbidity and mortality.[30] These proteins are useful prognostic indicators of severity of illness, but they should not be used routinely as the primary diagnostic marker of malnutrition. Synthesis of acute-phase proteins (eg, albumin, transferrin, prealbumin, and retinol-binding protein) decreases precipitously during inflammatory conditions. Positive acute-phase proteins (C-reactive protein) increase in concentration during acute and chronic inflammatory states. Elevation of C-reactive protein may be used to confirm inflammatory status.[30,65]

Nutrition Assessment Tools

Numerous tools are available for general assessment of nutritional status. In the clinical setting, one of the most commonly used and validated assessment tools is the subjective global assessment (SGA).

The SGA (see Figure 1.1) is a nutrition assessment tool used to measure nutritional status on the basis of weight, dietary intake, GI symptoms, functional capacity, and physical examination findings.[37] Nutritional status is categorized as well-nourished, moderately

FIGURE 1.1 The subjective global assessment

(Select appropriate category with a checkmark, or enter numerical value where indicated by "#.")

A. History
    1. Weight change
       Overall loss in past 6 months: amount = # _____ kg; % loss = # _____
       Change in past 2 weeks: _____increase,
              _____no change,
              _____decrease.

    2. Dietary intake change (relative to normal)
       _____No change,
       _____Change _____duration = #_____weeks
                     _____type: _____suboptimal liquid diet,_____full liquid diet
                                 _____hypocaloric liquids,   _____starvation.

    3. Gastrointestinal symptoms (that persisted for >2 weeks)
       _____none, _____nausea, _____vomiting, _____diarrhea, _____anorexia.

    4. Functional capacity
       _____No dysfunction (eg, full capacity),
       _____Dysfunction _____duration = # _____weeks.
                     _____type: _____working suboptimall
                                 _____ambulatory,
                                 _____bedridden.

    5. Disease and its relation to nutritional requirements
       Primary diagnosis (specify) _____
       Metabolic demand (stress): _____no stress, _____low stress,
              _____moderate stress, _____high stress.

B. Physical (for each trait specify: 0 = normal, 1+ = mild, 2+ = moderate, 3+ = severe).
    # _____loss of subcutaneous fat (triceps, chest)
    # _____   muscle wasting (quadriceps, deltoids)
    # _____   ankle edema
    # _____   sacral edema
    # _____   ascites

C. SGA rating (select one)
    _____A = Well nourished
    _____B = Moderately (or suspected of being) malnourished
    _____C = Severely malnourished

Adapted with permission from Detsky AJ, McLaughlin JR, Baker JP, et al. What is subjective global assessment of nutritional status? *JPEN J Parenter Enteral Nutr.* 1987;11:8-14.[37]

malnourished (or suspected of being malnourished), or severely malnourished. The SGA was originally developed for patients with GI disease.[14] It has since been validated and used clinically for many patient populations and is widely accepted as a practical and reliable tool for nutrition assessment.[66]

Documenting Malnutrition

Malnutrition is a diagnosis known to be associated with poor outcomes in individuals who are hospitalized and nonhospitalized. A joint task force of the Academy of Nutrition and Dietetics and ASPEN has recommended a standardized set of diagnostic characteristics to identify and document adult malnutrition (see Table 1.3).[67] A 2019 review evaluated the usability of these diagnostic characteristics in day-to-day practice and their association with clinical outcomes.[68] Many of the diagnostic characteristics are readily available to clinicians during nutrition assessment, and the use of this framework to assess the presence of malnutrition has been predictive of length of hospital stay, morbidity, and mortality. A large validation study led by the Academy of Nutrition and Dietetics is in progress.

Clinical characteristic	Malnutrition in the context of acute illness or injury				Malnutrition in the context of chronic illness				Malnutrition in the context of social or environmental circumstances			
	Moderate malnutrition		Severe malnutrition		Moderate malnutrition		Severe malnutrition		Nonsevere (moderate) malnutrition		Severe malnutrition	
(1) Energy intake Malnutrition is the result of inadequate food and nutrient intake or assimilation; thus, recent intake compared to estimated requirements is a primary criterion defining malnutrition. The clinician may obtain or review the food and nutrition history, estimate optimum energy needs, compare them with estimates of energy consumed, and report inadequate intake as a percentage of estimated energy requirements over time.	<75% of estimated energy requirement for >7 d		≤50% of estimated energy requirement for ≥5 d		<75% of estimated energy requirement for ≥1 mo		≤75% of estimated energy requirement for ≥1 mo		<75% of estimated energy requirement for ≥3 mo		≤50% of estimated energy requirement for ≥1 mo	
	%	Time	%	Time	%	Time	%	Time	%	Time	%	Time
(2) Interpretation of weight loss The clinician may evaluate weight in light of other clinical findings, including the presence of under- or overhydration. The clinician may assess weight change over time reported as a percentage of weight lost from baseline.	1-2	1 wk	>2	1 wk	5	1 mo	>5	1 mo	5	1 mo	>5	1 mo

Physical findings:

Malnutrition typically results in changes to the physical examination. The clinician may perform a physical examination and document any one of the findings below as an indicator of malnutrition.

(3) Body fat Loss of subcutaneous fat (eg, orbital, triceps, fat overlying the ribs)	Mild		Moderate		Mild		Severe		Mild		Severe	

Table continues

TABLE 1.3 Clinical Characteristics That Support a Diagnosis of Malnutrition[a,67] (continued)

Clinical characteristic	Malnutrition in the context of acute illness or injury		Malnutrition in the context of chronic illness		Malnutrition in the context of social or environmental circumstances	
	Moderate malnutrition	Severe malnutrition	Moderate malnutrition	Severe malnutrition	Nonsevere (moderate) malnutrition	Severe malnutrition
(4) **Muscle mass** Muscle loss (eg, wasting of the temples [temporalis muscle]; clavicles [pectoralis and deltoids]; shoulders [deltoids]; interosseous muscles; scapula [latissimus dorsi, trapezius, deltoids]; thigh [quadriceps]; and calf [gastrocnemius])	Mild	Moderate	Mild	Severe	Mild	Severe
(5) **Fluid accumulation** The clinician may evaluate generalized or localized fluid accumulation evident on examination (extremities; vulvar or scrotal edema or ascites). Weight loss is often masked by generalized fluid retention (edema), and weight gain may be observed.	Mild	Moderate to severe	Mild	Severe	Mild	Severe
(6) **Reduced grip strength** The clinician should consult normative standards supplied by the manufacturer of the measurement device.	N/A[b]	Measurably reduced	N/A	Measurably reduced	N/A	Measurable reduced

[a] The presence of at least two of the six characteristics is recommended for diagnosis of either severe or nonsevere malnutrition. Height and weight should be measured rather than estimated to determine body mass index. Usual weight should be obtained to determine the percentage and interpret the significance of weight loss. Basic indicators of nutritional status, (eg, body weight, weight change, and appetite) may substantively improve with refeeding in the absence of inflammation. Refeeding or nutrition support, or both, may stabilize but not significantly improve nutrition parameters in the presence of inflammation. The National Center for Health Statistics defines a chronic disease or condition as one lasting 3 months or longer. Serum proteins, such as albumin and prealbumin, are not included as defining characteristics of malnutrition because recent evidence analysis shows that serum levels of these proteins do not change in response to changes in nutrient intake.

[b] N/A = not applicable.

Adapted with permission from White JV, Guenter P, Jensen G, et al. Consensus statement of the Academy of Nutrition and Dietetics/American Society for Parenteral and Enteral Nutrition: characteristics recommended for the identification and documentation of adult malnutrition (undernutrition). *J Acad Nutr Diet.* 2012;112(5):730-738.[67]

A modified tool for assessing malnutrition has been developed by a working group spearheaded by ASPEN and the European Society for Clinical Nutrition and Metabolism.[69] The group found that there was no framework for identifying malnutrition that was accepted on a global scale. The members evaluated various malnutrition criteria to develop a simplified framework for identifying malnutrition that was then developed and accepted by a global group of clinical nutrition experts. The key characteristics include the evaluation of phenotypic criteria (weight change, BMI, and reduced muscle mass) and etiologic criteria (reduced food intake or assimilation, and inflammation). After identifying the initial phenotypic and etiologic criteria, clinicians can then determine severity of malnutrition (See Boxes 1.11 and 1.12). Validation studies are in progress to determine if this assessment framework can identify such clinically relevant outcomes as prolonged length of hospital stay, morbidity, and mortality on a global scale.[70]

BOX 1.11

Global Leadership Initiative in Malnutrition: Phenotypic and Etiologic Criteria for the Diagnosis of Malnutrition[69]

Phenotypic criteria

Weight loss (%)

More than 5% within past 6 months or more than 10% beyond 6 months

Low BMI

Less than 20 if aged 70 years or less, or less than 22 if aged more than 70 years

Asian populations: Less than 18.5 if aged 70 years or less, or less than 20 if aged more than 70 years

Reduced muscle mass

Reduced by validated body composition measuring techniques

Etiologic criteria

Reduced food intake or assimilation

50% or less of energy requirements for more than 1 week, or any reduction for more than 2 weeks, or any chronic gastrointestinal condition that adversely affects food assimilation or absorption

Inflammation

Acute disease or injury, or chronic disease-related

BOX 1.12

Thresholds for Severity Grading of Malnutrition Into Stage 1 (Moderate) and Stage 2 (Severe) Malnutrition[69]

[a] One phenotypic criterion is required to meet a particular grade of malnutrition.
[b] Further research is needed to secure consensus reference BMI data for Asian populations in clinical settings.

Stage 1 (moderate)	Phenotypic criteria[a]
Weight loss (%)	5% to 10% within the past 6 months, or 10% to 20% beyond 6 months
Low BMI[b]	Less than 20 if aged 70 years or less or less than 22 if aged 70 years or more
Reduced muscle mass	Mild-to-moderate deficit (using validated assessment methods)

Stage 2 (severe)	
Weight loss (%)	More than 10% within the past 6 months, or more than 20% beyond 6 months
Low BMI[b]	Less than 18.5 if aged 70 years or less, or less than 10 if aged 70 years or more
Reduced muscle mass	Severe deficit (using validated assessment methods)

Summary

The GI tract is essential for the absorption and digestion of foods, and disorders of the GI system can have a significant impact on dietary intake and nutritional status. Nutrition assessment plays a vital role in identifying nutrition-related problems in patients with GI disorders and in developing appropriate nutrition interventions. A complete nutrition assessment includes evaluating dietary data, biochemical test and procedure results, anthropometric measures, nutrition focused physical findings, and the personal, medical, and social history, with an ultimate goal of improving clinical outcomes in patients with GI disorders.

References

1. Fisher RL. Wasting in chronic gastrointestinal diseases. *J Nutr.* 1999;129 (1S suppl):252S-255S.
2. Correia MI, Waitzberg DL. The impact of malnutrition on morbidity, mortality, length of hospital stay and costs evaluated through a multivariate model analysis. *Clin Nutr.* 2003;22(3):235-239.
3. Goiburu ME, Goiburu MM, Bianco H, et al. The impact of malnutrition on morbidity, mortality and length of hospital stay in trauma patients. *Nutr Hosp.* 2006;21:(5)604-610.
4. Mogensen KM, Robinson MK, Casey JD, et al. Nutritional status and mortality in the critically ill. *Crit Care Med.* 2015;43(12):2605-2615.
5. Robinson MK, Mogensen KM, Casey JD, et al. The relationship among obesity, nutritional status, and mortality in the critically ill. *Crit Care Med.* 2015;43(1):87-100.
6. Mogensen KM, Horkan CM, Purtle SW, et al. Malnutrition, critical illness survivors, and post-discharge outcomes: a cohort study. *JPEN J Parenter Enteral Nutr.* 2018;42(3):557-565.
7. Mueller C, Compher C, Druyan ME, et al. A.S.P.E.N. Clinical guidelines: nutrition screening, assessment, and intervention in adults. *JPEN J Parenter Enteral Nutr.* 2011;35(1):16-24.
8. Academy of Nutrition and Dietetics. Electronic Nutrition Care Process Terminology (eNCPT). Accessed January 31, 2021. www.ncpro.org/pubs/2020 -encpt-en?

9. Robinson D, Walker R, Adams SC, et al. American Society for Parenteral and Enteral Nutrition (ASPEN) definitions of terms, style, and conventions used in ASPEN Board of Directors–approved documents. May 2018. Accessed April 30, 2021. www.nutritioncare.org /uploadedFiles/Documents/Guidelines_and_Clinical _Resources/ASPEN%20Definition%20of%20Terms ,%20Style,%20and%20Conventions%20Used%20in %20ASPEN%20Board%20of%20Directors%E2%80 %93Approved%20Documents.pdf

10. Academy of Nutrition and Dietetics. Definition of terms list. February 2021. Accessed April 30, 2021. www.eatrightpro.org/-/media/eatrightpro -files/practice/scope-standards-of-practice /academydefinitionoftermslist.pdf?la=en&hash =9C69653783C7F39EA2E0E4F9E6745A6D9343D32A

11. Skipper A, Coltman A, Tomesko J, et al. Position of the Academy of Nutrition and Dietetics: Malnutrition (undernutrition) screening for all adults. *J Acad Nutr Diet*. 2020;120(4):709-713.

12. McClave SA, Taylor BE, Martindale RG, et al. Guidelines for the provision and assessment of nutrition support therapy in the adult critically ill patient: Society of Critical Care Medicine (SCCM) and American Society for Parenteral and Enteral Nutrition (ASPEN). *JPEN J Parenter Enteral Nutr*. 2016;40(2):159-211.

13. Ferguson M, Capra S, Bauer J, Banks M. Development of a valid and reliable malnutrition screening tool for adult acute care hospitals. *Nutrition*. 1999;15(6);458-464.

14. Kondrup J, Allison SP, Elia M, Vellas B, Plauth M. ESPEN guidelines for nutrition screening 2002. *Clin Nutr*. 2003;22(4):415-421.

15. Heyland DK, Dhaliwal R, Jiang X, Day AG. Identifying critically ill patients who benefit the most from nutrition therapy: the development and initial validation of a novel risk assessment tool. *Crit Care*. 2011;15(6):R268.

16. Rahman A, Hasan RM, Agarwala R, Martin C, Day AG, Heyland DK. Identifying critically-ill patients who will benefit most from nutritional therapy: further validation of the "modified NUTRIC" nutrition risk assessment tool. *Clin Nutr*. 2016;35(1):158-162.

17. Jie B, Jiang ZM, Nolan MT, Zhu SN, Yu K, Kondrup J. Impact of preoperative nutritional support on clinical outcome in abdominal surgical patients at nutritional risk. *Nutrition*. 2012;28(10):1022-1027.

18. Maciel LRMA, Franzosi OS, Nunes DLS, et al. Nutrition Risk Screening 2002 cut-off to identify high-risk is a good predictor of ICU mortality in critically ill patients. *Nutr Clin Pract*. 2019;34(1):137-141.

19. Mendes R, Policarpo S, Fortuna P, et al. Nutritional risk assessment and cultural validation of the modified NUTRIC score in critically ill patients—a multicenter prospective cohort study. *J Crit Care*. 2017;37:45-49.

20. Mayr U, Pfau J, Lukas M, et al. NUTRIC and modified NUTRIC are accurate predictors of outcome in end-stage liver disease: a validation in critically ill patients with liver cirrhosis. *Nutrients*. 2020;12(7):2134.

21. Schaefer EJ, Augustin JL, Schaefer MM, et al. Lack of efficacy of a food frequency questionnaire in assessing dietary macronutrient intakes in subjects consuming diets of known composition. *Am J Clin Nutr*. 2000;71(3):746-751.

22. Willett WC, ed. *Nutritional Epidemiology*. 2nd ed. Oxford University Press; 1998.

23. Buzzard IM, Faucett CL, Jeffery RW, et al. Monitoring dietary change in a low-fat diet intervention study: advantages of using 24-hour dietary recalls vs food records. *J Am Diet Assoc*. 1996;96(6):574-579.

24. Buzzard M. 24-hour recall and food record methods. In: Willett WC, ed. *Nutritional Epidemiology*. 2nd ed. Oxford University Press; 1998:50-73.

25. Zhang L, Misir A, Boshuizen H, Ocke M. A systematic review and meta-analysis of validation studies performed on dietary record apps. *Adv Nutr*. 021;12(6)2321-2332.

26. Ferrara G, Kim J, Lin S, Hua J, Seto E. A focused review of smartphone diet-tracking apps: usability, functionality, coherence with behavior change theory, and comparative validity of nutrient intake and energy estimates. *JMIR Mhealth Uhealth*. 2019;7(5):e9232.

27. Kelly JT, Collins PF, McCamley J, Ball L, Roberts S, Campbell KL. Digital disruption of dietetics: are we ready? *J Hum Nutr Diet*. 2021;34(1):134-146.

28. Chen J, Gemming L, Hanning R, Allman-Farinelli M. Smartphone apps and the nutrition care process: current perspectives and future considerations. *Patient Educ Couns*. 2018;101(4):750-757.

29. Sullivan SC, Bopp MM, Weaver DL, et al. Innovations in calculating precise nutrient intake of hospitalized patients. *Nutrients*. 2016;8:412.

30. Evans DC, Corkins MR, Malone A, et al. The use of visceral proteins as nutrition markers: an ASPEN position paper. *Nutr Clin Pract*. 2021;36(1):22-28.

31. Mordarski B. *Nutrition Focused Physical Exam*. 3rd ed. Academy of Nutrition and Dietetics; 2022.

32. Clark FS. Vitamin and trace elements. In: Gottschlich MM, ed. *The ASPEN Nutrition Support Core Curriculum: A Case-Based Approach—The Adult Patient*. American Society for Parenteral and Enteral Nutrition; 2007:129-159.

33. Pesce-Hammond K, Wessel J. Nutrition assessment and decision making. In: Merrit R, ed. *The ASPEN Nutrition Support Practice Manual*. American Society for Parenteral and Enteral Nutrition; 2005.

34. McKeever L. Vitamins and trace elements. In: Mueller CM, ed. *The ASPEN Adult Nutrition Support Core Curriculum*. 3rd ed. American Society for Parenteral and Enteral Nutrition; 2017:139-182.

35. Hamwi G. Changing dietary concepts. In: Danowski TS, ed. *Diabetes Mellitus: Diagnosis and Treatment*. American Diabetes Association; 1964.

36. Kyle UG, Genton L, Pichard C. Hospital length of stay and nutritional status. *Curr Opin Clin Nutr Metab Care*. 2005;8(4):397-402.

37. Detsky AS, McLaughlin JR, Baker JP, et al. What is subjective global assessment of nutritional status? *JPEN J Parenter Enteral Nutr*. 1987;11:8-14.

38. Blackburn GL, Bisttian BR, Maini BS, et al. Nutritional and metabolic assessment of the hospitalized patient. *JPEN J Parenter Enteral Nutr.* 1977;11(1):11-22.

39. Schneider AG, Baldwin I, Freitag E, et al. Estimation of fluid status changes in critically ill patients: fluid balance chart or electronic bed weight? *J Crit Care.* 2012;27:745.e7-745.e12.

40. Schneider AG, Thorpe C, Dellbridge K, et al. Electronic bed weighing vs daily fluid balance changes after cardiac surgery. *J Crit Care.* 2013;28:1113.e1-1113.e5.

41. NHLBI Obesity Education Initiative Expert Panel on the Identification, Evaluation, and Treatment of Obesity in Adults (US). *Clinical Guidelines on the Identification, Evaluation, and Treatment of Overweight and Obesity in Adults: The Evidence Report.* National Heart, Lung, and Blood Institute; 1998.

42. WHO Expert Committee. *Physical Status: The Use and Interpretation of Anthropometry.* WHO Technical Report Series 854. World Health Organization; 1995.

43. Sheehan P, Gonzalez C, Prado CM, et al. American Society for Parenteral and Enteral Nutrition clinical guidelines: the validity of body composition assessment in clinical populations. *JPEN J Parenter Enteral Nutr.* 2020;44(1):12-43.

44. Earthman CP. Body composition tools for assessment of adult malnutrition at the bedside: a tutorial on research considerations and clinical applications. *JPEN J Parenter Enteral Nutr.* 2015;39:(7)787-822.

45. Chan JM, Rimm EB, Colditz GA, Stampfer MJ, Willett WC. Obesity, fat distribution, and weight gain as risk factors for clinical diabetes in men. *Diabetes Care.* 1994;17(9):961-969.

46. Streat SJ, Beddoe AH, Hill GL. Aggressive nutritional support does not prevent protein loss despite fat gain in septic intensive care patients. *J Trauma.* 1987;27(3):262-266.

47. Martindale RG, Patel JJ, Herron TJ, Codner PA. Sepsis and critical illness. In: Mueller CM, ed. *The ASPEN Adult Nutrition Support Core Curriculum.* 3rd ed. American Society for Parenteral and Enteral Nutrition; 2017:457-472.

48. Evans DC, Collier BR. Trauma, surgery, and burns. In: Mueller CM, ed. *The ASPEN Adult Nutrition Support Core Curriculum.* 3rd ed. American Society for Parenteral and Enteral Nutrition; 2017:473-488.

49. Haugen HA, Chan LN. Indirect calorimetry: a practical guide for clinicians. *Nutr Clin Pract.* 2007;22(4):377-388.

50. Academy of Nutrition and Dietetics. 2012 Critical illness evidence-based nutrition practice guideline. Evidence Analysis Library. 2012. Accessed January 31, 2021. www.andeal.org/topic.cfm?menu=4800

51. Frankenfield D, Smith S, Cooney RN. Validation of 2 approaches to predicting resting metabolic rate in critically ill patients. *JPEN J Parenter Enteral Nutr.* 2004;28(4):259-264.

52. Frankenfield D. Validation of an equation for resting metabolic rate in older obese critically ill patients. *JPEN J Parenter Enteral Nutr.* 2011;35(2):264-269.

53. Mogensen, KM, Andrew BY, Corona JC, Robinson MK. Validation of the Society of Critical Care Medicine and American Society for Parenteral and Enteral Nutrition recommendations for caloric provision to critically ill patients: a pilot study. *JPEN J Parenter Enteral Nutr.* 2016;40(5):713-721.

54. Compher C, Nicolo M, Chittams J, et al. Clinical outcomes in critically ill patients associated with the use of complex vs weight-only predictive equations. *JPEN J Parenter Enteral Nutr.* 2015;39(7):864-869.

55. Harris JA, Benedict FG. *Biometric Studies of Basal Metabolism in Man.* Carnegie Institution of Washington; 1919.

56. Mifflin MD, St. Jeor ST, Hill LA, Scott BJ, Daugherty SA, Koh YO. A new predictive equation for resting energy expenditure in healthy individuals. *Am J Clin Nutr.* 1990;51(2):241-247.

57. Frankenfield DC, Roth-Yousey L, Compher C. Comparison of predictive equations for resting metabolic rate in healthy nonobese and obese individuals, a systematic review. *J Am Diet Assoc.* 2005;105(5):775-789.

58. Institute of Medicine. *Dietary Reference Intakes for Energy, Carbohydrate, Fiber, Fat, Fatty Acids, Cholesterol, Protein, and Amino Acids.* National Academies Press; 2005:589.

59. ASPEN Board of Directors and Clinical Guidelines Task Force. Guidelines for the use of parenteral and enteral nutrition in adult and pediatric patients. *JPEN J Parenter Enteral Nutr.* 2002;26(1 suppl):1SA-138SA.

60. Lentner C. *Geigy Scientific Tables: Units of Measurement, Body Fluids, Composition of the Body, Nutrition.* Vol 1. 8th ed. Ciba-Geigy Corporation; 1981.

61. Heimburger DC. Malnutrition and nutrition assessment. In: Fauci AS, Kasper DL, Longo DL, Braunwald E, Hauser SL, Jameson JL, eds. *Harrison's Principles of Internal Medicine.* 17th ed. Mcgraw-Hill; 2008:451.

62. Hansen RD, Raja C, Allen BJ. Total body protein in chronic diseases and in aging. *Ann N Y Acad Sci.* 2000;904:345-352.

63. Meesters RJ, Wolfe RR, Deutz NE. Application of liquid chromatography-tandem mass spectrometry (LC-MS/MS) for the analysis of stable isotope enrichments of phenylalanine and tyrosine. *J Chromatogr B Analyt Technol Biomed Life Sci.* 2009; 877(1/2):43-49.

64. Tuvdendorj D, Chinkes DL, Zhang XJ, et al. Adult patients are more catabolic than children during acute phase after burn injury: a retrospective analysis on muscle protein kinetics. *Intensive Care Med.* 2011;37(8):1317-1322.

65. Empana JP, Jouven X, Canouï-Poitrine F, et al. C-reactive protein, interleukin 6, fibrinogen and risk of sudden death in European middle-aged men: the PRIME study. *Arterioscler Thromb Vasc Biol.* 2010;30(10):2047-2052.

66. Baker JP, Detsky AS, Wesson DE, et al. Nutritional assessment: a comparison of clinical judgment and objective measures. *N Engl J Med.* 1982;306(16):969-973.

67. White JV, Guenter P, Jensen G, et al. Consensus statement of the Academy of Nutrition and Dietetics/ American Society for Parenteral and Enteral Nutrition: characteristics recommended for the identification and documentation of adult malnutrition (undernutrition). *J Acad Nutr Diet.* 2012;112(5):730-738.

68. Mogensen KM, Malone A, Becker P, et al. Academy of Nutrition and Dietetics/American Society for Parenteral and Enteral Nutrition consensus malnutrition characteristics: usability and association with outcomes. *Nutr Clin Pract.* 2019;34(5):657-665.

69. Jensen GL, Cederholm T, Correia MITD, et al. GLIM criteria for the diagnosis of malnutrition: a consensus report from the global clinical nutrition community. *JPEN J Parenter Enteral Nutr.* 2019;43(1):32-40.

70. Keller H, de van der Schueren MAE, Jensen GL, et al. Global Leadership Initiative on Malnutrition (GLIM): guidance on validation of the operational criteria for diagnosis of protein-energy malnutrition in adults. *JPEN J Parenter Enteral Nutr.* 2020;44(6):992-1003.

Gastrointestinal Tests and Procedures

Gerard E. Mullin, MD, AGAF, FACG, FACN
Amy K. Fischer, MS, RD, CDN

KEY POINTS

- Knowledge of tests and procedures used to diagnose and treat gastrointestinal disorders is essential to the practice of gastrointestinal nutrition.
- Endoscopic procedures require conscious sedation and carry risks that vary by procedure type and patient comorbidity. Risks and potential benefits must be weighed in each case.
- Endoscopic procedures that provide enteral access for feeding carry a higher risk, as the comorbidities tend to be higher and the surgical incision used for placement of the feeding tube device carries a risk of infection and sepsis. Ethical considerations must be weighed with each patient.

Introduction

This chapter reviews the relevance and importance of gastrointestinal (GI) tests for the diagnosis and treatment of GI nutritional disorders. Disorders relating to the GI tract are considered digestive disorders. "Good" digestive health is an ability to process nutrients through properly functioning GI organs, including the stomach, intestine, liver, pancreas, and gallbladder. When these organs do not function properly, patients may need to consult a gastroenterologist for further testing and diagnosis.

Digestive disorders are one of the most common reasons people seek medical advice, and many digestive problems are multifactorial. Diagnosis and treatment generally involve GI tests and procedures. The following tests and procedures are summarized in this chapter along with their indications, preparation, and risks:

- upper endoscopy
- colonoscopy
- flexible sigmoidoscopy
- capsule procedures, including wireless capsule, SmartPill capsule, and Bravo pH capsule
- enteroscopy, including push enteroscopy, single-balloon enteroscopy, and double-balloon enteroscopy
- endoscopic retrograde cholangiopancreatography
- motility procedures, including esophageal motility study, anorectal motility study, and gastric emptying study
- feeding tubes, including percutaneous endoscopic gastrostomy and percutaneous endoscopic jejunostomy

Box 2.1 on page 28 summarizes additional tests that may be used in the diagnosis and monitoring of various GI conditions.

Examples of Other Diagnostic Gastrointestinal Tests

General gastrointestinal (GI) tests

7AC4, bile acid synthesis, serum

Galactose-α-1,3-galactose (α-gal), immunoglobulin E, serum

Galactose-α-1,3-galactose (α-gal) mammalian meat allergy profile, serum

Celiac disease comprehensive cascade, serum and whole blood

Celiac disease serology cascade, serum

Celiac disease gluten-free cascade, serum, whole blood

Celiac-associated *HLA-DQA1* and *HLA-DQB1* DNA typing, blood

GI pathogen panel, polymerase chain reaction (PCR), feces

QuantiFERON-TB Gold Plus (QFT-Plus), blood

Autoimmune GI dysmotility evaluation, serum

Helicobacter pylori breath test

H pylori with clarithromycin resistance prediction, molecular detection, PCR, feces

Disaccharidase activity panel, tissue

Liver disease tests

Wilson disease, full gene analysis, varies

Nonalcoholic steatohepatitis (NASH)-FibroTest, serum and plasma

FibroTest-ActiTest, serum

Autoimmune liver disease panel, serum

Hepatocellular carcinoma risk panel with GALAD score,[a] serum

α1-Antitrypsin proteotype S/Z by liquid chromatography with tandem mass spectrometry (LC-MS/MS), serum

Lysosomal acid lipase, blood

Inflammatory bowel disease tests

Adalimumab quantitative with reflex to antibody, serum

Infliximab quantitation with reflex to antibodies to infliximab, serum

Ustekinumab quantitation with antibodies, serum

Vedolizumab quantitation with reflex to antibodies, serum

Vedolizumab quantitation with antibodies, serum

Thiopurine methyltransferase (TPMT) and Nudix hydrolase (NUDT15) genotyping, varies

TPMT activity profile, erythrocytes

Thiopurine metabolites, whole blood

Calprotectin, feces

Box continues

Inflammatory bowel disease serology panel, serum

C-reactive protein, serum

Celiac-associated *HLA-DQA1* and *HLA-DQB1* DNA typing, blood

Inflammatory bowel disease primary immunodeficiency panel, varies

Pancreatic tests

Pancreatic elastase, feces

Hereditary pancreatitis panel, varies

ᵃ GALAD stands for gender, age, α-fetoprotein-L3, α-fetoprotein, des-γ-carboxy prothrombin

Upper Endoscopy

An upper endoscopy (also known as an endoscopy, gastroscopy, or esophagogastroduodenoscopy) is a procedure that allows a physician to examine the lining of the upper GI tract, including the esophagus, stomach, and duodenum (first portion of the small intestine).[1] The procedure is used to visually examine the upper digestive system by passing a flexible tube (with a light and tiny camera on the distal end) into the esophagus. This tube, known as an endoscope, can view, photograph, and biopsy and identify inflammation, erosions, ulcerations, changes in blood vessels, and the destruction of surface cells.

Upper endoscopy procedures are used for many different indications, including the following[1]:

- removal of stuck objects, including food
- detection of ulcers, abnormal growths, precancerous conditions, small bowel inflammation, and hiatal hernias
- treatment of bleeding ulcers
- tissue biopsy
- determination of the cause of abdominal pain, nausea, vomiting, swallowing difficulties, gastric reflux, unexplained weight loss, or bleeding in the upper GI tract

Preparation and Procedure

The upper GI tract must be empty before the procedure; patients should not eat anything during the 8 hours before the test. Anesthesia guidelines for fasting of liquids can vary, but generally small amounts of clear liquids (less than 4 oz) are permitted up to 4 hours prior to the procedure. Patients should discuss all health conditions, medications, and vitamins they are taking with their physicians in advance. The patient is sedated before the procedure with fast-acting intravenous anesthesia. To decrease intravenous anesthetic requirements, the physician may numb the patient's throat with a local anesthetic spray.[2]

During the procedure, the patient lies on their back or side on an examining table. The endoscope is carefully passed through the mouth and down the esophagus into the stomach and duodenum under direct visualization. The camera on the endoscope transfers images of the intestinal lining to a monitor. More commonly, carbon dioxide is pumped through the endoscope to inflate the stomach and duodenum. During this procedure, the physician can perform biopsies, stop bleeding, and sample or remove abnormal growths.

Risks

Risks associated with upper endoscopy can range from none to death, depending on a patient's comorbidities. Direct procedure-related complications include adverse reactions to sedatives, aspiration pneumonia, cardiac arrhythmias, bleeding from the biopsy site, and accidental puncture of the GI tract.

Colonoscopy

Colonoscopy enables physicians to see inside the colon and detect inflamed tissue, abnormal growths, and early signs of colorectal cancer.[3] It also facilitates the investigation of potential causes of changes in bowel habits, abnormal pain, bleeding from the anus, and weight loss. Colonoscopy is considered the gold standard for detecting colorectal cancers and adenoma.[4]

Preparation and Procedure

To prepare for a colonoscopy, patients typically follow a clear liquid diet for 1 day, unless there is a history of constipation and known slow gut transit, in which case the recommended duration of bowel preparation is 2 days. After preparation, all solids must be emptied from the GI tract before the procedure. Acceptable liquids include fat-free bouillon, strained fruit juice, water, plain coffee, plain tea, sports drinks, and gelatin. The day before the procedure, patients must consume only clear liquids and then ingest some form of purgative (low-volume sodium phosphate purge or high-volume polyethylene glycol purge). A laxative or enema may be required the night before a colonoscopy. Because sedation is administered, patients cannot drive after the procedure and should be accompanied by another individual to escort them home. Recovery time is approximately 30 minutes to 1 hour unless a complication occurs.[5]

During a colonoscopy, the patient is placed on their left side. A long, flexible, lighted tube known as a colonoscope is inserted into the anus and slowly guided through the rectum into the colon. The scope inflates the large intestine with carbon dioxide gas, and a camera is mounted on the scope. Once the tubular camera reaches the cecum with the appendiceal in view, it is slowly withdrawn, and the large intestine is examined again slowly. The recommended withdrawal time is no less than 6 minutes. During the procedure, the physician can remove growths and polyps to detect signs of colorectal cancer. Routine colonoscopy should typically begin at age 45; starting earlier may be recommended for people with a personal or family history of colorectal cancer or inflammatory bowel disease.[4]

Risks

Direct risks attributable to colonoscopy include severe abdominal pain, bowel perforation, fever, bloody bowel movements, dizziness, and weakness. The removal of polypoid growths increases these risks, as does the presence of widespread colonic diverticulosis or severe colitis. Rare complications include splenic or hepatic trauma and splenic rupture.[6]

Flexible Sigmoidoscopy

A flexible sigmoidoscopy is an internal examination of the rectum and sigmoid colon using a flexible sigmoidoscope. The test can help diagnose the cause of diarrhea; colon polyps; diverticulitis; inflammatory bowel disease; blood, mucus, or pus in stool; and colorectal cancer. Normal findings show that the lining of the sigmoid colon, rectal mucosa rectum, and anus are normal in color, texture, and size. Abnormal results may indicate anal fissures,

anal-rectal abscesses, bowel obstruction, cancer, colorectal polyps, diverticulitis, hemorrhoids, inflammatory bowel disease, inflammation, and proctitis.[7]

Preparation and Procedure

On the morning of the procedure, the patient should consume a light breakfast. One hour
before the procedure, one to two saline enemas are required. The examination can be done
in a physician's office or the hospital. Sedation is not administered, and patients usually
experience some tolerable abdominal pain.[8]

During a sigmoidoscopy, the patient lies on their left side with the knees drawn
toward the chest. First, the physician performs a digital rectal examination to enlarge
the anus for the sigmoidoscope. Next, a 60-cm flexible sigmoidoscope is inserted into
the rectum; air or carbon dioxide gas is introduced into the colon to expand the area and
may cause the patient to experience the feeling of an urge to have a bowel movement if
awake for the procedure. The sigmoidoscope is usually inserted into the sigmoid colon or
descending colon. The scope is used to observe the bowel lining, and a hollow channel in
the center of the scope allows the physician to take biopsies. The procedure usually takes
7 to 15 minutes. Patients may return to ordinary daily activities immediately after the
procedure unless given an intravenous anesthetic, in which case they may return to usual
activities the following day.

Risks

The risk for complications is very low. Rare side effects include bowel perforation and bleeding
at the biopsy site. However, anxiety is common if the patient is awake during the procedure.[9]

Capsule Procedures

Wireless Capsule Endoscopy

Wireless capsule endoscopy uses a miniature wireless camera that the patient swallows. As
the camera makes its way through the digestive tract, it captures pictures of the GI mucosa.
Wireless capsule endoscopy is used for the following[10,11]:

- investigating the potential cause of obscure GI bleeding following a negative upper
  and lower endoscopy (diagnostic yield is 65% for detecting the cause of occult GI
  bleeding)[12]
- diagnosing small bowel Crohn's disease (see Chapter 3)[13,14]
- assessing the extent and activity of celiac disease throughout the small intestine
  (see Chapter 6)
- screening for and surveilling small intestinal polyps in familial polyposis
  syndromes[15]
- screening for small bowel tumors

Preparation and Procedure

Patient preparation for an endoscopy is similar to preparation for a colonoscopy except
that the patient uses one-half of the dose of purgative. The procedure is done using an
11×26-mm capsule endoscope consisting of an optical dome, four light-emitting electrodes,
a sensor, two batteries, and a microtransmitter.[11]

The capsule acquires and transmits digital images at the rate of two images per second
to a sensor array attached to the patient's abdomen. The capsule endoscope can directly
capture video images of the mucosal surface of the entire length of the small intestine. The

procedure is virtually pain-free because the capsule is propelled forward through the GI tract by peristalsis.

Patients can engage in normal daily activities after the procedure. Also, they can eat a regular diet 4 hours after ingesting the capsule; however, if a patient has delayed gastric emptying, which can interfere with the test, a solid meal should be postponed until the 8-hour mark.[11]

Risks

There is a risk of capsule retention or entrapment in strictures or diverticula. The presence of intestinal obstruction, fistulas, or strictures may impede the passage of the capsule. It can cause retention of the capsule in the gut, which can be silent or cause symptomatic intestinal obstruction. Capsules that are retained can be removed by a lengthy endoscope procedure called enteroscopy. Enteroscopy can be done regardless of the location of the capsule in the small bowel capsule. Capsule endoscopy is contraindicated in patients with known strictures or swallowing disorders. Patients with extensive small bowel Crohn's disease, those who chronically use nonsteroidal anti-inflammatory drugs, and those with abdominal radiation injury are at higher risk for capsule retention.[16]

Clinicians have used small bowel series to look for strictures and determine whether the capsule will safely pass through the small intestine and into the colon. However, a negative small bowel series does not exclude a stricture and has been associated with several capsule retentions. A solid, sugarcoated pill containing a tiny metallic radiofrequency identification device (RFID) can be given to the patient to determine if the capsule is safe to administer. Passage of the RFID is confirmed by abdominal radiography and correlates with the safe passage of the capsule.[17] The history of obstructive symptoms or a prior history of intestinal surgery is more predictive of capsule retention than a negative small bowel series.[18]

SmartPill Capsule

The SmartPill is a wireless, ingestible capsule that measures pressure, pH, and temperature data at regular intervals as it travels through the GI tract. Gastric emptying and whole-tract transit can be assessed. The information gathered also helps diagnose gastroparesis and other GI motility disorders, such as slow transit constipation.[19]

Preparation and Procedure

The preparation for the SmartPill is a standard overnight fast. On the study day, the patient is given a standardized SmartBar (255 kcal, 75% carbohydrate, 21% protein, 3% fat, and 3% fiber) just before ingesting the SmartPill. The patient is then expected to fast for 6 hours, except for drinking small quantities of water (up to ½ cup, or 120 ml).[20]

Risks

The only potential risk is capsule retention in the setting of a stricture in the GI tract.

Bravo pH Monitoring Test

The Bravo pH monitoring test is a catheter-free pH test used to measure and monitor acid reflux in the setting of gastroesophageal reflux disease (GERD). With the Bravo system, during standard upper endoscopy a small pH capsule is attached to the esophageal wall. The capsule transmits pH data every 12 seconds to a small receiver unit via radiofrequency telemetry for 48 hours.[21] The Bravo test is used to diagnose GERD or determine whether medical therapy is working to prevent acid reflux.

Preparation and Procedure

Preparation for a Bravo pH test is the same as for a standard upper endoscopy—the patient fasts overnight. During the procedure, the patient either sits or lies down while the physician places the capsule into the esophagus. After the capsule is in place, suction is applied, drawing a small amount of tissue into the capsule and locking it in place. The pH recording starts immediately after the capsule is attached and continues for 48 hours, transmitting pH measurements wirelessly to a small receiver on a waistband or belt. Patients are instructed to keep a diary and record mealtimes, position changes, and the time and type of their symptoms. They are encouraged to pursue their daily activities and diet. Upon completing the procedure, the patient returns the recording device to the physician, who uploads the data. The capsule is disposable and passes naturally through a bowel movement within a few days after the test.[22]

Risks

Risks of this procedure include premature detachment of the pH capsule; failure of the capsule to detach from the esophagus within a few days after placement; tears in the mucosal and submucosal layers of the esophagus, causing bleeding; and perforation.[22]

Enteroscopy

The small bowel can be a difficult area to examine due to its anatomy, location, and relative tortuosity. Conventional endoscopy cannot provide adequate visualization because the small intestine is 18 to 22 ft long. Enteroscopy is the use of scopes to examine the small intestine.[23] There are several different types of enteroscopy.

Push Enteroscopy

Push enteroscopy is one of the most frequently used endoscopic methods for small bowel examination. It is usually considered the next diagnostic step in evaluating patients with obscure GI bleeding after negative endoscopy and colonoscopy.[24] Indications for push enteroscopy include the following:

- determining the cause of malabsorption
- determining the cause of unexplained diarrhea
- diagnosing refractory celiac disease
- determining the cause of unexplained GI bleeding

Preparation and Procedure

Patients should not take products containing aspirin for 1 week before a push endoscopy and should tell their physicians about any blood thinners they are taking (eg, warfarin or clopidogrel) because these medications can interfere with the test. The patient should follow a liquid diet the day before the procedure and may consume clear liquids up to 4 hours before the examination. Numbing medication is usually administered to reduce gagging feelings when the tube is inserted into the mouth.

A thin, flexible tube (endoscope) is inserted through the mouth and advanced into the proximal jejunum. Push enteroscopy is an outpatient procedure done under conscious sedation and lasts from 15 to 45 minutes. The patient may experience mild cramping.[24]

Risks

Risks are rare and include excessive bleeding at the biopsy site, bowel perforation, infection of the biopsy site, and vomiting.[25,26]

Double-Balloon and Single-Balloon Enteroscopy

The primary uses for balloon enteroscopy are to visualize the small bowel and perform diagnostic and therapeutic procedures. The double-balloon enteroscopy, also known as the push-and-pull enteroscopy, allows for visualization of the entire small intestine, tissue sampling, and therapeutic intervention. Single-balloon enteroscopy was designed to mimic the functions of double-balloon enteroscopy.[25,26] The single-balloon system looks just like the double-balloon system except that it lacks a balloon at the tip of the endoscope.

Preparation and Procedure

Patient preparation for this procedure is the same as for capsule endoscopy and colonoscopy. During a double-balloon enteroscopy, balloons are attached to the endoscope and are inflated to allow the physician to view the large part of the small intestine.

Risks

The main risks for balloon enteroscopy procedures are anesthesia-related risks, possible perforation of the intestine, and bleeding.

Endoscopic Retrograde Cholangiopancreatography

Endoscopic retrograde cholangiopancreatography (ERCP) is used to diagnose and treat problems in the liver, gallbladder, bile ducts, and pancreas, including gallstones, inflammatory strictures (scars), leaks (from trauma and surgery), and cancer.[27]

Preparation and Procedure

The stomach and duodenum must be empty to obtain accurate results. Patients should not consume any food or beverages after midnight the night before the procedure or 6 to 8 hours beforehand.

X-rays and an endoscope are used in the procedure. The patient lies on their left side on an examining table in an x-ray room. Medication is administered to numb the back of the throat, and a sedative is given before the examination. The patient swallows the endoscope, and the physician guides the scope through the esophagus, stomach, and duodenum until it reaches the location where the ducts of the biliary tree and pancreas open into the duodenum. At this time, the patient is turned to lie flat on the stomach, and the physician passes a small plastic tube through the scope. Dye is injected into the ducts to allow visualization by x-ray. X-rays are taken immediately after the dye injection. If a gallstone is obstructing the ducts, instruments can be inserted into the scope to remove or relieve the obstruction. A biopsy can be done for further testing.

ERCP requires 30 minutes to 2 hours to complete. The patient may experience discomfort when air is blown into the duodenum and dye is injected into the ducts. This discomfort can generally be managed with sedation and mild pain medication. Tenderness or lump at the site of sedative injection usually subsides within a few days.[28]

Risks

Risks associated with ERCP are usually mild but can be moderate-to-severe requiring hospitalization, and may include pancreatitis and (less commonly) infection, bleeding, and perforation of the duodenum.[28]

Motility Procedures

Disorders of gastric motor function include impaired accommodation, gastroparesis, and dumping syndrome.[17-19] The symptoms that occur in patients with gastric motor disorders are nonspecific, and they include poor appetite, postprandial fullness, bloating, nausea, vomiting, epigastric pain, and early satiety (inability to finish a normal-size meal).

GI motility and functional bowel diseases include achalasia, scleroderma, mixed connective tissue disease, GERD, gastroparesis, functional dyspepsia, irritable bowel syndrome, colonic inertia, pelvic floor dyssynergia, and fecal incontinence.

Esophageal Motility Study

Esophageal motility study, or esophageal manometry, is used to evaluate lower- and upper-esophageal sphincter pressure, esophageal body contraction amplitude, and peristaltic sequence. The procedure helps evaluate patients with dysphagia, unexplained or noncardiac chest pain, or symptoms suggestive of GERD. It is also used to assess patients before antireflux surgery. The two manometric methods employed are the low-compliance water-perfused catheter system and the solid-state pressure system.[29]

Preparation and Procedure
The preparation for this procedure is an overnight fast.

Risks
The main risk associated with an esophageal motility study is discomfort to the patient during the procedure.

Anorectal Motility Study

Anorectal manometry is a test to evaluate patients with fecal incontinence and constipation. The test measures the pressure of the anal sphincter muscles and assesses rectal sensation, anorectal reflexes, and rectal compliance.[30]

Preparation and Procedure
The patient should use one or two enemas 2 hours before the procedure and consume no food or liquids during those 2 hours. Regular medications and water are allowed up to 2 hours before the examination. Patients who are allergic to latex should inform the physician of this allergy before the test so that a latex-free balloon can be used.

The procedure lasts approximately 30 minutes. The patient lies on their left side. A small flexible tube with a balloon on the end is inserted into the rectum. The balloon is attached to a catheter that may inflate the rectum to assess the normal reflex pathways. The physician or nurse may ask the patient to squeeze, relax, and push at various times throughout the examination to measure the anal sphincter muscle pressures.[31]

Two other tests may be done: (1) anal sphincter electromyography (EMG) to evaluate the nerve supply to the anal muscles, and (2) a balloon expulsion test to measure the time it takes to expel a balloon from the rectum.[31] Anal sphincter EMG is recorded with a small plug electrode placed in the anal canal. The patient is asked to relax, squeeze, and push at different times. The electrical activity of the anal sphincter muscle is recorded and displayed on a computer screen. Anal sphincter EMG confirms the proper muscle contractions during squeezing and proper muscle relaxation during pushing. Normal anal EMG activity with low anal-squeeze pressures on manometry may indicate a torn sphincter muscle that can be repaired.[32] The test is used to look for defects in anal sphincter smooth-muscle dysfunction.

In a balloon expulsion test, a small balloon is inserted into the rectum and inflated with water. The patient then tries to defecate (expel) the small balloon from the rectum. The amount of time it takes to expel the balloon is recorded. Prolonged balloon expulsion suggests a dysfunction in the anorectum area.[33,34] The patient can drive after the procedure and resume normal activities.

Risks

Anorectal manometry is a safe procedure with minimal risk and is unlikely to cause any pain. The main risk is discomfort to the patient during the procedure and possible anxiety. Rare complications include a perforation (tearing) or bleeding of the rectum.[35]

Gastric Emptying Studies

Gastroparesis is impaired gastric motility that results in delayed or irregular contractions of the stomach leading to various GI symptoms, such as early satiety, bloating, nausea, vomiting, diarrhea, and constipation. Tests used to evaluate a patient with impaired gastric emptying include upper endoscopy, barium x-ray, and ultrasound, to rule out obstructions or mucosal or structural disorders. Once other causes are ruled out, SmartPill tests, gastric emptying scintigraphy, and breath tests can be done to diagnose gastroparesis.[36]

Preparation and Procedure

As described earlier, the SmartPill is a small wireless device in capsule form that can be swallowed. For gastric emptying scintigraphy, the patient eats a meal consisting of eggs that contain a small amount of radioisotope, a radioactive substance that shows up on scans. The scan measures the rate of gastric emptying at 1, 2, 3, and 4 hours. When more than 10% of the meal is still in the stomach at 4 hours, the diagnosis of gastroparesis is confirmed.[37]

For a breath test, the patient ingests a meal containing a small amount of isotope; breath samples are then taken to measure the presence of the isotope in exhaled carbon dioxide. The results reveal how fast the stomach is emptying.

Risks

No risks. Patient may express concerns about ingesting isotopes that pass through the body, but these are typically short-lived.

Feeding Tubes

Feeding tubes provide nutrition support to patients who cannot take food by mouth or eat enough to support their nutritional needs (see Chapter 19 for more information on tube feeding, or enteral nutrition). Percutaneous endoscopic gastrostomy (PEG), jejunal extension through a PEG (gastrojejunostomy), or direct endoscopic jejunostomy is appropriate when nutrition support is required for more than 3 weeks. Short-term tube feeding is generally managed by placing a nasoenteric tube.[38]

Percutaneous Endoscopic Gastrostomy

PEG is a nonsurgical procedure in which a feeding tube (called a PEG tube or gastrostomy tube) is placed through the skin and abdominal wall directly into the stomach with an endoscope. Appropriate indications for PEG tube placement include esophageal obstruction, head and neck cancer, dysphagia, and supplemental nutrition during chemotherapy or radiation.[39]

Preparation and Procedure

Patients prepare for this procedure by fasting overnight, as for an upper endoscopy, and receive a dose of intravenous antibiotics according to physician preference.

During an upper endoscopy, the endoscopist must demonstrate the transillumination of light across the abdominal wall to ensure no overlying bowel is present. After successful transillumination, an incision is made on the abdominal wall under sterile conditions after local anesthesia. A thin wire is introduced through the incision and into the stomach under visualization and then delivered externally through the oral cavity. The gastrostomy tube is provided over the wire and placed via a push-and-pull technique. A successful placement is confirmed via visualization with the endoscope. The gastrostomy tube is externally secured to the abdominal wall with a fastener and then dressed in gauze after the procedure. The procedure takes 15 to 20 minutes.[39]

The gastrostomy tube can be used once the patient is discharged from the endoscopy unit. Use of a PEG feeding tube can be temporary or permanent, depending on the medical condition. The life span of the tube is about 1 year. Replacement gastrostomy tubes that use a balloon inflation system can be used when the original tube needs to be replaced.[39]

Protocols for immediate postplacement care of the tube should be implemented to ensure that the feeding tube site is kept clean and the feeding tube is kept patent. If the tube is accidentally dislodged, the physician should be contacted immediately, and the tube should be replaced within 24 hours to prevent the incision from closing.[40]

Risks

Minor complications include leakage of food or fluid around the tube. Mild bleeding or infection may occur at the incision site.[40]

Percutaneous Endoscopic Jejunostomy

A percutaneous endoscopic jejunostomy (PEJ) tube, also known as a jejunostomy tube, is surgically implanted in the upper section of the small intestine (jejunum) just below the stomach. The PEJ tube bypasses the stomach, and food is delivered directly into the patient's intestinal tract. The placement of a PEJ tube is indicated in patients with the following[41,42]:

- unsuitable stomach access
- high risk for aspiration
- gastric resection (partial or total)
- gastric pull-up, gastric outlet obstruction, or obstructed or nonfunctioning gastrojejunostomy
- gastric dysmotility
- gastroparesis
- stenosis
- previous esophageal surgery

Preparation and Procedure

Preparation is the same as for upper endoscopy (an overnight fast). Although it is similar to PEG tube placement, direct PEJ tube placement is considerably more difficult. If necessary, the tube can be secured in place with sutures by a physician. The skin surrounding the tube should be kept clean, dry, and covered with a gauze dressing.[43]

Risks

Risks of PEJ are the same as described for PEG, which includes bleeding from the incision site, anesthesia, aspiration, and infection.

Summary

Digestive disorders are one of the most common reasons people seek medical advice, and many digestive problems are multifactorial. Diagnosis and treatment generally involve GI tests and procedures.

References

1. Miller AT, Sedlack RE; ACE Research Group. Competency in esophagogastroduodenoscopy: a validated tool for assessment and generalizable benchmarks for gastroenterology fellows. *Gastrointest Endosc.* 2019;90(4):613-620.e1.

2. Benzoni T, Cascella M. Procedural sedation. In: *StatPearls* (online). StatPearls Publishing; 2021. NCBI Bookshelf. Accessed September 20, 2021. www.ncbi.nlm .nih.gov/books/NBK551685

3. Ahmed M. Colon cancer: a clinician's perspective in 2019. *Gastroenterology Res.* 2020;13(1):1-10.

4. Karatzas PS, Rosch T, Papanikolaou IS, de Heer J, Schachschal G, Groth S. Recognizing post-endoscopy complications: a database filter reduces quality assurance workload for inpatients. *Dig Dis.* 2021;39(2):171-178.

5. ASGE Standards of Practice Committee; Saltzman JR, Cash BD, et al. Bowel preparation before colonoscopy. *Gastrointest Endosc.* 2015;81(4):781-794.

6. Kothari ST, Huang RJ, Shaukat A, et al. ASGE review of adverse events in colonoscopy. *Gastrointest Endosc.* 2019;90(6):863-876.e33.

7. Ko MS, Rudrapatna VA, Avila P, Mahadevan U. Safety of flexible sigmoidoscopy in pregnant patients with known or suspected inflammatory bowel disease. *Dig Dis Sci.* 2020;65(10):2979-2985.

8. Travis E, Ashley L, Pownall M, O'Connor DB. Barriers to flexible sigmoidoscopy colorectal cancer screening in low uptake socio-demographic groups: a systematic review. *Psychooncology.* 2020;29(8):1237-1247.

9. Yang C, Sriranjan V, Abou-Setta AM, Poluha W, Walker JR, Singh H. Anxiety associated with colonoscopy and flexible sigmoidoscopy: a systematic review. *Am J Gastroenterol.* 2018;113(12):1810-1818.

10. Gressot P, Chatelanat O, Frossard JL. Vidéocapsule endoscopique. *Rev Med Suisse.* 2021;17(748):1437-1442.

11. Bolwell JG, Wild D. Indications, contraindications, and considerations for video capsule endoscopy. *Gastrointest Endosc Clin N Am.* 2021;31(2):267-276.

12. Romeo S, Neri B, Mossa M, et al. Diagnostic yield of small bowel capsule endoscopy in obscure gastrointestinal bleeding: a real-world prospective study. *Intern Emerg Med.* Published online June 27, 2021. doi:10.1007/s11739-021 -02791-z

13. Leighton JA, Helper DJ, Gralnek IM, et al. Comparing diagnostic yield of a novel pan-enteric video capsule endoscope with ileocolonoscopy in patients with active Crohn's disease: a feasibility study. *Gastrointest Endosc.* 2017;85(1):196-205.e1.

14. Leighton JA, Gralnek IM, Cohen SA, et al. Capsule endoscopy is superior to small-bowel follow-through and equivalent to ileocolonoscopy in suspected Crohn's disease. *Clin Gastroenterol Hepatol.* 2014;12(4):609-615.

15. Tacheci I, Kopacova M, Bures J. Peutz-Jeghers syndrome. *Curr Opin Gastroenterol.* 2021;37(3):245-254.

16. Wang YC, Pan J, Liu YW, et al. Adverse events of video capsule endoscopy over the past two decades: a systematic review and proportion meta-analysis. *BMC Gastroenterol.* 2020;20(1):364.

17. Cebrian Garcia A, Elosua Gonzalez A, Fernandez-Urien Sainz I. Use of patency capsule in daily practice. *Rev Esp Enferm Dig.* 2019;111(6):491-492.

18. Kopylov U, Nemeth A, Cebrian A, et al. Symptomatic retention of the patency capsule: a multicenter real life case series. *Endosc Int Open.* 2016;4(9):E964-969.

19. Chander Roland B, Mullin GE, Passi M, et al. A prospective evaluation of ileocecal valve dysfunction and intestinal motility derangements in small intestinal bacterial overgrowth. *Dig Dis Sci.* 2017;62(12):3525-3535.

20. Roland BC, Lee D, Miller LS, et al. Obesity increases the risk of small intestinal bacterial overgrowth (SIBO). *Neurogastroenterol Motil.* 2018;30(3).

21. Moore MD, Gray KD, Panjwani S, et al. Impact of procedural multimedia instructions for pH BRAVO testing on patient comprehension: a prospective randomized study. *Dis Esophagus.* 2020;33(1):doz068.

22. Butt I, Kasmin F. Esophageal pH monitoring. In: *StatPearls* (online). StatPearls Publishing; 2021. NCBI Bookshelf. Accessed Sept 20, 2021. www.ncbi.nlm.nih.gov/books/NBK553089

23. Safatle-Ribeiro AV, Ribeiro U, Jr. Impact of enteroscopy on diagnosis and management of small bowel tumors. *Chin J Cancer Res.* 2020;32(3):319-333.

24. Perez-Cuadrado Martinez E, Perez-Cuadrado Robles E. Advanced therapy by device-assisted enteroscopy. *Rev Esp Enferm Dig.* 2020;112(4):273-277.

25. May A. Double-balloon enteroscopy. *Gastrointest Endosc Clin N Am.* 2017;27(1):113-122.

26. Lenz P, Domagk D. Single-balloon enteroscopy. *Gastrointest Endosc Clin N Am.* 2017;27(1):123-131.

27. ASGE Standards of Practice Committee; Buxbaum JL, Abbas Fehmi SM, et al. ASGE guideline on the role of endoscopy in the evaluation and management of choledocholithiasis. *Gastrointest Endosc.* 2019;89(6):1075-1105.e15.

28. ASGE Standards of Practice Committee; Chandrasekhara V, Khashab MA, et al. Adverse events associated with ERCP. *Gastrointest Endosc.* 2017;85(1):32-47.

29. DeLay K, Yadlapati R, Pandolfino JE. Chicago Classification of esophageal motility disorders: past, present, and future. *Indian J Gastroenterol.* 2021;40(2):120-130.

30. Ortengren AR, Ramkissoon RA, Chey WD, et al. Anorectal manometry to diagnose dyssynergic defecation: systematic review and meta-analysis of diagnostic test accuracy. *Neurogastroenterol Motil.* 2021;33(11):e14137.

31. Rao SSC, Tetangco EP. Anorectal disorders: an update. *J Clin Gastroenterol.* 2020;54(7):606-613.

32. Grasland M, Turmel N, Pouyau C, et al. External anal sphincter fatigability: an electromyographic and manometric study in patients with anorectal disorders. *J Neurogastroenterol Motil.* 2021;27(1):119-126.

33. Pannemans J, Masuy I, Tack J. Functional constipation: individualising assessment and treatment. *Drugs.* 2020;80(10):947-963.

34. Neshatian L, Williams MOU, Quigley EM. Rectal distension increased the rectoanal gradient in patients with normal rectal sensory function. *Dig Dis Sci.* 2021;66(7):2345-2352.

35. Lamparyk K, Mahajan L, Debeljak A, Steffen R. Anxiety associated with high-resolution anorectal manometry in pediatric patients and parents. *J Pediatr Gastroenterol Nutr.* 2017;65(5):e98-e100.

36. Roland BC, Ciarleglio MM, Clarke JO, et al. Low ileocecal valve pressure is significantly associated with small intestinal bacterial overgrowth (SIBO). *Dig Dis Sci.* 2014;59(6):1269-1277.

37. Ziessman HA, Okolo PI, Mullin GE, Chander A. Liquid gastric emptying is often abnormal when solid emptying is normal. *J Clin Gastroenterol.* 2009;43(7):639-643.

38. Epp LM, Salonen BR, Hurt RT, Mundi MS. Cross-sectional evaluation of home enteral nutrition practice in the United States in the context of the new enteral connectors. *JPEN J Parenter Enteral Nutr.* 2019;43(8):1020-1027.

39. Hitawala AA, Mousa OY. Percutaneous gastrostomy and jejunostomy. In: *StatPearls* (online). StatPearls Publishing; 2021. NCBI Bookshelf. Accessed Sept 19, 2021. www.ncbi.nlm.nih.gov/books/NBK559215

40. Arvanitakis M, Gkolfakis P, Despott EJ, et al. Endoscopic management of enteral tubes in adult patients—part 1: definitions and indications. European Society of Gastrointestinal Endoscopy (ESGE) guideline. *Endoscopy.* 2021;53(1):81-92.

41. Wang ZM, Jiang ZW, Diao YQ, et al. [Clinical application of percutaneous endoscopic gastrostomy/jejunostomy]. *Zhongguo Yi Xue Ke Xue Yuan Xue Bao.* 2008;30(3):249-252.

42. Dibba P, Ludwig E, Calo D, et al. Bevacizumab does not increase risk of perforation in patients undergoing percutaneous endoscopic gastrostomy or jejunostomy placement. *Surg Endosc.* 2021;35(6):2976-2980.

43. Barrera R, Schattner M, Nygard S, et al. Outcome of direct percutaneous endoscopic jejunostomy tube placement for nutritional support in critically ill, mechanically ventilated patients. *J Crit Care.* 2001;16(4):178-181.

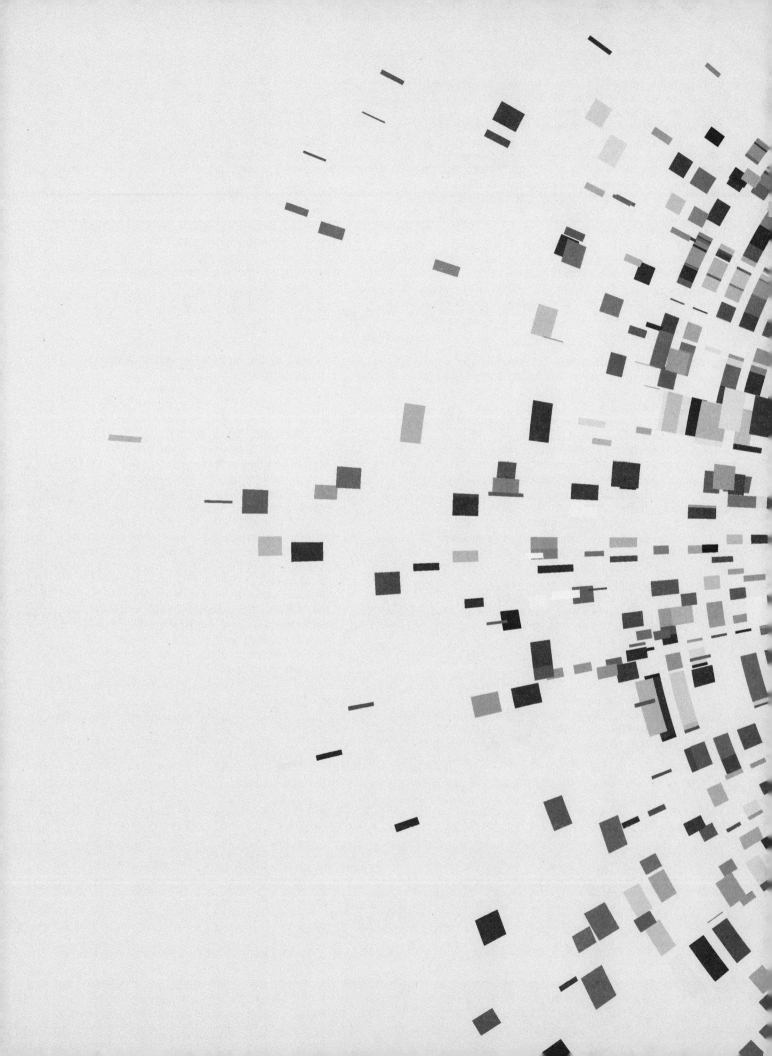

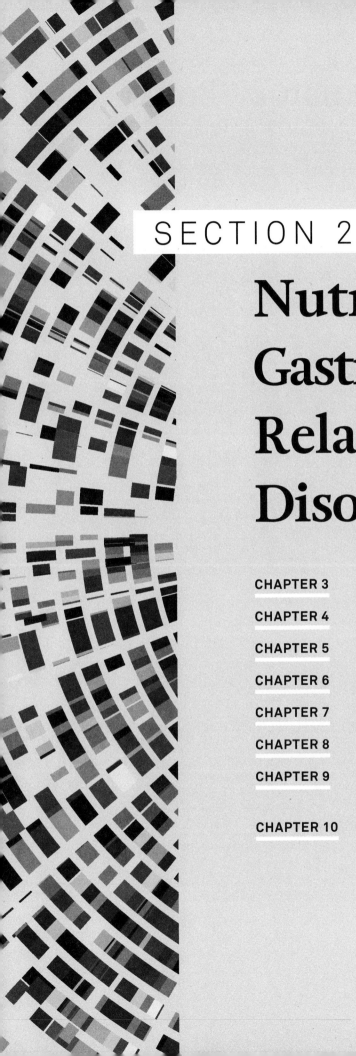

Nutrition and Gastrointestinal- Related Disorders

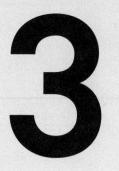

CHAPTER 3

Inflammatory Bowel Disease

Anoushka Dua, MD
Natalie Manitius, MPH, RDN
Berkeley N. Limketkai, MD, PhD

KEY POINTS

- Inflammatory bowel disease is a relapsing and remitting condition characterized by chronic intestinal inflammation.
- As a result of ongoing intestinal injury and loss of absorptive surface area, numerous nutritional complications can arise from inflammatory bowel disease, including micronutrient deficiencies and protein-energy malnutrition.
- Diet may play a role in the development of inflammatory bowel disease and may be used in combination with traditional medical therapy to minimize adverse effects and promote favorable disease outcomes.

Introduction

Inflammatory bowel disease (IBD) is a relapsing and remitting condition characterized by chronic intestinal inflammation.[1] The two most common subtypes of IBD are Crohn's disease and ulcerative colitis. As a result of ongoing intestinal injury and loss of absorptive surface area, nutritional complications can arise from IBD, including micronutrient deficiencies and protein-energy malnutrition. Moreover, as IBD is a disorder of the gastrointestinal (GI) tract, nutrition plays an important—albeit not well-defined—role in the risk for developing IBD. This chapter reviews the data that support identification of the specific dietary components that represent potential risk factors in the development of IBD, describes the impact of IBD on nutritional status, and provides an overview of the role of established and investigational dietary interventions in the delivery of care for patients with IBD.

Pathogenesis of Inflammatory Bowel Disease

The specific factors that contribute to the pathogenesis of IBD are not well defined; however, the current paradigm of pathogenesis is thought to involve a combination of underlying genetic risk, gut microbiota, and environmental factors.[2] Crohn's disease and ulcerative colitis can occur at any age, but the onset is most often between the ages of 15 and 30 years.

Population-based studies suggest that the risk of IBD may be in part attributable to genetics. If an individual has IBD, that person's family members have an eight- to 10-fold increased risk of developing IBD. Twin studies have also demonstrated that children who have a sibling with IBD have an increased risk of developing IBD. Genetics is, therefore, one component of an individual's risk factors for development of the disease.[2]

As for environmental factors, studies have hypothesized luminal antigens in the diet to be an important factor in the immunopathogenesis of IBD. By triggering an immune response or exerting changes on the gut microbiota, luminal antigens may indirectly increase the risk of IBD. For example, a possible relationship between hypersensitivity to cow's milk early in life and the subsequent development of ulcerative colitis was postulated in a 1990 retrospective study[3]; since then, investigators have found that lactose sensitivity occurs in a much higher proportion of adult patients with IBD (approximately 70%) than was previously thought.[4] Other studies have established a potential link between not breast-feeding and increased risk of Crohn's disease or ulcerative colitis.[5,6] In addition to dietary antigens having the capability of directly modifying the inflammatory response, they also play a strong role in shaping the composition of the intestinal microbiome, an entity that is strongly implicated in the pathogenesis of IBD.[7,8]

Global trends in IBD incidence and prevalence shed light on the interaction between diet and IBD pathogenesis. The incidence of Crohn's disease in North America is approximately 20 per 10,000 person-years compared with 13 per 100,000 person-years in Europe, and there is a generally lower incidence in Asia and the Middle East.[9] However, IBD prevalence and incidence have been rising in Asia and the Middle East, and immigrants from these regions into North America or Europe experience an increased risk of developing IBD.[10,11] These incidence rates and increase in risk based on migration patterns may be attributable to the westernization of lifestyles and diets, often characterized as a shift toward processed foods that are higher in fats, sugars, and refined carbohydrates and lower in nutrients.[12]

Several studies report that a higher dietary intake of refined sugar and carbohydrates often precedes IBD development, although this outcome is more often associated with Crohn's disease than ulcerative colitis.[13-17] Also, high levels of fat intake have been associated with an increased risk of IBD, and high fast-food consumption has been shown to predate both ulcerative colitis and Crohn's disease.[18] Moreover, a high ratio of omega-6 to omega-3 fatty acids and increased meat intake have been reported in immigrants to the Western world,[11] and a 2011 systematic review reported increased risk of developing both Crohn's disease and ulcerative colitis with a high intake of polyunsaturated fatty acids, omega-6 fatty acids, and meat.[19] A high intake of animal protein (excluding fish protein) is the strongest independent factor associated with the development of IBD.[20]

Increasingly, data suggest that diet and lifestyle may play an important role, independent of genetic risk factors, in the onset of IBD. Despite these findings, there is currently no consensus as to the role that dietary patterns play and the degree of risk they represent in the development of IBD.[21] Known risk factors for IBD are listed in Table 3.1.[22-31]

TABLE 3.1 Risk Factors for Inflammatory Bowel Disease[22-31]

Risk factor	Crohn's disease	Ulcerative colitis
Smoking	↑	↓
Family history of disease	↑	↑
Use of oral contraceptive pills	↔	↑
Antibiotic use	↑	↔
Use of nonsteroidal anti-inflammatory drugs	↑?	↑?
Low vitamin D level	↑?	↑?
Air pollution	↑	↑

Symbols key: ↑, increases risk; ↓, decreases risk; ↔, equivocal; ?, questionable risk.

Clinical Presentation of Inflammatory Bowel Disease

Inflammation in Crohn's disease can be present anywhere along the GI tract from the mouth to the anus. The most commonly affected areas are the small intestine and the colon; the rectum is usually spared. Inflammation can appear with a patchy distribution and have transmural involvement (affecting multiple or all layers of the intestine). Distinguishing features of Crohn's disease may include stricturing (narrowing) of the intestinal lumen and fistulas (tunnels) that connect the intestine to neighboring organs or the skin. Patients with Crohn's disease can experience significant weight loss and generalized malnutrition through several mechanisms. Ongoing intestinal inflammation and injury lead to loss of the absorptive lining; small bowel involvement in Crohn's disease, particularly higher in the GI tract, can compromise the sites most critical for nutrient absorption. Surgical resection resulting in a loss of bowel length similarly compromises nutrient absorption. Strictures can lead to obstructive symptoms of nausea, vomiting, abdominal discomfort, and distention that deter patients from eating. Fistula output may be high in protein and electrolytes and can place patients at risk for protein-energy malnutrition.

By contrast, ulcerative colitis is characterized by inflammation limited to the mucosal lining of the colon and rectum. It usually extends proximally from the rectum in a symmetrical, uninterrupted pattern to involve part or all of the colon. Unlike patients with Crohn's disease, patients with ulcerative colitis may achieve definitive disease remission through surgical removal of the colon, rectum, or both colon and rectum. Diarrhea, abdominal pain, and hematochezia (passage of blood in or with stools) represent typical symptoms of ulcerative colitis. Patients with ulcerative colitis are more likely than those with Crohn's disease to experience anemia due to overt blood loss during defecation. Nutritional deficiencies typically arise from symptoms-associated food aversion, compromised colonic absorption, and the catabolic nature of inflammation.

Nutrition Management of Inflammatory Bowel Disease

IBD is episodic in nature, alternating between flaring and remission. As such, nutritional management for patients with IBD will change according to the severity of their disease course, as well as the symptoms they face at a given point in time.

Patients with IBD often report alterations in bowel habits and may present with diarrhea or constipation. During periods of more active disease, individuals may experience stools that are bloody or greasy and have accompanying symptoms such as abdominal pain, bloating, or gas. During acute episodes with greater inflammation, increased catabolism, and significant stool output, patients are at increased risk of malnutrition, dehydration, and micronutrient deficiencies. Additionally, certain medications used in the management of IBD may affect micronutrient status in patients with IBD. Given the episodic nature of the disease, many individuals may exhibit fears or fraught relationships with food, and it is important that the registered dietitian nutritionist (RDN) be aware of these dynamic needs in the IBD patient.

Prevalence and Mechanisms of Malnutrition

The prevalence of malnutrition in IBD ranges from 6% to 16%. Compared with the general population, individuals with IBD have a fivefold increased risk of malnutrition.[32] When compared with other chronic diseases, patients with IBD have an increased risk of malnutrition. In a 2003 study of 502 hospitalized patients with various chronic medical conditions, the prevalence of malnutrition in IBD was 40%, the highest rate of malnutrition among all nonmalignant diseases.[33] Among outpatients with IBD, no significant difference has been found in the prevalence of malnutrition in patients with Crohn's disease and ulcerative colitis. Weight loss, however, is more common in patients with Crohn's disease than in those with ulcerative colitis; as many as 20% of patients with Crohn's disease in clinical remission have a significantly reduced lean body mass and weigh 10% below their ideal body weight.[32,34]

Taken together, patients with IBD across the health care continuum remain at increased risk of weight loss and malnutrition.

The etiology of malnutrition in IBD is multifactorial, with contributions from increased catabolism, nutrient malabsorption, impaired dietary intake, and iatrogenic mechanisms. Increases in both nutrient needs and losses in the affected mucosa are primary contributors to malnutrition in patients with this disease. The secretion of proinflammatory cytokines during the inflammatory process results in increased catabolism, thereby increasing nutritional needs. As active IBD is overall catabolic, the inflammatory process and its sequelae of vomiting, diarrhea, blood loss, and accompanying intestinal protein loss contribute to rapid weight loss, particularly of lean mass. Given these alterations in metabolism during acute stages of the disease, increasing the patient's nutrient and energy intake is crucial when symptoms are active.[35]

Nutrient malabsorption also contributes to increased risk of malnutrition in IBD. Inflammatory cytokines released in the gut mucosa may alter epithelial transport and compromise mucosal integrity, resulting in malabsorption.[36] Terminal ileal disease in Crohn's disease and small bowel resection can lead to reduced absorptive surface area and lack of bile salt recycling.[34,35] Patients who undergo small bowel resections because of ileal involvement are at increased risk of nutrient deficiencies, particularly fat-soluble vitamins, as a result of diminished bile salt recycling. Moreover, small bowel resections as a whole may affect nutritional status, as the small bowel is a primary site of absorption for various micronutrients (see Managing Nutritional Deficiencies later in this chapter).

Poor dietary intake commonly occurs in IBD and is another etiology of malnutrition. Owing to GI symptoms (eg, abdominal pain, nausea, vomiting, and diarrhea), dietary intake in IBD is often decreased. Research reveals that many patients with IBD engage in self-imposed food restriction behaviors that result in reduced caloric intake; in a large study of 1,271 patients, 76% avoided eating some food groups in order to prevent a disease flare, and 86% avoided eating some food groups when they had disease activity out of fear of worsening symptoms.[32] Many patients report beliefs about foods triggering their symptoms, and such beliefs may lead to maladaptive behaviors, including eating disorders. The prevalence of eating disorders in IBD has not been well characterized; however, risk factors include fear of abdominal discomfort from eating, disease severity, and challenges with body image and weight changes that often occur with the disease.[36] These behaviors highlight the importance of nutrition counseling and interventions to mitigate factors that contribute to malnutrition.

Medications and surgery are iatrogenic mechanisms of malnutrition. For example, sulfasalazine, an anti-inflammatory drug used in IBD management, blocks folate from metabolizing to its active form (tetrahydrofolate), thereby minimizing the absorption of folic acid. Corticosteroids also have an indirect inhibitory effect on intestinal calcium absorption by suppressing the transcription of calcium-transport genes.[37,38] Corticosteroids also alter the protein metabolism that causes muscle wasting.[39,40] Cholestyramine alleviates diarrhea by binding bile acids, but because these acids are also important for adequate digestion of fat and fat-soluble vitamins, deficiencies of these vitamins can occur.[41] Moreover, the diminished bile acid pool results in the retention of free long-chain fatty acids in the gut, which are saponified by calcium, resulting in decreased absorption of calcium. For optimal care of the malnourished patient with IBD, collaboration between the RDN and prescribing physician is important.

Undiagnosed and untreated malnutrition in IBD has important implications in the course and treatment of the disease. In general, systemic inflammation often interferes with the clinical response to medical therapy, and nutrition therapy can be a critical supportive intervention to assist in the effective medical treatment of chronic disease.[42] In malnourished patients with long-standing Crohn's disease, loss of visceral protein mass and impaired cellular immunity increases the risk of infection and poor wound healing.[43] Growth impairments may also occur because of malnutrition in IBD. In children with Crohn's disease, approximately 40% to 50% experience reduced growth velocity, linear growth retardation, and delayed pubertal growth.[40] In addition, malnutrition itself has been associated with a variety of poor outcomes, including longer hospital stays, higher frequency of postoperative complications, and decreased function and quality of life.[44,45] Improving a patient's nutritional status is central not only to optimizing the disease course but also to improving quality of life.

Bone Health

Bone health may be adversely affected by the course of IBD and the medications used to treat it. The prevalence of osteopenia and osteoporosis in IBD are 50% and 15%, respectively, and the risk of fractures among patients with IBD is 40% higher than age- and sex-matched controls.[41,46-49] Pediatric patients with this disease are particularly at risk of decreased bone density. In a cross-sectional cohort study of 80 patients with IBD, childhood IBD was associated with low bone mineral density and reduced bone mass accrual relative to muscle mass.[50] Bone thinning associated with IBD is often attributed to corticosteroid use; however, in 2002, researchers demonstrated the presence of osteopenia in patients newly diagnosed with IBD before any steroid therapy was initiated.[51] Age, BMI, serum magnesium, and a history of bowel resections may be better predictors than corticosteroid use for low bone mineral density.[52,53]

Bone health is best supported by calcium and vitamin D supplementation. These nutrients are highly recommended for use in preventing and treating decreased bone density in patients with IBD.[54] Although preventive measures are especially important in the pediatric patient, ongoing monitoring of bone health is warranted in all patients with IBD, regardless of age.

Managing Nutritional Deficiencies

Micronutrient deficiencies are relatively common in patients with IBD, particularly in those with Crohn's disease who have active small bowel disease or multiple resections, or both. Associated complications in such patients include anemia (iron, folate, and vitamin B12 deficiencies), bone disease (calcium, vitamin D, and possibly vitamin K deficiencies), hypercoagulability (folate, vitamin B6, and vitamin B12 deficiencies), poor wound healing (zinc, vitamin A, and vitamin C deficiencies), and colorectal cancer risk (folate and possibly vitamin D and calcium deficiencies). Patients with IBD—particularly those with Crohn's disease—are significantly affected by micronutrient deficiencies even when the disease is quiescent.[55-57] See Table 3.2 for information on micronutrient supplementation.

Anemia

Reported prevalence of anemia in patients with IBD ranges widely because of significant heterogeneity in study designs; the changing prevalence in more recent studies may be the result of increased awareness and early intervention.[58] The etiologies of anemia in IBD are multifactorial and include iron deficiency (resulting from decreased absorption, poor intake, and, commonly, chronic GI blood loss), anemia of chronic disease (resulting from systemic inflammation), and, less frequently, vitamin B12 or folate deficiency. Anemia may also be induced by medications. This effect is associated with mesalazine, sulfasalazine, azathioprine, and mercaptopurine. Iron therapy was reported to normalize elevated platelet counts in patients with IBD-associated anemia.[59]

Vitamin B12 and folate deficiencies—often detected among patients with IBD—may also lead to megaloblastic anemia.[58] Insufficient levels of folic acid are typically found in patients with IBD, so levels of that nutrient should be monitored at least annually for all patients with IBD.[60] Medications (eg, sulfasalazine, methotrexate) that interfere with the transport of folic acid potentially contribute to low levels of folate. Loss of surface area related to the primary disease or surgery may also play a role. Bacterial overgrowth, a complication of IBD, can result in depletion of vitamin B12 because bacteria preferentially

TABLE 3.2 Nutrient Deficiencies in Inflammatory Bowel Disease

| Deficiency | Approximate frequency of deficiency | | Treatment |
	Crohn's disease	Ulcerative colitis	
Negative nitrogen balance	69%	Unknown	Adequate energy and protein
Vitamin B12	48%	5%	1,000 mcg/d for 7 d then once monthly
Folate	67%	30%-40%	1 mg/d
Vitamin A	11%	Unknown	5,000-10,000 IU/d
Vitamin D	75%	35%	2,000-4,000 IU/d
Calcium	13%	Unknown	1,000-1,200 mg/d
Potassium	5%-20%	Unknown	Variable
Iron	39%	81%	65-200 mg/d elemental iron (many formulations, including ferrous sulfate, ferrous gluconate)[a] Intravenous iron for moderate to severe inflammatory bowel disease activity, severe anemia, or poor response to oral iron
Zinc	50%	Unknown	50 mg elemental zinc once or twice daily

[a] Alternate-day dosing has been shown to result in greater absorption.
Courtesy of Gerard E. Mullin, MD.

consume vitamin B12. Distal ileal resection or active disease of the ileum can also result in vitamin B12 deficiency because vitamin B12 is absorbed in the last 60 cm of ileum. Because in Crohn's disease the terminal ileum lacks a functional absorptive area, vitamin B12 usually must be delivered subcutaneously, intramuscularly, or sublingually (daily).

Deficiencies in Fat-Soluble Vitamins

Decreased bile acid absorption may occur when ileal disease is present. Solubilization to facilitate absorption of lipids and fat-soluble vitamins (A, D, E, and K) is normally aided by bile acids. Malabsorption of bile acids results in poor absorption of lipids and fat-soluble vitamins.

Vitamin D represents the fat-soluble vitamin most commonly deficient among patients with IBD.[61] A combination of vitamin D deficiency and calcium malabsorption—particularly when taking corticosteroids—has the potential to significantly alter bone density. Vitamin D levels are inversely associated with inflammatory markers, and normalization of vitamin D levels has been correlated with decreased use of the health care system.[61]

Deficiencies in vitamin A are more likely in patients with Crohn's disease than in healthy controls. Vitamin A is converted to its active form in the proximal intestine, and mouse models indicate its role in modulating intestinal inflammation and the immune response.[61] Research examining the benefits of vitamin A supplementation in IBD is limited at this time and remains to be clarified.

Vitamin K deficiency is estimated to occur in 31% of patients with IBD.[61] Its multiple roles in the body include blood clotting, maintenance of bone, and modulating inflammatory signaling—particularly interleukin-6, a proinflammatory cytokine. Vitamin K can be obtained through diet and through production by the commensal gut bacteria, and alterations in fat absorption and intestinal bacteria may affect a patient's vitamin K status.

Zinc Deficiency

Zinc is an important cofactor for antioxidant defenses. Patients with severe diarrhea, intestinal fistulas, and high-output ostomies are especially at risk for zinc deficiency. Zinc deficiency may occur in IBD regardless of these factors. A cohort study of nearly 1,000 patients with IBD indicated an increased risk of adverse outcomes with zinc deficiency in IBD, but further studies are needed to understand zinc's role in inflammatory signaling.[62]

Enteral Nutrition in the Treatment of Inflammatory Bowel Disease

Enteral nutrition (EN) encompasses liquid formulations delivered orally or through nasogastric or gastrostomy tubes. A wide range of commercial formulas are available, but the optimal formula for achieving a strong clinical response in IBD is not known.[63] EN formulations can be polymeric, semielemental, or elemental. Polymeric formations contain intact macronutrients (approximately 45%–60% carbohydrate, 12%–20% protein, and 30%–40% fat)[63] and, therefore, are best for patients with normal digestive and absorptive capabilities. Semielemental formulations consist of partially digested macronutrients (oligopeptides, dipeptides, or tripeptides, and medium-chain triglycerides), and elemental formulations consist of fully digested macronutrients (amino acids and simple sugars, with a low fat content). These formulations are designed for patients with dysfunctional digestion and absorption; however, for reasons of cost and availability, they are typically not used until after the patient has been tried, unsuccessfully, on a polymeric formulation. Exclusive EN has been studied as primary therapy for the management of Crohn's disease in both adults and children.[63] One meta-analysis found that EN and corticosteroids were equally effective in inducing remission in pediatric cases of Crohn's disease (relative risk, 0.95; 95% confidence intervial, 0.67–1.34).[64] Exclusive EN is thought to decrease intestinal permeability, modify the gut flora, possibly modulate inflammatory signaling and possibly improve growth in the pediatric population.[65] Research interventions typically employ exclusive EN over the course of 6 to 8 weeks, followed by a reintroduction of the oral diet. Of note, data suggest that there is no significant difference between EN formulations in their ability to induce Crohn's disease remission.[66]

As such, the mainstay of treatment for active Crohn's disease in pediatric patients is EN. In fact, the European Crohn's and Colitis Organisation, European Society for Paediatric Gastroenterology, Hepatology, and Nutrition, and European Society for Clinical Nutrition and Metabolism (ESPEN) recommend exclusive EN as a first-line choice for inducing remission in pediatric Crohn's disease.[67,68] Given the challenges associated with exclusive EN, including palatability and mode of delivery, partial EN has been explored. A 2019 randomized controlled trial demonstrated that partial EN in combination with the Crohn's disease exclusion diet (CDED; a whole-food diet designed to reduce exposure to dietary antigens) was equally efficacious to exclusive EN in inducing Crohn's disease remission and was actually better tolerated by patients.[69] These findings establish a role for CDED plus partial EN in treating children with Crohn's disease.

Although the evidence demonstrates that exclusive EN has shown efficacy in the maintenance of Crohn's disease remission in adults,[69] it does not support EN as the sole therapy in treating adult patients with the disease. A Cochrane meta-analysis and other meta-analyses demonstrated higher rates of efficacy of steroid administration compared with EN in adults.[66,71,72] In adults for whom corticosteroids may not be feasible, however, ESPEN guidelines do recommend exclusive EN as a primary therapy in adults.[68] In adults with Crohn's disease, long-term use of partial EN appears to be more feasible than exclusive EN, and multiple studies have demonstrated benefit for the maintenance of disease remission in addition to standard maintenance therapies.[73-76]

In contrast to the medical treatment of Crohn's disease in the United States, the first-line medical treatment for adult patients with Crohn's disease in Japan is EN therapy, which is covered by the Japanese national health insurance plan.[73] In general, approximately 3 to 5 weeks of treatment induces remission in approximately 85% of patients with active Crohn's disease, and EN is often used in research to achieve remission before a new treatment is tested.[74,75] Once remission is reached, patients begin the "slide method," in which a low-fat diet slowly replaces an elemental diet, nasogastric tube feeding during the night at home, and a low-fat diet (20–30 g fat per day) during the day.[77] Possible side effects of liquid elemental diets are osmolar diarrhea, abdominal distension, colic, cholelithiasis, and pneumonia (due to pulmonary aspiration).[78]

There are no compelling data to identify the precise role of EN in treating patients with Crohn's disease, but it is potentially useful as an auxiliary treatment for inducing and maintaining remission. Before EN can be definitively identified as truly effective in this line of treatment for Crohn's disease, large randomized controlled trials are necessary. In the patient population with active ulcerative colitis, EN has not been extensively evaluated.[79,80]

Parenteral Nutrition in the Treatment of Inflammatory Bowel Disease

Parenteral nutrition (PN) consists of a mixture of macronutrients (carbohydrates, proteins, and lipids), micronutrients (vitamins and minerals), and electrolytes that are administered intravenously. Since PN was first used in the treatment of IBD, its role has evolved. In the early years, PN, along with complete bowel rest, was the primary treatment for IBD. The rationale for its use has been that dietary antigens may stimulate the mucosal immune system and stimulate motor and transport functions of the diseased bowel, hypothetically worsening inflammation and disease. Although some small studies have shown bowel rest with PN to be effective at inducing remission, the benefits of PN appear to be short-lived.[81,82] Moreover, PN carries many associated risks, including bloodstream infections, PN-associated liver disease, and venous thromboses. For all these reasons, it is not used as primary therapy for IBD today.

The role of PN in IBD management is typically limited to select scenarios. As mentioned, PN is commonly used with bowel rest to induce remission, though studies have shown that bowel rest is not a major factor in achieving remission during nutritional support.[82] Another common use of PN in IBD is in patients with short bowel syndrome resulting from extensive intestinal resection (see Chapter 4).[83] Other indications include fistulous disease of the intestine or leaks resulting from surgical complications; malabsorption causing failure to thrive from extensive small intestinal Crohn's disease; and severe Crohn's disease in which standard drug therapy is not improving outcomes as anticipated or EN is not tolerated.[84] When extensive stenosing Crohn's disease is present, short-term use of PN and bowel rest may be indicated to limit the extent of resection or to deliver nutrition support until the disease responds to drug therapy. At this time, the use of PN as primary therapy in ulcerative colitis is not supported by data.

Modified Diets in the Treatment of Inflammatory Bowel Disease

Diet and nutrition have emerged as a growing area of interest in IBD treatment. The premise that diets play a role in IBD management stems from the belief that nutrients both shape the intestinal microbiome and modify the inflammatory response, which in turn may influence IBD activity. Many patients report subjective improvement in symptoms and quality of life with various dietary interventions, and though emerging literature describes the utility of specific dietary interventions, a systematic dietary approach in IBD has yet to be supported by GI or nutrition societies in the form of practice guidelines. Various diets and their impacts on IBD symptoms and disease activity have been investigated and are summarized in Box 3.1 on page 50.[69,85-97]

BOX 3.1

Evaluation of Diets in the Treatment of Inflammatory Bowel Disease[69,85-97]

Specific carbohydrate diet (SCD)

This diet excludes complex carbohydrates in favor of monosaccharides, which are more readily absorbed and reduce the burden of carbohydrates in the gut available for bacterial growth and dysbiosis.

Excluded foods

All grains, potatoes, yams, corn, all legumes, milk

Allowed foods

Unprocessed meats, poultry, eggs, fish

Fresh fruits, vegetables (with a high amylose-to-amylopectin ratio)

Lactose-free yogurt

All fats and oils

Possible benefits

In children: improvement in clinical symptoms when treated with SCD for 5 to 30 months; some with improvement in intestinal inflammation on endoscopy

In adults: 42% to 66% reported clinical remission in survey-based studies; research studies are small and limited for adult populations

Low-FODMAP diet

A diet low in fermentable oligosaccharides, disaccharides, monosaccharides, and polyols (FODMAPs) limits short-chain carbohydrates that are poorly absorbed in the small intestine. This reduces the following effects: water secretion, bacterial fermentation, and gas production, all of which contribute to luminal distension, abdominal discomfort, and mucosal inflammation.

Excluded foods[a]

Vegetables—garlic, onion, cauliflower, mushrooms

Fruits—blackberries, peaches, watermelon

Allowed foods[a]

Vegetables—carrots, cucumbers, green beans, lettuce, potatoes, tomatoes

Fruits (avoid large amounts)—bananas, cantaloupe, grapes, kiwi, lemons, oranges, strawberries, raspberries

Dairy—butter, lactose-free milk or yogurt, hard (aged) cheeses

Dairy alternatives—almond milk, coconut yogurt, hemp milk

Grains—wheat-free grains and flours, gluten-free products, popcorn, rice, tortilla chips

Beverages—coffee, green tea, peppermint tea, black tea

Proteins—chicken, eggs, firm tofu, peanut or almond butter, tempeh, turkey, fish, beef, pork, lamb

Sweeteners—granulated sugar, brown sugar, pure maple syrup, stevia

BOX 3.1 (CONTINUED)

Possible benefits

Primarily studied in patients with irritable bowel syndrome (IBS)

Can significantly improve abdominal pain and diarrhea in inflammatory bowel disease (IBD)

Caveats:

- Symptom benefit may be derived from the fact that IBS is present in more than 30% of people with IBD
- Does not affect clinical markers of intestinal inflammation (eg, fecal calprotectin)

Gluten-free diet

Gliadin protein, found in wheat, barley, rye, and oats (if cross-contaminated), may have a negative effect on the integrity of the intestinal barrier; a gluten-free diet restricts gliadin protein.

Excluded foods

Any foods made with wheat, rye, or barley, including pasta, breads, bread crumbs, cream of wheat, crackers, pretzels, matzo

Soy sauce

Beer, malted beverages

Oats (unless labeled gluten-free)

Possible benefits

Primarily studied and used in patients with celiac disease

Research ongoing on nonceliac wheat sensitivity vs nonceliac gluten sensitivity

May improve some gastrointestinal (GI) symptoms (eg, bloating, diarrhea, abdominal pain, nausea, fatigue)

Caveat: No studies link consumption of gluten with inflammation in IBD

Anti-inflammatory diet for IBD (IBD-AID)

This diet derived from SCD is divided into three phases that correlate with symptoms and are based on food textures.

Dietary components

Increase amounts of fruits, vegetables, plant-based protein, lean animal protein, fatty fish, and fiber

Restrict carbohydrates (lactose, refined or processed complex carbohydrates)

Reduce saturated fat

Focus on prebiotics and probiotics

Include omega-3 and other unsaturated fatty acids

Possible benefits

Can help reduce the intensity of medication-based therapy

May improve clinical scores indicating IBD severity (components such as general well-being, abdominal pain, diarrhea)

ᵃ This list is not exhaustive.

Box continues

BOX 3.1 (CONTINUED)

Crohn's disease exclusion diet (CDED)

This whole-food diet limits exposure to foods that may adversely affect the microbiome or alter intestinal barrier function. CDED is coupled with partial enteral nutrition (EN).

Dietary components

Phase 1 (weeks 0 to 6): 50% of kcal from partial EN; 50% from allowed foods

Phase 2 (weeks 6 through 12): 25% of kcal from partial EN; 75% from allowed foods

---

Allowed foods[a]

Lean fish (1 portion per week)

Fresh chicken breast

Potatoes, tomatoes, onion, garlic, ginger

Apples, bananas, avocados, strawberries, melon, fresh-squeezed lemon juice

Rice and rice flour or noodles

Olive and canola oils only

Eggs

Allowed foods after week 6 only[a]

Whole grain bread (1 slice per day)

Oatmeal (½ c dry per week)

Sweet potatoes, yams, red peppers, zucchini, mushrooms, broccoli, cauliflower

Pears, peaches, kiwis, blueberries

Quinoa; almonds or walnuts (8 per day)

Excluded foods[a]

Seafood other than fish

Processed meat

Dairy

Seeds

Artificial sweeteners

Cocoa, coffee, alcohol

Possible benefits

Effective in inducing remission by week 6 in children with mild to moderate Crohn's disease

Increased tolerability compared to exclusive EN

Box continues

BOX 3.1 (CONTINUED)

High-fiber diet

Dietary fiber (carbohydrates that are not broken down by small-intestinal enzymes) is fermented by intestinal bacteria into short-chain fatty acids which exert anti-inflammatory properties, improve intestinal barrier function, and positively alter intestinal microbiome.

Dietary components

Increased amounts of high-fiber foods, such as:

- Fruits—apples and pears with skin, bananas, oranges, strawberries, raspberries
- Whole grains—barley, bran flakes, popcorn, brown rice, oatmeal
- Vegetables—green peas, broccoli, turnip greens, artichokes, brussels sprouts, avocados
- Proteins—lentils, black beans, kidney beans

Possible benefits

May reduce length of hospital stay or hospitalization in general

May reduce odds of having a Crohn's disease flare

Caveat: Possible poor tolerance of high dietary fiber intake in patients with severe disease, history of strictures or bowel obstructions, diverticular disease, chronic diarrhea, high output ileostomies

Low-residue diet

Avoiding poorly digested nutrients, such as fiber, helps minimize stool production and reduces exposure of the intestine to food antigens. However, "low-residue" is poorly defined; it refers generally to nondigestible food components or foods that may increase stool output. It is used interchangeably with "low-fiber diet," but components vary.

Allowed foods

Dairy—nonfat, low-fat, reduced fat, or whole milk, yogurt, cottage cheese

Protein—tender-cooked meats, fish without bones

Grains—enriched bread with finely milled whole-grain or refined flour; plain rolls, muffins, and crackers; strained oatmeal

Vegetables—asparagus, beets, carrots, green beans, winter squash, white or sweet potatoes without skin

Fruits without seeds and skins

Possible benefits

May be helpful for patients with Crohn's disease who have stricturing disease or who undergo abdominal surgery, but data are not sufficient

ᵃ This list is not exhaustive.

Box continues

BOX 3.1 (CONTINUED)

Mediterranean diet

A diet high in nutrients such as fiber, mono- and polyunsaturated fatty acids, vitamin C, vitamin E, and carotenoids has anti-inflammatory and immune-modulating effects.

Dietary components

Plant-forward diet high in fruits, vegetables, beans, legumes, whole grains, nuts, seeds

Olive oil as main source of fat

Dairy, wine, fish, and poultry in low to moderate amounts

Red meat allowed only for infrequent consumption

Avoid processed meats, added sugar, and foods high in added sodium

---

Possible benefits

Best studied with respect to cardiovascular health

Limited data with IBD, but may improve clinical markers of inflammation

a This list is not exhaustive.

The foundation for the diets listed in Box 3.1 lies in their increased amounts of nutrients that are anti-inflammatory or are known to promote the growth of beneficial intestinal microorganisms and a reduction in nutrients that are proinflammatory or otherwise cause intestinal irritation and injury. For example, the Mediterranean diet and the anti-inflammatory diet for IBD strongly promote foods rich in omega-3 fatty acids. The clinical usefulness of omega-3 fatty acids for patients with IBD is that they regulate transcription factors, including peroxisome proliferator-activated receptors; inhibit nuclear factor κB; suppress the signaling of T cells; reduce the recruitment of inflammatory cells; and decrease the release of the proinflammatory cytokines interleukin-1β and tumor necrosis factor α.[98-100] Tissue cultures derived from biopsy specimens of patients with Crohn's colitis suggest that butyrate and other short-chain fatty acids decrease tumor production of necrosis factor α and nuclear factor κB as well as cytokine messenger RNA expression and may have an anti-inflammatory effect.[101,102]

One caveat of employing treatment strategies that involve dietary modification is that, with any restrictive diet, one needs to consider the risks of undernutrition and the development of maladaptive food-restrictive behaviors. This is a critical caveat, as it is well known that the IBD population is at high risk for malnutrition. When recommending a diet that limits consumption to a certain group of foods, the beneficial effects on clinical symptoms mentioned in Box 3.1 must be weighed against these risks.

Despite the immense interest in these established diets for the treatment of IBD, evidence delineating their benefits with regard to intestinal inflammation and disease prognosis is lacking. Research in this realm appears to be limited to small, often observational or retrospective studies with heterogeneous methodologies describing the impact of dietary interventions on clinical symptom scores, with no outcomes focusing on objective markers of inflammation.[103] There is, without a doubt, a role for diet and nutrition in the treatment of IBD, but further research is needed to clarify the optimal nutritional approach. As a result, and because of the limited data on the effectiveness of any one specific diet, current practice tends to focus on helping patients adopt a nutritionally adequate diet while working with them to identify foods that exacerbate symptoms.

Summary

Researchers have been focusing increasingly on the role of diet in the development of IBD and how it may be used in combination with traditional medical therapy to minimize adverse effects and promote favorable disease outcomes. Because nutritional deficiencies and malnutrition are common in patients with IBD, these patients should receive ongoing care from an RDN, as well as their digestive care specialist.

References

1. Abraham C, Cho JH. Inflammatory bowel disease. *N Engl J Med*. 2009;361(21):2066-2078.
2. Loddo I, Romano C. Inflammatory bowel disease: genetics, epigenetics, and pathogenesis. *Front Immunol*. 2015;6:551. Published online November 2, 2015. doi:10.3389/fimmu.2015.00551
3. Glassman MS, Newman LJ, Berezin S, et al. Cow's milk protein sensitivity during infancy in patients with inflammatory bowel disease. *Am J Gastroenterol*. 1990;85:838-840.
4. Eadala P, Matthews SB, Waud JP, Green JT, Campbell AK. Association of lactose sensitivity with inflammatory bowel disease—demonstrated by analysis of genetic polymorphism, breath gases and symptoms. *Aliment Pharmacol Ther*. 2011;34(7):735-746.
5. Koletzko S, Sherman P, Corey M, et al. Role of infant feeding practices in development of Crohn's disease in childhood. *BMJ*. 1989;298:1617-1618.
6. Corrao G, Tragnone A, Caprilli R, et al. Risk of inflammatory bowel disease attributable to smoking, oral contraception and breastfeeding in Italy: a nationwide case-control study. Cooperative Investigators of the Italian Group for the Study of the Colon and the Rectum (GISC). *Int J Epidemiol*. 1998;27:397-404.
7. David LA, Maurice CF, Carmody RN, et al. Diet rapidly and reproducibly alters the human gut microbiome. *Nature*. 2014;505(7484):559-563.
8. Chapman-Kiddell CA, Davies PS, Gillen L, et al. Role of diet in the development of inflammatory bowel disease. *Inflamm Bowel Dis*. 2010;16(1):137-151.
9. Molodecky NA, Soon IS, Rabi DM, Ghali WA, Ferris M, Chernoff G, et al. Increasing incidence and prevalence of the inflammatory bowel diseases with time, based on systematic review. *Gastroenterology*. 2012;142:46-54.
10. Benchimol EI, Mack DR, Guttmann A, et al. Inflammatory bowel disease in immigrants to Canada and their children: a population-based cohort study. *Am J Gastroenterol*. 2015;110:553-563.
11. Pinsk V, Lemberg DA, Grewal K, Barker CC, Schreiber RA, Jacobson K. Inflammatory bowel disease in the South Asian pediatric population of British Columbia. *Am J Gastroenterol*. 2007;102:1077-1083.
12. Foster A, Jacobson K. Changing incidence of inflammatory bowel disease: environmental influences and lessons learnt from the South Asian population. *Front Pediatr*. 2013;1:34.
13. Thompson NP, Montgomery SM, Wadsworth ME, et al. Early determinants of inflammatory bowel disease: use of two national longitudinal birth cohorts. *Eur J Gastroenterol Hepatol*. 2000;12:25-30.
14. Thornton JR, Emmett PM, Heaton KW. Diet and Crohn's disease: characteristics of the pre-illness diet. *Br Med J*. 1979;2:762-764.
15. Mayberry JF, Rhodes J, Newcombe RG. Increased sugar consumption in Crohn's disease. *Digestion*. 1980;20:323-326.
16. Mayberry JF, Rhodes J, Allan R, et al. Diet in Crohn's disease: two studies of current and previous habits in newly diagnosed patients. *Dig Dis Sci*. 1981;26:444-448.
17. Tragnone A, Valpiani D, Miglio F, et al. Dietary habits as risk factors for inflammatory bowel disease. *Eur J Gastroenterol Hepatol*. 1995;7:47-51.

18. Reif S, Klein I, Lubin F, et al. Pre-illness dietary factors in inflammatory bowel disease. *Gut.* 1997;40:754-760.

19. Hou JK, Abraham B, El-Serag H. Dietary intake and risk of developing inflammatory bowel disease: a systematic review of the literature. *Am J Gastroenterol.* 2011;106(4):563-573.

20. Amre DK, D'Souza S, Morgan K, et al. Imbalances in dietary consumption of fatty acids, vegetables, and fruits are associated with risk for Crohn's disease in children. *Am J Gastroenterol.* 2007;102:2016-2025.

21. Huda-Faujan N, Abdulamir AS, Fatimah AB, et al. The impact of the level of the intestinal short chain fatty acids in inflammatory bowel disease patients versus healthy subjects. *Open Biochem J.* 2010;4:53-58.

22. Loftus EV. Clinical epidemiology of inflammatory bowel disease: incidence, prevalence, and environmental influences. *Gastroenterology.* 2004;126:1504-1517.

23. Abegunde AT, Muhammad BH, Bhatti O, Ali T. Environmental risk factors for inflammatory bowel diseases: evidence based literature review. *World J Gastroenterol.* 2016;22(27):6296-6317.

24. Del Pinto R, Pietropaoli D, Chandar AK, Ferri C, Cominelli F. Association between inflammatory bowel disease and vitamin d deficiency: a systematic review and meta-analysis. *Inflamm Bowel Dis.* 2015;21(11):2708-2717.

25. Mahid SS, Minor KS, Soto RE, Hornung CA, Galandiuk S. Smoking and inflammatory bowel disease: a meta-analysis. *Mayo Clin Proc.* 2006;81(11):1462-1471.

26. Higuchi LM, Khalili H, Chan AT, Richter JM, Bousvaros A, Fuchs CS. A prospective study of cigarette smoking and the risk of inflammatory bowel disease in women. *Am J Gastroenterol.* 2012;107(9):1399-1406.

27. Ben-Horin S, Avidan B, Yanai H, et al. Familial clustering of Crohn's disease in Israel: prevalence and association with disease severity. *Inflamm Bowel Dis.* 2009;15(2):171-175.

28. Cornish JA, Tan E, Simillis C, Clark SK, Teare J, Tekkis PP. The risk of oral contraceptives in the etiology of inflammatory bowel disease: a meta-analysis. *Am J Gastroenterol.* 2008;103(9):2394-2400.

29. Khalili H, Higuchi LM, Ananthakrishnan AN, et al. Hormone therapy increases risk of ulcerative colitis but not Crohn's disease. *Gastroenterology.* 2012;143(5):1199-1206.

30. Ekbom A, Montgomery SM. Environmental risk factors (excluding tobacco and microorganisms): critical analysis of old and new hypotheses. *Best Pract Res Clin Gastroenterol.* 2004;8(3):497-508.

31. Ungaro R, Bernstein CN, Gearry R, Hviid A, Kolho KL, Kronman MP, Shaw S, Van Kruiningen H, Colombel JF, Atreja A. Antibiotics associated with increased risk of new-onset Crohn's disease but not ulcerative colitis: a meta-analysis. *Am J Gastroenterol.* 2014;109(11):1728-1738.

32. Casanova MJ, Chaparro M, Molina B, et al. Prevalence of malnutrition and nutritional characteristics of patients with inflammatory bowel disease. *J Crohns Colitis.* 2017;11(12):1430-1439.

33. Danese S, Fiocchi C. Etiopathogenesis of inflammatory bowel diseases. *World J Gastroenterol.* 2006;12(30):4807-4812.

34. Filippi J, Al-Jaouni R, Wiroth JB, et al. Nutritional deficiencies in patients with Crohn's disease in remission. *Inflamm Bowel Dis.* 2006;12:185-191.

35. Seidman EG. Nutritional management of inflammatory bowel disease. *Gastroenterol Clin N Am.* 1989;18:129-155.

36. Scaldaferri F, Pizzoferrato M, Lopetuso LR, et al. Nutrition and IBD: malnutrition and/or sarcopenia? A practical guide. *Gastroenterol Res Pract.* 2017;2017:8646495.

37. Mohn ES, Kern HJ, Saltzman E, Mitmesser SH, McKay DL. Evidence of drug-nutrient interactions with chronic use of commonly prescribed medications: an update. *Pharmaceutics.* 2018;10(1):36.

38. Hahn TJ, Halstead LR, Baran DT. Effects off short term glucocorticoid administration on intestinal calcium absorption and circulating vitamin D metabolite concentrations in man. *J Clin Endocrinol Metab.* 1981;52(1):111-115.

39. Steiner SJ, Noe JD, Denne SC. Corticosteroids increase protein breakdown and loss in newly diagnosed pediatric Crohn disease. *Pediatr Res.* 2011;70:484-488.

40. Al-Jaouni R, Schneider SM, Piche T, Rampal P, Hebuterne X. Effect of steroids on energy expenditure and substrate oxidation in women with Crohn's disease. *Am J Gastroenterol.* 2002;97:2843-2849.

41. Sapone N, Pellicano R, Simondi D, et al. A 2008 panorama on osteoporosis and inflammatory bowel disease. *Minerva Med.* 2008;99(1):65-71.

42. Jensen GL, Mirtallo J, Compher C, et al. Adult starvation and disease-related malnutrition: a proposal for etiology-based diagnosis in the clinical practice setting from the International Consensus Guideline Committee. *JPEN J Parenter Enteral Nutr.* 2010;34:156-159.

43. Jahnsen J, Falch JA, Mowinckel P, et al. Body composition in patients with inflammatory bowel disease: a population-based study. *Am J Gastroenterol.* 2003;98(7):1556-1562.

44. Tinsley A, Ehrlich OG, Hwang C, et al. Knowledge, attitudes, and beliefs regarding the role of nutrition in IBD among patients and providers. *Inflamm Bowel Dis.* 2016;22(10):2474-2481.

45. Jensen, GL. Inflammation as the key interface of the medical and nutrition universes: a provocative examination of the future of clinical nutrition and medicine. *JPEN J Parenter Enteral Nutr.* 2006;30(5):453-463.

46. Silvennoinen JA, Karttunene TJ, Niemela SE, et al. A controlled study of bone mineral density in patients with inflammatory bowel disease. *Gut.* 1995;37:71-76.

47. Fries W, Dinca M, Luisetto G, et al. Calcaneal ultrasound bone densitometry in inflammatory bowel disease: a comparison with double energy x-ray absorptiometry. *Am J Gastroenterol.* 1998;93:2339-2344.

48. Bernstein CN. Calcium and bone issues in inflammatory bowel disease. *Gastroenterol Int.* 1997;10:71-77.

49. Compston JE. Review article: osteoporosis, corticosteroids and inflammatory bowel disease. *Aliment Pharmacol Ther.* 1995;9:237-250.

50. Jong DJ, Corstens FHM, Mannaerts L, et al. Corticosteroid induced osteoporosis: does it occur in patients with Crohn's disease? *Am J Gastroenterol.* 2002;97(8):2011-2015.

51. Robinson RJ, Iqbal SJ, Abrams K, et al. Increased bone resorption in patients with Crohn's disease. *Aliment Pharmacol Ther.* 1998;12:699-705.

52. Bernstein CN, Blanchard JF, Leslie W, et al. The incidence of fracture among patients with inflammatory bowel disease. *Ann Int Med.* 2000;133:795-799.

53. Lamb EJ, Wong T, Smith DJ, et al. Metabolic bone disease is present at diagnosis in patients with inflammatory bowel disease. *Aliment Pharmacol Ther.* 2002;16(11):1895-1902.

54. Habtezion A, Silverberg MS, Parkes R, et al. Risk factors for low bone density in Crohn's disease. *Inflamm Bowel Dis.* 2002;8(2):87-92.

55. Vaisman N, Dotan I, Halack A, Niv E. Malabsorption is a major contributor to underweight in Crohn's disease patients in remission. *Nutrition.* 2006;22(9):855-859.

56. Mijač DD, Janković GL, Jorga J, Krstić MN. Nutritional status in patients with active inflammatory bowel disease: prevalence of malnutrition and methods for routine nutritional assessment. *Eur J Intern Med.* 2010;21(4):315-319.

57. Hwang C, Ross V, Mahadevan U. Micronutrient deficiencies in inflammatory bowel disease: from A to zinc. *Inflamm Bowel Dis.* 2012;18(10):1961-1981.

58. Bergamaschi G, Di Sabatino A, Albertini R, et al. Prevalence and pathogenesis of anemia in inflammatory bowel disease: influence of anti-tumor necrosis factor-alpha treatment *Haematologica.* 2010;95(2):199-205.

59. Bayraktar UD, Bayraktar S. Treatment of iron deficiency anemia associated with gastrointestinal tract diseases. *World J Gastroenterol.* 2010;16(22):2720-2725.

60. Kulnigg-Dabsch S, Evstatiev R, Dejaco C, Gasche C. Effect of iron therapy on platelet counts in patients with inflammatory bowel disease-associated anemia. *PLoS One.* 2012;7(4):e34520.

61. Kilby K, Mathias H, Boisvenue L, Heisler C, Jones JL. Micronutrient absorption and related outcomes in people with inflammatory bowel disease: a review. *Nutrients.* 2019;11(6):1388.

62. Siva S, Rubin DT, Gulotta G, Wroblewski K, Pekow J. Zinc deficiency is associated with poor clinical outcomes in patients with inflammatory bowel disease. *Inflamm Bowel Dis*. 2017;23:152-157.

63. Hansen T, Duerksen DR. Enteral nutrition in the management of pediatric and adult Crohn's disease. *Nutrients.* 2018;10(5):537.

64. Messori A, Trallori G, D'Albasio G, et al. Defined-formula diets versus steroids in the treatment of active Crohn's disease: a meta-analysis. *Scand Gastroenterol.* 1996;31:267-272.

65. Durchschein F, Petritsch W, Hammer HF. Diet therapy for inflammatory bowel diseases: the established and the new. *World J Gastroenterol.* 2016;22(7):2179-2194.

66. Zachos M, Tondeur M, Griffiths AM. Enteral nutritional therapy for induction of remission in Crohn's disease. *Cochrane Database Syst Rev.* 2007;(1):CD000542.

67. Ruemmele FM, Veres G, Kolho KL, et al. Consensus guidelines of ECCO/ES- PGHAN on the medical management of pediatric Crohn's disease. *J Crohns Colitis.* 2014;8(10):1179-1207.

68. Bischoff SC, Escher J, Hebuterne X, et al. ESPEN practical guideline: clinical nutrition in inflammatory bowel disease. *Clin Nutr.* 2020;39(3):632-653.

69. Levine A, Wine E, Assa A, et al. Crohn's disease exclusion diet plus partial enteral nutrition induces sustained remission in a randomized controlled trial. *Gastroenterology.* 2019;157(2):440-450.e8.

70. Akobeng AK, Thomas AG. Enteral nutrition for maintenance of remission in Crohn's disease. *Cochrane Database Syst Rev.* 2007;(3):CD005984.

71. Fernandez-Banares F, Cabre E, Esteve-Comas M, et al. How effective is enteral nutrition in inducing clinical remission in active Crohn's disease? A meta-analysis of the randomized clinical trials. *JPEN J Parenter Enteral Nutr.* 1995;19:356-364.

72. Griffiths AM, Ohlsson A, Sherman PM, et al. Meta-analysis of enteral nutrition as a primary treatment of active Crohn's disease. *Gastroenterology.* 1995;10:1056-1067.

73. Matsui T, Sakurai T, Yao T. Nutritional therapy for Crohn's disease in Japan. *J Gastroenterol.* 2007;40(suppl 16):S25-S31.

74. Axelsson C, Jarnum S. Assessment of the therapeutic value of an elemental diet in chronic inflammatory bowel disease. *Scand J Gastroenterol.* 1977;12(1):89-95.

75. Göschke H, Buess H, Gyr K, et al. [Elementary diet as an alternative to parenteral feeding in severe gastrointestinal diseases.] *Schweiz Med Wochenschr.* 1977;107(2):43-49.

76. Yamamoto T, Nakahigashi M, Saniabadi AR. Review article: diet and inflammatory bowel disease—epidemiology and treatment. *Aliment Pharmacol Ther.* 2009;30(2):99-112.

77. Yamamoto T, Nakahigashi M, Saniabadi AR, et al. Impacts of long-term enteral nutrition on clinical and endoscopic disease activities and mucosal cytokines during remission in patients with Crohn's disease: a prospective study. *Inflamm Bowel Dis.* 2007;13:1493-1501.

78. Yamamoto T, Nakahigashi M, Umegae S, et al. Impact of long-term enteral nutrition on clinical and endoscopic recurrence after resection for Crohn's disease: a prospective, non-randomized, parallel, controlled study. *Aliment Pharmacol Ther.* 2007;25:67-72.

79. Klaassen J, Zapata R, Mella JG, et al. Enteral nutrition in severe ulcerative colitis. Digestive tolerance and nutritional efficiency [in Spanish with English abstract]. *Rev Med Chil.* 1998;126:899-904.

80. Gonzalez-Huix F, Fernandez-Banares F, Esteve-Comas M, et al. Enteral versus parenteral nutrition as adjunct therapy in acute ulcerative colitis. *Am J Gastroenterol.* 1993;88:227-232.

81. Müller JM, Keller HW, Erasmi H, Pichlmaier H. Total parenteral nutrition as the sole therapy in Crohn's disease—a prospective study. *Br J Surg.* 1983;70(1):40-43.

82. Greenberg GR, Fleming CR, Jeejeebhoy KN, Rosenberg IH, Sales D, Tremaine WJ. Controlled trial of bowel rest and nutritional support in the management of Crohn's disease. *Gut.* 1988;29(10):1309-1315.

83. Ekema G, Milianti S, Boroni G. Total parenteral nutrition in patients with short bowel syndrome. *Minerva Pediatr.* 2009;61(3):283-291.

84. Evans JP, Steinhart AH, Cohen Z, McLeod RS. Home total parenteral nutrition: an alternative to early surgery for complicated inflammatory bowel disease. *J Gastrointest Surg.* 2003;7(4):562-566.

85. Limketkai BN, Wolf A, Parian AM. Nutritional interventions in the patient with inflammatory bowel disease. *Gastroenterol Clin North Am.* 2018;47(1):155-177.

86. Suskind DL, Wahbeh G, Gregory N, et al. Nutritional therapy in pediatric Crohn disease: the specific carbohydrate diet. *J Pediatr Gastroenterol Nutr.* 2014;58(1):87-91.

87. Cohen SA, Gold BD, Oliva S, et al. Clinical and mucosal improvement with specific carbohydrate diet in pediatric Crohn's disease. *J Pediatr Gastroenterol Nutr.* 2014;59(4):516-521.

88. Kakodkar S, Farooqui AJ, Mikolaitis SL, Mutlu EA. The specific carbohydrate diet for inflammatory bowel disease: a case series. *J Acad Nutr Diet.* 2015;115(8):1226-1232.

89. Suskind DL, Wahbeh G, Cohen SA, et al. Patients perceive clinical benefit with the specific carbohydrate diet for inflammatory bowel disease. *Dig Dis Sci.* 2016;61(11):3255-3260.

90. Halpin SJ, Ford AC. Prevalence of symptoms meeting criteria for irritable bowel syndrome in inflammatory bowel disease: systematic review and meta-analysis. *Am J Gastroenterol.* 2012;107(10):1474-1482.

91. Herfarth HH, Martin CF, Sandler RS, et al. Prevalence of a gluten-free diet and improvement of clinical symptoms in patients with inflammatory bowel diseases. *Inflamm Bowel Dis.* 2014;20(7):1194-1197.

92. Heaton KW, Thornton JR, Emmett PM. Treatment of Crohn's disease with an unrefined-carbohydrate, fibre-rich diet. *Br Med J.* 1979;2(6193):764-766.

93. Brotherton CS, Martin CA, Long MD, Kappelman MD, Sandler RS. Avoidance of fiber is associated with greater risk of Crohn's disease flare in a 6-month period. *Clin Gastroenterol Hepatol.* 2016;14(8):1130-1136.

94. Casas R, Urpi-Sardà M, Sacanella E, et al. Anti-inflammatory effects of the Mediterranean diet in the early and late stages of atheroma plaque development. *Mediators Inflamm.* 2017;2017:3674390.

95. Shah N, Limketkai B. Low residue vs. low fiber diets in inflammatory bowel disease: evidence to support vs habit? Nutrition Issues in Gastroenterology, Series 143. *Pract Gastroenterol.* 2015;39(7):48, 50-52, 55-57.

96. Dinu M, Pagliai G, Casini A, Sofi F. Mediterranean diet and multiple health outcomes: an umbrella review of meta-analyses of observational studies and randomised trials. *Eur J Clin Nutr.* 2018;72(1):30-43.

97. Limketkai BN, Iheozor-Ejiofor Z, Gjuladin-Hellon T, et al. Dietary interventions for induction and maintenance of remission in inflammatory bowel disease. *Cochrane Database of Syst Rev.* 2019;(2):CD012839.

98. Andersen V, Olsen A, Carbonnel F, Tønneland A, Vogel U. Diet and risk of inflammatory bowel disease. *Dig Liver Dis.* 2012;44(3):185-194.

99. Whiting CV, Bland PW, Tarlton JF. Dietary n-3 polyunsaturated fatty acids reduce disease and colonic proinflammatory cytokines in a mouse model of colitis. *Inflamm Bowel Dis.* 2005;11(4):340-349.

100. Zhang P, Kim W, Zhou L, et al. Dietary fish oil inhibits antigen-specific murine Th1 cell development by suppression of clonal expansion. *J Nutr.* 2006;136(9):2391-2398.

101. Caughey GE, Mantzioris E, Gibson RA, et al. The effect on human tumor necrosis factor alpha and interleukin 1 beta production of diets enriched in n-3 fatty acids from vegetable oil or fish oil. *Am J Clin Nutr.* 1996;63(1):116-122.

102. Segain JP, Raingeard de la Bletiere D, Bourrelle A, et al. Butyrate inhibits inflammatory responses through NFkappaB inhibition: implications for Crohn's disease. *Gut.* 2000;47(3):397-403.

103. Limketkai BN, Gordon M, Mutlu EA, De Silva PS, Lewis JD. Diet therapy for inflammatory bowel diseases: a call to the dining table. *Inflamm Bowel Dis.* 2020;26(4):510-514.

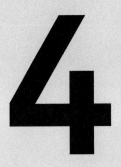

CHAPTER 4

Short Bowel Syndrome

Laura E. Matarese, PhD, RDN, LDN, FADA, FASPEN, FAND
Glenn Harvin, MD

KEY POINTS

- Short bowel syndrome is a debilitating disease and the most common form of intestinal failure.
- Patients with short bowel syndrome constitute a heterogenous patient population, and, as such, their care should be individualized to enhance intestinal adaptation, improve absorption, and reduce dependence on parenteral nutrition.
- Therapeutic strategies may include diet modification, medications, proadaptive therapies, reconstructive surgery, and intestinal transplantation.

Introduction

Intestinal failure is a condition resulting from obstruction, dysmotility, surgical resection, congenital defect, or disease-associated loss of absorption. Short bowel syndrome (SBS) is one of the most common forms of intestinal failure.[1] It is defined as the reduction of gut function below the minimum necessary for the absorption of macronutrients or the absorption of water and electrolytes, such that intravenous supplementation is required to maintain health, growth, or both.[2,3] The spectrum of SBS ranges from insufficiency to failure. The reduction of gut absorptive function that does not require intravenous supplementation to maintain health or growth can be considered "intestinal insufficiency."[3]

Pathogenesis of Short Bowel Syndrome

Estimates of the incidence and prevalence of SBS are difficult to make and, therefore, lacking. Most estimates are based on data describing patients who require long-term home parenteral nutrition for SBS, but these estimates do not take into account patients who have a shortened intestine and are maintained on intravenous fluids and other rehabilitation therapies. In the United Kingdom, the incidence of SBS requiring home parenteral nutrition was reported to be two patients per million population.[4] In the United States, approximately 10,000 to 20,000 patients receive home parenteral nutrition for SBS.[5]

SBS is associated with either the loss of portions of the intestine due to surgical resection (anatomical) or the loss of intestinal function despite adequate intestinal length (eg, pseudo-obstruction, dysmotility). The risk factors associated with SBS and the subsequent malabsorption are causally related to the length and health of the remnant bowel. The causes of SBS vary for adults and children (Box 4.1 on page 60). Regardless of the cause, the physiologic consequences result in an inability to maintain fluid, electrolyte, and nutrient balance from a normal diet such that intravenous fluids or nutrition is required. Because of the heterogeneity of patients with SBS—owing to variations in their remnant gastrointestinal (GI) anatomy, mucosa health, and nutritional status—treatment often requires a coordinated, multipronged, and dynamic approach.[6]

The etiology of the malabsorption that results from SBS is multifactorial and involves:

- reduced mucosal surface area,
- changes in motility,
- increased gastric secretions,

BOX 4.1

Causes of Short
Bowel Syndrome in
Children and Adults

Children

Abdominal tumors

Apple peel anomaly

Crohn's disease

Congenital short bowel syndrome

Gastroschisis

Hirschsprung disease

Intestinal atresia

Necrotizing enterocolitis

Radiation enteritis

Trauma

Adults

Crohn's disease

Chronic intestinal pseudo-obstruction

Complications of bariatric surgery

Extensive surgical resection

Hypercoagulable states

Malignancy

Radiation enteritis

Strangulated hernia

Small bowel fistulas

Surgical bypass

Trauma

Volvulus

- osmotic stimulation from hypertonic fluids and fatty acids,
- deconjugated bile salts,
- bacterial overgrowth,
- lactose intolerance, and
- fatty acid irritation of the colon.

The treatment of the patient with SBS is complex. Commonly, after bowel resection, the patient is on short-term parenteral nutrition (PN). If possible, bowel rehabilitation and surgical reconstruction should be considered to avoid long-term PN. Some patients on long-term PN may eventually become candidates for intestinal or multivisceral transplantation.

Factors Affecting Absorption

The severity of malabsorption in individuals with SBS is determined by the following:

- extent of intestinal resection
- site of the resection
- capability of the intestine to undergo adaptive hyperplasia
- health of the remaining intestinal mucosa

The classification and characterization of SBS is constantly evolving and is based on the result of the surgical intervention, remnant anatomy, and expected outcome. The metabolic and expected outcome criteria are classified into three types[7,8]:

- type I: an acute, short-term, and often self-limiting condition
- type II: a prolonged acute condition, often in metabolically unstable patients, requiring complex multidisciplinary care and intravenous supplementation over periods of weeks or months
- type III: a chronic condition, in metabolically stable patients, requiring intravenous supplementation over months or years; may be reversible or irreversible

The bowel begins to adapt both structurally and functionally immediately after a surgical resection. This generally occurs over a 2- to 3-year period.[9,10] The remnant bowel will compensate for a reduction in surface area both by increasing the length and diameter of the remaining intestine through villous hypertrophy and by altering the motility and hormonal response.

The length of the remaining healthy bowel is one of the most important factors for absorption—the more bowel that remains, the greater the absorption. Small bowel resections decrease transit time through the intestine and reduce the normal rate of mixing of food with digestive enzymes and the contact time of nutrients with the mucosal surface. The adult human small intestine ranges in length from 275 to 1,049 cm, as calculated from studies performed on cadavers, with the average length being approximately 600 cm.[11] The large bowel ranges in length from 80 to 313 cm. The minimum amount of intestine required to be autonomous from PN is estimated to be 60 to 90 cm of small bowel with a portion of the colon, or 150 cm of small bowel if the colon is absent.[12,13] This is largely due to the gut hormones produced in the intestinal mucosa, which are involved in motility and absorption. This also illustrates the importance of the colon and its role as an absorptive organ.

The site of the intestinal resection and length of remaining small bowel affects absorption and can be classified into three groups[13]:

- end-enterostomy, less than 100 cm
- jejunocolic anastomosis, less than 65 cm
- jejunoileocolic anastomosis, less than 30 cm

Resection of the jejunum will affect intestinal motility less than an equivalent length of ileal resection.[9] The more distal portions of the intestine tend to slow the transit of chyme through the previous segments of bowel. Motilin, which is secreted by M cells in the duodenum and jejunum, stimulates GI motility.[14] In the small bowel, this effect is most prominent in the ileum. Unless more than 75% of the jejunum has been resected, absorption of vitamin B12 is adequate because the ileum is intact,[5] and the patient will have preserved absorption of vitamin B12 and bile salts and good ileal adaptation.[10] Overall transit time is normal with a jejunal resection, but gastric emptying of liquids is increased.[10,12] Digestive secretions contribute to stool or stoma losses. Sodium and water losses may be high. Dietary sodium and oral rehydration solutions (ORS) can help control output. Fat absorption is constant. The consequences of an ileal resection are more severe.[7,10] Patients who have undergone an ileal resection may have the following:

- adequate calorie and fluid absorption but malabsorption of bile salts and vitamin B12
- poor jejunal adaptation and very rapid intestinal transit
- increased fluid losses and shorter transit times if the patient has an ileal resection and loss of the ileocecal valve
- bile acid malabsorption resulting in bile salt pool depletion, leading to fat and fatty acid malabsorption
- decreased calcium, zinc, and magnesium absorption

If the colon is in continuity, the potential exists for increased colonic oxalate absorption and increased colonic secretions caused by unabsorbed bile salts and fatty acids that can irritate the colonic lining. There is also an increased risk of small intestinal bacterial overgrowth (SIBO) if the ileocecal valve is absent.

When an intestinal resection results in an enterocolic anastomosis, sodium and water balance is often positive. Diarrhea may be due to unabsorbed fatty acids of bile salts if enterohepatic circulation is maintained. Carbohydrate malabsorption can cause osmotic diarrhea and D-lactic acidosis. Colonic fermentation of unabsorbed carbohydrates can result in energy absorption along with a reduced stool pH.

The extent of resection determines the degree of clinical severity. The physiologic consequences of extensive small bowel resection can be quite severe.[9,14] Patients with extensive resection often experience the following:

- substantial fluid and electrolyte losses
- nutrient malabsorption
- gastric acid hypersecretion
- vitamin B12 and bile salt malabsorption
- rapid gastric emptying and intestinal transit
- SIBO

The ileocecal valve and colon have an even greater tendency to increase (slow) intestinal transit time. The colon is important for the absorption of fluid, electrolytes, and nutrients such as short-chain fatty acids.[15-17]

An intact stomach, pancreas, and liver are all important for digestion; therefore, any previous surgeries or disease of these organs can affect absorption in patients with SBS. The health of the remaining intestinal mucosa also affects absorption. Patients with active Crohn's disease, ulcerative colitis, or radiation enteritis in the remnant bowel may not absorb fluid, electrolytes, and other nutrients as well as patients with healthy mucosa do. See Chapter 3 for more information on Crohn's disease and ulcerative colitis.

Nutrition Assessment

The initial evaluation of a patient with SBS should include a comprehensive nutrition assessment that is based on the history and physical examination, GI symptoms affecting oral intake, whether nutrient intake and absorption meet the nutrient requirements of an individual, and functional capacity (see Chapter 1). An assessment of weight before and after a surgical resection is important to help determine a functional weight for the patient. Signs and symptoms of micronutrient deficiencies should be noted, and the patient should be physically assessed for signs of dehydration and malnutrition. Symptoms that may affect oral intake or fluid loss should also be noted. The number and location of surgical resections and the length of the remnant bowel are extremely important. A thorough diet history provides insight to the amount and types of foods that trigger an increase in ostomy effluent or the number and consistency of bowel movements. For patients requiring nutrition support, a history should also be obtained regarding the enteral or central venous access device, the formula used, the route and method of administration, and any known prior complications. Finally, it is important to gather any information regarding medications and pertinent past medical and psychiatric history, as well as the level of motivation the patient requires to adhere to the dietary, fluid, and medical treatments.

Treatment and Management of Short Bowel Syndrome

Dietary Modification

Dietary modification is the cornerstone of management of SBS. The aim is to minimize GI symptoms, optimize absorption, and provide a stimulus to enhance intestinal adaptation while minimizing parenteral nutrient and fluid requirements.[18,19] The general tactics for dietary modification are as follows:

- Patients should consume small, frequent meals, minimize their intake of concentrated sugars, and maximize their intake of complex carbohydrates.
- In some circumstances, patients may find it helpful to limit their fluid intake with solids and take sips of fluids between meals.
- Commercial fiber supplementation (nondigestible, resistant starches) is used, as needed, to slow intestinal transit, gelatinize ostomy effluent, and provide a substrate to produce short-chain fatty acids in the colon.

- Patients should take vitamin and mineral supplements as dictated by remnant GI anatomy, degree of malabsorption, and laboratory monitoring.

The dietary modification plan is based on the presence or absence of the colon. Table 4.1 outlines the appropriate diet modification for patients with SBS depending on whether the colon is present or absent.[20] Table 4.2 on page 64 presents recommendations for oral vitamin and mineral supplements for patients with SBS.[6,18]

TABLE 4.1 Diet Modifications for Short Bowel Syndrome According to Gastrointestinal Anatomy[20]

Diet component	Colon present	Colon absent
Carbohydrate, % of kcal/d	50%-60% (limit simple sugars)	40%-50% (restrict simple sugars)
Protein, % of kcal/d	20%	20%
Fat, % of kcal/d	20%-30% (primarily essential fats)	30%-40% (primarily essential fats)
No. of meals/d	5-6	4-6
Oxalates	Limit intake	No restriction
Fluids	Isotonic or hypo-osmolar fluids	Isotonic, high-sodium fluids; rehydration solutions
Soluble fiber, g/d	5-10 (if stool output >3 L/d)	5-10 (if stool output >3 L/d)
Lactose	As tolerated	As tolerated

Management of Fluids

The typical volume of fluid entering the intestine is approximately 8.8 L/d and is derived from oral intake and endogenous GI secretions.[18] Most of the fluid that passes through the intestine is absorbed, and only about 150 to 200 mL is passed in stool. The small intestine's maximum resorptive capacity is 12 L, and the colon's is 5 L.[19] When the maximum resorptive capacity of the colon is exceeded, diarrhea is the result. In the case of SBS, this may be due to decreased intestinal fluid absorption, increased secretion, or both. An important component of the management of the patient with SBS is the optimization of fluids.[21]

The factors that determine the capacity of the bowel for intestinal fluid absorption include:

- surface area (residual length),
- mucosal integrity (residual healthy tissue vs damaged tissue),
- motility (contact time: faster motility means less contact time for absorption), and
- luminal osmolarity (unabsorbed solutes in lumen of the gut draw in water and electrolytes from the plasma).

Impairment of any one or all these factors can result in diarrhea. Positive fluid balance is generally achieved when the length of the small bowel approaches 90 cm and the colon is present.

TABLE 4.2 Oral Vitamin and Mineral Supplements for Patients With Short Bowel Syndrome[6,18]

Nutrient	Strength	Dose
Vitamins A, D, and E	Vitamin A: 25,000 IU/tablet Vitamin D: 1,000 IU/tablet Vitamin E: 400 IU/tablet	1 tablet/d
Calcium citrate	500-600 mg/tablet	1-2 tablets tid
Magnesium lactate	84 mg/tablet	1-2 tablets tid
Magnesium gluconate	1,000 mg/tablet (or liquid)	1-3 tablets tid
Potassium chloride	20 mEq/tablet	1-2 tablets/d
Phosphorus (eg, Neutra-Phos)	250 mg/package	1 package tid
Sodium bicarbonate	650 mg/tablet	1 tablet tid
Chromium	100 mcg/tablet	1-2 tablets tid
Copper	3 mg/tablet	1-2 tablets/d
Selenium	200 mcg/tablet	1 tablet/d
Zinc sulfate	220 mg/tablet	1-3 tablets/d

tid = three times a day.

The discovery of the sodium-glucose cotransporter and clinical studies in patients with cholera led to the development of ORS that are used to treat diarrhea in developing countries. Because the maximum absorption of sodium and water occurs from a solution with a sodium concentration of 90 to 120 mM/L and a glucose concentration of 56 mM/L, ORS solutions have been formulated to achieve these parameters.[22-24] Several ORS are commercially available (see Table 4.3), although the sodium and carbohydrate contents vary considerably. ORS can also be made with individual components or simple household ingredients (see Box 4.2).

TABLE 4.3 Examples of Commercially Available Oral Rehydration Solutions

	Carbohydrate, g/L	Sodium, mEq/L	Potassium, mEq/L	Bicarbonate, mEq/L	Osmolality, mOsm/L
World Health Organization oral rehydration solution (ORS)					
Standard formula	20	90	20	30	310
Reduced-osmolality formula	13.5	75	20	30	245
Rehydration solutions					
CeraLyte 70[a]	40	70	20	30	235
CeraLyte 90[a]	40	90	20	30	260
CVS Adult Electrolyte Solution	25	45	19		

Table continues

	Carbohydrate, g/L	Sodium, mEq/L	Potassium, mEq/L	Bicarbonate, mEq/L	Osmolality, mOsm/L
DripDrop[b]	40	30	20		235
Enfalyte[c]	30	50	25	33	160
Hydralyte[d]	20	60	20		
Jianas Brothers ORS[e]	20	90	20	10	300
Pedialyte[f]	25	45	20	10	250
Speedlyte[g]	25.5	45	20	8.7	
Sport drinks					
Gatorade[h]	60	20	3		340
G2[f] plus ½ tsp salt	29	63	3		254

[a] Cera Products
[b] Drip Drop
[c] Mead Johnson
[d] Hydration Pharmaceuticals
[e] Jianas Brothers
[f] Abbott
[g] Einsof Biohealth
[h] PepsiCo

BOX 4.2

Oral Rehydration Solution Recipes

[a] By prescription
[b] Potassium concentration: 7 to 14 mEq/g. Note 1 tsp weighs 5 g (0.17 oz) and, therefore, contains 35 to 70 mEq potassium.

Basic oral rehydration solution (ORS) recipe[25]

4½ c water

¾ tsp table salt

3 tbsp sugar (sucrose)

1 tsp baking powder (or ½ tsp baking soda)

½ tsp 20% potassium chloride[a] or salt substitute[b]

Sugar-free artificial flavoring or sweetener

Juice-based or sport beverage–based ORS recipes[26-28]

Grape or cranberry juice ORS

½ c 100% grape or cranberry juice

3½ c water

½ tsp table salt

Apple juice ORS

1 c apple juice

3 c water

½ tsp table salt

Orange juice ORS

½ tsp table salt

½ tsp baking soda

8 tsp sugar

1 c orange juice (unsweetened) without the pulp

4½ c water

Gatorade-based ORS

2 c Gatorade (do not use reduced-calorie products)

2 c water

½ tsp table salt

Most sport drinks are *not* appropriate for patients with SBS because of the high glucose content and low electrolyte content of these products. Other drinks that are low in sodium, such as water and fruit juices, will cause sodium to move from the blood into the lumen of the bowel. Hypertonic juices (which are rich in fructose) also draw water into the intestinal lumen, thereby increasing fluid loss. Because the bowel is shortened, sodium and water are lost in the ostomy effluent.

Medications

Adjunctive medical therapy is used to control symptoms and maximize absorption.[6,29,30] For a list of medications used to treat SBS, see Box 4.3.

BOX 4.3

Medications for Short Bowel Syndrome[6,29,30]

Medication	Dose and administration notes
Antidiarrheals	
Loperamide (Imodium) (OTC)	2 to 6 mg by mouth (PO), three times a day (tid) or four times a day (qid), 30 to 60 minutes before meals; minimal side effects
Diphenoxylate with atropine (Lomotil)	2.5 to 7.5 mg PO, tid or qid, 1 hour before meals; maximum daily dose, 20 to 25 mg
Codeine phosphate	15 to 60 mg PO, qid, 1 hour before meals
Opium tincture (1% morphine anhydrous)[a]	0.3 to 1 mL PO, qid, 1 hour before meals
H_2 receptor antagonists	
Famotidine (Pepcid)	20 to 40 mg PO or intravenous (IV), every day (qd)
Ranitidine (Zantac)	150 to 300 mg PO, two times per day (bid); or 300 mg PO, qd; or 50 mg IV, every 6 to 8 hours
Cimetidine (Tagamet)	200 to 400 mg PO or IV, qid
Proton pump inhibitors	
Omeprazole (Prilosec)	20 to 40 mg PO, bid
Lansoprazole (Prevacid)	15 to 30 mg PO, qd, for up to 7 days
Esomeprazole (Nexium)	20 to 40 mg PO, bid
Pantoprazole (Protonix)	20 to 40 mg IV or PO, qd or bid
Rabeprazole (AcipHex)	20 mg PO, bid
Dexlansoprazole (Dexilant)	30 to 60 mg PO, qd

Box continues

BOX 4.3 (CONTINUED)

Medication	Dose and administration notes
Somatostatin analogues	
Octreotide (Sandostatin)	50 to 250 mcg subcutaneous, tid
Octreotide LAR Depo (sandostatine injection)	10 mg, 20 mg, or 30 mg 1 injection per month
α$_2$-Adrenergic receptor antagonist	
Clonidine	0.1 to 0.3 mg PO, up to tid
Pancreatic enzyme	
Pancrelipase	500 lipase units per kg body weight per meal; maximum dose, 2,500 lipase units per kg body weight per meal or 10,000 lipase units per kg body weight per day. Use uncoated, rapid-release preparations, one to eight capsules with meals and snacks.
Choleretic	
Ursodeoxycholic acid (ursodiol) (Actigall)	300 mg PO, bid
Bile acid sequestrants	
Cholestyramine	2 to 4 g PO, up to qid
Colestipol	5 g packet or tablet, one to six times a day
Antibiotics	
Amoxicillin and clavulanic acid (Augmentin)	500 mg PO, bid for 7 to 14 days
Levofloxacin (Levaquin)	500 mg PO, qd
Metronidazole (Flagyl)	250 mg PO, tid for 7 to 14 days
Ciprofloxacin (Cipro)	500 mg PO, bid for 7 to 14 days
Rifaximin (Xifaxan)	200 to 550 mg PO, tid for 7 to 14 days
Tetracycline	250 to 500 mg PO, qid for 7 to 14 days
Doxycycline	100 mg PO, bid for 7 to 14 days
Neomycin	500 mg PO, bid for 7 to 14 days
Proadaptive therapies	
Glucagon-like peptide-2 analogues (Gattex)	0.05 mg/kg qd by subcutaneous injection

[a] Not to be confused with paregoric, which is much less concentrated.

Antidiarrheals

Antidiarrheal medications slow intestinal transit and are generally given 30 to 60 minutes before meals.

Acid Blockers

Acid blockers, including H_2 receptor antagonists and proton pump inhibitors, are used to reduce gastric hyperacidity that occurs within the first 6 months after a massive small bowel resection. They work by different mechanisms. H_2 antagonists inhibit histamine stimulation of the H_2 receptor in gastric parietal cells, which in turn reduces gastric acid secretion, gastric volume, and hydrogen concentrations. Proton pump inhibitors decrease gastric acid secretion by inhibiting the parietal-cell H^+/K^+-ATPase activity.

Octreotide

Octreotide, a somatostatin analogue, is an inhibitory hormone (somatostatin) produced by neuroendocrine cells throughout the GI tract and pancreas. It is effective in controlling hypersecretory states and severe diarrhea and slows jejunal transit. Significant side effects include increased risk for the following:

- cholelithiasis
- maldigestion
- pseudo-obstruction
- inhibition of intestinal adaptation (animal models)

Clonidine

Clonidine is an α_2-adrenergic receptor antagonist that has been shown to reduce output (fecal and stomal) in patients with SBS.[31,32]

Pancreatic Enzymes

Patients with SBS have rapid intestinal transit and, therefore, have reduced mixing of pancreatic enzymes with food. Theoretically, supplementing pancreatic enzymes may help with digestion.

Choleretics

Patients with SBS who are receiving PN may develop PN-associated liver disease (PNALD). Ursodeoxycholic acid (ursodiol) has been used to treat PNALD by changing bile composition and flow. However, optimal dosing, timing, duration of therapy, and long-term effects are unknown.

Bile Acid Sequestrants

Bile salts are absorbed primarily in the distal ileum. Some patients with ileal resections of less than 100 cm with the colon in circuit may secrete bile salts into the colon, resulting in diarrhea. This may be treated with bile acid–binding resins (eg, cholestyramine, colestipol, colesevelam), also called bile acid sequestrants. These resins bind and sequester bile acids in the intestine, producing an insoluble complex, which is excreted in the stool. The use of bile acid sequestrants also results in partial removal of bile acids from the enterohepatic circulation, which prevents reabsorption. These medications also bind and impede the absorption of a variety of nutrients, including the fat-soluble vitamins, and they may worsen diarrhea in some patients.

Antibiotics

As a result of rapid intestinal transit, malabsorption, hyperacidity, and anatomical changes following a massive resection, patients with SBS often experience small intestinal bacterial overgrowth, or SIBO. Correction of SIBO to restore the natural flora is attempted with antibiotics. Unfortunately, very few well-controlled clinical trials have been conducted for the treatment of SIBO, so recommendations are often based on clinical experience. In general, antibiotics are prescribed for short-term treatment (1–2 weeks). The use of antibiotics for treating SIBO has certain disadvantages, including[33]:

- recurrence of symptoms after treatment is discontinued;
- the need for a prolonged or repeated course of treatment in some patients; and
- long-term side effects of the antibiotics, such as diarrhea, impaired immunity, changes in gut microflora, and the emergence of bacteria that are resistant to the antibiotics.

Despite the current popularity of probiotics and a growing number of experimental studies demonstrating their potential benefits, the role of these agents in the management of SIBO remains unclear.[33] Probiotics are currently unregulated, so the exact quantity and quality of the bacteria cannot be guaranteed. Also, some data suggest that adding certain probiotics may actually limit intestinal adaptation and that prebiotics, such as fructo-oligosaccharide, may be more effective in stimulating adaptation through butyrate production.[34] In the face of a paucity of clinical studies evaluating the efficacy, appropriate strain, and dosage of probiotics in SBS, the use of these agents in this patient population should be considered only when strong scientific evidence supports it.[6]

Proadaptive Therapies

Some patients are candidates for pharmacologic proadaptive treatments such as glucagon-like peptide-2 (GLP-2) analogues. GLP-2 is naturally secreted from distal small intestine and proximal colonic mucosal L cells in response to a meal, which results in increased villus height and crypt depth by stimulating crypt cell proliferation and inhibiting enterocyte apoptosis. It also increases hexose and nutrient transporter activity, inhibits gastric acid secretion and gastric motility, increases intestinal blood flow, and decreases intestinal permeability. Native GLP-2 has a half-life of only 7 minutes, which limits its clinical utility. However, a longer-acting analogue (teduglutide) has an extended half-life of 1.3 hours. This was shown to be safe, well tolerated, and intestinotrophic, and it significantly increased intestinal wet weight absorption and reduced PN requirements.[34-36] Additionally, teduglutide restored the structural integrity of the mucosa, as evidenced by increased villus height, plasma citrulline concentration, and lean body mass. Teduglutide (GATTEX) is indicated for the treatment of adults and pediatric patients aged 1 year and older with SBS who are dependent on parenteral support. Although the drug is safe and well tolerated, teduglutide has been associated with acceleration of neoplastic growth, intestinal obstruction, biliary and pancreatic disease, fluid imbalance and fluid overload, and increased absorption of concomitant oral medication. Thus, the patient should be carefully monitored, particularly during the weaning phase.

Long-Term Parenteral Nutrition

When rehabilitation efforts fail, patients can also be supported with long-term home PN, which has been considered a standard life-saving therapy for more than 40 years. Long-term PN is costly and has appreciable risks, such as life-threatening bloodstream infections (Box 4.4 on page 70).[37-39] See Chapter 22 for information on home PN.

BOX 4.4

Complications of Parenteral Nutrition Dependency[37-39]

Catheter-related

Infection

Loss of vascular access

Central venous thrombosis

Liver-related

Steatosis

Cholestasis

Gallbladder sludge and stones

Metabolic

Fluid and electrolyte abnormalities

D-lactic acidosis

Weight loss

Bone-related

Metabolic bone disease: osteoporosis, osteomalacia

Gastrointestinal

Diarrhea

Gastric hypersecretion

Small intestinal bacterial overgrowth

Kidney-related

Nephrolithiasis

Quality of life–related

Depression, irritability, confusion

Reduced freedom

Disrupted sleep

Financial

High cost of care

Inability to work (in some patients)

Surgical Reconstruction

Attempts at intestinal rehabilitation with diet and adjunctive medication sometimes fail. In such cases, surgical options for preventing dehydration and malnutrition should be considered. Surgical intestinal rehabilitation or autologous GI reconstruction can restore intestinal continuity by reanastomosing isolated loops of bowel to provide more absorptive surface, lengthen and taper the bowel, or relieve obstructions.[40] In some instances, it may be necessary to slow transit by using a reversed segment of bowel. See Box 4.5 for a list of reconstructive procedures for the surgical management of SBS.

Only a small number of patients are candidates for these reconstructive procedures. However, for eligible patients, GI reconstruction may provide autonomy from PN. The decision to proceed with reconstructive surgery depends on the disease origin, remnant bowel length, degree of bowel dilation, and other residual anatomic characteristics, such as the presence of stomas, blind loops, or colonic remnant.[40,41]

Small Bowel Transplantation

Small bowel transplantation, with or without other viscera, should be considered in patients who are candidates and fail to improve with more conservative therapy. The Centers for Medicare & Medicaid Services approved intestinal transplantation for patients with irreversible intestinal failure and PN-related complications in 2000 and extended the approval

BOX 4.5

Surgical Procedures for Short Bowel Syndrome

Surgical reconstruction

Strictureplasty

Salvage of out-of-circuit bowel

Colon preservation

Fistula repair instead of excision

Procedures to slow intestinal motility of dilated bowel

Tapering enteroplasty

Longitudinal intestinal lengthening and tailoring (Bianchi procedure)

Transverse intestinal lengthening (Kimura and Georgeson procedure)

Serial transverse enteroplasty procedure (STEP)

Procedures to slow intestinal transit of nondilated bowel

Creation or repair of small bowel valves

Reverse segments of bowel

Colon interposition

Bowel replacement

Small bowel or multivisceral transplantation

---

to multivisceral transplantation the following year. PN failure was defined by any of the following[42]:

- presence of PN-associated liver disease
- loss of central venous access (defined as the loss of three to six central venous access sites in children or two to four sites in adults)
- recurrent catheter-related sepsis or a single episode of fungal sepsis
- recurrent bouts of severe dehydration or metabolic abnormalities

The Intestinal Transplant Registry has gathered information on intestine transplantation since 1985. Survival rates have been improving over the last decade. Current actuarial patient survival rates are 76%, 56%, and 43% at 1, 5, and 10 years, respectively.[43]

Monitoring, Follow-Up, and Complications

Regular and periodic follow-up is essential, especially during the adaptive and weaning phases of intestinal rehabilitation. The exact timing of these intervals varies. Patients in the active weaning phase may have to be seen weekly. During this period, patients may develop fluid and electrolyte abnormalities, nutrient deficiencies, and malnutrition. As intestinal absorption improves, the patient may also experience fluid overload from combined oral nutrition and PN. As the patient stabilizes, the time between follow-up visits can be prolonged. Patients receiving PN should be monitored for potential complications (see Box 4.4).

Summary

The management of SBS is complex and requires a comprehensive, multidisciplinary approach with meticulous attention to detail. Specific and meticulous personalized nutrition interventions can facilitate weaning from PN. The use of certain nutrients or nonnutritive components of foods may also benefit some patients. When nutritional autonomy cannot be achieved through efforts in a rehabilitation program and home PN is unsuccessful, small bowel transplantation should be considered. The ultimate goal is to improve the nutritional status of these patients through the safest, most efficacious method that will improve the quality of their lives.

References

1. Pironi L, Arends J, Bozzetti F, et al. ESPEN guidelines on chronic intestinal failure in adults. *Clin Nutr.* 2016;35(2):247-307.
2. O'Keefe SJ, Buchman AL, Fishbein TM, Jeejeebhoy KN, Jeppesen PB, Shaffer J. Short bowel syndrome and intestinal failure: consensus definitions and overview. *Clin Gastroenterol Hepatol.* 2006;4(1):6-10.
3. Pironi L, Arends J, Baxter J, et al. ESPEN endorsed recommendations: definition and classification of intestinal failure in adults. *Clin Nutr.* 2015;34(2):171-180.
4. Lennard-Jones JE. Indications and need for long-term parenteral nutrition: implications for intestinal transplantation. *Transplant Proc.* 1990;22(6):2427-2429.
5. Byrne TA, Persinger RL, Young LS, Ziegler TR, Wilmore DW. A new treatment for patients with short bowel syndrome: growth hormone, glutamine and a modified diet. *Ann Surg.* 1995;222(3):243-254.
6. Matarese LE, Harvin G. Nutritional care for patients with intestinal failure. *Gastroenterol Clin North Am.* 2021;50(1):201-216.
7. Lal S, Teubner A, Shaffer JL. Review article: intestinal failure. *Aliment Pharmacol Ther.* 2006;24(1):19-31.
8. Pironi L, Corcos O, Forbes A, et al. Intestinal failure in adults: recommendations from the ESPEN expert groups. *Clin Nutr.* 2018;37:1798-1809.
9. Jeppesen PB, Mortensen PB. Experimental approaches: dietary and hormone therapy. *Best Pract Res Clin Gastroenterol.* 2003;17(6):1041-1054.
10. Nightingale JM, Lennard-Jones JE. The short bowel syndrome: what's new and old? *Dig Dis.* 1993;11(1):12-31.
11. Hounnou G, Destrieux C, Desmé J, Bertrand P, Velut S. Anatomical study of the length of the human intestine. *Surg Radiol Anat.* 2002;24(5):290-294.
12. Carbonnel F, Cosnes J, Chevret S, et al. The role of anatomic factors in nutritional autonomy after extensive small bowel resection. *JPEN J Parenter Enteral Nutr.* 1996;20:275-280.
13. Messing B, Crenn P, Beau P, et al. Long-term survival and parenteral nutrition dependence in adult patients with the short bowel syndrome. *Gastroenterology.* 1999;117:1043-1050.
14. Chaudri O, Small C, Bloom S. Gastrointestinal hormones regulating appetite. *Phil Trans R Soc B.* 2006;361:1187-1209.
15. Nightingale JM, Kamm MA, van der Sijp JR, et al. Disturbed gastric emptying in the short bowel syndrome: evidence for a "colonic brake." *Gut.* 1993;34(9):1171-1176.
16. Royall D, Wolever TM, Jeejeebhoy KN. Evidence for colonic conservation of malabsorbed carbohydrate in short bowel syndrome. *Am J Gastroenterol.* 1992;87(6):751-756.
17. Jeppesen PB, Mortensen PB. The influence of a preserved colon on the absorption of medium chain fat in patients with small bowel resection. *Gut.* 1998;43(4):478-483.
18. Matarese LE, Steiger E. Dietary and medical management of short bowel syndrome in adult patients. *J Clin Gastroenterol.* 2006;40(suppl 2):S85-S93.
19. Matarese LE, O'Keefe SJ, Kandil HM, Bond G, Costa G, Abu-Elmagd K. Short bowel syndrome: clinical guidelines for nutrition management. *Nutr Clin Pract.* 2005;20(5):493-502.
20. Byrne TA, Veglia L, Camelio M, et al. Beyond the prescription: optimizing the diet of patients with short bowel syndrome. *Nutr Clin Pract.* 2000;15(6):306-311.

21. Matarese LE. Nutrition and fluid optimization for patients with short bowel syndrome. *JPEN J Parenter Enteral Nutr*. 2013;37(2):161-170.

22. Fordtran JS, Locklear TW. Ionic constituents and osmolality of gastric and small-intestinal fluids after eating. *Am J Dig Dis*. 1966;11(7):503-521.

23. Levitan R, Fordtran JS, Burrows BA, Ingelfinger FJ. Water and salt absorption in the human colon. *J Clin Invest*. 1962;41:1754-1759.

24. Lennard-Jones JE. Oral rehydration solutions in short bowel syndrome. *Clin Ther*. 1990;12(suppl A):129-137; discussion, 138.

25. Camilleri M, Prather CM, Evans MA, Andresen-Reid ML. Balance studies and polymeric glucose solution to optimize therapy after massive intestinal resection. *Mayo Clin Proc*. 1992;67(8):755-760.

26. Matarese LE, Harvin GK. Parenteral nutrition for short bowel syndrome: practical aspects. In: DiBaise J, Thompson J, Parrish C, eds. *Short Bowel Syndrome Practical Approach to Management*. CRC Press; 2016:196-204.

27. Parrish CR, DiBaise J. Part III: hydrating the adult patient with short bowel syndrome. *Pract Gastroenterol*. 2015;39(2):10.

28. Parrish CR. The clinician's guide to short bowel syndrome. *Pract Gastroenterol*. 2005;29(9):67.

29. Kumph VJ. Pharmacologic management of diarrhea in patients with short bowel syndrome. *JPEN J Parenter Enteral Nutr*. 2014;38(suppl 1):38S-44S.

30. Steiger E. Guidelines for pharmacotherapy, nutritional management, and weaning parenteral nutrition in adult patients with short bowel syndrome: introduction. *J Clin Gastroenterol*. 2006;40(suppl 2):S73-S74.

31. McDoniel K, Taylor B, Huey W, et al. Use of clonidine to decrease intestinal fluid losses in patients with high-output short-bowel syndrome. *JPEN J Parenter Enteral Nutr*. 2004;28(4):265-268.

32. Buchman AL, Fryer J, Wallin A, Ahn CW, Polensky S, Zaremba K. Clonidine reduces diarrhea and sodium loss in patients with proximal jejunostomy: a controlled study. *JPEN J Parenter Enteral Nutr*. 2006;30(6):487-491.

33. Johnson E, Vu L, Matarese LE. Bacteria, bones, and stones: managing complications of short bowel syndrome. *Nutr Clin Pract*. 2018;33(4):454-466.

34. Barnes JL, Hartmann B, Holst JJ, Tappenden KA. Intestinal adaptation is stimulated by partial enteral nutrition supplemented with the prebiotic short-chain fructooligosaccharide in a neonatal intestinal failure piglet model. *JPEN J Parenter Enteral Nutr*. 2012;36:524-537.

35. Jeppesen PB, Gilroy R, Pertkiewicz M, et al. Randomised placebo-controlled trial of teduglutide in reducing parenteral nutrition and/or intravenous fluid requirements in patients with short bowel syndrome. *Gut*. 2011;60:902-914.

36. Pironi L. Translation of evidence into practice with teduglutide in the management of adults with intestinal failure due to short-bowel syndrome: a review of recent literature. *JPEN J Parenter Enteral Nutr*. 2020;44(6):968-978.

37. Nightingale JMD. The short bowel. In: Nightingale JMD, ed. *Intestinal Failure*. Greenwich Medical Media; 2001:177-198.

38. Hofstetter S, Stern L, Willet J. Key issues in addressing the clinical and humanistic burden of short bowel syndrome in the US. *Curr Med Res Opin*. 2013;29(5):495-504.

39. Buchman AL, Scolapio J, Fryer J. AGA technical review on short bowel syndrome and intestinal transplantation. *Gastroenterology*. 2003;124(4):1111-1134.

40. Iyer K. Surgical management of short bowel syndrome. *JPEN J Parenter Enteral Nutr*. 2014;38(suppl 1):53S-59S.

41. Abu-Elmagd KM, Armanyous SR, Fujiki M, et al. Management of five hundred patients with gut failure at a single center: surgical innovation versus transplantation with a novel predictive model. *Ann Surg*. 2019;270:656-674.

42. Centers for Medicare and Medicaid Services. National Coverage Analysis. Intestinal and multivisceral transplantation. CMS.gov website. Accessed May 13, 2022. www.cms.gov/Medicare/Provider-Enrollment -and-Certification/CertificationandComplianc /Transplant

43. Grant D, Abu-Elmagd K, Mazariegos G, et al. Intestinal Transplant Registry report: global activity and trends. *Am J Transplant*. 2015;15:210-219.

Irritable Bowel Syndrome

Justin Brandler, MD
Eden Koo, MD
William D. Chey, MD
Amanda Lynett, MS, RDN

KEY POINTS

- Irritable bowel syndrome is a symptom-based disorder characterized by recurrent bouts of abdominal pain associated with altered bowel movements; it often has a negative impact on quality of life.
- It is a common disorder of diverse pathogenesis and clinical phenotype in which food is a critical trigger for gastrointestinal symptoms in most patients suffering from the disorder.
- Although diet plays a key role in managing the disorder, other novel therapies are on the horizon, such as biomarkers, which can leverage the microbiome, metabolome, and genetics to help providers choose the right diet intervention for the right patient.

Introduction

Irritable bowel syndrome (IBS) is a symptom-based disorder characterized by recurrent bouts of abdominal pain that are associated with altered bowel movements.[1] IBS affects 10% to 15% of the US population[2] and is reported roughly twice as often in females compared to males. Although IBS does not affect life span or predispose individuals to the development of organic diseases (eg, inflammatory bowel disease [IBD] or colon cancer), it often has a negative impact on quality of life and creates a significant societal and financial burden; it is associated with absenteeism from work and health care costs that measure in the billions of dollars annually.[3]

Diagnosis of Irritable Bowel Syndrome

The pathophysiology of IBS is heterogeneous: different patients may report similar symptoms, but the cause of the symptoms can vary from one patient to the next. Some factors that have been implicated in the pathophysiology of IBS include altered enteric neurotransmitters, imbalances in the small bowel and colonic microbiota, neuroendocrine cell dysregulation, altered intestinal permeability, gut immune activation, and psychosocial stressors. Combinations of these factors can enable changes in motility, visceral sensation, and bidirectional abnormalities in brain-gut interactions that can result in IBS symptoms.[4-8]

The current gold standard for the symptom-based diagnosis of IBS is the Rome IV criteria.[9] According to these criteria, a diagnosis of IBS is appropriate in individuals with the following:

- symptoms that have developed at least 6 months prior to diagnosis
- abdominal pain or discomfort that has been present for at least 1 day a week for the past 3 months, associated with two or more of the following:
  - related to defecation (increasing or improving the pain)
  - a change in stool frequency
  - a change in the form (appearance) of the stool

In addition to confirming the Rome IV criteria, providers should also exclude "alarm features," such as gastrointestinal (GI) bleeding, unintentional weight loss, nocturnal diarrhea, or a family history of organic diseases, such as colon cancer, IBD, or celiac disease.[10] Selected diagnostic tests can also aid in making a confident diagnosis of IBS.[1,11] In the past, many viewed IBS as a diagnosis of exclusion. In the strictest sense, this is true because nearly all of the currently recommended tests to confirm a diagnosis of IBS are performed to rule out diseases that can mimic IBS. At present, there are no adequately validated biomarkers that reliably "rule in" IBS. That said, labeling the disorder as a diagnosis of exclusion implies that a provider can only arrive at a diagnosis of IBS after exhaustive diagnostic testing to rule out a library of organic diseases. Multiple studies and clinical practice guidelines argue that such a strategy is neither necessary nor cost-effective.[12] In fact, only very limited diagnostic testing is recommended to arrive at a confident diagnosis of IBS (Figure 5.1).

FIGURE 5.1 Diagnostic testing to establish a confident diagnosis of irritable bowel syndrome[1,10,11]

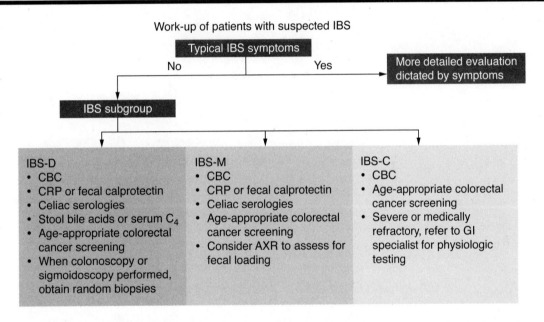

AXR = abdominal x-ray | C_4 = 7α-hydroxy-4-cholesten-3-one | CBC = complete blood count | CRP = C-reactive protein | GI = gastrointestinal | IBS = irritable bowel syndrome |
IBS-C = IBS with predominant constipation | IBS-D = IBS with predominant diarrhea | IBS-M = IBS with mixed bowel habits
Celiac serologies refers to tissue transglutaminase immunoglobulin A (IgA) test and IgA level

In recent years, the treatment of IBS has expanded beyond medications. Persuasive evidence now also supports important roles for diet and behavioral interventions in the treatment of IBS.[13] This has made clear the critical role that properly trained registered dietitians should play in the management of patients with IBS. Indeed, a pragmatic trial from Australia demonstrated improved clinical outcomes and reduced cost per cure with an integrated care model (including a collaborative team composed of a gastroenterologist, GI dietitian, GI psychologist, and psychiatrist) when compared to traditional care offered by a gastroenterologist.[14] This outcome is particularly important in an age of increasing awareness of disordered eating and eating disorders for which awareness, education, and vigilance are required. The remainder of this chapter provides a primer on the important role of food in the pathogenesis and management of patients with IBS.[15]

Dietary Etiology and Management of Irritable Bowel Syndrome

Food Allergies and Sensitivities

Approximately 90% of food allergies worldwide can be attributed to nine food groups: milk, eggs, peanuts, tree nuts, fish, shellfish, wheat, soy, and sesame.[16] Between 60% and 84% of patients report food-related IBS symptoms,[17,18] and more than half of gastroenterologists surveyed recommend dietary therapy to the majority of their patients with IBS.[18] Moreover, although 35% of patients with IBS self-reported food allergies,[19] only 3.6% of 2.7 million patients actually had a documented food reaction or validated testing in the electronic medical record.[20] This discrepancy demonstrates the crucial unmet need for validated food allergy testing to guide diagnosis and management, especially given that elimination diets can be expensive and needlessly reduce intake of important nutrients. Because of the lack of validated testing methodologies, routine ordering of food allergy or sensitivity panels is not currently recommended for patients with IBS.

If a patient experiences an adverse reaction to food, the causes for their symptoms can be categorized as immune-mediated or non–immune-mediated (or both). Non–immune-mediated reactions include those resulting from osmotic effects, mechanical effects, or carbohydrate or protein fermentation.[21] Immune-mediated food reactions (allergies) can be further classified as immunoglobulin E (IgE)–mediated, non–IgE-mediated, or a combination. Clinically, this becomes important because confirming IgE-mediated disease requires a battery of tests, including allergen-specific IgE serologies, skin prick tests, and supervised double-blind oral challenges. These tests are recommended by national societies,[22] but they can be expensive and nonspecific.[23] Thus, it is recommended to only perform these tests in patients after obtaining a detailed clinical history or if the physical examination is highly suggestive of an IgE-mediated food allergy.[21]

Testing for non–IgE-mediated food allergies has traditionally been controversial. One of the most popular approaches in patients with IBS is to use food elimination diets guided by IgG-antibody testing.[24-34] This approach has been associated with reducing both IBS global symptoms and quality of life in a small number of studies.[25,26,30,32-34] However, IgG-based elimination diets are currently marketed directly to consumers, and the testing methods used commercially and in research have not been harmonized or standardized. Also, relatively few randomized controlled trials have validated their value.[30,32,33] Thus, many professional societies recommend against ordering IgG-based food sensitivity testing.[12,35,36] To bridge this knowledge gap, a multicenter randomized controlled trial of IgG-based elimination diets in patients with IBS is underway in the United States (ClinicalTrials.gov identifier: NCT03459482).

Another emerging test for food allergy variants is leukocyte activation testing. A small randomized controlled trial showed improvement in global IBS symptoms in patients who followed an elimination diet guided by leukocyte activation testing vs a sham elimination diet.[37] Two other tests that have been explored in small studies are basophil activation assay[38] and confocal laser endomicroscopy (CLE), which can show magnified, real-time views of the gut mucosal changes, including cellular injury, changes in barrier structure, and increases in inflammatory cells. CLE has been used to characterize gut mucosal changes in patients with IBS who were exposed to various food extracts, correlating with symptom reductions after exclusion diets.[39,40]

If a patient has an adverse reaction to food, has minimal extraintestinal allergic symptoms, or tests negative for food allergies (using a validated food allergy testing method), it is prudent to consider whether the patient has a non–immune-mediated intolerance to components such as lactose, fructose, or other carbohydrates.

Lactose

Lactose is a disaccharide commonly found in dairy products (eg, milk, yogurt, and unaged cheese). It is normally digested into the monosaccharides glucose and galactose by lactase, a brush border enzyme in the small intestine.[41] Lactose malabsorption occurs when brush border lactase is absent or present in insufficient quantities to digest ingested lactose. In individuals with lactose malabsorption, undigested lactose is delivered to the colon where it is fermented by the native microbiota, producing short-chain fatty acids and gases including hydrogen, methane, and carbon dioxide.[42] These fermentation byproducts can trigger symptoms of what is widely referred to as lactose intolerance, including abdominal cramping, bloating, flatulence, and diarrhea. Delivery of lactose to the intestinal lumen may additionally exert an osmotic effect and result in more luminal water, increasing the liquidity of intestinal contents.

Because IBS and lactose intolerance share overlapping presentations, the relationship between IBS and lactose malabsorption has been extensively studied. A 4-month, double-blind, crossover, therapeutic clinical trial involving 12 individuals with IBS found that lactase supplementation does not improve symptoms in patients with IBS who ingest lactose products, suggesting that their IBS symptoms were independent of lactose malabsorption.[43] A Norwegian case-control study that included 82 participants with IBS and 105 healthy control subjects determined that 38% of the participants with IBS had symptoms after ingesting lactose products, compared with 20% of the healthy control subjects ($P = .01$).[44] The study, however, also concluded that IBS and lactose malabsorption are unrelated disorders in the Norwegian population.

On the other hand, it has been hypothesized that patients with IBS, who often harbor underlying abnormalities in gut motility and sensation, are more likely to manifest symptoms in the face of lactose malabsorption. A study of 60 participants with IBS and 60 control subjects found that following lactose ingestion, the patients with IBS experienced both more frequent and more severe GI symptoms than the control subjects did.[45] Other study results suggest that, in addition to hydrogen gas production, visceral hypersensitivity increases the severity of GI symptoms in patients with IBS following lactose ingestion.[46] This evidence implies that individuals with lactose malabsorption and IBS share a common pathological basis in which sensitive (or "irritable") bowels contribute to symptoms of lactose malabsorption. Moreover, a 2009 narrative review of the effect of diet on IBS symptoms in adults suggested that patients with IBS and known lactose intolerance show improvement with dietary restriction.[47] Individuals can reduce their lactose intake by consuming lactose-free dairy products or fortified dairy alternatives. Additionally, lactase digestive enzyme supplements available on the market can improve lactose digestion and associated GI symptoms.

Sucrose

Sucrose is the key ingredient of table sugar and accounts for about 30% of ingested carbohydrates in the Western diet.[48] It is a disaccharide that is hydrolyzed by the enzyme sucrase to the monosaccharides glucose and fructose. Sucrase-isomaltase is a specific form of the sucrase enzyme that may be variably expressed in individuals.[49] Sucrase-isomaltase deficiency is characterized by the absence, reduction, or dysfunction of sucrase or isomaltase enzyme with a subsequent inability to digest sucrose or maltose (a sugar found in grains), which can lead to symptoms that include diarrhea, flatulence, bloating, abdominal distention, and pain.[50] This deficiency can be of genetic etiology (congenital sucrase-isomaltase deficiency) or secondary to any disease that damages the brush border epithelium of the small intestine.

Studies have reported a number of rare and common variants in the sucrase-isomaltase gene, which have been linked to an increased risk of IBS.[51-53] In one study, gene variants for sucrase-isomaltase deficiency were found in 35% of patients with IBS, particularly in those with diarrhea-predominant IBS (IBS-D).[54] As with the mechanism of lactose intolerance, it is thought that sucrase-isomaltase deficiency causes undigested sucrose to reach the colon, where it is fermented by the microbiota, producing short-chain fatty acids and gases that can trigger symptoms in patients with IBS and underlying abnormalities in motility and visceral sensation. Another study reported that sucrase-isomaltase gene variations were associated with a threefold to fourfold reduction in the likelihood that patients with IBS-D would respond to a diet low in fermentable oligosaccharides, disaccharides, monosaccharides, and polyols (the low-FODMAP diet; see the section on FODMAPs).[55] Though it is likely that sucrase-isomaltase deficiency contributes to the development of gut symptoms in a subset of IBS sufferers, the prevalence of the deficiency in patients with IBS remains to be confidently defined. Patients in whom this deficiency is a concern should undergo diagnostic testing before being treated with sucrose- or maltose-restricted diets or enzyme replacement therapy. Sucrase-isomaltase deficiency can be confirmed by one of three methods: upper endoscopy (with biopsies of the small intestine for disaccharidase assay),[13,53] C-sucrose breath testing, or traditional hydrogen-methane breath testing for sucrose. Some practitioners have also advocated for a sucrose challenge when other diagnostic tests are unavailable. A combination of a reduction in sucrose and maltose in the diet and the use of oral sucrase enzyme replacement therapy (eg, sacrosidase) taken with meals can be used for symptom management in patients with a diagnosis of sucrase-isomaltase deficiency.[50]

Fructose

Key monosaccharides in the human diet include glucose, galactose, and fructose. Fructose is naturally found in honey, fruits, and table sugar, and it is present in many processed foods and beverages as high-fructose corn syrup. In the United States, individuals consume, on average, more than 50 g fructose daily.[56] Being a monosaccharide, fructose does not require enzymatic digestion before absorption in the small intestine. Rather, it relies in part on glucose transporters for absorption, which can become overwhelmed with a large fructose load (more than 25 g), leading to malabsorption, colonic fermentation, and the development of GI symptoms in some individuals.

In a case-control study of 25 women with IBS and 25 healthy control subjects, fructose intolerance was observed more frequently in the women with IBS than in the control subjects (52% vs 16%; $P = .01$), and patients clearly benefited from dietary restriction.[57] A double-blind, randomized, quadruple-arm, placebo-controlled rechallenge trial concluded that, in some patients with IBS, restriction of fructose and fructans was beneficial in resolving symptoms.[58]

FODMAPs

Fermentable oligosaccharides, disaccharides, monosaccharides, and polyols (FODMAPs) represent a family of poorly absorbed, short-chain carbohydrates that are highly fermentable in the presence of gut bacteria. The fermentation of FODMAPs by the gut microbiota produces gases and osmotically active short-chain fatty acids. These cause luminal distension and changes in stool viscosity that can trigger abdominal pain, flatulence, bloating, and, to a lesser extent, diarrhea in individuals with IBS, who often have underlying abnormalities in motility and visceral sensation. The major FODMAPs consumed in the standard American diet are fructans and galacto-oligosaccharides (oligosaccharides); lactose (a disaccharide); fructose (a monosaccharide); and sorbitol, mannitol, isomalt, xylitol, and glycerol (polyols).

Fructose is primarily absorbed by glucose transporter 5, located on the luminal surface of the brush border epithelium.[59] Fructose is considered a FODMAP only when it is present in excess of glucose in a given food or beverage. For example, sucrose, which is exactly 50% fructose, is considered a suitable component of a low-FODMAP diet.

Oligosaccharides are chains of monosaccharides linked together. Fructans are long polymers of fructose with a glucose terminal end. Fructans with 10 or more molecules of fructose in a chain are known as inulins, and those with fewer than 10 fructose molecules in a chain are called fructo-oligosaccharides (FOS), or oligofructose. Wheat-based products and onions account for most fructan intake in typical Western diets.

Galacto-oligosaccharides (GOS) are polymerized galactose molecules that behave similarly to fructans. Foods rich in GOS include legumes (eg, kidney beans, baked beans, pinto beans), soy beans, soy milk, and green peas. A study found that oral α-galactosidase digestive enzymes, when coingested with foods high in GOS, can reduce symptoms in individuals with IBS and GOS-sensitivity.[60] For efficacy, patients should take half of the α-galactosidase enzyme treatment right before eating and the other half midway through the meal.

Polyols or sugar alcohols, such as sorbitol and mannitol, are present in fruits (eg, apricots, peaches) and vegetables (eg, cauliflower, mushrooms). They do not require digestion and are slowly, and often incompletely, absorbed via passive diffusion. Polyols are osmotically active in the intestinal lumen and are subsequently fermented by the gut microbiota.[61]

Since its development by researchers at Monash University in Australia, a diet low in FODMAPs has been found to be effective and safe in patients with IBS in numerous randomized controlled trials.[62] Although one meta-analysis notes that the quality of evidence for the low-FODMAP diet in IBS is "very low," the totality of the evidence favors a benefit to the low-FODMAP diet over a wide range of other interventions.[62] In a single-blind, crossover intervention trial involving 15 patients with IBS and 15 healthy control subjects, individuals who ingested a diet high in FODMAPs had higher levels of breath hydrogen and methane, reflecting bacterial fermentation.[63] A 2020 review of studies concerning the low-FODMAP diet found that, overall, 52% to 86% of patients with IBS reported a significant improvement in overall IBS symptoms with restriction of dietary FODMAPs.[64] Additionally, a 2021 systematic review and meta-anaylsis concluded that the diet reduces GI symptoms and improves the quality of life in patients with IBS compared to control diets.[65] Foods higher and lower in FODMAPs are shown in Figure 5.2.

A randomized controlled trial compared the efficacy of the low-FODMAP diet to a diet based on modified National Institute for Health and Care Excellence guidelines (mNICE) in American adults with IBS-D.[66] The researchers found that 40% to 50% of patients experienced adequate relief of their overall IBS symptoms with either diet, but the low-FODMAP diet led to greater improvements than the mNICE diet in important individual symptoms, including abdominal pain and bloating.

In 2021, a practice guideline released by the American College of Gastroenterology (ACG) recommended a limited trial of a low-FODMAP diet in patients with IBS to improve

FIGURE 5.2 FODMAP content of foods

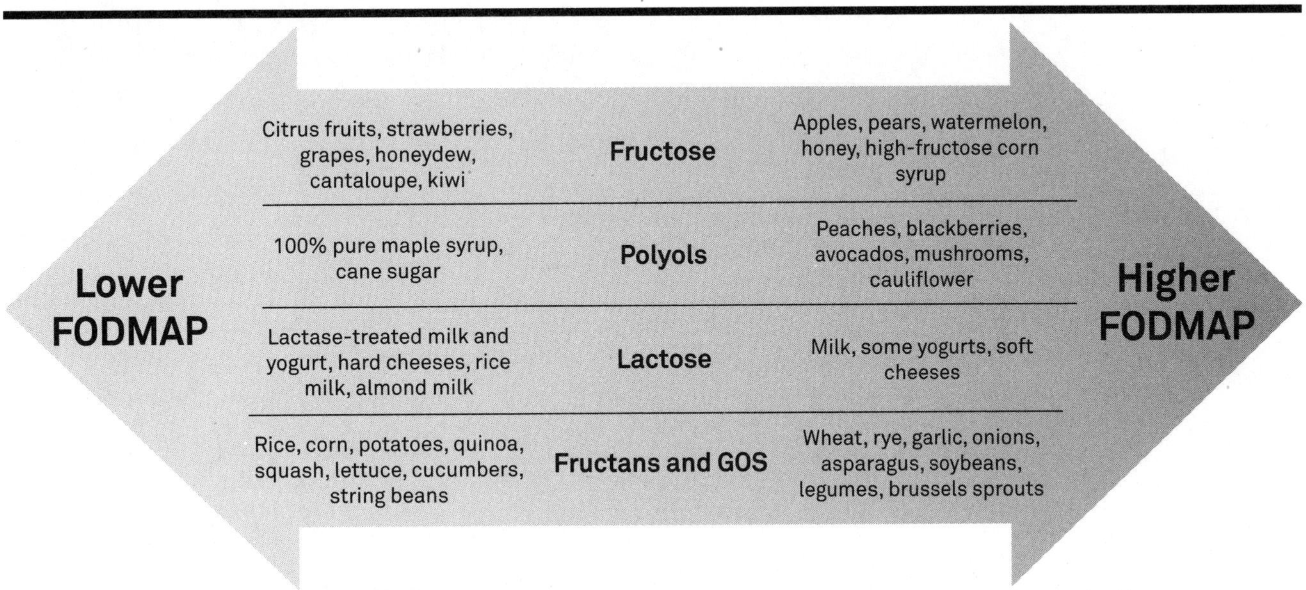

FODMAP = fermentable oligosaccharides, disaccharides, monosaccharides, and polyols | GOS = galacto-oligosaccharides
Portion size is important when determining the suitability of specific foods for a low FODMAP diet. Certain foods can be lower in FODMAPs depending on the portion size.

global IBS symptoms.[12] The low-FODMAP diet consists of three separate phases. An initial elimination phase that lasts 2 to 6 weeks helps determine whether or not a patient with IBS is sensitive to FODMAPs.[67] If the patient does not respond to the elimination phase, the low-FODMAP diet should be discontinued. If the patient does respond, foods containing individual FODMAPs are reintroduced over 6 to 8 weeks to determine sensitivities and tolerances. This information is then used to customize a personalized plan for the individual patient.

Given the complexity of the diet and the need for three phases, it is highly recommended that the low-FODMAP diet be administered with the assistance of a trained GI dietitian. A GI dietitian can help implement the diet and can also assist with a general nutritional assessment, screening for eating disorders, and assuring that diet interventions are nutritionally adequate. Recent studies have found significantly reduced daily intakes of key nutrients, compared with recommended daily intakes, in patients with IBS, even before they start the low-FODMAP diet.[13]

Wheat and Gluten

Wheat and gluten have a complex relationship with IBS physiology. Although a standard IBS evaluation excludes celiac disease, patients with IBS may still react to gluten-containing grains (which compose 80% to 85% of wheat grain).[68] This condition has recently been named nonceliac gluten sensitivity (NCGS). Patients with NCGS can have symptoms nearly identical to those of celiac disease but with negative serologies and normal small intestinal histology, and they frequently have prominent extraintestinal symptoms including fatigue, "brain fog," and headache.[69] Several studies have shown immune activation occurring in the small bowel mucosa of these wheat-sensitive, celiac-negative patients.[39,70,71] Subsequent elimination of wheat can result in long-term improvement in symptoms, especially in patients with NCGS who have the HLA-DQ2 or HLA-DQ8 haplotypes, the genetic markers for celiac disease.[72] Despite the widespread acceptance of the concept of gluten sensitivity, it should be noted that true sensitivity to gluten in patients without celiac disease is uncommon, as determined by studies using a double-blind gluten challenge.[73]

Thus, it is important to ask whether gluten or something else is the main culprit in patients who test negative for celiac disease but develop GI symptoms after eating wheat. The answer is likely multifactorial, with contributions coming from carbohydrates (eg, fructan) and nongluten proteins (eg, amylase-trypsin inhibitors [ATIs]). Wheat is high in fructans and, therefore, is a high-FODMAP food. Although previous double-blind, placebo-controlled trials involving wheat-filled capsules[73] and gluten-enriched bread[74] provoked IBS-like GI symptoms, a 2017 randomized crossover controlled trial that included 59 patients with NCGS and IBS symptoms found that ingesting fructan bars caused more GI symptoms, fatigue, and weakness than ingesting gluten or placebo bars.[75] In addition to fructans, ATIs are another potential culprit in wheat. These plant proteins are highly resistant to intestinal degradation and have been found to induce low-level intestinal inflammation in vivo in rats.[76] Given the heterogeneous pathophysiology of symptoms in patients who consume wheat, most experts recommend abandoning the antiquated term *gluten sensitivity* in favor of more holistic terms, such as *wheat sensitivity* or *wheat intolerance*.

Restrictive diets, such as a gluten-free diet or a low-FODMAP diet, can reduce the intake of healthful foods such as whole grains, which are important for cardiovascular health.[77,78] Given the complexities of balancing the medical, nutritional, and behavioral issues in patients with GI symptoms, many authorities recommend a team-based, collaborative, multidisciplinary approach to the management of IBS. Ideally, this approach would include a gastroenterologist, pathologist, allergist, dietitian, and psychologist familiar with the nuances surrounding these disease entities.[79]

Dietary Supplement Use in Irritable Bowel Syndrome

A diet to manage IBS can eliminate potential triggers or provide foods or food-based supplements that offer a therapeutic benefit. The following dietary supplements may provide symptomatic improvement in patients with IBS.

Fiber

Multiple systematic reviews and meta-analyses have been published on fiber as a treatment for IBS.[80-85] The most recently published meta-analysis compiled results from 14 randomized controlled trials and determined that patients with IBS predominantly benefit from soluble rather than insoluble fiber,[84] especially those with constipation. The most recent ACG guidelines for IBS strongly recommend soluble fiber over insoluble fiber to treat global IBS symptoms, with the most studied soluble fiber being psyllium (or ispaghula) husk.[12] The ideal soluble fiber is viscous (to increase stool water content) and poorly fermentable (to minimize gas formation). Insoluble fiber, however, is often nonviscous, which can harden stool (particularly when particle size is small) and, if fermentable, exacerbate problems with bloating and flatulence. Not all soluble fiber is created equal, however, as some patients with IBS can develop symptoms after consuming highly fermentable soluble fibers found in short-chain carbohydrates. These include the FOS and GOS found in legumes, wheat, onions, and garlic, mentioned previously in the discussion of FODMAP food groups.[85]

Examples of advisable dietary soluble fibers that cause moderate gas formation include psyllium, acacia, guar gum, kasha, barley, and beans. Insoluble fibers that cause high gas production are present in some vegetables and fruits, whole-meal pasta, and defatted ground flax seed. Oat bran is a 50-50 mixture of soluble and insoluble fiber. Examples of commercially available fiber preparations include psyllium, wheat dextrin, and inulin, which can be purchased under brand names such as Metamucil, Benefiber, and Quaker Oats, respectively. Insoluble fiber formulations that are nonfermentable include methylcellulose (Citrucel) and karaya gum, or sterculia (Normacol).[85] Various factors affect personalized patient recommendations for fiber preparations. Gas and bloating can complicate the use of fiber supplements. For some patients, this can be more prominent with psyllium than with methylcellulose or sterculia, though head-to-head studies are not available. Nevertheless, more-robust efficacy data exists for psyllium than for other fiber preparations. Thus, when initiating fiber in patients with IBS, the clinical axiom of "start low and go slow" remains highly applicable.

Prebiotics and Probiotics

Prebiotics are indigestible, fermentable food components that result in the selective growth or activity of one or a limited number of microbial genuses or species in the gut microbiota that confer health benefits to the host. The most commonly used prebiotics are known as inulin-type fructans (inulin, oligofructose, FOS) and GOS, because the human GI tract does not contain enzymes to digest these carbohydrates. Therefore, they reach the colon and are fermented by microbiota. A 2018 systematic review[86] found three randomized controlled trials that evaluated prebiotics in IBS.[87-89] The first two compared powders of short-chain FOS against placebo, and although both groups had symptomatic improvements, these did not reach statistical significance.[87,88] The third, a crossover trial, compared low-dose GOS (3.5 g), high-dose GOS (7 g), and placebo in 44 patients. Patients in both the low-dose and high-dose groups had a significant reduction in their global-symptoms scores compared to those taking the placebo, and adverse events were similar in all three groups.[89]

Whereas prebiotics feed the gut microbiota, probiotics are dietary supplements containing microorganisms themselves that, when ingested, have a beneficial effect on the host. Among the most commonly used and studied genuses and species are *Lactobacillus*,

Bifidobacterium, Saccharomyces boulardii, Escherichia coli, Streptococcus faecium, and multistrain combinations. Probiotics may improve IBS by modulating the gut microbiota, immune function, intestinal permeability, enteric nervous system function, and bidirectional gut-brain interactions.[90] A 2018 meta-analysis found that combination formulations improved the persistence of IBS symptoms, global symptoms, and abdominal pain, whereas individual-strain formulations often did not.[86] However, because of the significant variation among strain combinations, doses, and durations, the most recent American Gastroenterological Association guidelines on probiotics only suggest probiotics for IBS within the context of a clinical trial.[91] The AGC, in its clinical practice guideline, also recommends against the routine use of probiotics as a treatment for patients with IBS.[12] Furthermore, some experts are concerned that probiotics may worsen small intestinal bacterial overgrowth through increased microbiota in the proximal GI tract.[92] See Chapters 15 and 16 for more information on prebiotics and probiotics.

Complementary and Alternative Supplements

Most patients with IBS use at least one form of complementary and alternative medicine (CAM). Dietary supplements are the CAM modality most commonly used by patients with IBS.[93,94] Dietary supplements that have been studied for IBS management include prebiotics and probiotics, peppermint oil, STW 5 (a liquid extract of nine Western-based herbs that is formulated in Germany and sold under the brand name Iberogast), turmeric (containing the active ingredient curcumin), glutamine, berberine, *Aloe vera*, artichoke leaf extract, and melatonin. Table 5.1 highlights dosing and safety profile of these supplements.

Peppermint Oil

Peppermint oil has various mechanisms that are believed to improve IBS symptoms; these mechanisms include blocking smooth muscle spasms in the gut[95,96] and acting on the 5-HT$_3$ serotonin receptor to help with nausea.[97] A 2019 meta-analysis examined the role of enteric-coated peppermint oil in 835 patients with IBS from 12 randomized controlled trials. It found that only three patients needed to be treated for one patient to have improvement in global IBS symptoms, and only four patients to have improvement in abdominal pain.[98]

Though the results from this meta-analysis were promising for the efficacy of peppermint oil in IBS, a more recent randomized controlled trial not included in this meta-analysis evaluated 190 patients with IBS and did not find significant relief for abdominal pain from either small bowel–release or ileocolonic-release preparations over placebo. However, the small bowel–release form did achieve some benefits over placebo in providing moderate relief of abdominal pain and discomfort.[99] The most common commercial enteric-coated peppermint oil supplement is IBgard, which is triple-enteric-coated and timed to release in the small bowel. Caution should be taken if pills are not enteric-coated, as this can increase reflux symptoms.

STW 5 (Iberogast)

STW 5 typically is used for the treatment of functional dyspepsia,[93] but it has also been studied in patients with IBS with limited—but promising—results. A multicenter, randomized, double-blind, placebo-controlled trial found that both traditional STW 5 (nine herb extracts) and a research formulation, STW 5-II (STW 5 without three herbs), modestly reduced IBS symptoms and abdominal pain compared to placebo.[100] Though these results are promising, more data are emerging regarding possible liver toxicity leading to liver transplant in one case report.[101] This was reported again in another patient and confirmed with reexposure and in vitro cellular testing and histology.[102] Therefore, if patients are not

TABLE 5.1 Supplement Dosing and Safety in Irritable Bowel Syndrome

Supplement	Recommended dose	Possible adverse effects
Peppermint oil[98,99]	Two 90-mg capsules, PO, qd	Increased acid reflux
STW 5 (Iberogast)[100-102]	1 mL PO, tid	Liver toxicity, drug-drug interactions
Curcumin[103-108]	2 g PO, qd, in divided doses	No toxicity found up to 12 g/d
Glutamine[109]	5 mg PO, tid	Similar to placebo
Berberine[111,112]	400 mg PO, bid	Similar to placebo
Aloe vera[113-120]	1-2 tbsp to ⅓ c, qd	Liver toxicity, drug-drug interactions, possible colorectal cancer correlation
Artichoke leaf extract[120-123]	Two 320-mg capsules, tid (studied in functional dyspepsia)	Similar to placebo
Melatonin[124-130]	3 mg nightly	Similar to placebo

bid = twice a day | PO = by mouth | qd = every day | tid = three times a day

responding to initial therapy with STW 5, or develop signs of liver toxicity, the therapy should be promptly discontinued.

Turmeric

Turmeric is a member of the ginger family and contains a chemical called curcumin. While frequently used as a spice in Eastern cuisine, it is also felt to have medicinal properties through antinociceptive effects and reduction of low-grade inflammation.[103] It may also increase GI transit in the small bowel, as indirectly measured through hydrogen breath tests.[104] Most studies on the effect of turmeric in GI disease have focused on IBD. A 2018 meta-analysis[105] found it also modestly improved IBS symptoms in two of three randomized controlled trials,[106,107] though study methodologies significantly varied. Frequently, curcumin is given as 2 g/d in divided doses and administered as capsules, fresh root, or dried spices. It has been found to be safe in single doses as high as 12 g/d.[108]

Glutamine

Another promising dietary supplement is the amino acid glutamine, especially in patients with postinfection IBS. It has been suggested that glutamine can restore normal intestinal permeability after epithelial damage has occurred after an infection, thus theoretically decreasing bacterial and toxin translocation across the gut epithelium. In a randomized controlled trial that included 54 patients with postinfection IBS-D, glutamine administered as 5-mg pills three times daily for 8 weeks was found to significantly reduce IBS symptom severity via a validated scale. The clinical improvement was striking (a 79.6% improvement with glutamine vs a 5.8% improvement with placebo). It also significantly reduced daily bowel movement frequency, thickened stool consistency, and made the gut less "leaky" via standardized, though poorly validated, tests of intestinal permeability. Adverse events were not significantly different between groups.[109] Though promising for postinfection IBS-D, in which there is a significant gap in effective therapeutics, glutamine therapy requires further validation in larger studies.

Berberine

Another supplement gaining interest in IBS treatment is berberine. This extract, found in a variety of plants, possibly increases the pain threshold via nitrous oxide–mediated pathways[110] and while potentially increasing fluid absorption in the gut by increasing expression of the Na^+/H^+ exchanger3 and aquaporin4 channels.[111] It has been studied in a randomized controlled trial that included 196 patients with IBS-D. Although berberine hydrochloride, 400 mg delivered twice daily, showed initial improvement over placebo at 8 weeks for diarrhea frequency, fecal urgency, and reduction of abdominal pain, this effect did not persist to 12 weeks.[112] Berberine is being studied in a variety of disorders, including diabetes, obesity, bacterial overgrowth, and inflammatory conditions, and thus further data are likely forthcoming.

Aloe Vera

Rat models suggest that *Aloe vera* could have healing and anti-inflammatory effects within the stomach after ulcer damage.[113,114] Furthermore, barbaloin, a major component of *Aloe vera*, can have a stimulant laxative effect.[115] A 2018 meta-analysis of three randomized trials with a total of 151 patients with IBS found that *Aloe vera* provided short-term benefit for decreasing the severity of IBS symptoms at 1 month, but this effect did not persist at 3-month follow-up.[116] *Aloe vera* extract can be ingested in the amount of 1 to 2 tablespoons to ⅓ cup daily. Caution should be taken in patients on anticoagulants or glucose-lowering medications because the cathartic effect theoretically could reduce absorption. A case series from Korea has also raised concern for aloe-induced acute hepatitis, which resolved after discontinuation.[117] Furthermore, some studies have found the two active components of *Aloe vera* extracts, aloin and aloesin, are associated with colorectal cancer physiology in mice.[118,119] Data from further, high-quality clinical trials are clearly needed.

Artichoke Leaf

Artichoke leaf extract possibly possesses antioxidant and liver-protective properties.[120] Although it has traditionally been investigated in patients with functional dyspepsia,[121] these patients frequently also have IBS. Thus, investigators have done post hoc analyses to extrapolate for the effects of artichoke leaf extract on IBS symptoms. Taking data from an uncontrolled 6-week open-label study on the effects of artichoke leaf extract in patients with functional dyspepsia, investigators retrospectively evaluated IBS symptoms also reported by these patients. Artichoke leaf extract reduced abdominal pain and constipation, and 96% of patients rated it as better or at least equal to prior therapies they had taken.[122] Another post hoc analysis of data from an open-label dyspepsia study found that a statistically significant portion of patients changed to "normal" bowel movements after 8 weeks of treatment with artichoke leaf extract, compared to their "alternating constipation/diarrhea" bowel movements at baseline.[123] Adverse events were similar between extract and placebo in a previous dyspepsia trial.[121] Thus, artichoke leaf extract appears promising for IBS, but further confirmatory placebo-controlled trials are needed.

Melatonin

Melatonin is a hormone produced by the pineal gland and is a precursor to serotonin, a neurotransmitter with a prominent role in modulating GI motility and visceral sensation. Melatonin is broken down into the urinary metabolite 6-hydroxymelatonin sulfate (6-HMS). Previous studies have shown that patients with both IBS-D and IBS with predominant constipation (IBS-C) have higher urinary excretion of 6-HMS compared to control subjects, especially in postmenopausal women with IBS-D.[124,125] This suggests that patients with IBS may be melatonin-deficient, and thus repletion could potentially be therapeutic.

Several small randomized controlled trials of melatonin in patients with IBS have shown promising results. One study of 40 patients with IBS showed mildly decreased mean abdominal pain scores, but this study had only a 2-week follow-up.[126] A different randomized controlled trial involving 18 patients found that 3 mg melatonin nightly for 8 weeks reduced overall IBS symptoms and improved quality of life compared to placebo.[127] A cross-over trial in 17 women found that the same dose and duration improved IBS symptoms without changing mean sleep, anxiety, or depression scores.[128] A larger trial that included 80 postmenopausal women reported that a higher dose of melatonin—3 mg daily and 5 mg nightly—led to a statistically significant decrease in visceral pain and bloating in 70% of patients with IBS-C. These benefits were also found in 45% of women with IBS-D, but this did not meet statistical significance.[129] There may also be a correlation between the probiotic medical food VSL#3 and melatonin. In a randomized controlled trial in 42 patients with IBS, VSL#3 led to an increase in salivary melatonin levels in the morning, which mildly correlated with the patients' endorsing improved satisfaction in bowel habits after 6 weeks of treatment.[130] Melatonin could also be used to treat comorbidities that commonly occur with IBS, such as sleep disorders, depression, and anxiety.[131] Note that, owing to a lack of quality control, there is tremendous variability in the true melatonin content of products vs the content listed on product labels; one study reported that actual content could range anywhere from 83% to 478% of the labeled content.[132]

Summary

IBS is a common disorder of diverse pathogenesis and clinical phenotype. A confident diagnosis can be established by identifying the characteristic symptoms of abdominal pain and altered bowel habits, excluding alarm features, and performing selected tests to rule out organic diseases that can mimic IBS, such as celiac disease, chronic infections, IBD, and bacterial overgrowth.

In the vast majority of patients suffering from IBS, food is a critical trigger for their GI symptoms. Food can cause GI symptoms in a variety of ways, and diet interventions are becoming an increasingly important part of the IBS treatment armamentarium. The low-FODMAP diet may be the first evidence-based diet intervention for IBS, but it certainly will not be the last. In addition to methodologically rigorous studies to identify other novel diet therapies for IBS, future research should also aim to identify biomarkers, leveraging the microbiome, metabolome, and genetics, which will allow providers to choose the right diet intervention for the right patient. The identification of multiple diet options, coupled with the ability to map specific diet therapies to specific patients, opens the door to the aspirational goal of "precision nutrition."

The future of diet therapies for IBS and other GI conditions is indeed bright but demands imagination and commitment on the part of the scientific community. Only then can we make available the largest range of scientifically valid and safe diet solutions for our patients with IBS.

References

1. Chey WD, Kurlander J, Eswaran S. Irritable bowel syndrome: a clinical review. *JAMA*. 2015;313(9):949-958.
2. Choung RS, Locke GR. Epidemiology of IBS. *Gastroenterol Clin North Am*. 2011;40(1):1-10.
3. Maxion-Bergemann S, Thielecke F, Abel F, Bergemann R. Costs of irritable bowel syndrome in the UK and US. *Pharmacoeconomics*. 2006;24(1):21-37.
4. Feng B, La JH, Schwartz ES, Gebhart GF. Irritable bowel syndrome: methods, mechanisms, and pathophysiology. Neural and neuro-immune mechanisms of visceral hypersensitivity in irritable bowel syndrome. *Am J Physiol Gastrointest Liver Physiol*. 2012;302(10):G1085-G1098.

5. Camilleri M, Lasch K, Zhou W. Irritable bowel syndrome: methods, mechanisms, and pathophysiology. The confluence of increased permeability, inflammation, and pain in irritable bowel syndrome. *Am J Physiol Gastrointest Liver Physiol.* 2012;303(7):G775-G785.

6. Zhou Q, Verne GN. New insights into visceral hypersensitivity—clinical implications in IBS. *Nat Rev Gastroenterol Hepatol.* 2011;8(6):349-355.

7. O'Malley D, Quigley EM, Dinan TG, Cryan JF. Do interactions between stress and immune responses lead to symptom exacerbations in irritable bowel syndrome? *Brain Behav Immun.* 2011;25(7):1333-1341.

8. Hasler WL. Traditional thoughts on the pathophysiology of irritable bowel syndrome. *Gastroenterol Clin North Am.* 2011;40(1):21-43.

9. Mearin F, Lacy BE, Chang L, et al. Bowel disorders. *Gastroenterology.* Published online February 18, 2016:S0016-5085(16)00222-5. doi:10.1053/j.gastro.2016.02.031

10. Brandler J, Chey WD. Fishing for irritable bowel syndrome: which alarm features weave the best net? *Clin Gastroenterol Hepatol.* Published online November 18, 2020;S1542-3565(20)31554-8. doi:10.1016/j.cgh.2020.11.020

11. Carrasco-Labra A, Lytvyn L, Falck-Ytter Y, Surawicz CM, Chey WD. American Gastroenterology Association Institute technical review on the evaluation of functional diarrhea and diarrhea predominant irritable bowel disease in adults (IBS-D). *Gastroenterol.* 2019;157:859-880.

12. Lacy BE, Pimentel M, Brenner D, Chey WD, Keefer L, Moshiree B. ACG clinical guideline: management of irritable bowel syndrome. *Am J Gastroenterol.* 2021;116:17-44.

13. Chey WD, Keefer L, Whelan K, Gibson PR. Behavioral and diet therapies in integrated care for patients with irritable bowel syndrome. *Gastroenterology.* 2021;160(1):47-62.

14. Basnayake C, Kamm MA, Stanley A, et al. Standard gastroenterologist versus multidisciplinary treatment for functional gastrointestinal disorders (MANTRA): an open-label, single-centre, randomised controlled trial. *Lancet Gastroenterol Hepatol.* 2020;5(10):890-899.

15. Eswaran S, Tack J, Chey WD. Food: the forgotten factor in the irritable bowel syndrome. *Gastroenterol Clin North Am.* 2011;40(1):141-162.

16. National Academies of Sciences, Engineering, and Medicine (US); Health and Medicine Division; Food and Nutrition Board; Committee on Food Allergies: Global Burden, Causes, Treatment, Prevention, and Public Policy. *Finding a Path to Safety in Food Allergy: Assessment of the Global Burden, Causes, Prevention, Management, and Public Policy.* Stallings VA, Oria M, eds. National Academies Press; 2017.

17. Lenhart A, Ferch C, Shaw M, Chey WD. Use of dietary management in irritable bowel syndrome: results of a survey of over 1500 United States gastroenterologists. *J Neurogastro Motil.* 2018;24(3):437-446.

18. Bohn L, Storsrud S, Tornblom H, Bengtsson U, Simren M. Self-reported food-related gastrointestinal symptoms in IBS are common and associated with more severe symptoms and reduced quality of life. *Am J Gastro.* 2013;108(5):634-41.

19. Rona RJ, Keil T, Summers C, et al. The prevalence of food allergy: a meta-analysis. *J Allergy Clin Immunol.* 2007;120:638-646.

20. Acker WW, Plasek JM, Blumenthal KG, et al. Prevalence of food allergies and intolerances documented in electronic health records. *J Allergy Clin Immunol.* 2017;140:1587-1591.

21. Onyimba F, Crowe SE, Johnson S, Leung J. Food allergies and intolerances: a clinical approach to the diagnosis and management of adverse reactions to food. *Clin Gastroenterol Hepatol.* 2021;19(11):2230-2240.

22. NIAID-Sponsored Expert Panel; Boyce JA, Assa'ad A, et al. Guidelines for the diagnosis and management of food allergy in the United States: report of the NIAID-sponsored expert panel. *J Allergy Clin Immunol.* 2010;126(suppl 6):S1-58.

23. Soares-Weiser K, Takwoingi Y, Panesar SS, et al. The diagnosis of food allergy: a systematic review and meta-analysis. *Allergy.* 2014;69(1):76-86.

24. Yang CM, Li YQ. [The therapeutic effects of eliminating allergic foods according to food-specific IgG antibodies in irritable bowel syndrome]. *Zhonghua Nei Ke Za Zhi.* 2007;46(8):641-643.

25. Drisko J, Bischoff B, Hall M, McCallum R. Treating irritable bowel syndrome with a food elimination diet followed by food challenge and probiotics. *J Am Coll Nutr.* 2006;25(6):514-522.

26. Zar S, Mincher L, Benson MJ, Kumar D. Food-specific IgG4 antibody-guided exclusion diet improves symptoms and rectal compliance in irritable bowel syndrome. *Scand J Gastroenterol.* 2005;40(7):800-807.

27. Hunter JO. Food elimination in IBS: the case for IgG testing remains doubtful. *Gut.* 2005;54(8):1203.

28. Zar S, Benson MJ, Kumar D. Food-specific serum IgG4 and IgE titers to common food antigens in irritable bowel syndrome. *Am J Gastroenterol.* 2005;100(7):1550-1557.

29. Floch MH. Use of diet and probiotic therapy in the irritable bowel syndrome: analysis of the literature. *J Clin Gastroenterol.* 2005;39(5 suppl 3):S243-S246.

30. Atkinson W, Sheldon TA, Shaath N, Whorwell PJ. Food elimination based on IgG antibodies in irritable bowel syndrome: a randomised controlled trial. *Gut.* 2004;53(10):1459-1464.

31. Zar S, Kumar D, Kumar D. Role of food hypersensitivity in irritable bowel syndrome. *Minerva Med.* 2002;93(5):403-412.

32. Aydinlar EI, Dikmen PY, Tiftikci A, et al. IgG-based elimination diet in migraine plus irritable bowel syndrome. *Headache.* 2013;53(3):514-525.

33. Xie Y, Zhou G, Xu Y, et al. Effects of diet based on IgG elimination combined with probiotics on migraine plus irritable bowel syndrome. *Pain Res Manag.* 2019;2019:7890461.

34. Cappelletti M, Tognon E, Vona L, et al. Food-specific serum IgG and symptom reduction with a personalized, unrestricted-calorie diet of six weeks in irritable bowel syndrome (IBS). *Nutr Metab (Lond)*. 2020;17(1):101.

35. Collins SC. Practice paper of the Academy of Nutrition and Dietetics: role of the registered dietitian nutritionist in the diagnosis and management of food allergies. *J Acad Nutr Diet*. 2016;116(10):1621-1631.

36. American Academy of Allergy, Asthma, and Immunology. The myth of IgG food panel testing. Accessed August 13, 2021. www.aaaai.org/conditions-and-treatments/library/allergy-library/IgG-food-test

37. Ali A, Weiss TR, McKee D, et al. Efficacy of individualised diets in patients with irritable bowel syndrome: a randomised controlled trial. *BMJ Open Gastroenterol*. 2017;4(1):e000164.

38. Carroccio A, Brusca I, Mansueto P, et al. A cytologic assay for diagnosis of food hypersensitivity in patients with irritable bowel syndrome. *Clin Gastroenterol Hepatol*. 2010;8:254-260.

39. Fritscher-Ravens A, Schuppan D, Ellrichmann M, et al. Confocal endomicroscopy shows food-associated changes in the intestinal mucosa of patients with irritable bowel syndrome. *Gastroenterology*. 2014;147:1012-1020.e4.

40. Fritscher-Ravens A, Pflaum T, Mösinger M, et al. Many patients with irritable bowel syndrome have atypical food allergies not associated with immunoglobulin E. *Gastroenterology*. 2019;157(1):109-118.e5.

41. Skovbjerg H, Norén O, Sjöström H, Danielsen EM, Enevoldsen BS. Further characterization of intestinal lactase/phlorizin hydrolase. *Biochimica et biophysica acta*. 1982;707(1):89-97.

42. Misselwitz B, Butter M, Verbeke K, Fox MR. Update on lactose malabsorption and intolerance: pathogenesis, diagnosis and clinical management. *Gut*. 2019;68(11):2080-2091.

43. Lisker R, Solomons NW, Perez Briceno R, Ramirez Mata M. Lactase and placebo in the management of the irritable bowel syndrome: a double-blind, cross-over study. *Am J Gastroenterol*. 1989;84(7):756-762.

44. Farup PG, Monsbakken KW, Vandvik PO. Lactose malabsorption in a population with irritable bowel syndrome: prevalence and symptoms. A case-control study. *Scand J Gastroenterol*. 2004;39(7):645-649.

45. Yang J, Deng Y, Chu H, et al. Prevalence and presentation of lactose intolerance and effects on dairy product intake in healthy subjects and patients with irritable bowel syndrome. *Clin Gastroenterol Hepatol*. 2013;11(3):262-268.

46. Zhu Y, Zheng X, Cong Y, et al. Bloating and distention in irritable bowel syndrome: the role of gas production and visceral sensation after lactose ingestion in a population with lactase deficiency. *American J Gastroenterol*. 2013;108(9):1516-1525.

47. Heizer WD, Southern S, McGovern S. The role of diet in symptoms of irritable bowel syndrome in adults: a narrative review. *J Am Diet Assoc*. 2009;109(7):1204-1214.

48. Sibley E. Carbohydrate digestion and absorption. In: Johnson L, ed. *Encyclopedia of Gastroenterology*. Elsevier; 2004:275-278.

49. Hunziker W, Spiess M, Semenza G, Lodish HF. The sucrase-isomaltase complex: primary structure, membrane-orientation, and evolution of a stalked, intrinsic brush border protein. *Cell*. 1986;46(2):227-234.

50. Boney A, Elser HE, Sliver HJ. Relationships among dietary intakes and persistent gastrointestinal symptoms in patients receiving enzyme treatment for genetic sucrase-isomaltase deficiency. *J Acad Nutr Diet*. 2018;118(3):440-447.

51. Henström M, Diekmann L, Bonfiglio F, et al. Functional variants in the sucrase-isomaltase gene associate with increased risk of irritable bowel syndrome. *Gut*. 2018;67:263-270.

52. Thingholm L, Rühlemann M, Wang J, et al. Sucrase-isomaltase 15Phe IBS risk variant in relation to dietary carbohydrates and faecal microbiota composition. *Gut*. 2019;68(1):177-178.

53. Garcia-Etxebarria K, Zheng T, Bonfiglio F, et al. Increased prevalence of rare sucrase-isomaltase pathogenic variants in irritable bowel syndrome patients. *Clin Gastroenterol Hepatol*. 2018;16:1673-1676.

54. Kim SB, Calmet FH, Garrido J, Garcia-Buitrago MT, Moshiree B. Sucrase-isomaltase deficiency as a potential masquerader in irritable bowel syndrome. *Dig Dis Sci*. 2020;65(2):534-540.

55. Zheng T, Eswaran S, Photenhauer AL, Merchant JL, Chey WD, D'Amato M. Reduced efficacy of low FODMAPs diet in patients with IBS-D carrying sucrase-isomaltase (*SI*) hypomorphic variants. *Gut*. 2020;69(2):397-398.

56. Vos MB, Kimmons JE, Gillespie C, Welsh J, Blanck HM. Dietary fructose consumption among US children and adults: the Third National Health and Nutrition Examination Survey. *Medscape J Med*. 2008;10(7):160.

57. Reyes-Huerta JU, de la Cruz-Patino E, Ramirez-Gutierrez de Velasco A, Zamudio C, Remes-Troche JM. [Fructose intolerance in patients with irritable bowel syndrome: a case-control study]. *Rev Gastroenterol Mex*. 2010;75(4):405-411.

58. Shepherd SJ, Parker FC, Muir JG, Gibson PR. Dietary triggers of abdominal symptoms in patients with irritable bowel syndrome: randomized placebo-controlled evidence. *Clin Gastroenterol Hepatol*. 2008;6(7):765-771.

59. Ferraris R, Choe JY, Patel CR. Intestinal absorption of fructose. *Ann Rev Nutr*. 2019;38:41-67.

60. Tuck CJ, Taylor KM, Gibson PR, Barrett JS, Muir JG. Increasing symptoms in irritable bowel symptoms with ingestion of galacto-oligosaccharides are mitigated by α-galactosidase treatment. *Am J Gastroenterol*. 2018;113(1):124-134.

61. Lenhart A, Chey WD. A systematic review of the effects of polyols in gastrointestinal health and irritable bowel syndrome. *Adv Nutrition*. 2017;8:587-596.

62. Dionne J, Ford AC, Yuan Y, et al. A systematic review and meta-analysis evaluating the efficacy of a gluten-free diet and a low FODMAPs diet in treating symptoms of irritable bowel syndrome. *Amer J Gastroenterol.* 2018;113(9):1290-1300.

63. Ong DK, Mitchell SB, Barrett JS, et al. Manipulation of dietary short chain carbohydrates alters the pattern of gas production and genesis of symptoms in irritable bowel syndrome. *J Gastroenterol Hepatol.* 2010;25(8):1366-1373.

64. Liu J, Chey WD, Haller E, Eswaran S. Low-FODMAP diet for irritable bowel syndrome: what we know and what we have yet to learn. *Annu Rev Med.* 2020;71(1):303-314.

65. Van Lanen AS, de Bree A, Greyling A. Efficacy of a low-FODMAP diet in adult irritable bowel syndrome: a systematic review and meta-analysis. *Eur J Nutr.* 2021;60(6):3505-3522.

66. Eswaran SL, Chey WD, Han-Markey T, Ball S, Jackson K. A randomized controlled trial comparing the low FODMAP diet vs. modified NICE guidelines in US adults with IBS-D. *Amer J Gastroenterol.* 2016;111(12):1824-1832.

67. Tuck CJ, Barrett JS. Re-challenging FODMAPs: the low FODMAP diet phase two. *J Gastroenterol Hepatol.* 2017;32:11-15.

68. Catassi C, Alaedini A, Bojarski C, et al. Overlapping area of non-celiac gluten sensitivity (NCGS) and wheat-sensitive irritable bowel syndrome (IBS): an update. *Nutrients.* 2017;9(11):1268.

69. Leonard MM. Celiac disease and nonceliac gluten sensitivity: a review. *JAMA Review.* 2017;318(7):647-656.

70. Volta U, Caio G, Karunaratne TB, et al. Non-coeliac gluten/wheat sensitivity: advances in knowledge and relevant questions. *Expert Rev Gastroenterol Hepatol.* 2017;11(1):9-18.

71. Di Liberto D, Mansueto P, D'Alcamo A, et al. Predominance of type 1 innate lymphoid cells in the rectal mucosa of patients with non-celiac wheat sensitivity: reversal after a wheat-free diet. *Clin Transl Gastroenterol.* 2016;7:e178.

72. Vasques Roque MI, Camilleri M, Smyrk T, et al. A controlled trial of gluten-free diet in patients with irritable bowel syndrome-diarrhea: effects on bowel frequency and intestinal function. *Gastroenterology.* 2013;144(5):903-911.e3.

73. Carroccio A, Mansueto P, Iacono G, et al. Non-celiac wheat sensitivity diagnosed by double-blind placebo-controlled challenge: exploring a new clinical entity. *Am J Gastroenterol.* 2012;107(12):1898-1906.

74. Biesiekierski JR, Newnham ED, Irving PM, et al. Gluten causes gastrointestinal symptoms in subjects without celiac disease: a double-blind randomized placebo-controlled trial. *AmJ Gastroenterol.* 2011;106(3):508-514.

75. Skodje GI, Sarna VK, Minelle IH, et al. Fructan, rather than gluten, induces symptoms in patients with self-reported non-celiac gluten sensitivity. *Gastroenterology.* 2018;154:529-539.e2.

76. Zevallos VF, Raker V, Tenzer S, et al. Nutritional wheat amylase-trypsin inhibitors promote intestinal inflammation via activation of myeloid cells. *Gastroenterology.* 2017;152:1100-1113.

77. Chen GC et al. Whole-grain intake and total, cardiovascular, and cancer mortality: a systematic review and meta-analysis of prospective studies. *Am J Clin Nutr.* 2016;104(1):164-172.

78. Zhong G et al. Whole grain intake and mortality from all causes, cardiovascular disease, and cancer: a meta-analysis of prospective cohort studies. *Circulation.* 2016;133(24):2370-2380.

79. Khan A, Suarez MG, Murray JA. Nonceliac gluten and wheat sensitivity. *Clin Gastroenterol Hepatol.* 2020;18(9):1913-1922.e1.

80. Ruepert L, Quartero AO, de Wit NJ, et al. Bulking agents, antispasmodics and antidepressants for the treatment of irritable bowel syndrome. *Cochrane Database Syst Rev.* 2011;(8):CD003460.

81. Quartero AO, Meineche-Schmidt V, Muris J, Rubin G, de Wit N. Bulking agents, antispasmodic and antidepressant medication for the treatment of irritable bowel syndrome. *Cochrane Database Syst Rev.* 2005;(2):CD003460.

82. Bijkerk CJ, de Wit NJ, Muris JW, Whorwell PJ, Knottnerus JA, Hoes AW. Soluble or insoluble fibre in irritable bowel syndrome in primary care? Randomised placebo controlled trial. *BMJ.* 2009;339:b3154.

83. Ford AC, Talley NJ, Spiegel BM, et al. Effect of fibre, antispasmodics, and peppermint oil in the treatment of irritable bowel syndrome: systematic review and meta-analysis. *BMJ.* 2008;337:a2313.

84. Moayyedi P, Quigley EM, Lacy BE, et al. The effect of fiber supplementation on irritable bowel syndrome: a systematic review and meta-analysis. *Am J Gastroenterol.* 2014;109(9):1367-1374.

85. Eswaran S, Muir J, Chey WD. Fiber and functional gastrointestinal disorders. *Am J Gastroenterol.* 2013;108(5):718-727.

86. Ford AC, Harris LA, Lacy BE, et al. Systematic review with meta-analysis: the efficacy of prebiotics, probiotics, synbiotics and antibiotics in irritable bowel syndrome. *Aliment Pharmacol Ther.* 2018;48:1044-1060.

87. Olesen M, Gudmand-Hoyer E. Efficacy, safety, and tolerability of fructooligosaccharides in the treatment of irritable bowel syndrome. *Am J Clin Nutr.* 2000;72:1570-1575.

88. Azpiroz F, Dubray C, Bernalier-Donadille A, et al. Effects of scFOS on the composition of fecal microbiota and anxiety in patients with irritable bowel syndrome: a randomized, double blind, placebo controlled study. *Neurogastroenterol Motil.* 2017;29(2). 10.1111/nmo.12911. doi:10.1111/nmo.12911

89. Silk DB, Davis A, Vulevic J, Tzortzis G, Gibson GR. Clinical trial: the effects of a trans-galactooligosaccharide prebiotic on faecal microbiota and symptoms in irritable bowel syndrome. *Aliment Pharmacol Ther.* 2009;29:508518.

90. Marteau P. Probiotics in functional intestinal disorders and IBS: proof of action and dissecting the multiple mechanisms. *Gut.* 2010;59(3):285-286.

91. Su GL, Ko CW, Bercik P, et al. AGA clinical practice guidelines on the role of probiotics in the management of gastrointestinal disorders. *Gastroenterology.* 2020;159(2):697-705.

92. Mullin GE. Probiotics and digestive disease. *Nutr Clin Pract.* 2012;27(2):300-302.

93. Deutsch JK, Levitt J, Hass DJ. Complementary and alternative medicine for functional gastrointestinal disorders. *Am J Gastroenterol.* 2020;115(3):350-364.

94. Shapiro JM, Deutsch JK, Chey WD. An evidence-based narrative review of oral supplements for the treatment of patients with irritable bowel syndrome. *NeuroGastroLATAM Rev.* 2020;4(1):1-13.

95. Hills JM, Aaronson PI. The mechanism of action of peppermint oil on gastrointestinal smooth muscle: an analysis using patch clamp electrophysiology and isolated tissue pharmacology in rabbit and guinea pig. *Gastroenterology.* 1991;101:55-65.

96. Forster HB, Niklas H, Lutz S. Antispasmodic effects of some medicinal plants. *Planta Med.* 1980;40:309-319.

97. Heimes K, Hauk F, Verspohl EJ. Mode of action of peppermint oil and (-)-menthol with respect to 5-HT$_3$ receptor subtypes: binding studies, cation uptake by receptor channels and contraction of isolated rat ileum. *Phytother Res.* 2011;25:702-708.

98. Alammar N, Wang L, Saberi B, et al. The impact of peppermint oil on the irritable bowel syndrome: a meta-analysis of the pooled clinical data. *BMC Complement Altern Med.* 2019;19(1):21.

99. Weerts ZZRM, Masclee AAM, Witteman BJM, et al. Efficacy and safety of peppermint oil in a randomized, double-blind trial of patients with irritable bowel syndrome. *Gastroenterology.* 2020;158(1):123-136.

100. Madisch A, Holtmann G, Plein K, Hotz J. Treatment of irritable bowel syndrome with herbal preparations: results of a double-blind, randomized, placebo-controlled, multi-centre trial. *Aliment Pharmacol Ther.* 2004;19(3):271-279.

101. Sáez-González E, Conde I, Díaz-Jaime FC, Benlloch S, Prieto M, Berenguer M. Iberogast-induced severe hepatotoxicity leading to liver transplantation. *Am J Gastroenterol.* 2016;111(9):1364-1365.

102. Gerhardt F, Benesic A, Tillmann HL, et al. Iberogast-induced acute liver failure-reexposure and in vitro assay support causality. *Am J Gastroenterol.* 2019;114(8):1358-1359.

103. Hewlings SJ, Kalman DS. Curcumin: a review of its effects on human health. *Foods.* 2017;6:92.

104. Shimouchi A, Nose K, Takaoka M, Hayashi H, Kondo T. Effect of dietary turmeric on breath hydrogen. *Dig Dis Sci.* 2009;54(8):1725-1729.

105. Ng QX, Soh AY, Loke W, Venkatanarayanan N, Lim DY, Yeo WS. A meta-analysis of the clinical use of curcumin for irritable bowel syndrome (IBS). *J Clin Med.* 2018;7:298.

106. Alt F, Chong PW, Teng E, Uebelhack R. Evaluation of benefit and tolerability of IQP-CL-101 (Xanthofen) in the symptomatic improvement of irritable bowel syndrome: a double-blinded, randomised, placebo-controlled clinical trial. *Phytother Res.* 2017;31:1056-1062.

107. Bundy R, Walker AF, Middleton RW, Booth J. Turmeric extract may improve irritable bowel syndrome symptomology in otherwise healthy adults: a pilot study. *J Altern Complement Med.* 2004;10:1015-1018.

108. Lao CD, Ruffin MT, Normolle D, et al. Dose escalation of a curcuminoid formulation. *BMC Complement Altern Med.* 2006;6:10.

109. Zhou Q, Verne ML, Fields JZ, et al. Randomised placebo-controlled trial of dietary glutamine supplements for postinfectious irritable bowel syndrome. *Gut.* 2019;68(6):996-1002.

110. Tang QL, Lai ML, Zhong YF, Wang AM, Su JK, Zhang MQ. Antinociceptive effect of berberine on visceral hypersensitivity in rats. *World J Gastroenterol.* 2013;19(28):4582-4589.

111. Zhang Y, Wang X, Sha S, et al. Berberine increases the expression of NHE3 and AQP4 in sennosideA-induced diarrhoea model. *Fitoterapia.* 2012;83(6):1014-1022.

112. Chen C, Tao C, Liu Z, et al. A randomized clinical trial of berberine hydrochloride in patients with diarrhea-predominant irritable bowel syndrome. *Phytother Res.* 2015;29(11):1822-1827.

113. Eamlamnam K, Patumraj S, Visedopas N, Thong-Ngam D. Effects of *Aloe vera* and sucralfate on gastric microcirculatory changes, cytokine levels and gastric ulcer healing in rats. *World J Gastroenterol.* 2006;12:2034-2039.

114. Werawatganon D, Rakananurak N, Sallapant S, et al. *Aloe vera* attenuated gastric injury on indomethacin-induced gastropathy in rats. *World J Gastroenterol.* 2014;20:18330-18337.

115. Ishii Y, Tanizawa H, Takino Y. Studies of aloe: V. Mechanism of cathartic effect. (4). *Biol Pharm Bull.* 1994;17(5):651-653.

116. Hong SW, Chun J, Park S, Lee HJ, Im JP, Kim JS. *Aloe vera* is effective and safe in short-term treatment of irritable bowel syndrome: a systematic review and meta-analysis. *J Neurogastroenterol Motil.* 2018;24(4):528-535.

117. Yang HN, Kim DJ, Kim YM, et al. Aloe-induced toxic hepatitis. *J Korean Med Sci.* 2010;25(3):492-495.

118. Peng C, Zhang W, Dai C, et al. Study of the aqueous extract of *Aloe vera* and its two active components on the Wnt/β-catenin and Notch signaling pathways in colorectal cancer cells. *J Ethnopharmacol.* 2019;243:112092.

119. Peng C, Zhang W, Shen X, et al. Post-transcriptional regulation activity through alternative splicing involved in the effects of *Aloe vera* on the Wnt/β-catenin and Notch pathways in colorectal cancer cells. *J Pharmacol Sci.* 2020;143(3):148-155.

120. Ben Salem M, Affes H, Ksouda K, et al. Pharmacological studies of artichoke leaf extract and their health benefits. *Plant Foods Hum Nutr.* 2015;70:441-453.

121. Holtmann G, Adam B, Haag S, et al. Efficacy of artichoke leaf extract in the treatment of patients with functional dyspepsia: a six-week placebo-controlled, double-blind, multicentre trial. *Aliment Pharmacol Ther.* 2003;18:1099-1105.

122. Walker AF, Middleton RW, Petrowicz O. Artichoke leaf extract reduces symptoms of irritable bowel syndrome in a post-marketing surveillance study. *Phytother Res.* 2001;15:58-61.

123. Bundy R, Walker AF, Middleton RW, Marakis G, Booth JC. Artichoke leaf extract reduces symptoms of irritable bowel syndrome and improves quality of life in otherwise healthy volunteers suffering from concomitant dyspepsia: a subset analysis. *J Altern Complement Med.* 2004;10:667-669.

124. Radwan P, Skrzydlo-Radomanska B, Radwan-Kwiatek K, Burak-Czapiuk B, Strzemecka J. Is melatonin involved in the irritable bowel syndrome? *J Physiol Pharmacol.* 2009;60(suppl 3):67-70.

125. Wisniewska-Jarosinska M, Chojnacki J, Konturek S, et al. Evaluation of urinary 6-hydroxymelatonin sulphate excretion in women at different age with irritable bowel syndrome. *J Physiol Pharmacol.* 2010;61(3):295-300.

126. Song GH, Leng PH, Gwee KA, Moochhala SM, Ho KY. Melatonin improves abdominal pain in irritable bowel syndrome patients who have sleep disturbances: a randomised, double blind, placebo controlled study. *Gut.* 2005;54:1402-1407.

127. Saha L, Malhotra S, Rana S, Bhasin D, Pandhi P. A preliminary study of melatonin in irritable bowel syndrome. *J Clin Gastroenterol.* 2007;41:29-32.

128. Lu WZ, Gwee KA, Moochhalla S, Ho KY. Melatonin improves bowel symptoms in female patients with irritable bowel syndrome: a double-blind placebo-controlled study. *Aliment Pharmacol Ther.* 2005;22:927-934.

129. Chojnacki C, Walecka-Kapica E, Lokieć K, et al. Influence of melatonin on symptoms of irritable bowel syndrome in postmenopausal women. *Endokrynol Pol.* 2013;64:114-120.

130. Wong RK, Yang C, Song GH, Wong J, Ho KY. Melatonin regulation as a possible mechanism for probiotic (VSL#3) in irritable bowel syndrome: a randomized double-blinded placebo study. *Dig Dis Sci.* 2015;60:186-194.

131. Lei WY, Chang WC, Wong MW, et al. Sleep disturbance and its association with gastrointestinal symptoms/diseases and psychological comorbidity. *Digestion.* 2019;99(3):205-212.

132. Erland LA, Saxena PK. Melatonin natural health products and supplements: presence of serotonin and significant variability of melatonin content. *J Clin Sleep Med.* 2017;13:275-281.

CHAPTER 6

Celiac Disease

Dennis Kumral, MD
Mallory Foster, RD, CNSC, CCTD
Sheila Crowe, MD, FRCPC, FACP, FACG, AGAF

KEY POINTS

- Celiac disease (gluten-sensitive enteropathy) is an immune-mediated disorder that is triggered by the dietary ingestion of gluten in genetically susceptible individuals.
- The immune response in patients with celiac disease leads to inflammation, villous atrophy, and crypt hyperplasia in the small intestine and may also include notable systemic manifestations, such as micronutrient deficiencies, low bone density, and dermatitis herpetiformis.
- Dietary elimination of all sources of gluten is the backbone for treatment of celiac disease.

Introduction

Celiac disease (gluten-sensitive enteropathy) is an immune-mediated disorder that is triggered by the dietary ingestion of gluten in genetically susceptible individuals. Gluten—the main storage protein of the grains wheat, barley, and rye—is common in diets across the world.[1] The immune response in patients with celiac disease leads to inflammation, villous atrophy, and crypt hyperplasia in the small intestine. However, the sequelae are not limited to small bowel enteropathy, as celiac disease has several notable systemic manifestations (micronutrient deficiencies, low bone density, dermatitis herpetiformis, and others). Dietary elimination of all sources of gluten is the backbone for treatment of celiac disease. In recent years, accessibility to gluten-free dietary options has increased, but this is mainly due to their popularity among people without celiac disease who choose to avoid gluten.[2]

Epidemiology of Celiac Disease

Celiac disease is a global disease affecting approximately 1% of the world's population. A cross-sectional study of duodenal biopsies submitted to a national laboratory found an overall celiac disease prevalence of 1.7% in the United States. Ethnic variations were notable: celiac disease was most common in patients from the Punjab region of India (3.08%), and there was a lower incidence in patients of East Asian (0.15%) or Hispanic (1.06%) ancestry.[3] Additionally, incidence remains common in Europe, particularly in Scandinavian countries, but is rare in sub-Saharan Africa.[4] As with other immune-mediated disorders, incidence is higher in females than in males at a ratio of 2.9 to 1.[5] A 2014 study found that the gender disparity in diagnosis was greatest between ages of 18 and 29 years, with only 18% of patients diagnosed with celiac disease in that age range were male. This disparity may be due to milder symptoms or to factors that contribute to lower utilization of health care by this population.[6]

There is lag time between symptom onset and diagnosis of celiac disease. Some studies have reported a lag time of as high as 11 years, particularly in patients with nonclassical manifestations.[5] More recently, however, the diagnostic delay was found to be more modest—a 2018 study reported a median duration of symptoms before celiac disease diagnosis of 3 years (range, 0-50 years). This diagnostic delay was consequential, as it was associated with reduced self-perceived health and psychological well-being in patients with diagnostic delay.[7]

For every case of celiac disease diagnosed on clinical suspicion, many more remain undiagnosed. The prevalence of celiac disease has been increasing, in part because of the improved sensitivity of diagnostic testing and also because of improved screening of individuals for conditions that increase the risk of celiac disease.[8-10]

Pathogenesis of Celiac Disease

Celiac disease develops as a result of altered mucosal immune responses in genetically susceptible individuals who are exposed to dietary gluten.

Genetic Factors

Celiac disease inheritance involves complex genetic factors involving the human leukocyte antigen (HLA) class II genes *HLA-DQ2* and *HLA-DQ8*, which increase susceptibility.[11] These genes are necessary but not sufficient for a diagnosis of celiac disease, because 30% of the general population encode *HLA-DQ2* and *HLA-DQ8* but only 1% have celiac disease.[12] *HLA-DQ2* homozygosity confers the greatest risk for celiac disease (28%), whereas *HLA-DQ8* heterozygotes have lower risk (2.8%).[13] Least common is the genetic type called *HLA-DQ2.2*, which includes only half the gene pair encoding *HLA-DQ2*.[9]

The Role of Gluten

Gluten is the main storage protein in wheat, barley, and rye. The gluten matrix is heat stable and provides elasticity, texture, flavor, and moisture retention in cooking. Immunogenic peptides within the gliadin fraction of the gluten protein trigger the host immune response, leading to the clinical phenotype of celiac disease.[1] The gliadin molecules that have not been digested can enter the lamina propria and interact with antigen-presenting cells (APCs).

Mucosal Immune Responses

Celiac disease involves both innate and adaptive immune responses.[14] Figure 6.1 presents the immunologic processes that cause celiac disease–associated mucosal damage. Gluten is first broken down into gliadin. Gliadin moves from the lumen into the mucosa via tight but leaky junctions between the epithelial cells. An enzyme called tissue transglutaminase (tTG) is responsible for deamidation, which is the conversion of glutamine residues on the gliadin protein to glutamic acid, thereby facilitating the binding of gliadin to APCs. Once gliadin binds to APCs, deamidated gliadin is presented by HLA-DQ2 or HLA-DQ8 molecules (or both) to CD4 T cells. This process yields cytokines,[14] which induce the production of antibodies to gliadin, tTG, and endomysium, and the eventual development of mucosal damage—villous atrophy, crypt hyperplasia—which defines patients with celiac disease.[15]

Clinical Manifestations of Celiac Disease

The spectrum of clinical presentations in celiac disease is wide, necessitating a high index of suspicion among clinicians to uncover "hidden" undiagnosed individuals with this disease.

Celiac disease can be classified into the following clinical subtypes, depending on the presence or absence of symptoms:

- classical (typical)
- nonclassical (atypical or silent)
- potential

FIGURE 6.1 Pathophysiology of celiac disease

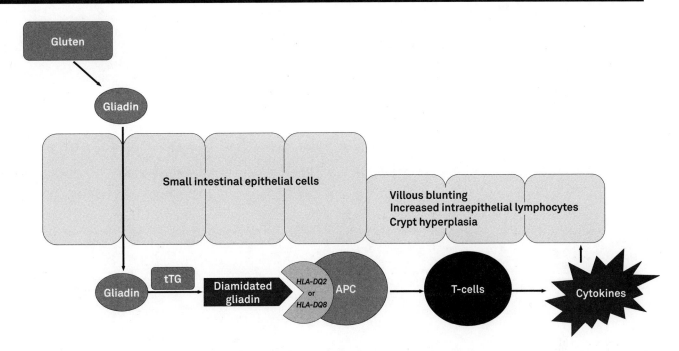

APC = antigen-presenting cells | tTG = tissue transglutaminase | HLA = human leukocyte antigen
Celiac disease develops when gliadin molecules that have not been digested enter the lamina propria and interact with APCs. A T-cell–mediated response is mounted in genetically predisposed individuals, resulting in malabsorption caused by villous atrophy and crypt hyperplasia.

Patients with *classical celiac disease* present with malabsorption symptoms, including chronic diarrhea, steatorrhea, weight loss, bloating, flatulence, and micronutrient deficiencies. Patients with *nonclassical celiac disease* may present without symptoms but are diagnosed because of extraintestinal manifestations (eg, iron deficiency anemia or low bone density) or screening tests place them in high-risk groups (eg, people who have first-degree relatives with celiac disease, people with type 1 diabetes mellitus [T1DM], or people with autoimmune thyroid disease).[16] Conditions associated with celiac disease are listed in Box 6.1 on page 94. Patients with *potential celiac disease* screen positive for the disease based on serologic test results but do not yet exhibit histologic findings of villous blunting or increased intraepithelial lymphocytosis.[17]

Hematologic Manifestations

Iron deficiency is the most common etiology of anemia in patients with celiac disease. In a study from India, 66% of patients with celiac disease had iron deficiency at the time of diagnosis; mixed nutritional deficiencies (folate, vitamin B12) and anemia of chronic disease were also found in 16.5% and 3.9% of patients, respectively.[18] Following a strict gluten-free diet typically addresses these nutrient deficiencies, though deficiencies in vitamin B12 and folate can persist with a gluten-free diet in some individuals.[19] Persistent vitamin B12 deficiency may be explained by malabsorption due to pancreatic insufficiency, comorbid small intestinal bacterial overgrowth, and, less commonly, distal ileal enteropathy.

BOX 6.1

Disorders Associated With Celiac Disease

Endocrine

Addison disease

Alopecia areata

Autoimmune thyroid disorders

Reproductive disorders

Type 1 diabetes mellitus

Neurologic

Cerebellar ataxia

Epilepsy

Migraine

Neuropathy

Cardiac

Autoimmune myocarditis

Idiopathic dilated cardiomyopathy

Hepatic

Autoimmune cholangitis

Autoimmune hepatitis

Primary biliary cirrhosis

Other

Autoimmune atrophic gastritis

Bone loss and osteoporosis

Delayed growth or short stature

Dental enamel defects

Dermatitis herpetiformis

Down syndrome

Immunoglobulin A deficiency

Intestinal lymphoma

Iron deficiency anemia

Psoriasis

Recurrent aphthous stomatitis

Sjögren syndrome

Turner syndrome

Dermatologic Manifestations

Dermatitis herpetiformis—an inflammatory skin condition that presents with pruritic papules involving extensor surface, buttocks, neck, trunk, or scalp—may present as an extraintestinal manifestation of celiac disease; diagnostic delay has been reported to be up to 2 years.[20] As with celiac disease, dietary ingestion of gluten triggers this condition.[21] Dapsone, an antibiotic agent with anti-inflammatory properties, can be used initially to treat patients with dermatitis herpetiformis.[22] It is typically well tolerated, but notable hematologic adverse reactions include hemolytic anemia and rare agranulocytosis.[23] Dapsone may also cause drug-induced liver injury; therefore, monitoring with a periodic hepatic function panel while the patient is on therapy is prudent.[24] Because of these potential toxicities of dapsone and the efficacy of dietary therapy, long-term management of dermatitis herpetiformis involves a gluten-free diet.[25]

Neurologic Manifestations

Gluten ataxia—a neurologic disorder characterized by dysarthria, dysphonia, and disorders of gaze—may occur in patients with celiac disease (or nonceliac gluten sensitivity).[26] As with celiac disease, gluten ataxia is caused by an immune response to gluten ingestion; but in this case, the cerebellum is particularly affected. Patients with this disorder often have a mild enteropathy.[27] A systematic review concluded that a gluten-free diet may improve the course of gluten ataxia.[28]

Gluten neuropathy is the gluten-related autoimmune damage to the peripheral nervous system. It accounts for up to a quarter of neurologic symptoms in patients with celiac disease. Symptoms may respond to a gluten-free diet, but the diet has not been shown to prevent the development of or completely reverse the neuropathy.[29]

Other neurologic symptoms associated with celiac disease that may respond to a gluten-free diet include migraine headaches, impaired cognition, and seizure disorders.[30]

Hepatic Manifestations

Celiac hepatitis is a gluten-dependent liver injury that frequently occurs in patients with untreated celiac disease.[31] Undetected celiac disease may be the cause of cryptogenic elevated transaminases in 3% to 4% of patients.[32] Nonspecific histologic changes may be seen if a biopsy is pursued, but biopsy is often unwarranted, as the liver injury resolves with a strict gluten-free diet.

Coexistent autoimmune liver disease (primary sclerosing cholangitis and primary biliary cirrhosis) has been reported in celiac disease.[33] Recently, there has been an uptick in the diagnosis of celiac disease in patients with a normal or high BMI, and coexistent nonalcoholic fatty liver disease should be considered in patients with celiac disease and elevated transaminases.[34]

Bone Disease

Low bone mineral density, a condition of impaired bone microarchitecture with increased fragility and fracture risk, is found in up to 75% of patients with celiac disease.[35] Bone density is compromised in celiac disease, owing to both local and systemic causes. Mucosal enteropathy in the small bowel limits calcium absorption, and the resultant secondary hyperparathyroidism stimulates osteoclasts to degrade bones, which leads to bone loss and osteoporosis. Additionally, inflammatory cytokines play a role in increased osteoclastic bone resorption.[36] Bone density is reduced in patients with nonclassical (atypical) celiac disease,[37] but the risk of fracture appears to be associated with classical (symptomatic) clinical presentation and male sex.[37] The management of low bone density includes following a gluten-free diet to improve enteropathy and reduce inflammation, and supplementing the diet with 1,000 to 1,500 mg calcium per day and vitamin D to maintain a serum 25-hydroxyvitamin D level of approximately 30 ng/mL.[38] The European Society for the Study of Coeliac Disease recommends a baseline bone density scan (dual-energy x-ray absorptiometry [DXA]) at the time of diagnosis of celiac disease in adults with malabsorption or in those at increased risk of low bone density because of a long delay in diagnosis. In others with celiac disease, they recommend DXA no later than at age 30 to 35 years, with repeat scans every 5 years when the results are normal, and every 2 to 3 years in cases of low bone mineral density, ongoing villous atrophy, or poor compliance with a gluten-free diet.[8] In patients with diagnosed osteoporosis, comanagement with an endocrinologist may be advised to assist with intravenous bisphosphonate therapy.[8]

Endocrine Disorders

T1DM, the leading form of diabetes in children and adolescents, has been associated with celiac disease. The coprevalence of T1DM and celiac disease ranges from 1.9% to 7.7%, and diabetes is often diagnosed at a younger age in patients with celiac disease than in those without.[39] The association between celiac disease and T1DM is due to shared susceptibility alleles in the HLA region.[40] Similarly, autoimmune thyroid disease has a high prevalence in patients with celiac disease because of increased genetic susceptibility.[41] A multicenter prospective study in Italy found that patients with celiac disease were three times more likely to be diagnosed with autoimmune thyroid disease than the general population.[42]

Pregnancy Outcomes

Celiac disease may be discovered in the evaluation of infertility. Untreated celiac disease has also been implicated in pregnancy-related complications, including recurrent spontaneous abortion and infants who are small for gestational age.[43] A gluten-free diet leads to favorable pregnancy outcomes with a lower risk of preterm birth, intrauterine growth restriction, stillbirth, low birth-weight, and small for gestational age.[44]

Diagnosis of Celiac Disease

The diagnosis of celiac disease is a two-step process involving blood serologic tests and endoscopy with duodenal biopsy for histologic confirmation.

Serologic Testing

The serologic tests for celiac disease (see Table 6.1[45]) can be broadly separated into those that measure antibodies directed toward connective tissue components (tTG antibodies and endomysial antibodies) and those that measure antibodies directed toward gluten components (deamidated gliadin peptide [DGP] antibodies).[46] Previously, the antigliadin antibody had been the serologic test for celiac disease; however, it has been shown to have lower sensitivity (approximately 80%) and specificity (80%-90%) and, therefore, is no longer a first-line test.[47] Traditionally, it has been recommended that serologic testing for celiac disease be done while the patient is still on a gluten-containing diet,[48] though serology is a poor surrogate marker for gluten exposure and does not accurately predict short-term gluten exposure or mucosal healing.[49]

tTG, the autoantigen in celiac disease, is an enzyme responsible for the process of deamidation of gliadin (conversion of a glutamine to glutamate).[50] Testing for immunoglobulin A (IgA) anti-tTG antibodies is the initial test of choice in celiac disease because

TABLE 6.1 Serum Tests Used for the Diagnosis of Celiac Disease[45]

Test	Suggested use	Sensitivity (range)	Specificity (range)
IgA anti-tTG antibodies	Use as first-level screening test	>95.0% (73.9%-100%)	>95.0% (77.8%-100%)
IgG anti-tTG antibodies	Use for patients with IgA deficiency	Widely variable (12.6%-99.3%)	Widely variable (86.3%-100%)
IgA antiendomysial antibodies	Use for patients with an uncertain diagnosis	>90% (82.6%-100%)	98.2% (94.7%-100%)
IgG DGP	Use for patients with IgA deficiency and in young children	>90.0% (80.1%-98.6%)	>90.0% (86.0%-96.9%)
HLA-DQ2 or HLA-DQ8	Use for at-risk patients or to confirm diagnosis	91.0% (82.6%-97.0%)	54.0% (12.0%-68.0%)

Ig = immunoglobulin | tTG = tissue transglutaminase | DGP = deamidated gliadin peptides | HLA = human leukocyte antigen

of its availability in clinical laboratories and high sensitivity and specificity (95%–98%).[51] IgA antiendomysial antibody tests have a similarly high sensitivity and specificity but are technically more difficult to perform and are not as widely available in community practice.[52]

Selective IgA deficiency is rare in the general population (0.002% prevalence) but is diagnosed in 2% to 3% of patients with celiac disease.[53] Assessment of total IgA concurrently with IgA anti-tTG ensures that celiac disease diagnosis is not missed in patients with concurrent selective IgA deficiency. In these individuals, immunoglobulin G (IgG)–based testing, particularly the IgG anti-DGP antibody test, has a diagnostic accuracy of up to 90%.[54]

Genetic Testing

Genetic tests for celiac disease assess for the presence of the HLA class II genes *HLA-DQ2* and *HLA-DQ8*. This testing has a high negative predictive value, which means that the disease is unlikely to develop in those who are negative for both *HLA-DQ2* and *HLA-DQ8*. Celiac disease inheritance is complex and is not passed on with a Mendelian inheritance pattern. Up to 40% of the population carry these susceptibility alleles, whereas only 1% have celiac disease.[55] Genetic testing should not be incorporated into the first-line testing but instead should be reserved for equivocal cases to rule out celiac disease or for patients who already strictly adhere to a gluten-free diet, in which case serologic testing would not be of value.[11] Genetic testing may be used as a first-line test in relatives of patients with celiac disease to determine which individuals should be monitored for development of the disease.[8]

Endoscopic and Histologic Assessment

Although the serologic tests have become widely accessible in routine clinical practice, and positive serologies are supportive for a diagnosis of celiac disease, they are not diagnostic. Approximately 5% of patients with celiac disease have seronegative disease and receive their diagnosis based solely on histology.[56] The gold standard confirmatory test for the diagnosis of celiac disease in adults remains upper endoscopy with histologic assessment of duodenal biopsies.[51] Adult patients with elevated celiac serologies should undergo upper endoscopy with six duodenal biopsies to account for patchy disease (at least four from the second portion of the duodenum and two from the duodenal bulb).[57] A systematic review showed that adding duodenal bulb biopsies improved the diagnostic yield for celiac disease by 5%.[58]

Endoscopic features may be suggestive of celiac disease, but the diagnosis relies on histology. Macroscopic endoscopic markers include the absence of villi, scalloping of mucosal folds, the absence or reduction of folds, mosaicism or evidence of a submucosal vascular pattern, and fissure of the mucosa.[59] Water immersion in the duodenum during endoscopy has been shown to highlight macroscopic features of celiac disease and may allow for targeted biopsy.[60]

The cardinal histologic features of celiac disease include crypt hyperplasia (elongation of crypts), loss of villous height, chronic inflammatory cell infiltration, and surface intraepithelial lymphocytosis.[61] The Marsh-Oberhuber classification of histologic findings in celiac disease accounts for these features. Marsh type 1 findings demonstrate only increased surface intraepithelial lymphocytes and alone are not diagnostic for celiac disease. Type 3 findings include increased intraepithelial lymphocytes, crypt hyperplasia, and villous blunting, which together form the histologic diagnosis of celiac disease.[62] The diagnosis must be made in the right clinical context, as there are a number of histologic mimickers, including the effects of certain medications (eg, nonsteroidal anti-inflammatory drugs, olmesartan), infections (eg, small intestinal bacterial overgrowth, *Helicobacter pylori* infection, giardiasis, tropical sprue), autoimmune conditions (eg, Crohn's disease, autoimmune enteropathy, collagenous sprue, Whipple disease), and malignancy (eg, enteropathy-associated T-cell lymphoma).[63]

A nonbiopsy approach to the diagnosis of celiac disease has been recommended in pediatric patients by the European Society for Paediatric Gastroenterology, Hepatology, and Nutrition (ESPGHAN). Specifically, the 2020 ESPGHAN guideline for diagnosing celiac disease recommends a nonbiopsy approach in children with a serum IgA anti-tTG antibody level of more than 10 times the upper limit of normal and a positive test for IgA antiendomysial antibody on a second serum sample. A prior requirement for HLA testing is no longer included in the 2020 guideline because emerging data suggest that HLA-typing does not add to the certainty of diagnosis. Additionally, the guideline makes the conditional recommendation that celiac disease can be diagnosed in asymptomatic children meeting serologic criteria.[64] An international study applying the ESPGHAN nonbiopsy guidelines to pediatric practice found a positive predictive value of more than 99% for the nonbiopsy approach and suggested that more than 50% of children and adolescents with celiac disease could be diagnosed without a biopsy, thus avoiding procedural risks and associated costs.[65] To date, the nonbiopsy approach to celiac disease diagnosis has not been recommended by societal guidelines for adult patients. A 2020 study of adult patients in a Finnish celiac disease registry assessed four commercial IgA anti-tTG antibody assays and demonstrated a positive predictive value of 100% for celiac disease when applying the cutoff of 10 times the upper limit of normal.[66] Further validation will be required for adult patients in the future before employing this practice.

Video capsule endoscopy provides high-resolution imaging of the entire small bowel and has been shown to have high sensitivity and specificity for detection of villous atrophy in patients suspected of having celiac disease.[67] The primary role of video capsule endoscopy in celiac disease is to diagnose complications and direct the need for deep enteroscopy in patients thought to have ulcerative jejunoileitis or malignancy.[8] Video capsule endoscopy has also been proposed for diagnostic purposes in patients suspected of having celiac disease who are unable or unwilling to undergo upper endoscopy and in equivocal cases.[68] See Chapter 2 for more on diagnostic tests and procedures.

Treatment of Celiac Disease

Gluten-Free Diet

Although other treatment options are being researched and pursued, the only currently accepted treatment for celiac disease is strict, lifelong adherence to a gluten-free diet.[69] Gluten is a protein found in wheat (all types, including spelt, einkorn, emmer, kamut, and durum), rye, and barley. Patients with celiac disease must entirely eliminate these grains as well as any ingredients derived from these grains from their diet. However, patients with suspected celiac disease should not start a gluten-free diet until the diagnosis is confirmed on serologic testing and small bowel biopsy because adhering to a gluten-free diet can yield false negative results when testing for celiac disease.[70]

Oats do not naturally contain gluten, but they are often contaminated with gluten-containing grains.[71] There continues to be ambiguity regarding oat consumption in celiac disease, and more randomized controlled trials are needed on this topic. A 2017 systematic review concluded that uncontaminated oats are tolerated by the majority of patients with celiac disease and can safely be incorporated into the diets of patients with the disease.[72]

Nutrition Education

The registered dietitian nutritionist (RDN), in collaboration with the multidisciplinary team, plays a key role in the care of patients with celiac disease. An RDN specializing in celiac disease should provide comprehensive education on the gluten-free diet at the time of diagnosis, as well as ongoing nutrition follow-up and review of the gluten-free diet.[73,74] Patients with celiac disease should be monitored regularly by both the physician and RDN to monitor symptoms and dietary compliance and to reinforce the importance of maintaining a strict, lifelong, gluten-free diet.[75]

Adhering to a gluten-free diet can be challenging for patients at first; therefore, nutrition education should focus on the foods that the patient can still eat. The patient should be encouraged to consume naturally gluten-free foods, as these tend to be more cost-effective and palatable. Naturally gluten-free foods include the following:

- vegetables
- fruits
- meats, poultry, and seafood (made without gluten-containing breading, spices, or marinades)
- dairy
- beans, legumes, unseasoned nuts, and seeds

Note that bags of lentils can sometimes contain foreign grains. Gluten Free Watchdog, an independent gluten-testing program, generally recommends lentils that are labeled gluten-free. Patients should be instructed to carefully inspect lentils for foreign grains and rinse lentils under running water.[76]

Some gluten-free starches include:

- potato
- corn
- rice
- oats (if labeled gluten-free)
- millet
- buckwheat
- amaranth
- wild rice
- quinoa
- sorghum
- teff
- tapioca

Naturally gluten-free grains and flours can be contaminated with wheat, rye, or barley; therefore, patients should be advised to choose products that are labeled gluten-free.[77]

It is important for RDNs to discuss with their patients the wide variety of foods that are gluten-free and can still be enjoyed. The RDN should obtain a diet history to determine the patient's typical diet pattern and food preferences. Then, gluten-free diet education can be tailored to the individual patient's food preferences, comorbidities, food allergies or intolerances, lifestyle, culture, and social situation. The RDN should identify the patient's readiness to change and work in collaboration with the patient to identify strategies to increase diet compliance.[73]

Some patients may experience a decreased quality of life as a result of celiac disease and the need for a gluten-free diet.[78,79] They may find that they can no longer eat their favorite foods, dine at their favorite restaurants, or enjoy gluten-containing staples of their culture's diet. RDNs should work with their patients to identify similar gluten-free items to substitute for foods that they typically enjoy. Adolescents and young adults may also struggle with feeling left out at social events because they cannot enjoy gluten-containing foods such as pizza. These situations can lead to feelings of isolation, shame, and fear, along with hypervigilance regarding the risk of ingesting gluten.[80] The RDN should discuss strategies with patients for accommodating these situations, such as packing gluten-free meals for themselves or bringing gluten-free dishes to share with the group. Local or online support groups can also be helpful; in these groups, patients can hear from others with celiac disease, learn to normalize eating a gluten-free diet, and gain confidence in talking with their peers about celiac disease and the gluten-free diet.

Often, patients feel overwhelmed by dining out, traveling, or eating at someone else's home.[80,81] Patients with celiac disease should be taught strategies for following a gluten-free diet when dining outside the home. The following are some tips for patients:

- Patients can plan ahead by choosing a restaurant with gluten-free options on the menu. Patients should read reviews from others with celiac disease who have dined there before. They can call the restaurant to ask questions and make sure that they are able to accommodate a gluten-free diet.
- Instruct patients to briefly inform the server or host that they have celiac disease and require a gluten-free diet. Discuss the importance of the food being completely free of gluten.
- Remind patients to ask lots of questions. They can ask how foods are prepared, whether there are any gluten-containing ingredients in the dishes they are ordering, whether the meal will have contact with gluten-containing items in the kitchen, and so on.
- Remind patients to stick with foods that are naturally gluten-free, such as plain meats, fruits, plain rice, and baked potatoes.

Although adhering to a gluten-free diet is of paramount importance for those with celiac disease, it is also important that patients not become hypervigilant, as hypervigilance can lead to increased anxiety and fatigue and poorer quality of life. Patients should be encouraged to balance following the gluten-free diet with maintaining their social and emotional health. Celiac disease should not become something that prevents affected individuals from attending social gatherings, going to events, or spending time with loved ones.[83]

Patients may experience weight gain as enteropathy improves and caloric absorption increases on the gluten-free diet. Also, some commercially available gluten-free foods have higher calorie content than gluten-containing options.[74] The RDN should discuss weight management, an overall healthy diet, and increased physical activity as appropriate.

Patients should also be informed of hidden sources of gluten. Gluten can be found in communion wafers, soups, gravies, soy sauce, marinades, salad dressings, processed meats (eg, sausage), medications, herbal supplements,[84] and lip balm or other cosmetics used near the mouth.[85]

Patients with a new diagnosis of celiac disease often ask how much gluten they can eat safely. Recommendations in the literature about how much gluten a person with celiac disease can safely ingest vary widely, ranging from 10 to 100 mg/d. A conservative threshold of 50 mg/d is prudent.[70] A typical slice of sandwich bread contains 3,515 mg gluten, meaning 1/70 of a slice of sandwich bread (which amounts a single crumb) contains enough gluten to cause enteropathy.[86] For this reason, patients should be educated on the importance of strict diet adherence using real-world examples.

Cross-contact occurs when a gluten-free food comes in contact with gluten-containing ingredients or foods. Cross-contact can occur when shopping, storing and preparing foods, and eating out. Common sources of cross-contact include toasters, condiment containers (such as those for shared butter, mayonnaise, or jelly), fryers in restaurants (where gluten-containing items have been fried in the same oil as items that should be gluten-free), cutting boards, and grills. The importance of some casual kitchen cross-contact has been called into question after a recent study suggested that gluten-transfer using a shared toaster was limited.[87] The authors did note that the degree of cross-contact would inevitably vary in different kitchen environments. As many patients still report gastrointestinal side effects as a result of cross-contact, and some patients have had positive serologies as a result of cross-contact, the Academy of Nutrition and Dietetics continues to recommend that RDNs educate their patients about the risks of cross-contact.[73]

Label Reading

RDNs should also assist patients in learning label-reading skills that will help them avoid gluten-containing ingredients.[73] Wheat is considered a major food allergen under the Food Allergen Labeling and Consumer Protection Act of 2004 (FALCPA). When any ingredient in a food contains protein from wheat, the manufacturer is required to clearly indicate this fact on the label, either by including wheat in the ingredients list or by providing a "contains" statement that lists wheat (and any of the other eight major food allergens). This way, if a product's ingredients list includes wheat, the patient can know to avoid that food.[88] However, patients also need to understand that the omission of the word *wheat* does *not* guarantee that the food is gluten-free.[88,89] Because FALCPA does not include barley and rye as major food allergens, a food may contain gluten even though it does not contain wheat. Additionally, FALCPA only regulates ingredients; therefore, a food may contain wheat through cross-contact during the manufacturing process.

In August 2013, the US Food and Drug Administration passed a final rule regarding the use of the phrases *gluten-free*, *without gluten*, *free of gluten*, or *no gluten* on food product labels. The rule dictates that any foods labeled with these phrases must limit the unavoidable presence of gluten to less than 20 parts per million.[70,90] Patients should also understand that the labeling of products as gluten-free is voluntary; therefore, the absence of such labeling on a food product does not necessarily mean that the product contains gluten.

Treatment of Nutritional Deficiencies

Malabsorption of iron, folate, calcium, fat-soluble vitamins (A, D, E, and K), vitamins B12 and B6, zinc, and copper is linked to untreated celiac disease.[91-93] Iron deficiency is the most common micronutrient deficiency at the time of celiac disease diagnosis. Additional micronutrient deficiencies are more often seen in patients who present with diarrhea. A micronutrient assessment is essential at the time of celiac disease diagnosis. If deficiencies are present, the patient should receive vitamin or mineral supplementation (or both) as appropriate to correct any identified nutrient deficiencies.[73] Vitamin and mineral levels are generally assessed yearly if a patient requires vitamin or mineral supplementation, and all recommended supplements should be labeled gluten-free.

Nutritional deficiencies can also be related to the gluten-free diet itself (see Box 6.2 on page 102), because thiamin, riboflavin, niacin, folate, and iron are not found in many of the gluten-free grains.[74,89] The gluten-free diet is typically lower in fiber, and gluten-free processed foods are often higher in saturated fat, contain more sodium, and have a higher glycemic index.[19,90,93] In addition, because they have higher rates of lactose intolerance (due to brush-border lactase deficiency), patients with celiac disease often avoid dairy products and, consequently, eat fewer foods that are high in calcium and vitamin D.[94] Some patients on the gluten-free diet may require supplementation with a gluten-free multivitamin.[73]

Nonresponsive Celiac Disease

Clinical improvement in patients with celiac disease is possible within weeks to months of initiating the gluten-free diet. Histologic recovery may take months to years to improve enteropathy. Even with stringent adherence to a gluten-free diet, some patients may achieve incomplete mucosal recovery.[95]

If a patient is having no improvement in clinical or histological manifestations of celiac disease, the first step is to confirm the initial diagnosis. As noted previously, the absence of the *HLA-DQ2* and *HLA-DQ8* alleles essentially rules out a celiac disease diagnosis, so HLA-typing could be a beneficial assessment in this situation. The next step is to determine

BOX 6.2

Potential Nutritional Consequences of a Gluten-Free Diet

Potential consequence	Contributing factors
↑[a] Fat	Decreased intake of grain-food servings
	Substituting foods that are high in fat for grain foods
	Higher fat content of many gluten-free grain foods compared to similar gluten-containing products (because manufacturers may add extra fat to improve the texture and "mouth feel" of foods)
↓[b] Carbohydrate	Decreased intake of grain-food servings
	Historically, poor palatability of grain foods, especially some bread products
	High cost of many gluten-free grain foods
↓ Fiber	Low overall intake of carbohydrates, especially whole-grain carbohydrates
	Overuse of refined grains and starches in the manufacture of gluten-free grain foods such as bread products, pastas, and breakfast cereals
↓ Calcium	Decreased intake of milk-based products, owing to secondary lactose intolerance (usually a temporary condition that resolves as the intestine heals)
↓ Iron	Low overall intake of grain foods
	Low intake of gluten-free whole grains
	Lack of iron enrichment and fortification of gluten-free grain foods (eg, bread products, pastas, and breakfast cereals)
↓ Folate	Low overall intake of grain foods
	Low intake of gluten-free whole grains
	Lack of folate enrichment and fortification of gluten-free grain foods such as bread products, pastas, and breakfast cereals
↓ Niacin	Low overall intake of grain foods
	Low intake of gluten-free whole grains
	Lack of niacin enrichment and fortification of gluten-free grain foods such as bread products, pastas, and breakfast cereals
↓ Vitamin B12	Decreased intake of milk-based products, owing to secondary lactose intolerance
	Lack of vitamin and mineral fortification (including vitamin B12) of most gluten-free breakfast cereals
↓ Phosphorus	Decreased intake of milk-based products, owing to secondary lactose intolerance
↓ Zinc	Low overall intake of grain foods
	Low intake of gluten-free whole grains

[a] ↑ = increase
[b] ↓ = decrease

Adapted with permission from: Thompson T. *Academy of Nutrition and Dietetics Pocket Guide to Gluten-Free Strategies for Clients With Multiple Diet Restrictions. 2nd ed. Academy of Nutrition and Dietetics; 2016:42-43.*[89]

the patient's true level of adherence to the gluten-free diet. Often, refractory symptoms are due to nonadherence to the gluten-free diet or inadvertent intake of gluten through hidden sources, cross-contact, or the need for more education.[90] In many cases, unrecognized gluten intake is the cause of nonresponsive celiac disease.[69] An RDN with expertise in gluten-free diets should be consulted to determine whether the patient is closely adhering to the gluten-free diet and to identify any potential sources of gluten intake.[70] Gluten immunogenic peptides measured in urine or stool samples may provide a biomarker to assess compliance with the gluten-free diet.[96] Further study is needed to determine whether early identification of gluten immunogenic peptides affects outcomes in patients with nonresponsive celiac disease.

After the diagnosis of celiac disease is confirmed and the ingestion of any type of gluten is ruled out, additional diagnoses should be considered. Figure 6.2 shows diagnoses to consider if the clinical diagnosis of celiac disease is certain and the patient has not been ingesting gluten.

FIGURE 6.2 Diagnoses to consider in patients with confirmed celiac disease who do not respond to the gluten-free diet

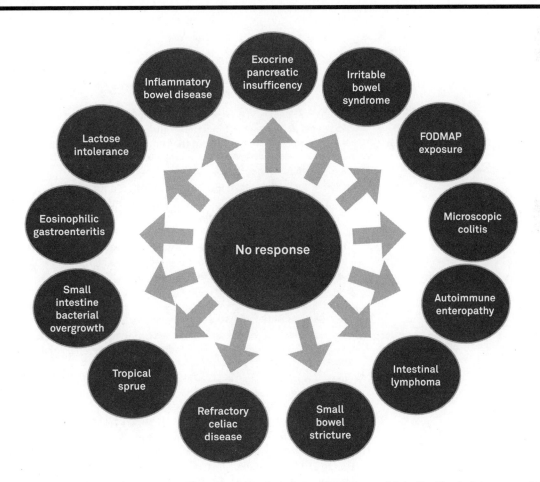

Differential diagnoses are numerous for nonresponders to a gluten-free diet and include small intestinal bacterial overgrowth (SIBO), eosinophilic gastroenteritis, lactose intolerance, inflammatory bowel disease, exocrine pancreatic insufficiency, irritable bowel syndrome, fermentable oligosaccharides, disaccharides, monosaccharides, and polyols (FODMAP) exposure, microscopic colitis, autoimmune enteropathy, intestinal lymphomas, small bowel stricture, and tropical sprue, among others. These conditions must be excluded before making a diagnosis of refractory celiac disease in a patient with confirmed celiac disease who presents with refractory symptoms despite following a strict gluten-free diet.

If the patient continues to have clinical manifestations of celiac disease despite strict adherence to a gluten-free diet, and if no other medical diagnoses have been identified, further steps should be taken to distinguish between nonresponsive disease and true refractory celiac disease. The gluten contamination elimination diet may be useful in these situations.[97] This modified diet aims to eliminate any possible sources of gluten cross-contamination in an already strict gluten-free diet. Patients who respond to the gluten contamination elimination diet likely had inadvertent gluten exposure that caused nonresponsive celiac disease rather than true refractory celiac disease.[98] In severe cases of refractory celiac disease, enteral or parenteral nutrition may be required, as well as corticosteroids or other immunosuppressive therapy.[99]

Summary

Celiac disease is a common immune-mediated enteropathy with systemic manifestations. The pathogenesis of celiac disease involves a disordered immune response to dietary gluten. With the increasing availability of serologic tests for celiac disease, as well as a heightened awareness of nonclassical or atypical presentations, all health care practitioners are likely to encounter celiac disease in their practices. Currently, the management of celiac disease relies on the strict gluten-free diet. Thus, a team-based approach involving the patient, the clinician, and an RDN is imperative to providing the patient with an accurate diagnosis and necessary support through the prescribed course of treatment.

References

1. Biesiekierski JR. What is gluten? *J Gastroenterol Hepatol*. 2017;32(suppl 1):78-81. doi:10.1111/jgh.13703
2. Choung RS, Unalp-Arida A, Ruhl CE, Brantner TL, Everhart JE, Murray JA. Less hidden celiac disease but increased gluten avoidance without a diagnosis in the United States: findings from the National Health and Nutrition Examination Surveys from 2009 to 2014. *Mayo Clin Proc*. 2017;92(1):30-38. doi:10.1016/j.mayocp.2016.10.012
3. Krigel A, Turner KO, Makharia GK, Green PHR, Genta RM, Lebwohl B. Ethnic variations in duodenal villous atrophy consistent with celiac disease in the United States. *Clin Gastroenterol Hepatol*. 2016;14(8):1105-1111. doi:10.1016/j.cgh.2016.04.032
4. Kang JY, Kang AHY, Green A, Gwee KA, Ho KY. Systematic review: worldwide variation in the frequency of coeliac disease and changes over time. *Aliment Pharmacol Ther*. 2013;38(3):226-245. doi:10.1111/apt.12373
5. Green PHR, Stavropoulos SN, Panagi SG, et al. Characteristics of adult celiac disease in the USA: results of a national survey. *Am J Gastroenterol*. 2001;96(1):126-131. doi:10.1111/j.1572-0241.2001.03462.x
6. Dixit R, Lebwohl B, Ludvigsson JF, Lewis SK, Rizkalla-Reilly N, Green PHR. Celiac disease is diagnosed less frequently in young adult males. *Dig Dis Sci*. 2014;59(7):1509-1512. doi:10.1007/s10620-014-3025-6
7. Fuchs V, Kurppa K, Huhtala H, Mäki M, Kekkonen L, Kaukinen K. Delayed celiac disease diagnosis predisposes to reduced quality of life and incremental use of health care services and medicines: a prospective nationwide study. *United Eur Gastroenterol J*. 2018;6(4):567-575. doi:10.1177/2050640617751253
8. Al-Toma A, Volta U, Auricchio R, et al. European Society for the Study of Coeliac Disease (ESsCD) guideline for coeliac disease and other gluten-related disorders. *United Eur Gastroenterol J*. 2019;7(5):583-613. doi:10.1177/2050640619844125
9. Ludvigsson JF, Murray JA. Epidemiology of celiac disease. *Gastroenterol Clin North Am*. 2019;48(1):1-18. doi:10.1016/j.gtc.2018.09.004

10. Catassi C, Gatti S, Fasano A. The new epidemiology of celiac disease. *J Pediatr Gastroenterol Nutr*. 2014;59(suppl 1):S7-S9. doi:10.1097/01.mpg.0000450393.23156.59

11. Brown NK, Guandalini S, Semrad C, Kupfer SS. A clinician's guide to celiac disease HLA genetics. *Am J Gastroenterol*. 2019;114(10):1587-1592. doi:10.14309/ajg.0000000000000310

12. Megiorni F, Mora B, Bonamico M, et al. HLA-DQ and risk gradient for celiac disease. *Hum Immunol*. 2009;70(1):55-59. doi:10.1016/j.humimm.2008.10.018

13. Pietzak MM, Schofield TC, McGinniss MJ, Nakamura RM. Stratifying risk for celiac disease in a large at-risk United States population by using HLA alleles. *Clin Gastroenterol Hepatol*. 2009;7(9):966-971. doi:10.1016/j.cgh.2009.05.028

14. Iacomino G, Marano A, Stillitano I, et al. Celiac disease: role of intestinal compartments in the mucosal immune response. *Mol Cell Biochem*. 2016;411(1-2):341-349. doi:10.1007/s11010-015-2596-7

15. Green PHR, Cellier C. Celiac disease. *N Engl J Med*. 2007;357(17):1731-1743. doi:10.1056/NEJMra071600

16. Kumral D, Syed S. Celiac disease screening for high-risk groups: are we doing it right? *Dig Dis Sci*. 2020;65(8):2187-2195. doi:10.1007/s10620-020-06352-w

17. Ludvigsson JF, Leffler DA, Bai JC, et al. The Oslo definitions for coeliac disease and related terms. *Gut*. 2013;62(1):43-52. doi:10.1136/gutjnl-2011-301346

18. Berry N, Basha J, Varma N, et al. Anemia in celiac disease is multifactorial in etiology: a prospective study from India. *JGH Open*. 2018;2(5):196-200. doi:10.1002/jgh3.12073

19. Vici G, Belli L, Biondi M, Polzonetti V. Gluten free diet and nutrient deficiencies: a review. *Clin Nutr*. 2016;35(6):1236-1241. doi:10.1016/j.clnu.2016.05.002

20. Mansikka E, Salmi TT, Kaukinen K, et al. Diagnostic delay in dermatitis herpetiformis in a high-prevalence area. *Acta Derm Venereol*. 2018;98(2):195-199. doi:10.2340/00015555-2818

21. Bolotin D, Petronic-Rosic V. Dermatitis herpetiformis: part I. epidemiology, pathogenesis, and clinical presentation. *J Am Acad Dermatol*. 2011;64(6):1017-1024. doi:10.1016/j.jaad.2010.09.777

22. Zhu YI, Stiller MJ. Dapsone and sulfones in dermatology: overview and update. *J Am Acad Dermatol*. 2001;45(3):420-434. doi:10.1067/mjd.2001.114733

23. Salmi TT. Dermatitis herpetiformis. *Clin Exp Dermatol*. 2019;44(7):728-731. doi:10.1111/ced.13992

24. Devarbhavi H, Raj S, Joseph T, Singh R, Patil M. Features and treatment of dapsone-induced hepatitis, based on analysis of 44 cases and literature review. *Clin Gastroenterol Hepatol*. 2017;15(11):1805-1807. doi:10.1016/j.cgh.2017.05.031

25. Garioch JJ, Lewis HM, Sargent SA, Leonard JN, Fry L. 25 years' experience of a gluten-free diet in the treatment of dermatitis herpetiformis. *Br J Dermatol*. 1994;131(4):541-545. doi:10.1111/j.1365-2133.1994.tb08557.x

26. Trovato CM, Raucci U, Valitutti F, et al. Neuropsychiatric manifestations in celiac disease. *Epilepsy Behav*. 2019;99:106393. doi:10.1016/j.yebeh.2019.06.036

27. Mitoma H, Adhikari K, Aeschlimann D, et al. Consensus paper: neuroimmune mechanisms of cerebellar ataxias. *Cerebellum*. 2016;15(2):213-232. doi:10.1007/s12311-015-0664-x

28. Hadjivassiliou M, Davies-Jones GAB, Sanders DS, Grünewald RA. Dietary treatment of gluten ataxia. *J Neurol Neurosurg Psychiatry*. 2003;74(9):1221-1224. doi:10.1136/jnnp.74.9.1221

29. Mearns ES, Taylor A, Craig KJT, et al. Neurological manifestations of neuropathy and ataxia in celiac disease: a systematic review. *Nutrients*. 2019;11(2):380. doi:10.3390/nu11020380

30. Nikpour S. Neurological manifestations, diagnosis, and treatment of celiac disease: a comprehensive review. *Iran J Neurol*. 2012;11(2):59-64.

31. Rubio-Tapia A, Murray JA. The liver and celiac disease. *Clin Liver Dis*. 2019;23(2):167-176. doi:10.1016/j.cld.2018.12.001

32. Sainsbury A, Sanders DS, Ford AC. Meta-analysis: coeliac disease and hypertransaminasaemia. *Aliment Pharmacol Ther*. 2011;34(1):33-40. doi:10.1111/j.1365-2036.2011.04685.x

33. Ludvigsson JF, Elfström P, BroomÉ U, Ekbom A, Montgomery SM. Celiac disease and risk of liver disease: a general population-based study. *Clin Gastroenterol Hepatol*. 2007;5(1):63-69.e1. doi:10.1016/j.cgh.2006.09.034

34. Valvano M, Longo S, Stefanelli G, Frieri G, Viscido A, Latella G. Celiac disease, gluten-free diet, and metabolic and liver disorders. *Nutrients*. 2020 Mar 28;12(4):940. doi:10.3390/nu12040940

35. Lucendo AJ, García-Manzanares A. Bone mineral density in adult coeliac disease: an updated review. *Rev Esp Enfermedades Dig*. 2013;105(3):154-162. doi:10.4321/S1130-01082013000300006

36. Zanchetta MB, Longobardi V, Bai JC. Bone and celiac disease. *Curr Osteoporos Rep*. 2016;14(2):43-48. doi:10.1007/s11914-016-0304-5

37. Sánchez MIP, Mohaidle A, Baistrocchi A, et al. Risk of fracture in celiac disease: gender, dietary compliance, or both? *World J Gastroenterol*. 2011;17(25):3035-3042. doi:10.3748/wjg.v17.i25.3035

38. Pantaleoni S, Luchino M, Adriani A, et al. Bone mineral density at diagnosis of celiac disease and after 1 year of gluten-free diet. *Sci World J*. 2014;2014:173082. doi:10.1155/2014/173082

39. Kylökäs A, Kaukinen K, Huhtala H, Collin P, Mäki M, Kurppa K. Type 1 and type 2 diabetes in celiac disease: prevalence and effect on clinical and histological presentation. *BMC Gastroenterol*. 2016;16(1):76. doi:10.1186/s12876-016-0488-2

40. Smigoc Schweiger D, Mendez A, Kunilo Jamnik S, et al. High-risk genotypes HLA-DR3-DQ2/DR3-DQ2 and DR3-DQ2/DR4-DQ8 in co-occurrence of type 1 diabetes and celiac disease. *Autoimmunity*. 2016;49(4):240-247. doi:10.3109/08916934.2016.1164144

41. Kahaly GJ, Frommer L, Schuppan D. Celiac disease and endocrine autoimmunity—the genetic link. *Autoimmun Rev*. 2018;17(12):1169-1175. doi:10.1016/j.autrev.2018.05.013

42. Sategna-Guidetti C, Volta U, Ciacci C, et al. Prevalence of thyroid disorders in untreated adult celiac disease patients and effect of gluten withdrawal: an Italian multicenter study. *Am J Gastroenterol*. 2001;96(3):751-757. doi:10.1111/j.1572-0241.2001.03617.x

43. Casella G, Orfanotti G, Giacomantonio L, et al. Celiac disease and obstetrical-gynecological contribution. *Gastroenterol Hepatol from Bed to Bench*. 2016;9(4):241-249. doi:10.22037/ghfbb.v0i0.1013

44. Saccone G, Berghella V, Sarno L, et al. Celiac disease and obstetric complications: a systematic review and metaanalysis. *Am J Obstet Gynecol*. 2016;214(2):225-234. doi:10.1016/j.ajog.2015.09.080

45. Fasano A, Catassi C. Clinical practice. Celiac disease. *N Engl J Med*. 2012;367(25):2419-2426. doi:10.1056/NEJMcp1113994

46. Lebwohl B, Rubio-Tapia A, Assiri A, Newland C, Guandalini S. Diagnosis of celiac disease. *Gastrointest Endosc Clin N Am*. 2012;22(4):661-677. doi:10.1016/j.giec.2012.07.004

47. Rostom A, Dubé C, Cranney A, et al. The diagnostic accuracy of serologic tests for celiac disease: a systematic review. *Gastroenterology*. 2005;128(4 suppl 1):S38-S46. doi:10.1053/j.gastro.2005.02.028

48. Leffler D, Schuppan D, Pallav K, et al. Kinetics of the histological, serological and symptomatic responses to gluten challenge in adults with coeliac disease. *Gut*. 2013;62(7):996-1004. doi:10.1136/gutjnl-2012-302196

49. Sharkey LM, Corbett G, Currie E, Lee J, Sweeney N, Woodward JM. Optimising delivery of care in coeliac disease—comparison of the benefits of repeat biopsy and serological follow-up. *Aliment Pharmacol Ther*. 2013;38(10):1278-1291. doi:10.1111/apt.12510

50. Dieterich W, Ehnis T, Bauer M, et al. Identification of tissue transglutaminase as the autoantigen of celiac disease. *Nat Med*. 1997;3(7):797-801. doi:10.1038/nm0797-797

51. Rubio-Tapia A, Hill ID, Kelly CP, Calderwood AH, Murray JA. ACG clinical guidelines: diagnosis and management of celiac disease. *Am J Gastroenterol*. 2013;108(5):656-676. doi:10.1038/ajg.2013.79

52. Grodzinsky E, Hed J, Skogh T. IgA antiendomysium antibodies have a high positive predictive value for celiac disease in asymptomatic patients. *Allergy*. 1994;49(8):593-597. doi:10.1111/j.1398-9995.1994.tb00124.x

53. McGowan KE, Lyon ME, Butzner JD. Celiac disease and IgA deficiency: complications of serological testing approaches encountered in the clinic. *Clin Chem*. 2008;54(7):1203-1209. doi:10.1373/clinchem.2008.103606

54. Villalta D, Tonutti E, Prause C, et al. IgG antibodies against deamidated gliadin peptides for diagnosis of celiac disease in patients with IgA deficiency. *Clin Chem*. 2010;56(3):464-468. doi:10.1373/clinchem.2009.128132

55. Almeida LM, Gandolfi L, Pratesi R, et al. Presence of DQ2.2 associated with DQ2.5 increases the risk for celiac disease. *Autoimmune Dis*. 2016;2016:5409653. doi:10.1155/2016/5409653

56. Cichewicz AB, Mearns ES, Taylor A, et al. Diagnosis and treatment patterns in celiac disease. *Dig Dis Sci*. 2019;64(8):2095-2106. doi:10.1007/s10620-019-05528-3

57. Kurien M, Evans KE, Hopper AD, Hale MF, Cross SS, Sanders DS. Duodenal bulb biopsies for diagnosing adult celiac disease: is there an optimal biopsy site? *Gastrointest Endosc*. 2012;75(6):1190-1196. doi:10.1016/j.gie.2012.02.025

58. McCarty TR, O'Brien CR, Gremida A, Ling C, Rustagi T. Efficacy of duodenal bulb biopsy for diagnosis of celiac disease: a systematic review and meta-analysis. *Endosc Int Open*. 2018;06(11):E1369-E1378. doi:10.1055/a-0732-5060

59. Ianiro G, Gasbarrini A, Cammarota G. Endoscopic tools for the diagnosis and evaluation of celiac disease. *World J Gastroenterol*. 2013;19(46):8562-8570. doi:10.3748/wjg.v19.i46.8562

60. Cammarota G, Pirozzi GA, Martino A, et al. Reliability of the "immersion technique" during routine upper endoscopy for detection of abnormalities of duodenal villi in patients with dyspepsia. *Gastrointest Endosc*. 2004;60(2):223-228. doi:10.1016/S0016-5107(04)01553-6

61. Dai Y, Zhang Q, Olofson AM, Jhala N, Liu X. Celiac disease. *Adv Anat Pathol*. 2019;26(5):292-312. doi:10.1097/PAP.0000000000000242

62. Marsh MN. Gluten, major histocompatibility complex, and the small intestine: a molecular and immunobiologic approach to the spectrum of gluten sensitivity ("celiac sprue"). *Gastroenterology*. 1992;102(1):330-354. doi:10.1016/0016-5085(92)91819-P

63. Kamboj AK, Oxentenko AS. Clinical and histologic mimickers of celiac disease. *Clin Transl Gastroenterol*. 2017;8(8):e114. doi:10.1038/ctg.2017.41

64. Husby S, Koletzko S, Korponay-Szabó I, et al. European Society [for] Paediatric Gastroenterology, Hepatology and Nutrition guidelines for diagnosing coeliac disease 2020. *J Pediatr Gastroenterol Nutr*. 2020;70(1):141-156. doi:10.1097/MPG .0000000000002497

65. Werkstetter KJ, Korponay-Szabó IR, Popp A, et al. Accuracy in diagnosis of celiac disease without biopsies in clinical practice. *Gastroenterology*. 2017;153(4):924-935. doi:10.1053/j.gastro.2017.06 .002

66. Ylönen V, Lindfors K, Repo M, et al. Non-biopsy serology-based diagnosis of celiac disease in adults is accurate with different commercial kits and pre-test probabilities. *Nutrients*. 2020;12(9):1-9. doi:10.3390 /nu12092736

67. Rondonotti E, Spada C, Cave D, et al. Video capsule enteroscopy in the diagnosis of celiac disease: a multicenter study. *Am J Gastroenterol*. 2007;102(8):1624-1631. doi:10.1111/j.1572-0241 .2007.01238.x

68. Rondonotti E, Paggi S. Videocapsule endoscopy in celiac disease: indications and timing. *Dig Dis*. 2015;33(2):244-251. doi:10.1159/000369510

69. Samasca G, Lerner A, Girbovan A, et al. Challenges in gluten-free diet in coeliac disease: Prague consensus. *Eur J Clin Invest*. 2017;47(5):394-397. doi:10.1111/eci .12755

70. Itzlinger A, Branchi F, Elli L, Schumann M. Gluten-free diet in celiac disease—forever and for all? *Nutrients*. 2018;10(11):1796. doi:10.3390/nu10111796

71. Smulders MJM, van de Wiel CCM, van den Broeck HC, et al. Oats in healthy gluten-free and regular diets: a perspective. *Food Res Int*. 2018;110:3-10. doi:10.1016 /j.foodres.2017.11.031

72. Pinto-Sánchez MI, Causada-Calo N, Bercik P, et al. Safety of adding oats to a gluten-free diet for patients with celiac disease: systematic review and meta-analysis of clinical and observational studies. *Gastroenterology*. 2017;153(2):395-409.e3. doi:10 .1053/j.gastro.2017.04.009

73. Cheng FW, Handu D. Nutrition assessment, interventions, and monitoring for patients with celiac disease: an Evidence Analysis Center scoping review. *J Acad Nutr Diet*. 2020;120(8):1381-1406. doi:10.1016 /j.jand.2019.09.019

74. Theethira TG, Dennis M. Celiac disease and the gluten-free diet: consequences and recommendations for improvement. *Dig Dis*. 2015;33(2):175-182. doi:10 .1159/000369504

75. National Institutes of Health Consensus Development Program. NIH Consensus Development Conference on Celiac Disease: National Institutes of Health Consensus Development Conference statement, June 28-30, 2004. NIH Consensus Development Program Archive. Accessed March 24, 2021. https://consensus .nih.gov/2004/2004CeliacDisease118html.htm

76. Thompson T. General product warning: check your lentils (including certified gluten-free lentils) for foreign grain. Gluten Free Watchdog. December 13, 2016. Accessed March 24, 2021. www .glutenfreewatchdog.org/news/general-product -warning-check-your-lentils-including-certified -gluten-free-lentils-for-foreign-grain

77. Thompson T, Lee AR, Grace T. Gluten contamination of grains, seeds, and flours in the United States: a pilot study. *J Am Diet Assoc*. 2010;110(6):937-940. doi:10 .1016/j.jada.2010.03.014

78. Roos S, Kärner A, Hallert C. Psychological well-being of adult coeliac patients treated for 10 years. *Dig Liver Dis*. 2006;38(3):177-180. doi:10.1016/j.dld.2006.01 .004

79. Zysk W, Głąbska D, Guzek D. Social and emotional fears and worries influencing the quality of life of female celiac disease patients following a gluten-free diet. *Nutrients*. 2018;10(10):1414. doi:10.3390 /nu10101414

80. Sverker A, Hensing G, Hallert C. "Controlled by food"—lived experiences of coeliac disease. *J Hum Nutr Diet*. 2005;18(3):171-180. doi:10.1111/j.1365-277X.2005 .00591.x

81. Lee A, Newman JM. Celiac diet: its impact on quality of life. *J Am Diet Assoc*. 2003;103(11):1533-1535. doi:10 .1016/j.jada.2003.08.027

82. Lee AR, Ng DL, Diamond B, Ciaccio EJ, Green PHR. Living with coeliac disease: survey results from the USA. *J Hum Nutr Diet*. 2012;25(3):233-238. doi:10.1111 /j.1365-277X.2012.01236.x

83. Wolf RL, Lebwohl B, Lee AR, et al. Hypervigilance to a gluten-free diet and decreased quality of life in teenagers and adults with celiac disease. *Dig Dis Sci*. 2018;63(6):1438-1448. doi:10.1007/s10620-018-4936-4

84. Thompson T, Dennis M, Emerson L. Gluten-free labeling: are growth media containing wheat, barley, and rye falling through the cracks? *J Acad Nutr Diet*. 2018;118(11):2025-2028. doi:10.1016/j.jand.2017.07 .004

85. Thompson T, Grace T. Gluten in cosmetics: is there a reason for concern? *J Acad Nutr Diet*. 2012;112(9):1316. doi:10.1016/j.jand.2012.07.011

86. Thompson T. What does 10 mg of gluten look like? Gluten Free Watchdog. October 9, 2019. Accessed January 10, 2021. www.glutenfreewatchdog.org/news /what-does-10-mg-of-gluten-look-like

87. Weisbrod VM, Silvester JA, Raber C, McMahon J, Coburn SS, Kerzner B. Preparation of gluten-free foods alongside gluten-containing food may not always be as risky for celiac patients as diet guides suggest. *Gastroenterology*. 2020;158(1):273-275. doi:10.1053/j .gastro.2019.09.007

88. Food Allergen Labeling and Consumer Protection Act of 2004 (FALCPA). Public Law 108-282, Title II. US Food and Drug Administration. Accessed January 10, 2021. www.fda.gov/food/food-allergensgluten-free-guidance -documents-regulatory-information/food-allergen -labeling-and-consumer-protection-act-2004-falcpa

89. Thompson T. *Academy of Nutrition and Dietetics Pocket Guide to Gluten-Free Strategies for Clients With Multiple Diet Restrictions*. 2nd ed. Academy of Nutrition and Dietetics; 2016.

90. Rostami K, Bold J, Parr A, Johnson MW. Gluten-free diet indications, safety, quality, labels, and challenges. *Nutrients*. 2017;9(8):846. doi:10.3390/nu9080846

91. Reinken L, Zieglauer H. Vitamin B-6 absorption in children with acute celiac disease and in control subjects. *J Nutr*. 1978;108(10):1562-1565. doi:10.1093 /jn/108.10.1562

92. Meyer D, Stavropolous S, Diamond B, Shane E, Green PHR. Osteoporosis in a North American adult population with celiac disease. *Am J Gastroenterol*. 2001;96(1):112-119. doi:10.1111/j.1572-0241.2001 .03507.x

93. Melini V, Melini F. Gluten-free diet: gaps and needs for a healthier diet. *Nutrients*. 2019;11(1):170. doi:10 .3390/nu11010170

94. Ojetti V, Nucera G, Migneco A, et al. High prevalence of celiac disease in patients with lactose intolerance. *Digestion*. 2005;71(2):106-110. doi:10.1159 /000084526

95. Haines ML, Anderson RP, Gibson PR. Systematic review: the evidence base for long-term management of coeliac disease. *Aliment Pharmacol Ther*. 2008;28(9):1042-1066. doi:10.1111/j.1365-2036.2008 .03820.x

96. Comino I, Segura V, Ortigosa L, et al. Prospective longitudinal study: use of faecal gluten immunogenic peptides to monitor children diagnosed with coeliac disease during transition to a gluten-free diet. *Aliment Pharmacol Ther*. 2019;49(12):1484-1492. doi:10.1111 /apt.15277

97. Leonard MM, Cureton P, Fasano A. Indications and use of the gluten contamination elimination diet for patients with non-responsive celiac disease. *Nutrients*. 2017;9(10):1129. doi:10.3390/nu9101129

98. Hollon JR, Cureton PA, Martin ML, Puppa ELL, Fasano A. Trace gluten contamination may play a role in mucosal and clinical recovery in a subgroup of diet-adherent non-responsive celiac disease patients. *BMC Gastroenterol*. 2013;13(1):40. doi:10.1186/1471-230X -13-40

99. Nasr I, Nasr I, Beyers C, Chang F, Donnelly S, Ciclitira P. Recognising and managing refractory coeliac disease: a tertiary centre experience. *Nutrients*. 2015;7(12):9896-9907. doi:10.3390/nu7125506

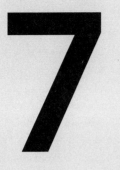

CHAPTER

7

Liver Disease

Jeanette M. Hasse, PhD, RD, LD, CNSC, CCTC, FASPEN, FADA
Sumeet K. Asrani, MD, MSc

KEY POINTS

- Malnutrition and nutritional disorders are common in individuals with chronic liver disease.
- A nutrition assessment is necessary to determine the degree of malnutrition, sarcopenia, and frailty, and to identify nutrient deficits to develop a nutrition plan.
- Nutrition interventions for patients may include measures such as eating frequent meals and snacks, eating high-protein foods, limiting sodium intake, avoiding alcohol, exercising, and avoiding dietary or herbal supplements. In some instances, nutrition support may be necessary.

Introduction

Liver disease accounts for approximately 2 million deaths worldwide per year—1 million due to complications of cirrhosis, and 1 million due to viral hepatitis and hepatocellular carcinoma.[1,2] Chronic liver disease and cirrhosis are, together, the 12th leading cause of death in the United States.[3] However, the true burden of liver disease may be underestimated and may be increasing.[4,5] The economic impact to society and individuals is also high, and quality-of-life indices are low in patients with chronic liver disease.[6,7] Among gastrointestinal (GI)-related hospitalizations, those for chronic liver disease have the highest inpatient mortality.[8,9]

Pathogenesis of Liver Disease

Liver disease comprises a continuum of disease progression. Globally, there are several types of liver disease, including viral hepatitis (eg, hepatitis B and C), nonalcoholic fatty liver disease (NAFLD), alcohol-associated liver disease, cholestatic liver disease, autoimmune disease, and several others. Over time, some affected individuals will develop chronic liver disease that can lead to permanent scarring of the liver, which is called cirrhosis. Compensated cirrhosis (the presence of liver scarring without complications) can progress, leading to decompensated cirrhosis, in which complications are prevalent. In 2017, there were 112 million cases of compensated cirrhosis and 10.6 million cases of decompensated cirrhosis worldwide.[5] In patients with decompensated cirrhosis, malnutrition, sarcopenia, and frailty are common and associated with premature mortality.

Etiology

Although there are several disease states that can lead to chronic liver disease and cirrhosis, the most commonly encountered liver disease states are alcohol-associated liver disease, NAFLD, and viral hepatitis.

Alcohol-Associated Liver Disease

Globally, about 2 billion people consume alcohol and more than 75 million are diagnosed with alcohol-use disorders that put them at risk for alcohol-associated liver disease. In 2016, global alcohol use was associated with 3 million deaths (5.3% of all deaths), surpassing the number of deaths from hypertension and diabetes combined.[10,11] Specifically, alcohol-attributable liver cirrhosis causes approximately 550,000 to 610,000 deaths annually and, together with rising rates of liver cancer, causes 1% of worldwide mortality.[11]

Nonalcoholic Fatty Liver Disease

Approximately 2 billion adults around the world are obese or overweight, and more than 400 million have diabetes. Obesity and type 2 diabetes mellitus are major risk factors for NAFLD. The prevalence of NAFLD within a population varies from 8% to 45%, depending on the definition of NAFLD used.[12,13] The global prevalence of NAFLD is 25.2%, with higher prevalence in the Middle East and South America.[14] NAFLD is more prevalent in patients with diabetes mellitus (59%), patients undergoing bariatric surgery, patients with morbid obesity, and Hispanic patients.[15-17] In the United States, according to data from the National Health and Nutrition Examination Survey (NHANES), the prevalence of NAFLD is between 18% and 24%, with over 30 million people diagnosed with NAFLD.[18] The prevalence of NAFLD among lean patients (ie, with a BMI of less than 25 in the West and less than 22 in Asia) is approximately 7% to 20%.[19]

Viral Hepatitis

Approximately 5% of the world's population suffers from chronic hepatitis B or C. Hepatitis, or inflammation of the liver, can occur for a variety of reasons, but it is most commonly caused by viruses. Worldwide, an estimated 248 million people are chronically infected with the hepatitis B virus. Among those infected, approximately 600,000 die annually from hepatitis B virus–related sequelae (principally hepatocellular carcinoma and cirrhosis-related complications).[20,21] Three to 4 million people are infected with hepatitis C virus each year. The global prevalence of viral hepatitis was estimated to be 185 million in 2005 (compared with 122 million in 1990).[22,23]

Clinical Presentation and Diagnosis of Liver Disease

Medical Presentation and Diagnosis

Patients with liver disease can be asymptomatic (compensated) or present with complications (decompensated). All diagnoses of liver disease can lead to compensated or decompensated cirrhosis, but some patients will be asymptomatic while others will have more severe symptoms.

Asymptomatic Liver Disease

Often, asymptomatic liver disease is identified through routine blood tests that note elevated liver enzyme levels (though they can be normal). Imaging can also incidentally detect the presence of liver disease. In addition, screening for hepatitis C among adults is now universal in the United States. In patients with risk factors for liver disease, blood tests such as a hepatic function panel, a complete blood count, and an abdominal ultrasound may help assess for liver disease. Although liver biopsy was common in the past as a first-line test to establish the presence of cirrhosis, now several noninvasive tests (blood-based and imaging-based) can help in risk stratification.[24] These include the aspartate aminotransferase-to-platelet ratio index, fibrosis-4 score, and NAFLD fibrosis score, which combine results of routine blood tests with relevant patient characteristics. Online calculators are readily available. Alternatively, imaging-based tests include ultrasound-based and magnetic resonance-based elastography.

Decompensated Cirrhosis

Often, patients present with complications of liver disease and cirrhosis. These include hepatic encephalopathy, jaundice, infection (sepsis, spontaneous bacterial peritonitis), kidney dysfunction (hyponatremia, hepatorenal syndrome), complications of portal hypertension (variceal bleeding, ascites), and liver cancer. Blood tests to establish disease severity include a hepatic function panel, a comprehensive metabolic panel, and the international normalized ratio (INR). The Model for End Stage Liver Disease–Sodium score is a composite score (INR; serum levels of bilirubin, creatinine, and sodium) that allows for assessment of disease severity and prognosis; it is used in the decision-making process for liver transplantation.[25] The score ranges from 6 to 40, with higher scores implying a higher risk of short-term mortality.

Nutritional Status Presentation

The prevalence of malnutrition in patients with liver disease is related to the severity of liver disease. Several nutrition assessment parameters are used to determine malnutrition. Patients with chronic liver disease should undergo a nutrition screening and assessment by a registered dietitian nutritionist (RDN) or other team member (see Figure 7.1).[26] Nutrition assessment is best accomplished using a variety of parameters (see Box 7.1 on page 112) and is further described in two recent reviews.[27,28] Because obesity itself is a risk factor for

FIGURE 7.1 Nutritional screening and assessment in patients with cirrhosis

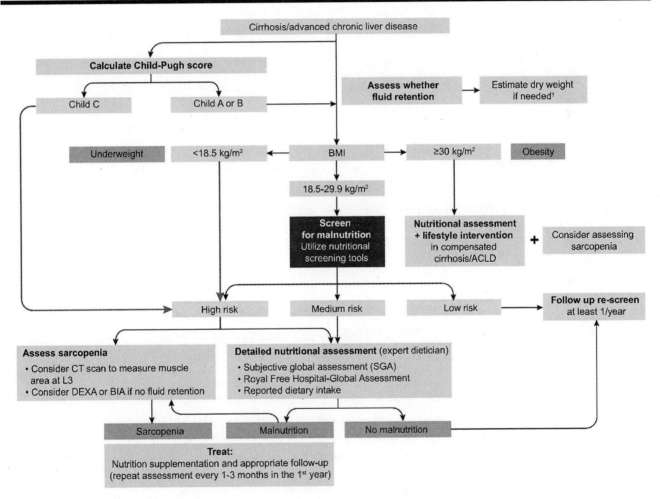

ACLD = advanced chronic liver disease | BIA = bioelectrical impedance analysis | CT = computed tomography | DEXA = dual-energy x-ray absorptiometry

All patients should undergo a rapid screening of malnutrition using validated, accepted tools. A liver specific screening tool which takes into consideration fluid retention may be advisable (eg, Royal Free Hospital Nutritional Prioritizing Tool [RFH-NPT]). Patients found to be at high risk of malnutrition should undergo a detailed nutritional assessment, and based on the findings they should receive either supplementation or regular follow-up.

†In a case of fluid retention, body weight should be corrected by evaluating the patient's dry weight by post-paracentesis body weight or weight recorded before fluid retention if available, or by subtracting a percentage of weight based upon severity of ascites (mild, 5%; moderate, 10%; severe, 15%), with an additional 5% subtracted if bilateral pedal oedema is present.

Reprinted with permission from European Association for the Study of the Liver. EASL Clinical Practice Guidelines on nutrition in chronic liver disease. *J Hepatol.* 2019;70(1):172-193.[26]

NAFLD, there is a prevalence of obesity among patients with NAFLD. However, patients with liver disease can display loss of muscle mass and function (sarcopenia) despite adequate fat stores, a condition often referred to as sarcopenic obesity. As discussed in a 2019 review, independent of liver function, sarcopenia in individuals with chronic liver disease is associated with increased mortality, infection, length of hospital stay, prevalence of malnutrition, and cost, as well as reduced quality of life.[29]

BOX 7.1

Parameters for Nutrition Assessment of Patients With Chronic Liver Disease

Parameter	Comments
Nutrition focused physical assessment	Look for signs of muscle wasting and fat loss.
	Examine the skin, hair, and nails for signs of macro- and micronutrient deficiencies.
Subjective global assessment	Obtain a history of gastrointestinal side effects and their duration, severity, and effect on intake (eg, nausea, vomiting, diarrhea, constipation, early satiety, dysgeusia, dysphagia).
	Perform a physical assessment (see above), looking for fat and muscle stores, as well as the presence and severity of edema and ascites.
	Assess nutrient intake via 24-hour diet recall, 3-day food record, or other methods.
	Determine the effect of the disease state on metabolism.
Anthropometric measurements	Evaluate body weight in view of the patient's usual body weight, current body weight, and the presence of fluid retention; weight or BMI is often not an accurate indicator by itself of nutritional status.
	Consider midarm muscle circumference and triceps skinfold measurements if the patient is not retaining fluid, as they may be useful if performed serially by the same observer over time.
Functional measurements	Use validated tools such as the Liver Frailty Index (liverfrailtyindex.ucsf.edu) to determine functional capacity; high frailty scores are associated with worsened outcomes.
	Assess hand-grip strength as an adjunct to other nutrition assessment tools; hand-grip strength is one of the measurements used in the Liver Frailty Index.
Body composition tools	Computed tomography (CT) and magnetic resonance imaging (MRI) have been used to determine sarcopenia, usually at the third lumbar spine vertebra level; sarcopenia is defined as skeletal muscle index less than 50 in men and skeletal muscle index less than 39 in women.
	Dual-energy x-ray absorptiometry (DXA) can be used to measure bone density as well as fat and fat-free mass.
	Single- and multiple-frequency bioelectrical impedance analysis approaches use a regression-derived equation to predict whole-body volumes and assume a linear relationship; bioimpedance spectroscopy devices use an approach based on biophysical modeling. Both are unproven in measuring fat and fat-free mass in the presence of fluid retention. A phase angle measurement may be predictive of outcomes in patients with liver disease; research suggests that a phase angle of 5.6 or lower in males and 5.4 or lower in females or 4.9 or less for any patient is associated with sarcopenia in patients with cirrhosis.[30]

Treatment of Chronic Liver Disease

Medical Management

Medical therapy for chronic liver disease aims to treat the underlying condition. As applicable, this may include alcohol cessation, weight loss (for those who are overweight or obese), treatment of viral hepatitis, and directed therapy for treatment of cholestatic liver disease or autoimmune liver disease. A loss of at least 3% to 5% of body weight appears necessary to improve steatosis, but a greater weight loss (up to 10%) may be needed to improve necroinflammation. Guidelines from the American Association for the Study of Liver Diseases provide up-to-date information on the treatment of specific conditions.[31] In select conditions, such as primary sclerosing cholangitis, advanced endoscopy is required (endoscopic retrograde cholangiopancreatography) for the management of bile duct strictures or cholangitis. In addition, several common strategies—varices surveillance, hepatocellular surveillance, and vaccination—target the complications of cirrhosis.

Varices Surveillance

Patients with cirrhosis should undergo screening for and treatment of esophageal varices at regular intervals. Esophageal varices are caused by reduced blood flow through the liver due to scarring. The blood is instead directed to the veins in the esophagus. Treatment includes nonselective β-blockers, endoscopic variceal ligation, or both.

Hepatocellular Carcinoma Surveillance

Patients with cirrhosis should also undergo screening for hepatocellular carcinoma every 6 months with an ultrasound and measurement of serum α-fetoprotein level. If cancer is suspected, multidisciplinary care should be initiated.

Vaccination

Patients with cirrhosis should be vaccinated against the hepatitis A and B viruses if indicated.

Surgical Management

General surgery is not a mainstay of the management of cirrhosis complications. However, often patients with decompensated cirrhosis may require surgery for management of symptomatic umbilical hernias or cholecystitis. The model for end-stage liver disease (MELD) score may assist in risk stratification and help assess the patient's risk of mortality. Predictive scores, such as the Mayo risk score and the VOCAL-Penn score (www.vocalpennscore.com), may serve as helpful guides.[32,33] Liver transplantation is the final surgical treatment for decompensated cirrhosis in selected individuals, and it requires referral to a transplant center.

Nutrition Management

Malnutrition is present in roughly 20% to 50% of patients with advanced liver disease, owing to inadequate nutrient intake often in the face of increased needs and malabsorption (see Figure 7.2 on page 114).[34] As discussed earlier, malnutrition and sarcopenia are associated with poor outcomes in patients with chronic liver disease and those awaiting liver transplantation as well as in posttransplant patients.[26,29] Providing adequate nutrition is essential for preventing and treating malnutrition, and nutrition can be delivered orally, enterally (tube feeding), or, sometimes, parenterally. Recent guidelines from the European Association for the Study of the Liver and the European Society for Clinical Nutrition and Metabolism offer recommendations for the management of nutrition in chronic liver disease.[26,35]

FIGURE 7.2 Causes of malnutrition in end-stage liver disease

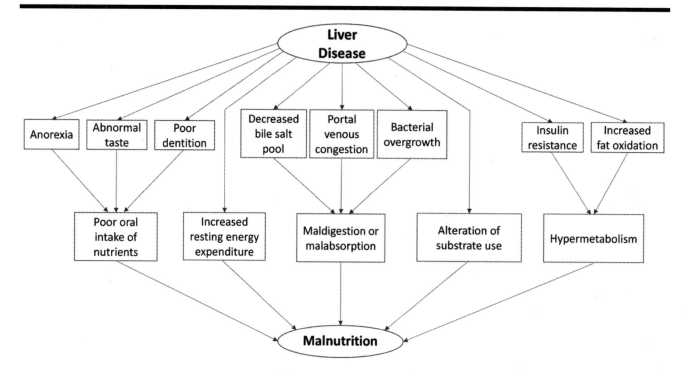

Reprinted with permission from Fallahzadeh MA, Rahimi RS. Hepatic encephalopathy and nutrition influences: a narrative review. *Nutr Clin Pract.* 2020;35(1):36-48.[34]

Nutrition Delivery

Oral nutrition is the first line of nutrition delivery for patients with chronic liver disease. The diet should be individualized to the patient based on the patient's presentation and symptoms, as well as on energy and protein needs in accordance with the patient's weight and nutritional status. Clinicians need to consider several factors, including barriers to food access and preparation, difficulties with GI symptoms (eg, nausea, vomiting, diarrhea, or constipation), early satiety, taste changes, and difficulties with chewing or swallowing. Once such factors have been identified, a comprehensive nutrition plan can be developed with the patient. In addition to diet, oral supplements in the form of shakes, bars, and commercial beverages can be recommended and are available in a variety of nutrient concentrations.

Whether because of nutrition or disease complications, if patients are unable to take adequate nutrient intake orally, enteral nutrition (EN) is the preferred form of nutrition support. Nasoenteric feeding tubes are usually the first choice for EN in patients with liver disease, certainly for short-term use, but also because gastrostomy and jejunostomy tubes are contraindicated in patients with decompensated cirrhosis and ascites. Box 7.2 describes EN access considerations for patients with chronic liver disease. A variety of EN formulas are available for use in this patient population, as summarized in Box 7.3 on page 116.[36]

BOX 7.2

Enteral Nutrition Access Options Specific to Patients With Chronic Liver Disease

Short-term (<30 d)

Nasogastric tube

Features	Available in a variety of sizes (usually 10 to 16 French [Fr] for adults)
	Can be used for delivery of medication, especially large-bore tubes
	Can also be used for suctioning stomach
	Can provide intermittent bolus feedings or continuous feedings
	Can provide larger volumes or osmolality in stomach vs small intestine
Cautions	Contraindicated in cases of high aspiration risk (eg, hepatic encephalopathy), gastrointestinal (GI) bleed, epistaxis, and severe esophagitis
	Not appropriate in cases of gastroparesis
	Caution with tube placement in cases of severe thrombocytopenia
	May cause irritation to nares

Nasointestinal tube

Features	Available in a variety of sizes (usually 10 to 12 Fr for adults) and lengths
	May reduce aspiration risk vs gastric delivery of feeding
	Requires pump infusion of formula
	Can be used in patients with gastroparesis
Cautions	Contraindicated in cases of GI bleed, epistaxis, and severe esophagitis
	Caution for tube placement in cases of severe thrombocytopenia
	Adequate water flushes and reduction or elimination of medication delivery via tube needed to maintain patency of small-bore tubes
	Possible contraindications to providing into small bowel if used for medication delivery
	Small intestine sensitive to volume and osmolality of formula
	Cannot provide bolus feedings into small intestine; must be continuous feeding
	May cause irritation to nares

Long-term (>30 d)

Gastrostomy

Features	Can be used for delivery of medication, especially larger bore tubes
	Can also be used for suctioning stomach
	May provide improved patient comfort compared with tubes inserted in nasal passage
	Can provide intermittent bolus feedings or continuous feedings
	Can provide larger volumes or osmolality in stomach vs small intestine

Box continues

BOX 7.2 (CONTINUED)

Cautions	Contraindicated with ascites, GI bleed
	Caution for use in cases of high aspiration risk (eg, hepatic encephalopathy)
	Caution for tube placement in cases of severe thrombocytopenia
	Risk of infection around gastrostomy site
	Not appropriate in cases of gastroparesis

Jejunostomy

Features	May reduce aspiration risk vs gastric delivery of feeding
	Requires pump infusion of formula
	Can be used in patients with gastroparesis
Cautions	Contraindicated with ascites, GI bleed
	Caution for tube placement in cases of severe thrombocytopenia
	Cannot provide bolus feedings into small intestine; must be continuous feeding

Gastrojejunostomy

Features	Gastrostomy port: useful for delivery of medications or gastric suctioning
	Jejunostomy port: useful for continuous feedings in cases of high-aspiration risk or gastroparesis; requires pump
Cautions	Contraindicated with ascites, GI bleed
	Caution for tube placement in cases of severe thrombocytopenia

BOX 7.3

Enteral Nutrition Formula Options for Patients With Chronic Liver Disease

Standard intact protein (polymeric)

Requires normal digestion

Available in a variety of protein and calorie concentrations

Low cost

Nutrient-dense polymeric

Requires normal digestion

Generally available as 1.5 to 2.0 kcal/mL concentrations

Useful in patients requiring fluid restriction (eg, patients with hypervolemic hyponatremia, fluid retention, reduced urine output, early satiety issues, high nutritional requirements)

Low cost

Box continues

BOX 7.3 (CONTINUED)

Semi-elemental or partially hydrolyzed

Useful in patients with impaired digestion

Available in a variety of protein and calorie concentrations

Often contains peptides or medium-chain triglycerides, or both

Moderate cost

Elemental

Useful when digestion is impaired or a very low-fat formula is preferred

Contains amino acids and dextrose (vs whole proteins and starches)

Usually high in carbohydrates, which could contribute to hyperglycemia in patients with insulin impairment

Usually hypertonic, which can reduce tolerance

High cost

Renal

Requires normal digestion

Useful in patients with renal dysfunction and hyperkalemia or hyperphosphatemia

Usually fluid-restricted with reduced amounts of potassium and phosphorus

Available in formulations for patients requiring dialysis and for patients with renal failure not undergoing dialysis

Moderate cost

Immuno-enhancing

Requires normal digestion

Has not been shown to be beneficial in patients with liver disease

Usually contains immune-enhancing nutrients, such as fish oil, arginine, RNA

May affect insulin sensitivity and satiety

May temporarily increase serum ammonia levels but does not worsen symptoms of hepatic encephalopathy

High cost

Branched-chain amino acid (BCAA)

Controversial as to benefit, but American and European guidelines suggest consideration of BCAA formulas in patients with encephalopathy refractory to other treatments or with a protein intolerance

Contains higher proportion of BCAAs and reduced amounts of aromatic amino acids and methionine

Usually with reduced electrolyte content

High cost

Adapted with permission from Hasse JM, DiCecco SR. Enteral nutrition in chronic liver disease: translating evidence into practice. Nutr Clin Pract. 2015;30(4):474-487.[36]

Parenteral nutrition (PN) is restricted to patients with dysfunctional GI tracts, such as with GI bleed, ileus, fistulas, short bowel syndrome, or other conditions warranting avoidance of EN. Alternative intravenous lipid emulsions, such as those containing either a mixture of soybean oil, medium-chain triglycerides, olive oil, and fish oil or a mixture of olive oil and soybean oil, can be preferentially used, as they tend to be less inflammatory and perhaps less harmful to the liver than traditional omega-6 fatty acid intravenous lipid emulsions.[37] PN can be concentrated and given via a central venous catheter for patients requiring fluid restriction; nutrients should be individualized to the patient's requirements and conditions. Because peripheral PN has a limit on osmolarity (usually approximately 900 mOsm/L),[38] it typically requires an increased volume that may not be suitable for patients with liver disease and fluid overload.

Nutrient Requirements

Regardless of the delivery route of nutrition, nutrient needs are altered with chronic liver disease. The macronutrient and micronutrient requirements of patients with chronic liver disease depend on the type of liver disease, comorbid conditions, nutritional status, goals of care, level of metabolic stress, and presence of malabsorption. Patients who have had weight reduction surgery are at risk for nutrient losses depending on the type of surgery they underwent. Clinicians may want to evaluate nutrient levels in any patient at risk of deficiencies before prescribing vitamin or mineral therapies.

In general, a daily energy intake of 30 to 35 kcal/kg of body weight (for nonobese patients) and a daily protein intake of 1 to 1.5 g/kg of body weight should be targeted, based on individual tolerance and needs. Periodic meals are recommended along with a late evening snack. The importance of maintaining muscle mass should be discussed, along with the associated recommendations for increased physical activity and exercise. In patients with suspected or established deficiencies, micronutrients and vitamins should be supplemented. Box 7.4 summarizes the general macronutrient requirements for individuals with chronic liver disease.[39] Box 7.5 lists the micronutrient (vitamin and mineral) deficits associated with decompensated liver disease.[40]

BOX 7.4

General Macronutrient Considerations for Individuals With Chronic Liver Disease

Protein

Estimated needs	1.0 to 1.5 g/kg/d Up to 2 g/kg/d for critical illness
Comments	Estimated need depends on nutritional status and comorbidities. Consider using dry weight or ideal body weight if patient is fluid-overloaded. Protein restriction is *not* recommended, as it leads to muscle loss and does not improve outcomes. Protein can be lost with paracentesis.

Energy

Estimated needs	Usually 20% to 50% above basal energy expenditure 30 to 35 kcal/kg/d (for individuals who are nonobese)
Comments	Estimated need depends on nutritional status and losses. Indirect calorimetry is the most accurate way to determine actual energy needs. Energy-intake restriction may be required for weight loss in patients with obesity.

Box continues

BOX 7.4 (CONTINUED)

Fat

Estimated needs	As needed to provide adequate energy
Comments	Patients with cholestatic liver disease may experience fat malabsorption.

Carbohydrate

Estimated needs	Controlled carbohydrate intake if patient has diabetes mellitus or insulin resistance; carbohydrate-restricted diet as an alternative for weight loss, especially in patients with nonalcoholic fatty liver disease Frequent meals and late-evening snack to prevent hypoglycemia
Comments	Patients with liver disease or obesity may have insulin resistance and hyperglycemia. In patients with severe or acute liver failure, hypoglycemia may ensue if the liver is unable to store glycogen or undergo gluconeogenesis.

Sodium

Estimated needs	2 g/d
Comments	Use if the patient has fluid retention.

Fluid

Estimated needs	Restrict to 1,000 to 1,500 mL/d
Comments	Use if the patient has hypervolemic hyponatremia.

Adapted with permission from Hasse JM, Gautam M. Nutrition support of patients with cirrhosis. In: Eghtesad B, Fung F, eds. Surgical Procedures on the Cirrhotic Patient. Springer International; 2017:71-88.39

BOX 7.5

Vitamin and Mineral Deficits Associated With Decompensated Liver Disease

	Predisposing factors	Signs of deficiency
Vitamin A	Steatorrhea, neomycin use, cholestyramine use, alcoholism	Night blindness, increased infection risk
Vitamin B1 (thiamin)	Alcoholism, high-carbohydrate diet	Neuropathy, ascites, edema, central nervous system dysfunction

Box continues

BOX 7.5 (CONTINUED)

	Predisposing factors	Signs of deficiency
Vitamin B3 (niacin)	Alcoholism	Dermatitis, dementia, diarrhea, inflammation of mucous membranes
Vitamin B6 (pyridoxine)	Alcoholism	Mucous membrane lesions, seborrheic dermatitis, glossitis, angular stomatitis, blepharitis, peripheral neuropathy, microcytic anemia, depression
Vitamin B12 (cyanocobalamin)	Alcoholism, cholestyramine use	Megaloblastic anemia, glossitis, central nervous system dysfunction
Folate	Alcoholism	Megaloblastic anemia, glossitis, irritability
Vitamin D	Steatorrhea, glucocorticoid use, cholestyramine use	Osteomalacia, rickets (in children), possible link to cancer or autoimmune disorders
Vitamin E	Steatorrhea, cholestyramine use	Peripheral neuropathy, ataxia, skeletal myopathy, retinopathy, immune system impairment
Vitamin K	Steatorrhea, antibiotic use, cholestyramine use	Excessive bleeding, bruising
Iron	Chronic bleeding	Stomatitis, microcytic anemia, malaise
Magnesium	Alcoholism, diuretic use	Neuromuscular irritability, hypokalemia, hypocalcemia
Phosphorus	Anabolism, alcoholism	Anorexia, weakness, cardiac failure, glucose intolerance
Selenium	Hepatitis C, impaired metabolism of selenomethionine	Insulin resistance, cardiomyopathy
Zinc	Diarrhea, diuretic use, alcoholism	Immunodeficiency, impaired taste acuity, delayed wound healing, impaired protein synthesis

Adapted with permission from Hasse JM, Matarese LE. Medical nutrition therapy for hepatobiliary and pancreatic disorders. In: Mahan LK, Raymond JL, eds. Krause's Food and the Nutrition Care Process. 14th ed. Elsevier; 2017:560-585.[40]

Patients should be cautioned against taking dietary or herbal supplements because many supplements may create drug-nutrient interactions or cause harm due to the hepatotoxic effects of ingredients. Some herbal supplements have been studied for their benefits in liver disease. S-adenosyl-L-methionine (SAMe) acts as a methyl donor for methylation reactions and participates in glutathione (an antioxidant) synthesis. Although SAMe may improve liver function, it has not been shown to improve chronic liver disease outcomes.[41] Milk thistle, with the active component being a flavonoid called silymarin, is the most popular and extensively studied herb in relation to liver disease. It is purported to have anti-inflammatory, antioxidant, and antifibrotic properties; however, meta-analyses have not found benefit in liver disease other than to lower liver function levels.[42,43] See Chapter 24 for more on nutraceuticals and dietary supplements.

Complications of Liver Disease and Suggested Treatments

Selected subsets of patients require further attention. Nutrition therapies, nutrient requirements, and delivery of nutrition may need to be adjusted according to the complications from chronic liver disease that are present.

Esophageal Varices and Gastrointestinal Bleed

Patients with cirrhosis are at risk for portal hypertension, esophageal varices, and variceal bleeding. Oral nutrition and EN should be withheld during active GI bleeding. Patients who have undergone endoscopic variceal ligation may have some difficulty swallowing, in which case they may best tolerate soft and liquid foods. Nasoenteric feeding tube placement usually needs to be deferred for several days after ligation. In patients who have not had ligation, the placement of a nasoenteric feeding tube is acceptable.

Fluid Retention

A low-sodium diet (<2,000 mg/d) is a mainstay of the nutrition treatment of ascites and edema. Restricting sodium any further can be counterproductive in that it may overly restrict energy and protein intakes. Adequate protein is needed to maintain normal oncotic pressure and to replace protein that may be lost in ascitic fluid removed during paracentesis. In addition, patients with fluid retention may need potassium restriction or supplementation, depending on their diuretic use. In cases of ascites that are not controlled with dietary modifications, scheduled large-volume paracentesis may be needed. Patients with refractory ascites may require a transjugular intrahepatic portosystemic shunt.[44]

Hepatic Encephalopathy

The management of hepatic encephalopathy involves identifying and managing the precipitants and treating the patient with lactulose and rifaximin. Protein restriction is *not* recommended for patients with hepatic encephalopathy. In fact, protein restriction often leads to loss of muscle mass, which limits the conversion of ammonia to glutamine in the muscle (see Figure 7.3 on page 122).[34] In addition, prolonged periods of fasting should be avoided to reduce proteolysis. Small frequent meals along with a late nighttime snack may be helpful.[45]

Branched-chain amino acid (BCAA; ie, leucine, isoleucine, and valine) supplementation has been purported to ameliorate hepatic encephalopathy. Elevated serum levels of aromatic amino acids (AAAs) have been observed in patients with chronic liver disease, whereas BCAA levels fall. A BCAA-to-AAA ratio of less than three increases the transfer of AAAs across the blood-brain barrier, where they act as false neurotransmitters.[34] A Cochrane

FIGURE 7.3 Hepatic encephalopathy interaction with frailty and sarcopenia

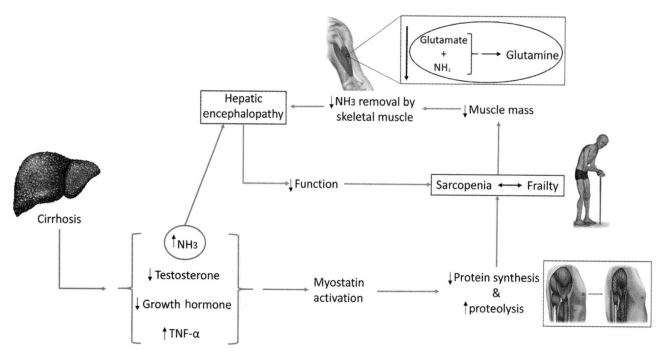

NH$_3$ = ammonia

TNF-α = tumor necrosis factor α

Reprinted with permission from Fallahzadeh MA, Rahimi RS. Hepatic encephalopathy and nutrition influences: a narrative review. *Nutr Clin Pract*. 2020;35(1):36-48.[34]

review of BCAA supplementation concluded that, compared with no intervention, the use of BCAA supplements may improve hepatic encephalopathy but does not affect nutritional status, quality of life, or mortality.[46] Barriers to their use include poor long-term compliance and high cost.

The administration of prebiotics and probiotics may play a role in reducing hepatic encephalopathy as well.[47,48] Finally, zinc supplementation should be considered, especially for patients with a zinc deficiency, as zinc acts as a cofactor for two urea-cycle enzymes and glutamine synthetase, which contribute to ammonia removal in muscle and liver. In hospitalized patients with hepatic encephalopathy who require prolonged intubation, EN should be considered.

Hyponatremia

Hyponatremia, which is determined by a serum sodium level below 135 mEq/L, may have multiple causes in patients in cirrhosis. On one hand, patients with cirrhosis are prone to volume depletion, which can lead to hypovolemic hyponatremia. In this case, expansion of fluid status and temporarily stopping any offending agents (eg, diuretics) may be crucial. On the other hand, as liver disease advances, patients may develop hypervolemic hyponatremia. In this case, restricting fluids to 1 to 1.5 L/d may be required, in addition to sodium restriction. The focus should be on restricting nonnutritional "free water" items, such as water, coffee, tea, juices, lemonade, and soft drinks. Allowing nutrient-dense oral nutrition supplements outside of the fluid restriction is often necessary to ensure adequate nutrient intake.

Glucose Abnormalities

Many patients with NAFLD, as well as patients with hepatitis C, develop insulin resistance and hyperglycemia. In patients with severe or acute liver failure, hypoglycemia may ensue as a result of the inability of the liver to store glycogen or undergo gluconeogenesis. Carbohydrate-controlled diets are appropriate for patients with hyperglycemia or diabetes mellitus and can be carefully considered for patients who need to lose weight. Small, frequent meals lessen hypoglycemic events and reduce proteolysis.

Kidney Dysfunction and Metabolic Alterations

If a patient has kidney dysfunction or electrolyte disturbances, dietary restrictions of potassium may become necessary. Hyperphosphatemia can be addressed with the addition of phosphate binders. Fluid requirements should be individualized depending on each patient's fluid status.

Bone Disease

Bone loss and osteoporosis may be common in patients with chronic liver disease, especially in those with cholestatic liver disease or those receiving long-term corticosteroid therapy. After appropriate diagnosis using bone densitometry, supplementation with calcium (1,000–1,500 mg/d) and vitamin D (≥1,000–1,500 mg/d if the patient is deficient) should be considered, along with bisphosphonates in patients with osteoporosis. In addition, alcohol intake and smoking should be discouraged, and patients should be encouraged to engage in weight-bearing exercise.

Summary

Malnutrition and nutritional disorders are common in individuals with chronic liver disease; therefore, consultation with an RDN is essential. A nutrition assessment is necessary to determine the degree of malnutrition, sarcopenia, and frailty, and to identify nutrient deficits in order to develop a nutrition plan. Some of the main goals for patients with chronic liver disease are to eat frequent meals and snacks, include high-protein foods, limit sodium intake, avoid alcohol, implement an exercise plan, and avoid dietary or herbal supplements. Nutrition meal plans for patients with chronic liver disease have been described in the literature,[49] and nutrition support may be required when oral intake is not adequate.

References

1. Mokdad AA, Lopez AD, Shahraz S, et al. Liver cirrhosis mortality in 187 countries between 1980 and 2010: a systematic analysis. *BMC Med.* 2014;12:145. doi:10.1186/s12916-014-0145-y
2. Asrani SK, Devarbhavi H, Eaton J, Kamath PS. Burden of liver diseases in the world. *J Hepatol.* 2019;70(1):151-171. doi:10.1016/j.jhep.2018.09.014
3. Asrani SK, Larson JJ, Yawn B, Therneau TM, Kim WR. Underestimation of liver-related mortality in the United States. *Gastroenterology.* 2013;145(2):375-382.e1-2. doi:10.1053/j.gastro.2013.04.005
4. Tapper EB, Parikh ND. Mortality due to cirrhosis and liver cancer in the United States, 1999-2016: observational study. *BMJ.* 2018;362:k2817. doi:10.1136/bmj.k2817
5. GBD 2017 Cirrhosis Collaborators. The global, regional, and national burden of cirrhosis by cause in 195 countries and territories, 1990-2017: a systematic analysis for the Global Burden of Disease Study 2017. *Lancet Gastroenterol Hepatol.* 2020;5(3):245-266. doi:10.1016/S2468-1253(19)30349-8

6. Stepanova M, De Avila L, Afendy M, et al. Direct and indirect economic burden of chronic liver disease in the United States. *Clin Gastroenterol Hepatol*. 2017 May;15(5):759-766.e5. doi:10.1016/j.cgh.2016.07.020

7. Onakpoya IJ, Heneghan CJ, Aronson JK. Post-marketing withdrawal of 462 medicinal products because of adverse drug reactions: a systematic review of the world literature. *BMC Med*. 2016;14:10. doi:10.1186/s12916-016-0553-2

8. Peery AF, Crockett SD, Barritt AS, et al. Burden of gastrointestinal, liver, and pancreatic diseases in the United States. *Gastroenterology*. 2015;149:1731-1741. e1733. doi:10.1053/j.gastro.2018.08.063

9. Chalasani N, Bjornsson E. Risk factors for idiosyncratic drug-induced liver injury. *Gastroenterology*. 2010;138:2246-2259. doi:10.1053/j.gastro.2010.04 .001

10. GBD 2016 Alcohol Collaborators. Alcohol use and burden for 195 countries and territories, 1990-2016: a systematic analysis for the Global Burden of Disease Study 2016. *Lancet*. 2018;392:1015-1035. doi:10.1016 /S0140-6736(18)31310-2

11. World Health Organization. *Global Status Report on Alcohol and Health 2018*. World Health Organization; 2018. Accessed March 5, 2021. https://apps.who.int /iris/handle/10665/274603

12. Browning JD, Szczepaniak LS, Dobbins R, et al. Prevalence of hepatic steatosis in an urban population in the United States: impact of ethnicity. *Hepatology*. 2004;40:1387-1395. doi:10.1002/hep.20466

13. Kanwal F, Kramer JR, Duan Z, Yu X, White D, El-Serag HB. Trends in the burden of nonalcoholic fatty liver disease in a United States cohort of veterans. *Clin Gastroenterol Hepatol*. 2016;14:301-308.e1-2. doi:10 .1016/j.cgh.2015.08.010

14. Younossi ZM, Koenig AB, Abdelatif D, Fazel Y, Henry L, Wymer M. Global epidemiology of nonalcoholic fatty liver disease: meta-analytic assessment of prevalence, incidence, and outcomes. *Hepatology*. 2016;64:73-84. doi:10.1002/hep.28431

15. Seki Y, Kakizaki S, Horiguchi N, et al. Prevalence of nonalcoholic steatohepatitis in Japanese patients with morbid obesity undergoing bariatric surgery. *J Gastroenterol*. 2016;51:281-289. doi:10.1007/s00535 -015-1114-8

16. Forlani G, Giorda C, Manti R, et al. The burden of NAFLD and its characteristics in a nationwide population with type 2 diabetes. *J Diabetes Res*. 2016;2016:2931985. doi:10.1155/2016/2931985

17. Zhang X, Heredia NI, Balakrishnan M, Thrift AP. Prevalence and factors associated with NAFLD detected by vibration controlled transient elastography among US adults: Results from NHANES 2017-2018. *PLoS One*. 2021;16(6):e0252164. doi:10 .1371/journal.pone.0252164

18. Lazo M, Hernaez R, Eberhardt MS, et al. Prevalence of nonalcoholic fatty liver disease in the United States: the Third National Health and Nutrition Examination Survey, 1988-1994. *Am J Epidemiol*. 2013;178(1):38-45. doi:10.1093/aje/kws448

19. Albhaisi S, Chowdhury A, Sanyal AJ. Non-alcoholic fatty liver disease in lean individuals. *JHEP Rep*. 2019;1(4):329-341. doi:10.1016/j.jhepr.2019.08.002

20. Elliott TR, Symes T, Kannourakis G, Angus P. Resolution of norfloxacin-induced acute liver failure after *N*-acetylcysteine therapy: further support for the use of NAC in drug-induced ALF? *BMJ Case Rep*. 2016;2016:bcr2015213189. doi:10.1136/bcr-2015 -213189

21. Blum HE. History and global burden of viral hepatitis. *Dig Dis*. 2016;34:293-302. doi:10.1159/000444466

22. Platt L, Easterbrook P, Gower E, et al. Prevalence and burden of HCV co-infection in people living with HIV: a global systematic review and meta-analysis. *Lancet Infect Dis*. 2016;16:797-808. doi:10.1016/S1473 -3099(15)00485-5

23. Stanaway JD, Flaxman AD, Naghavi M, et al. The global burden of viral hepatitis from 1990 to 2013: findings from the Global Burden of Disease Study 2013. *Lancet*. 2016;388:1081-1088. doi:10.1016/S0140 -6736(16)30579-7

24. European Association for Study of Liver; Asociacion Latinoamericana para el Estudio del Higado. EASL-ALEH Clinical Practice Guidelines: non-invasive tests for evaluation of liver disease severity and prognosis. *J Hepatol*. 2015;63(1):237-264. doi:10.1016/j.jhep .2015.04.006

25. Kim WR, Biggins SW, Kremers WK, et al. Hyponatremia and mortality among patients on the liver-transplant waiting list. *N Engl J Med*. 2008;359:1018-1026. doi:10 .1056/NEJMoa0801209

26. European Association for the Study of the Liver. EASL Clinical Practice Guidelines on nutrition in chronic liver disease. *J Hepatol*. 2019;70(1):172-193. doi:10.1016/j .jhep.2018.06.024

27. Tandon P, Raman M, Mourtzakis M, Merli M. A practical approach to nutritional screening and assessment in cirrhosis. *Hepatology*. 2017;65:1044-1057. doi:10.1002 /hep.29003

28. Mazurak VC, Tandon P, Montano-Loza AJ. Nutrition and the transplant candidate. *Liver Transpl*. 2017;23:1451-1464. doi:10.1002/lt.24848

29. Ebadi M, Bhanji RA, Mazurak VC, et al. Sarcopenia in cirrhosis: from pathogenesis to interventions. *J Gastroenterol*. 2019;54:845–859. doi:10.1007 /s00535-019-01605-6

30. Ruiz-Margáin A, Xie JJ, Román-Calleja BM, et al. Phase angle from bioelectrical impedance for the assessment of sarcopenia in cirrhosis with or without ascites. *Clin Gastroenterol Hepatol*. 2021;19(9):1941-1949.e2. doi:10.1016/j.cgh.2020.08.066

31. American Association for the Study of Liver Disease. Practice Guidelines. Accessed January 25, 2022. www .aasld.org/publications/practice-guidelines

32. Mahmud N, Fricker Z, Hubbard RA, et al. Risk prediction models for post-operative mortality in patients with cirrhosis. *Hepatology*. 2021;73:204-218. doi:10.1002/hep.31558

33. Teh SH, Nagorney DM, Stevens SR, et al. Risk factors for mortality after surgery in patients with cirrhosis. *Gastroenterology.* 2007;132(4):1261-1269. doi:10.1053/j.gastro.2007.01.040

34. Fallahzadeh MA, Rahimi RS. Hepatic encephalopathy and nutrition influences: a narrative review. *Nutr Clin Pract.* 2020;35(1):36-48. doi:10.1002/ncp.10458

35. Bischoff SC, Bernal W, Dasarathy S, et al. ESPEN practical guideline: clinical nutrition in liver disease. *Clin Nutr.* 2020;39(12):3533-3562. doi:10.1016/j.clnu.2020.09.001

36. Hasse JM, DiCecco SR. Enteral nutrition in chronic liver disease: translating evidence into practice. *Nutr Clin Pract.* 2015;30(4):474-487.

37. Mirtallo JM, Ayers P, Boullata J, et al. ASPEN lipid injectable emulsion safety recommendations, part 1: background and adult considerations. *Nutr Clin Pract.* 2020;35(5):769-782. doi:10.1002/ncp.10496

38. Worthington P, Balint J, Bechtold M, et al. When is parenteral nutrition appropriate? *JPEN J Parenter Enteral Nutr.* 2017;41(3):324-377. doi:10.1177/0148607117695251

39. Hasse JM, Gautam M. Nutrition support of patients with cirrhosis. In: Eghtesad B, Fung F, eds. *Surgical Procedures on the Cirrhotic Patient.* Springer International; 2017:71-88.

40. Hasse JM, Matarese LE. Medical nutrition therapy for hepatobiliary and pancreatic disorders. In: Mahan LK, Raymond JL, eds. *Krause's Food and the Nutrition Care Process.* 14th ed. Elsevier; 2017:560-585.

41. Guo T, Chang L, Xiao Y, Liu Q. S-adenosyl-L-methionine for the treatment of chronic liver disease: a systematic review and meta-analysis. *PLoS One.* 2015;10(3):e0122124. doi:10.1371/journal.pone.0122124

42. de Avelar CR, Pereira EM, de Farias Costa PR, de Jesus RP, de Oliveira LPM. Effect of silymarin on biochemical indicators in patients with liver disease: systematic review with meta-analysis. *World J Gastroenterol.* 2017;23(27):5004-5017. doi:10.3748/wjg.v23.i27.5004

43. Zhong S, Fan Y, Yan Q, et al. The therapeutic effect of silymarin in the treatment of nonalcoholic fatty disease: a meta-analysis (PRISMA) of randomized control trials. *Medicine (Baltimore).* 2017;96(49):e9061. doi:10.1097/MD.0000000000009061

44. Tsien C, Shah SN, McCullough AJ, Dasarathy S. Reversal of sarcopenia predicts survival after a transjugular intrahepatic portosystemic stent. *Eur J Gastroenterol Hepatol.* 2013;25(1):85-93. doi:10.1097/MEG.0b013e328359a759

45. Tsien CD, McCullough AJ, Dasarathy S. Late evening snack: exploiting a period of anabolic opportunity in cirrhosis. *J Gastroenterol Hepatol.* 2012;27(3):430-441. doi:10.1111/j.1440-1746.2011.06951.x

46. Gluud LL, Dam G, Les I, et al. Branched-chain amino acids for people with hepatic encephalopathy. *Cochrane Database Syst Rev.* 2017;5(5):CD001939. doi:10.1002/14651858.CD001939.pub4

47. Dalal R, McGee RG, Riordan SM, Webster AC. Probiotics for people with hepatic encephalopathy. *Cochrane Database Syst Rev.* 2017;2(2):CD008716. doi:10.1002/14651858.CD008716.pub3

48. Holte K, Krag A, Gluud LL. Systematic review and meta-analysis of randomized trials on probiotics for hepatic encephalopathy. *Hepatol Res.* 2012;42(10):1008-1015. doi:10.1111/j.1872-034X.2012.01015.x

49. Shaw J, Tate V, Hanson J, Bajaj JS. What diet should I recommend my patient with hepatic encephalopathy? *Curr Hepatol Rep.* 2020;19(1):13-22. doi:10.1007/s11901-020-00510-4

8

Pancreatic Disease

Arlene Stein, MS, RD, CDN, CNSC
James H. Grendell, MD

KEY POINTS

- The pancreas is a complex organ that performs both endocrine and exocrine functions.
- Nutritional status and diet affect the function of the pancreas, and diseases of the pancreas generally require dietary interventions for symptom management.
- Nutrition interventions vary for acute or chronic pancreatitis but may include diet, enteral nutrition, or parenteral nutrition, along with probiotics and enzyme replacement.

Introduction

The pancreas, a gland lying posterior to the stomach and alongside the duodenum, performs both exocrine and endocrine functions. As a master digestive gland of the body, the pancreas secretes up to 2 L of protein-rich and bicarbonate-rich clear fluid into the duodenum each day. The pancreas is responsible for producing and secreting:

- the digestive enzymes necessary for the digestion of macronutrients into forms that can be either absorbed directly by enterocytes or acted upon further by enterocyte brush border enzymes;
- the bicarbonate that is necessary for the optimal environment in the small intestine for the activity of pancreatic digestive enzymes and bile salts; and
- the hormones insulin and glucagon, which are essential for glucose homeostasis.

The release of enzymes and bicarbonate secretions are controlled by various neuro-humoral factors, including the hormones gastrin and secretin. Neuropeptides involved in pancreatic function include somatostatin, vasopressin (vasoactive intestinal polypeptide), and gastrin-releasing peptide (bombesin). Endocrine functions involving the secretion of insulin and glucagon are critical for the metabolism of glucose, fatty acids, and amino acids. When the normal processes of digestion and absorption are interrupted, the resulting signs and symptoms of pancreatitis occur.

Pancreatitis can be classified as either acute or chronic and designated as mild, moderate, or severe using a variety of guidelines. Signs and symptoms include abdominal pain radiating to the back, nausea, vomiting, and steatorrhea. This chapter focuses on nutritional considerations for patients with acute pancreatitis and pancreatic exocrine insufficiency (PEI). PEI in cystic fibrosis is covered in depth in Chapter 9, and pancreatic cancer is addressed in Chapter 10.

The Role of Nutrition in Pancreatic Function

The pancreas depends on the overall nutritional state of the body for its growth and function. It grows in parallel to general body growth and atrophies in the absence of food.[1] Feeding increases the rate of synthesis and secretion of digestive enzymes. The content and secretion of major digestive enzymes change in proportion to the dietary content of their respective substrates (carbohydrate, fat, and protein) over 5 to 7 days, primarily because of changes in the mRNA levels for these enzymes. Ingestion of large amounts of amino acids or proteins stimulates pancreatic growth.[2,3]

Hormones (eg, cholecystokinin, secretin, gastrin, insulin, insulin-like growth factor 1) and neurotransmitters mediate trophic effects of feeding, whereas neuropeptide Y and somatostatin inhibit pancreatic growth. In response to injury or surgical resection, dietary protein, cholecystokinin, insulin, and insulin-like growth factor 1 seem to be of primary importance in pancreatic regeneration.[4] Box 8.1 summarizes the potential effects of nutrition on the pancreas.

BOX 8.1 Effects of Nutrition on the Pancreas	The pancreas atrophies in the absence of food. Ingesting large amounts of amino acids or proteins stimulates pancreatic growth. Feeding increases the rate of synthesis and secretion of digestive enzymes. The content and secretion of digestive enzymes change in response to diet composition. Dietary protein, cholecystokinin, insulin, and insulin-like growth factor 1 are of primary importance in pancreatic repair and regeneration after injury or surgery.

Clinical Presentation of Acute Pancreatitis

Acute pancreatitis is an acute inflammatory process of the pancreas with variable involvement of peripancreatic tissue or remote organ systems (eg, kidneys, lungs). It ranges in severity from a mild, self-limited disease to a catastrophic one with multiple severe complications and the risk of death. Although acute pancreatitis has a number of potential causes, biliary tract obstruction and chronic excessive alcohol use account for the majority of cases. Some medications, such as diuretics (furosemide) or antibiotics (tetracycline), trauma, or surgery can lead to acute pancreatitis. For patients with acute pancreatitis, the two immediate concerns are reducing the metabolic work of the pancreas and meeting the nutritional needs of the patient.

Oral Nutrition Management

The presence of gastric acid, fats, amino acids, and peptides in the proximal duodenum stimulates the pancreas to synthesize and secrete digestive enzymes, thus increasing the metabolic work of an already inflamed gland. For this reason, oral intake is initially prohibited for acute pancreatitis on hospital admission.[5,6]

Patients with mild acute pancreatitis may be able to resume oral feeding as early as 24 hours from the onset of symptoms.[7] However, they still require intravenous hydration and electrolytes. Oral feeding can resume once patients experience an improvement in symptoms (eg, a reduction in abdominal pain and nausea). Oral feeding can be initiated with a low-fat solid diet rather than with clear liquids, which will allow the patient to reach nutrition goals sooner and shorten the length of hospitalization.[5,6,8]

Patients with severe acute pancreatitis often have a prolonged course involving organ failure and other complications, leading to extended stays in an intensive care unit. Nutrition support is often required for these patients. See Box 8.2 on page 128 for a summary of nutrition care considerations in severe acute pancreatitis. The following sections elaborate on some of the main issues.

Nutrition Support

Historically, treatment for acute pancreatitis included *complete* bowel rest for an extended period of time and, therefore, parenteral nutrition (PN) was often required. However, enteral feeding into the jejunum provides minimal stimulation of pancreatic secretion because the hormonal and neural factors resulting in meal-related stimulation of the pancreas are primarily located in the proximal duodenum. Prospective, randomized studies have demonstrated no improvement in survival in patients receiving PN compared to those receiving enteral nutrition (EN) through a nasojejunal feeding tube. Patients receiving EN had fewer complications, particularly less line sepsis, and EN was considerably less costly than PN.[9-11]

Because EN is more physiologic and may decrease the translocation of bacteria from the gastrointestinal (GI) tract into areas of pancreatic necrosis, initiation of EN within 24 to 48 hours of hospital admission has been advocated with the goals of modulating the acute stress response, promoting more rapid resolution of the disease process, and maintaining the integrity of the intestinal mucosa.[12] A multicenter, randomized trial, however, did not show the superiority of early nasoenteric tube feeding, as compared with an oral diet after 72 hours, in reducing the rate of infection or death in patients with acute pancreatitis at high risk for complications.[13] PN should be reserved for patients who do not tolerate EN (eg, due to severe ileus), when an enteral feeding tube cannot be placed, or when nutrition goals cannot be met within 7 to 10 days of initiating EN.[14]

Jejunal and Gastric Feedings

If an operation is being performed for a major complication of acute pancreatitis, placement of a jejunal feeding tube is often beneficial because the duration of time until oral feeding can be resumed is often difficult to predict. Because nasojejunal feeding tubes are harder to place than nasogastric tubes and more likely to migrate, studies have been done to determine whether the same results could be obtained with nasogastric feeding as with jejunal feeding. A 2016 meta-analysis including a total of 446 participants showed no significant difference between groups receiving gastric feeding and groups receiving jejunal feeding in terms of risk of mortality, infectious complications, pain, diarrhea, need for surgical intervention, feeding intolerance, and energy balance.[15]

Elemental or Semielemental vs Polymeric Feeding Solutions

A meta-analysis involving up to 20 randomized controlled studies did not demonstrate a difference in feeding intolerance, infectious complications, or death for patients fed lower-cost polymeric formulas compared to patients fed elemental or semielemental formulas.[16] Current data are limited; however, a 2018 study from Japan suggests that there is no clinical benefit to using elemental formulas over semielemental and polymeric formulas.[17]

Resumption of Oral Feeding

Oral feeding for patients with severe acute pancreatitis should be initiated once complications have been successfully treated and the patient is no longer experiencing substantial pain or nausea. If oral feeding is not initially tolerated, it should be suspended for 1 to 2 days and then retried. If it is still not tolerated, it should again be suspended and an evaluation performed for potential problems (eg, walled-off pancreatic necrosis, pseudocyst) that may be preventing the patient from eating.

Probiotics and Immunonutrition

Probiotics have been studied as a way to reduce the incidence of infectious complications for patients with acute pancreatitis. However, one large randomized controlled study of a multispecies probiotic product demonstrated that patients treated with the probiotic had increased mortality due to bowel ischemia.[18] A more recent systematic review and meta-analysis looked at six trials, with a total of 536 patients analyzed. Probiotics showed neither beneficial nor adverse effects on the clinical outcomes of patients with severe acute pancreatitis. The authors concluded that carefully designed clinical trials are needed to validate the effects of particular probiotics given at specific dosages and for specific treatment durations.[19] Until there is more evidence, the use of probiotics in patients with acute pancreatitis cannot be recommended.

Immunomodulating diets are nutrition formulations supplemented with increased amounts of nutrients that have been shown to modulate inflammation and improve immune function. These nutrients include arginine, glutamine, omega-3 fatty acids (eg, fish oil), and antioxidants. The use of immunomodulating diets in critically ill patients is controversial.[5] These feeding formulas may seem theoretically appealing for the treatment of patients with acute pancreatitis, but a meta-analysis concluded that immunomodulating diets did not reduce infectious complications, mortality, or length of hospital stay.[20] Clinicians should also consider that immunonutrition formulas are substantially more expensive than standard enteral formulas. Current evidence does not support the use of immunoenhanced nutrients.[21]

Nutrient Needs

The nutrient needs of the patient with acute pancreatitis depend on the severity of the pancreatitis and other comorbidities. See Box 8.3 on page 130 for a summary of nutrient needs for patients with acute pancreatitis.

Energy

The patient's resting energy expenditure is substantially increased if there is sepsis or multi-organ failure. General guidelines for enteral or parenteral feeding are 25 to 35 kcal/kg of body weight per day. Overfeeding and underfeeding should be avoided, and indirect calorimetry, when available, can help assess needs more accurately.

Total energy: 25 to 35 kcal/kg/d

Protein: 1.2 to 1.5 g/kg/d (may approach 2 g/kg/d in some patients)

Fat: less than 2 g/kg/d, constituting 20% to 30% of the patient's daily energy intake (maintain serum triglyceride levels below 400 mg/dL)

Carbohydrate: 3 to 6 g/kg/d, constituting 50% to 60% of the patient's daily energy intake (maintain blood glucose levels below 180–200 mg/dL, or achieve tighter glucose control, depending on the clinical situation)

Protein

Protein needs are generally 1.2 to 1.5 g/kg/d. However, individual needs may approach 2 g/kg/d, depending on the clinical situation. On the other hand, less protein may be beneficial for patients with renal or hepatic failure.[22]

Lipids

For patients receiving PN, intravenous lipid does not stimulate pancreatic secretion and can be given to patients with acute pancreatitis as long as serum triglyceride concentrations are maintained below 400 mg/dL.[23] Traditional lipid solutions are 100% soy, but newer formulations available in the United States contain combinations of soybean oil, medium-chain triglycerides, olive oil, and fish oil (eg, SMOFlipid). These newer solutions have been found to reduce liver function test and triglyceride levels in patients receiving total PN.[24,25] For enteral feeding, as previously stated, no benefit has been found in using elemental over standard, intact formulas.[16,17] For patients eating by mouth, a regular, solid oral diet is recommended as tolerated.[15] No matter how the patient is fed, a fat intake of less than 2 g/kg/d, or no more than 20% to 30% of the daily energy load from lipids, is recommended.[6,26]

Carbohydrates

Carbohydrates can be provided at levels of 3 to 6 g/kg/d, or 50% to 60% of the daily energy load, to maintain blood glucose levels below 180 to 200 mg/dL.[6,26] Tighter glucose control may be desirable, depending on the clinical situation. Insulin may be helpful in attaining this goal.

Clinical Presentation of Pancreatic Exocrine Insufficiency

PEI occurs when the pancreas is unable to produce or secrete adequate digestive enzymes into the intestine to promote adequate digestion of macronutrients. Causes of PEI include chronic pancreatitis, pancreatic cancer, cystic fibrosis, surgery of the pancreas or GI tract, Zollinger-Ellison syndrome, lipase or colipase deficiency, Shwachman-Diamond syndrome, celiac disease, and type 1 diabetes mellitus. There are also two very rare causes in children: Pearson syndrome and Johanson-Blizzard syndrome.[27]

PEI should be suspected if a patient reports unexplained weight loss, yellow or clay-colored stools, oily stools, or stools with an unusually foul or offensive odor. Frequent bowel movements, abdominal bloating, gas, or cramping may also be present.[28] Patients using anti-diarrheal medications or consuming a low-fat diet may not present with these symptoms.

Historically, quantitative determination of fecal fat excretion in a 72-hour stool collection has been the gold standard for diagnosing PEI. A patient's PEI is clinically significant when the patient consumes a diet with 100 g fat per day and there is more than 15 g of fat per day in the stool.[27,29] Steatorrhea and weight loss are manifestations of PEI with malabsorption due to maldigestion. PEI resulting in steatorrhea requires the loss of 90% or more of the capacity of the pancreas to secrete digestive enzymes.[22,30] Because the 72-hour stool collection is a cumbersome and unpopular test for patients, other tests have been developed. The best of these in current practice is measurement in a random stool sample of fecal elastase concentration. Elastase is a pancreatic enzyme that is relatively resistant to degradation as it passes through the intestine; therefore, its concentration in stool is a reliable indicator of pancreatic exocrine secretory function. The normal value is more than 200 mcg elastase per gram of stool. Values between 100 and 200 mcg/g indicate mild-to-moderate insufficiency. A value of less than 100 mcg/g demonstrates severe PEI. A value between 200 and 250 mcg/g is sometimes considered "borderline."[31]

Nutrition Management

Although strict fat restriction had been recommended in the past, experimental studies of pancreatic insufficiency found that fat absorption was actually improved when a high-fat diet was ingested along with effective pancreatic enzyme replacement therapy (PERT).[30] Therefore, fat restriction may not be necessary for patients using effective PERT at appropriate doses. Fat restriction can lead to reduced energy intake and subsequent weight loss.

Dietary management of pancreatic insufficiency includes abstinence from alcohol if it is thought to be a contributing factor to the underlying disease process (eg, chronic pancreatitis) causing the pancreatic insufficiency. If serum values indicate a deficiency of fat-soluble vitamins (A, D, E, and K), supplementation is required.[22] Small, frequent meals that are low in fiber may be beneficial for patients who are not responding as expected to PERT, as fiber may inhibit pancreatic lipase activity.[22,27,32]

Medium-chain triglycerides can be used by patients who are unable to maintain or gain weight despite appropriate PERT. They are absorbed directly across the enterocyte brush border and pass into the bloodstream without the need for pancreatic enzymes.

Pancreatic Enzyme Replacement Therapy

Currently, in the United States, the available PERT products (ie, forms of pancrelipase) are derived from porcine pancreas; they are the primary treatment for pancreatic insufficiency. Although pancreatic enzyme supplements contain amylase, protease, and lipase, dosing is based on the amount of lipase units contained in a given product. See Box 8.4 for dosing guidelines that include starting at a low dose and titrating up as needed.[29]

BOX 8.4	500 to 2,500 lipase units per kilogram of body weight per meal per day; not to exceed 10,000 lipase units per kilogram of body weight per day
Pancreatic Enzyme Dosing Guidelines[29]	or
	25,000 to 80,000 lipase units per meal
	20,000 to 40,000 lipase units per snack
	or
	500 to 4,000 lipase units per gram of fat

When the appropriate dose is administered, PERT can substantially reduce steatorrhea and help the patient maintain or gain weight.[33,34]

Enzyme replacement should not be given in advance of meals, as it may leave the stomach before the food arrives and be degraded in the small intestine. Instead, pancreatic enzyme supplements work best if given during (starting at the beginning of the meal and throughout) and right after a meal.[35]

For patients on EN, there are numerous ways to effectively provide PERT. These include oral administration of enzyme products or feeding-tube administration of crushed, non–enteric-coated PERT or the contents of enteric-coated PERT capsules. Tube feedings can also be administered through a cartridge containing enzymes that mimic the function of pancreatic lipase to deliver absorbable fats to the intestine. More detailed discussions regarding this are available.[28]

Because pancreatic enzymes are inactivated or denatured at acidic pH levels, most are enteric-coated (ie, encapsulated in microspheres or microtablets that release their contents at a pH greater than 5.5, a situation normally encountered in the proximal small intestine).[36] Enzyme supplements that are not enteric-coated require concomitant use of an H_2 receptor antagonist or one of the proton pump inhibitors to prevent inactivation of the enzymes in the stomach.[36] Even some patients taking enteric-coated enzyme preparations may benefit from acid suppression because decreased bicarbonate secretion by the pancreas may lead to a pH in the proximal small intestine low enough to prevent appropriate release of the digestive enzymes from the enteric coating. To avoid unnecessary use of proton pump inhibitors, non–enteric-coated PERT is generally not standard treatment and should be reserved for patients with rapid GI transit or who are not responsive to enteric-coated enzymes.

A patient's baseline weight should be obtained just before starting PERT. The primary goal of therapy is weight stabilization or gain. Patients should be monitored for resolution of other symptoms of PEI, if present, such as diarrhea, stool findings associated with steatorrhea, or abdominal bloating. Subsequent weights are then assessed to determine whether the patient is benefiting from the treatment.

Pancreatic Enzyme Supplements in Cystic Fibrosis

For children with cystic fibrosis, pancreatic enzyme supplementation is crucial to growth and development because malabsorption leads to malnutrition and growth retardation as well as to an increased risk of pulmonary complications.[33,37] PERT leads to a better quality of life for patients with cystic fibrosis.

In the past, fibrosing colonopathy presenting with bloody diarrhea, symptoms of GI obstruction, or chylous ascites was observed in children treated with very large daily doses of pancreatic lipase (>24,000 lipase units per kilogram of body weight per day). This treatment used enzyme replacement capsules or tablets with much higher lipase content than is provided by currently available products. With the current enzyme products and dosing guidelines, this complication of PERT no longer occurs.[33,38] For additional information on cystic fibrosis and PERT, refer to Chapter 9.

Regulation of Pancreatic Enzyme Supplements

The use of pancreatic enzyme products antedated the creation of the US Food and Drug Administration (FDA). Consequently, studies to assess the safety, efficacy, stability, or bioavailability of these products before marketing were not required until 2010. The FDA now requires that manufacturers complete the standard new drug application process for any pancreatic enzyme products to be prescribed in the United States. All prescription pancreatic enzyme products currently available in the United States have passed the FDA approval requirements.[38,39]

Summary

The pancreas is a complex organ with both endocrine and exocrine functions. Pancreatitis is a complicated condition involving an inflammation of the pancreas. The condition can be acute or chronic, and it can range from mild to severe. In the case of PEI and chronic pancreatitis, it can take several years to evolve, and chronic malabsorption can lead to compromised nutritional status requiring intervention. Acute inflammation of the pancreas often requires periods of consuming nothing by mouth and may require nutrition support. Nutrition interventions for symptom management and ongoing treatment may include modification of the diet and use of PERT. The level of nutrition intervention required depends on both the severity and cause of the disease, and the nutritional status of the patient.

References

1. Baumler MD, Koopmann MC, Thomas DD, Ney DM, Groblewski GE. Intravenous or luminal amino acids are insufficient to maintain pancreatic growth and digestive enzyme expression in the absence of intact dietary protein. *Am J Physiol Gastrointest Liver Physiol*. 2010;299(2):G338-G347. doi:10.1152/ajpgi.00165.2010

2. Crozier SJ, D'Alecy LG, Ernst SA, Ginsburg LE, Williams JA. Molecular mechanisms of pancreatic dysfunction induced by protein malnutrition. *Gastroenterology*. 2009;137:1093-1101.

3. Corring T. The adaptation of digestive enzymes to the diet: its physiological significance. *Reprod Nutr Dev*. 1980;20:1217-1235.

4. Pap A. Effects of insulin and glucose metabolism on pancreatic exocrine function. *Int J Diabetes Metabol*. 2004;12:30-34.

5. Marik P. What is the best way to feed patients with pancreatitis? *Curr Opin Crit Care*. 2009;15:131-138.

6. Mirtallo JM, Forbes A, McClave SA, Jensen GL, Waitzberg DL, Davies AR; International Consensus Guideline Committee Pancreatitis Task Force. International consensus guidelines for nutrition therapy in pancreatitis. *JPEN J Parenter Enteral Nutr*. 2012;36(3):284-291.

7. Crockett SD, Wani S, Gardner TB, et al. American Gastroenterological Association Institute guideline on initial management of acute pancreatitis. *Gastroenterology*. 2018;154:1096-1101.

8. Lankisch PG, Apte M, Banks PA. Acute pancreatitis. *Lancet*. 2015;386:85-96.

9. McClave SA, Green LM, Snider HL, et al. Comparison of the safety of early enteral vs. parenteral nutrition in mild acute pancreatitis. *JPEN*. 1997;21:14-20.

10. Kalfarentzos F, Kehagias J, Mead N, et al. Enteral nutrition is superior to parenteral nutrition in severe acute pancreatitis: results of a randomized prospective trial. *Br J Surg*. 1997;84:1665-1669.

11. Marik PE, Zaloga GP. Meta-analysis of parenteral nutrition versus enteral nutrition in patients with acute pancreatitis. *BMJ*. 2004;328:1407-1410.

12. McClave SA, Chang WK, Dhaliwal R, et al. Nutrition support in acute pancreatitis: a systematic review of the literature. *JPEN*. 2006;30:143-156.

13. Bakker OJ, van Brunschot S, van Santvoort HC, et al. Early versus on-demand nasoenteric tube feeding in acute pancreatitis. *NEJM*. 2014;371:1983-1993.

14. McClave SA, Taylor BE, Martindale RG, et al. Guidelines for the provision and assessment of nutrition support therapy in the adult critically ill patient: SCCM and ASPEN. *JPEN*. 2016;40(2):159-211.

15. Ramanathan M, Aadam AA. Nutrition management in acute pancreatitis. *Nutr Clin Pract*. 2019;34(suppl 1):S7-S12.

16. Petrov MS, Loveday BP, Pylpchuk RD, et al. Systematic review and meta-analysis of enteral nutrition formulations in acute pancreatitis. *Br J Surg*. 2009;96:1243-1252.

17. Endo A, Shiraishi A, Fushimi K, et al. Comparative effectiveness of elemental formula in the early enteral nutrition management of acute pancreatitis: a retrospective cohort study. *Ann Intensive Care*. 2018;8:69-76.

18. Besselink MGH, Van Santvoort HC, Buskens E, et al. Probiotic prophylaxis in predicted severe acute pancreatitis: a randomized, double-blind, placebo-controlled trial. *Lancet*. 2008;371:651-659.

19. Gou S, Yang Z, Liu T, et al. Use of probiotics in the treatment of severe acute pancreatitis: a systematic review and meta-analysis of randomized controlled trials. *Crit Care*. 2014;18(2):R57.

20. Petrov MS, Atduev VA, Zagainov VE. Advanced enteral therapy in acute pancreatitis: is there room for immunonutrition? A meta-analysis. *Int J Surg*. 2008;6:119-124.

21. Olah A, Romics L. Enteral nutrition in acute pancreatitis: a review of the current evidence. *World J Gastroenterol*. 2014;20(43):16123-16131.

22. Meier RF, Beglinger C. Nutrition in pancreatic diseases. *Best Pract Res Clin Gastroenterol*. 2006;20:507-529.

23. Klein S, Kinney J, Jeejeebhoy K, et al. Nutrition support in clinical practice: review of published data and recommendations for future research directions. *JPEN*. 1997;21:133-156.

24. Piper SN, Schade I, Beschmann RB, et al. Hepatocellular integrity after parenteral nutrition: comparison of a fish-oil-containing lipid emulsion with an olive-soybean oil-based lipid emulsion. *Eur J Anaesthesiology*. 2009;26:1076-1082.

25. Tian H, Yao X, Zeng R, et al. Safety and efficacy of a new parenteral lipid emulsion (SMOF) for surgical patients: a systematic review and meta-analysis of randomized controlled trials. *Nutrition Reviews*. 2013;71(12):815-821.

26. McIsaac C, Helton WS. Intravenous nutrition in patients with acute pancreatitis. In: Rombeau JL, Rolandelli RH, ed. *Clinical Nutrition: Parenteral Nutrition*. 3rd ed. W. B. Saunders; 2001:230-257.

27. Dominguez-Munoz JE. Pancreatic enzyme therapy for pancreatic exocrine insufficiency. *Curr Gastroenterol Rep*. 2007;9:116-122.

28. Phillips, ME, Berry, AJ, Gettle LS. Pancreatic exocrine insufficiency and enteral feeding: a practical guide with case studies. *Practical Gastroenterol*. 2018;42(11):62-74.

29. Berry, AJ. Pancreatic enzyme replacement therapy during pancreatic insufficiency. *Nutr Clin Pract*. 2014;29:312-321.

30. Krishnamurty DK, Jagannath SB, Andersen DK. Delayed release pancrelipase for treatment of pancreatic exocrine insufficiency associated with chronic pancreatitis. *Ther Clin Risk Manag*. 2009;507-520.

31. Leeds, JS, Oppong K, Sanders DS. The role of fecal elastase-1 in detecting exocrine pancreatic disease. *Nat Rev Gastroenterol Hepatol*. 2011;8:405-415.

32. Ribichini E, Stigliano S, Rossi S, et al. Role of fibre in nutritional management of pancreatic diseases. *Nutrients*. 2019;11(9):2219.

33. Baker SS. Delayed release pancrelipase for the treatment of pancreatic exocrine insufficiency associated with cystic fibrosis. *Ther Clin Risk Manag*. 2008;4:1079-1084.

34. Layer P, Groger G. Fate of pancreatic enzymes in the human intestinal lumen in health and pancreatic insufficiency. *Digestion*. 1993;54(suppl 2):10-14.

35. Dimagno EP, Malagelada JR, Go VL, et al. Fate of orally ingested enzymes in pancreatic insufficiency: comparison of two dosage schedules. *N Engl J Med*. 1977;296:1318-1322.

36. Forsmark CE. Chronic pancreatitis and pancreatic insufficiency. In: Friedman SL, McQuaid KR, Grendell JH, eds. *Current Diagnosis and Treatment in Gastroenterology*. 2nd ed. Lange Medical Books/McGraw-Hill; 2003:496-509.

37. Borowitz DS, Grand RJ, Durie PR. Use of pancreatic enzyme supplements for patients with cystic fibrosis in the context of fibrosing colonopathy. *J Pediatr*. 1995;127(5):681-684.

38. Taylor JR, Gardner TB, Waljee AK, et al. Systematic review: efficacy and safety of pancreatic enzyme supplements for exocrine pancreatic insufficiency. *Aliment Pharmacol Ther*. 2010;31:57-72.

39. Nakajima K, Oshida H, Muneyuki T, Kakei M. Pancrelipase: an evidence-based review of its use for treating pancreatic insufficiency. *Core Evid*. 2012;7:77-91.

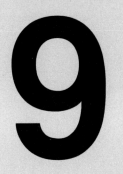

CHAPTER

9

Pediatric-Originating Gastrointestinal Disorders

M. Linley Harvie, MD
Anna Tuttle, MS, RD, LDN, CNSC
Kelly Green Corkins, MS, RD-AP, CSP, LDN, FAND, FASPEN
Mark R. Corkins, MD, CNSC, FASPEN, AGAF, FAAP

KEY POINTS

- Pediatric patients with certain pediatric-originating diseases develop related gastrointestinal disorders and cannot meet their nutrition needs orally, as evidenced by poor weight gain, decreased linear growth, or other signs of malnutrition. In such patients, enteral nutrition is indicated.
- When a birth mother's milk is not available for infant feeding, enteral nutrition should be initiated, taking into consideration factors such as the infant's age, clinical condition, and possible food allergies or intolerances.
- When enteral nutrition is not sufficient or has failed in a pediatric patient, parenteral nutrition should be considered early.

Introduction

Many diseases have their start at birth or during childhood (eg, coronary artery disease) but do not manifest until adulthood. However, some diseases have their onset during the early years of life and have important nutritional implications that affect childhood and adult health status. Fortunately, with advances in health care, many patients with such pediatric-originating diseases are now surviving into adulthood. This chapter provides an overview of and guidelines for the diagnosis, treatment, and nutrition management of several pediatric-originating diseases and their related gastrointestinal (GI) complications, as well as other GI disorders seen in the pediatric population.

Cystic Fibrosis

Cystic fibrosis (CF) is an autosomal recessive disorder that affects multiple organ systems, primarily the lungs. The defect is in the cystic fibrosis transmembrane conductance regulator gene (CFTR), which regulates ion flow across cell membranes, specifically the flow of chloride.[1] Disruption of the chloride flow leads to thicker secretions, which can cause mucus plugs in the tubes, passageways, and ducts of the lungs, pancreas, and liver. Resulting poor bile flow can cause liver disease, and the obstruction of pancreatic ducts leads to pancreatic insufficiency. Lung disease is the most severe CF-related health issue because patients are unable to clear thick mucus secretions from their lungs, which can cause airway obstruction and frequent respiratory infections. These patients require close nutrition management because of their increased metabolic requirements. In addition, the associated liver disease and pancreatic insufficiency can lead to malabsorption, which can result in poor growth.

Clinical Presentation and Diagnosis

CF is usually diagnosed shortly after birth. The majority of patients are identified on newborn screening by elevated levels of immunoreactive trypsinogen. The implementation of newborn screening has been a game changer for early diagnosis. Confirmatory testing includes a sweat test revealing elevated levels of chloride or a genetic test that is positive for abnormal mutations in the *CFTR* gene. Early diagnosis has led to improvements in overall nutritional status and survival.[1] If CF is not diagnosed in the newborn period, common presenting symptoms include frequent respiratory infections, persistent wheezing, poor growth, and greasy stools or constipation.

Performing a nutrition assessment and paying close attention to anthropometric patterns are vital steps to improving outcomes in young patients with CF. Regular weight, length, BMI, or weight-for-length measurements are needed to assess appropriate growth trends in these patients. A weight-for-length above the 50th percentile in children younger than 2 years has been linked to improved lung function. Following the same guidelines, a BMI greater than the 50th percentile is desired for children aged 2 to 18 years. A nutrition assessment should also include laboratory tests to evaluate for nutrient deficiencies, analyze regular dietary intake, and check for a history of steatorrhea.[2] A nutrition focused physical examination can help identify certain micronutrient deficiencies common in CF, such as deficiencies in fat-soluble vitamins, zinc, and iron. Many factors may contribute to growth deficits in this population, including inadequate intake, insufficient enzyme replacement, and micronutrient deficiency; therefore, a comprehensive assessment is critical.

Treatment and Nutrition Management

Nutrition Intervention

Roughly 85% of patients with CF have pancreatic insufficiency and require pancreatic enzyme replacement therapy (PERT). The goal of PERT is to replace the enzymes that patients with CF lack in order to help them digest nutrients in foods, such as fats. Enzyme dosing is usually done either in units of lipase per kilogram of body weight per meal, or units of lipase per kilogram of body weight per day; if the latter, then the dosage is divided into three meals and two snacks. Initially, the dosage for infants with CF was limited to a maximum of 10,000 lipase units per kilogram of body weight per day.[3] However, recent studies have shown that higher dosages of PERT are needed because of the high energy needs of these infants, and higher dosages lead to improved weight-for-age and weight-for-length *z* scores.[3] Patients with gastrostomy feeds can now use a PERT device that attaches to their enteral feeding tube. The formula passes through the enzyme cartridge (which contains lipase) to aid in the digestion of the formula.[3] Of note, patients who are pancreatic sufficient should continue to be monitored annually to assess for continued pancreatic sufficiency.

Because people with CF lose excessive amounts of salt through their skin, sodium chloride supplementation often needs to be added to feedings and to a regular diet. The Cystic Fibrosis Foundation recommends ⅛ tsp sodium chloride for infants younger than 6 months and ¼ tsp for children aged 6 months and older.[2] Fat-soluble vitamin deficiencies are common in patients with CF; therefore, regular assessment of vitamins A, D, E, and K are recommended to guide practitioners on the correct dosing of those supplements. CF-specific vitamins are available; however, individual dosing of each vitamin may be necessary to achieve optimal serum levels.[3]

Human milk is highly recommended for infants with CF. If human milk is not available, standard infant formula can be used unless the infant shows intolerance to intact formula. Increasing energy intake by adding extra fats and oils to foods should be encouraged, as fat loss is characteristic of CF. A high-fat diet should be initiated at a young age, with the addition of medium-chain triglycerides for improved absorption. Enteral feeding via nasogastric, gastrostomy, or gastrojejunal tubes may be necessary in patients with growth failure (weight and length <10th percentile). For these patients, the Cystic Fibrosis Foundation recommends nocturnal tube feedings so that patients can consume a regular diet during the day.[2]

Medical Management

Patients with CF typically require multiple medications to improve their overall lung function. These medications include anti-inflammatory agents (eg, ibuprofen and azithromycin), anti-infective agents (eg, inhaled tobramycin and inhaled aztreonam), and mucolytics (eg, DNAse and hypertonic saline). The newest drugs used to treat CF are CFTR modulators, which partially restore function of the CFTR protein. Ivacaftor is a potentiator CFTR modulator, which improves the function of the CFTR protein on the cell membrane. Lumacaftor and tezacaftor are known as corrector CFTR modulators, and they help the CFTR protein form the correct shape. The CFTR modulators are most effective in combination.[1] The newest combination therapy consists of elexacaftor, tezacaftor, and ivacaftor.

Other medications are directed toward complications outside of lung disease. These medications include osmotic softeners for constipation (eg, polyethylene glycol) and ursodeoxycholic acid for CF-associated liver disease.

Many patients also receive nonpharmacologic therapies (eg, manual chest physiotherapy or vest therapy) to improve their airway clearance and decrease the risk of lung infections. These techniques are often done at least once a day and sometimes multiple times per day.

Complications

Patients with CF can experience a variety of GI complications. Meconium, the thickened fecal material present in all newborns, may become congealed and cause obstruction of the terminal ileum in infants with CF. This is known as meconium ileus and can occur in up to 20% of infants with CF.[1] Most cases require surgical management, which can place the infant at risk for intestinal failure. More commonly, older children develop constipation due to intestinal dysmotility and altered intestinal fluid composition. This also increases the risk of rectal prolapse, which is sometimes the first presenting sign of CF. Similarly, patients can develop distal intestinal obstruction syndrome (DIOS), in which digested food, mucus, and intestinal secretions lodge in the ileum. Constipation and DIOS are usually treated with oral polyethylene glycol or an enema with diatrizoate meglumine and diatrizoate sodium solution.[1] Some severe cases of DIOS require surgical intervention.

CF-associated liver disease is another GI-related complication. Severe liver disease with cirrhosis and portal hypertension may develop in 5% to 10% of patients with CF. This usually occurs in the first 20 years of life.[4] These patients may require liver transplantation.

Immune-Mediated Gastrointestinal Disorders

Cow's Milk Protein Allergy

Cow's milk protein allergy (CMPA) is an immune reaction, either immunoglobulin E (IgE)–mediated or non–IgE-mediated, to cow's milk protein. The incidence has been reported to be between 2% to 7.5% in the first year of life. It is the most common food allergy in early childhood.[5] An infant is exposed to cow's milk protein either from drinking standard infant formula or as it passes through breast milk. Symptoms of non–IgE-mediated CMPA usually occur days after milk consumption, with the most common symptoms involving the skin and the GI tract. GI symptoms include vomiting, bloody stool, diarrhea, food aversion, and sometimes constipation. Occasionally, patients may present with poor growth or colic. Exclusively breastfed infants typically present with atopic dermatitis or blood in the stool from allergic proctocolitis, or both.[5] Diagnosis is made clinically and confirmed by the improvement of symptoms once cow's milk protein is eliminated from the diet. See Chapter 13 for more on food allergies.

Treatment and Nutrition Management

The treatment for CMPA is to alter the diet. Breastfeeding mothers should eliminate dairy from their diet. Once dairy has been eliminated, it can take 10 to 21 days for the breast milk to become entirely dairy-free. This is the recommended time frame to allow for an improvement of symptoms in the child. Studies have reported rates as low as 10% and as high as 43% for cross-reactivity to soy protein[6-8]; therefore, if symptoms do not improve within 21 days of dairy elimination, the breastfeeding mother may also need to eliminate soy protein from the diet.

For infants who are not exclusively breastfed, formula options include soy formula (for infants older than 6 months),[8] extensively hydrolyzed formula, or amino acid–based formula. Typically, for non-breastfed infants, an extensively hydrolyzed formula is the first-line therapy for CMPA.[9] If patients do not respond after 2 weeks on the extensively hydrolyzed formula, they are switched to an amino acid–based formula. However, if a patient is malnourished or presents with poor growth, an amino acid–based formula is considered first-line therapy.[9]

Food Protein–Induced Enterocolitis Syndrome

Food protein–induced enterocolitis syndrome (FPIES) is a non–IgE-mediated reaction to food. The most common presenting symptom is vomiting. There are two types of FPIES: acute (the most common form) and chronic. Acute FPIES usually presents in the first 7 months of life with multiple episodes of vomiting 1 to 4 hours after the infant ingests a trigger food. Diarrhea is also associated with acute FPIES and can occur up to 5 to 10 hours after food ingestion. Patients can become severely dehydrated and lethargic, almost appearing septic. Symptoms typically resolve after 24 hours from the time the offending food is removed from the diet. Chronic FPIES presents with a slower onset of symptoms, which include chronic vomiting, diarrhea, and even poor growth. It usually occurs in infants younger than 6 months who consume cow's milk–based or soy-based formula. Symptoms improve within days once the food-protein source is removed. The most common food-protein triggers for both acute and chronic FPIES are cow's milk and soy proteins. Solid-food triggers are more commonly seen in older infants and toddlers. Typical solid food-protein triggers include grains, such as rice and oats.[10] A food challenge test for the suspected trigger is the gold standard for the diagnosis of FPIES; however, if symptoms are most consistent with FPIES and removing the trigger improves the symptoms, the diagnosis can be made clinically.

Treatment and Nutrition Management

The primary therapy for FPIES is to eliminate the food-protein triggers from the diet. In many cases, an infant will have only one or two triggers. A hypoallergenic formula may need to be introduced if cow's milk is identified as a trigger, but breastfeeding mothers do not have to eliminate the trigger foods from their own diets, as long as the infant is not symptomatic. A trigger food should not be reintroduced until at least 12 months after the initial reaction. Depending on the severity of the infant's original reaction, the food challenge may need to be done in a supervised medical facility.[11] Parents of infants with FPIES are often leery of introducing new foods, for fear of another reaction. Foods less likely to cause FPIES should, therefore, be the focus of their child's diet. Lower-risk foods include broccoli, watermelon, avocado, strawberries, lamb, and millet.[12] Due to dietary limitations, infants with

FPIES can be at risk for specific nutrient deficiencies, such as protein, iron, zinc, B vitamins, and calcium. Working with a registered dietitian nutritionist (RDN) is essential to ensure that these children receive balanced nutrition.[12]

Eosinophilic Esophagitis

Eosinophilic esophagitis (EoE) is an immune-mediated inflammatory condition of the esophagus. The etiology is thought to be secondary to multiple factors, including genetic predisposition and an abnormal immune response to food antigens. This increased immune response leads to esophageal inflammation, dysmotility, and fibrosis if left untreated.[13]

Although EoE generally starts in childhood, it can occur at any age. The presentation can vary, with affected patients experiencing a wide array of symptoms, including vomiting, dysphagia, food getting stuck during swallowing, reflux, heartburn, or abdominal pain. EoE should be high on the list of differential diagnoses and investigated further in patients who report any of the following: other atopic conditions, such as asthma or eczema; a family history of food impaction or esophageal dilation; and any of the aforementioned GI symptoms at the time of presentation.[14] Some patients never report any symptoms but present for the first time with food impaction. If EoE is suspected, the patient should undergo an endoscopic evaluation, during which biopsies are taken from multiple areas and levels within the esophagus. Gross endoscopic findings of EoE include linear furrowing, white exudates, trachealization, strictures, or a narrow-caliber esophagus. However, some patients, especially those in whom EoE is diagnosed early, have a normal-appearing esophageal lining. The diagnosis is confirmed when patients have clinical symptoms of esophageal dysfunction and histologic findings of esophageal eosinophilia ($\geq$15 eosinophils per high-power field) from biopsies. Other disorders including eosinophilic gastritis, duodenitis, and gastroenteritis should be excluded with antral and duodenal biopsies. Other conditions that have been associated with esophageal eosinophilia include gastroesophageal reflux disease, hypereosinophilic syndrome, connective tissue disorders, Crohn's disease, and infections. These should be considered if the patient has other signs or symptoms that are not wholly explained by EoE.[14]

Treatment and Nutrition Management

Nutrition Interventions Dietary modification is appropriate when patients prefer to avoid pharmacologic interventions or when medications are not providing adequate treatment of EoE. In fact, elemental diets can be up to 90% effective in treating EoE; however, poor palatability of formulas, noncompliance, and the lack of food variety can limit the feasibility of a purely elemental diet for many young patients.[15] If a young child is put on an elemental diet, it is helpful to include one or two "safe" foods (apples, sweet potatoes) for some variety and to continue developing oral feeding skills.[16] Supplemental tube feeds may be needed in certain cases to promote growth while the child expands their diet. The six-food elimination diet eliminates the top allergens—dairy, wheat, eggs, soy, tree nuts and peanuts, fish and shellfish. The foods are reintroduced very gradually, and endoscopies with esophageal biopsies are done to evaluate for a histological response. The most commonly implicated allergens are cow's milk, wheat, eggs, soy, and peanuts. A test-directed elimination diet uses skin testing and atopy patch testing to guide the diet.[15] However, food atopy patch testing has not been validated in patients with EoE. The best way to ascertain what food is causing symptoms is to eliminate that food then reintroduce it to see if that leads to symptoms and increased eosinophil levels.[16] If it does, the patient will then know to eliminate that dietary allergen in the long term.

Medical Management Proton pump inhibitors (PPIs) are first-line therapy for patients with EoE. It is unclear why some patients respond to PPIs and others do not.

Experts believe that PPIs have some anti-inflammatory properties that may promote a stronger esophageal mucosal barrier in patients with EoE. If a patient does not respond or only partially responds to PPI therapy, further options include dietary management, as previously mentioned, and swallowed corticosteroids. The two corticosteroids used are fluticasone or viscous budesonide. Fluticasone comes in a metered-dose inhaler and is pumped into the mouth and swallowed instead of inhaled. Budesonide is made into a viscous slurry using sucralose (a 1-g packet of sucralose per 1 mg budesonide). Patients should not eat or drink for 30 minutes after swallowing the corticosteroids for this treatment to be effective. Biologic therapies are under investigation for use in EoE.[14]

Complications

Patients with poorly controlled EoE or who have trouble adhering to therapies are at risk for developing complications. The most common complication is fibrosis, which can lead to food impaction and strictures. Food impactions, while usually not life-threatening, can be traumatizing to patients and their families. Food impactions are considered urgent and sometimes emergent if patients are having difficulty handling their secretions. Patients typically need to be admitted to the hospital for urgent endoscopic removal of the food. Strictures usually require dilations, which can reduce dysphagia symptoms in patients with EoE.[17] Depending on the severity of the stricture, there is increased risk of perforation with dilation.

Monitoring and Follow-Up

Patients with EoE are typically monitored on a regular basis in a GI clinic for anywhere from 1 to 6 months, depending on the severity of the patient's symptoms. Once EoE is diagnosed, a patient is started on one of the aforementioned therapies, then reevaluated 2 to 3 months later with endoscopic and histologic testing. Patients in remission may have a follow-up endoscopy 1 year later and then less frequently. However, patients who are not in remission, as indicated by their clinical symptoms or histology, may require endoscopies more frequently until remission is established.

Inborn Errors of Metabolism

An inborn error of metabolism is an inherited disorder caused by a genetic defect. The congenital defect leads to the impaired production of an enzyme, cofactor, or transporter that is needed for a particular cellular pathway.[18] This metabolic disruption then leads to (1) the accumulation of a toxic metabolite, (2) the reduction of a required downstream metabolite, or (3) an abnormal alternative substrate metabolism, all of which can cause health issues.[19] GI manifestations of inborn errors of metabolism include abdominal pain, chronic vomiting, pancreatitis, diarrhea, constipation, and malabsorption.[20] With modern molecular biology techniques, scientists have been able to identify an extensive number of these disorders, which are cataloged in the lengthy *Online Metabolic and Molecular Bases of Inherited Disease*.[19,21] In-depth coverage of this topic is beyond the scope of this text, so a typical disorder that illustrates the general principles is presented.

Clinical Presentation and Diagnosis

Inborn errors of metabolism are, technically speaking, present at the moment of conception and, ipso facto, present at birth. The goal in newborns is to intervene before the metabolic disorder can result in long-term toxicities. To this end, the more common disorders are included in the newborn screening done for every infant shortly after birth.[19] Others are diagnosed based on the typical clinical manifestations of the metabolic defect. Although these disorders are usually diagnosed during childhood, they may not manifest in some individuals until adulthood.[20]

Treatment and Nutrition Management

The traditional approach to treating inborn errors of metabolism is dietary restriction. Other approaches for these disorders include substrate reduction or toxin removal. Substrate reduction often requires the supplementation of substances that are needed downstream for the cellular pathway.[18] A classic example of an inborn error of metabolism is maple syrup urine disease (MSUD). In this disorder, a defect in the branched-chain α-keto acid dehydrogenase complex blocks the metabolism of the branched-chain amino acids (BCAAs; ie, leucine, isoleucine, and valine). This causes BCAA levels to become elevated, which is toxic to the immune system, skeletal muscle, and central nervous system. MSUD is treated with dietary restriction of the BCAAs, although valine and isoleucine end up needing to be supplemented.[22] Routine follow-up by a multidisciplinary team that includes an RDN is necessary to ensure that patients with inborn errors of metabolism adhere to their diets, drink their prescribed formulas, maintain an appropriate growth trajectory, and avoid any nutrient deficiencies. Patients or their caregivers are often asked to keep a 3-day food log to help the team analyze the diet and provide insight into routine laboratory test results.[23]

The main goals of nutrition therapy for metabolic disorders are to maintain metabolic homeostasis and promote good growth. A special medical formula specific to the diagnosed inborn error of metabolism is a main component of treatment.[23] Patients with urea cycle disorder are prescribed a formula consisting of protein that is limited to essential amino acids (rather than whole protein) and mixed with standard infant formula. Patients with MSUD receive a blend of a BCAA-limiting formula and standard formula to meet their energy needs. The amount of standard infant formula used is based on the amount of BCAAs allowed in the diet. As mentioned previously, valine and isoleucine are dosed according to individual patient requirements to ensure good growth and development. Aside from the formula, a special diet is prescribed that is specific to the diagnosis. Patients with MSUD and patients with urea cycle disorder follow a prescription low-protein diet. Disorders such as glycogen storage disease and medium-chain acyl-CoA dehydrogenase deficiency require feedings, or meals or snacks, every 3 to 4 hours because of hypoglycemia concerns.[24] Adherence to the medical formula prescription and diet recommendations are crucial to these patients for their growth and to avoid hospitalizations.

Neurologic Impairments

Children with neurologic impairment typically have a wide variety of GI issues. Among the more common concerns are dysphagia, dysmotility, gastroesophageal reflux, and constipation.[25,26] These issues make the safe supply of nutrition an important concern.

Clinical Presentation and Diagnosis

Because of their neurologic impairment, these children have substantial developmental delays, and most require some sort of intervention to even administer their nutrition. Also, owing to their neurologic challenges, these children may not be able to express when they are hungry or full and generally cannot ask to be fed or report GI symptoms. The spectrum of interventions is very broad, ranging from supervised meals to the use of feeding tubes. One study found that 60% of children with cerebral palsy were totally dependent on their caregivers for all their nutritional intake.[25] The type and severity of neurologic impairment determines the level of nutrients needed. Some children will require an energy intake that exceeds the norm for their age, whereas others may need an energy intake far below the norm for their age.[27] Children with neurologic impairment may be brought to a physician initially for poor weight gain as a consequence of inadequate intake.[26] Others present with pulmonary symptoms because they have dysphagia and aspirate.[27]

The GI issues common in children with neurologic impairment negatively affect their nutritional intake, both orally and enterally, resulting in undernutrition and growth failure and contributing to multiple micronutrient deficiencies.[25,26,28-30] Micronutrient deficiencies common to these children include iron, zinc, magnesium, carnitine, calcium, vitamin D, vitamin E, vitamin B12, folate, and niacin deficiencies.[25,26] Even with supplementation, the levels of folate, iron, magnesium, vitamin D, selenium, and carnitine are consistently low in these patients.[25,26] This may be because the absorption and utilization of these nutrients is altered by the chronic use of certain medications.[27,31] Phenytoin, phenobarbital, carbamazepine, oxcarbazepine, valproate, and levetiracetam are all associated with low vitamin D levels.[32,33] Low carnitine and low selenium levels are associated with inadequate amounts of these nutrients in the enteral formula given or because the volume of formula given is inadequate, so nutrient intake is limited.[26]

Children with neurologic impairment tend to store fat centrally and can easily become overweight; thus, BMI tends to underestimate adiposity.[25] Misinterpretation of a low BMI or other anthropometric measurements may lead to overestimating needs and overfeeding, especially with children who are tube fed.[26]

Bone health is a common concern because children with neurological issues tend to be non–weight-bearing, have an inadequate intake of vitamin D and calcium, have limited exposure to sunlight, and take antiseizure medications that, with chronic use, alter nutrient absorption and bone turnover.[27,31]

Nutrition Assessment

Assessing the nutritional intake of a child with neurologic impairment is a crucial step in determining the child's nutritional status and concerns. Inadequate nutritional intake contributes not only to poor growth but also to multiple micronutrient deficiencies.[25,31] Oropharyngeal dysfunction, gastroesophageal reflux, constipation, and GI dysmotility all negatively affect the patient's oral intake and, potentially, the enteral regimen.[26,28-30]

Anthropometric measurements, although important when assessing the growth and nutritional status of children with neurologic impairment, may have limited value because they are difficult to perform on children with moderate or severe impairment and, as a result, may be inaccurate.[26] Spasticity, contracture, and scoliosis limit length or height measurements, so segmentally derived measures from knee height or tibial length may be used.[26,29,30] These derived measures can be plotted on the age-appropriate growth charts of normally developed children (the World Health Organization or Centers for Disease Control and Prevention growth charts) and on appropriate specialty charts. Clinical judgment is essential when using growth charts because (1) children with neurologic impairment do not develop normally, and (2) specialty growth charts show how the children do grow, not how they should grow.[28] When tracking growth using the growth charts, trending z scores may be more useful than absolute percentile because children with severe neurologic impairment may not fall within age-appropriate growth percentiles. Calculating BMI using the segmental derived measures is not recommended because these extrapolations can be off by 1 to 2 cm.[26]

Mid upper arm circumference and triceps skinfold thickness can be measured but should be interpreted with caution because most children with moderate to severe neurologic impairment store body fat centrally and not in their extremities.[26] With limitations on the objective measurements, subjective parameters may be more useful.[28] Subjective global assessment has been shown to better identify malnourished children with cerebral palsy than objective parameters.[29,30] In addition, a nutrition focused physical examination can identify potential micronutrient deficiencies.[34]

Treatment and Nutrition Management

Micronutrient needs for children with neurologic impairment are based on the Dietary Reference Intakes, as with normally developed children. Review of dietary intake and nutrient medication interactions guide the practitioner to what nutrients need to be supplemented. Estimating energy needs is challenging because the level of neurologic impairment varies from child to child.[25,26] Energy needs vary according to the patient's severity of neurologic impairment, physical activity, seizure activity, muscle tone, and severity of malnutrition.[25,26]

Oral nutrition is the preferred mode of nutrition intake and should be made safe and stress-free. Inadequate oral intake is usually secondary to GI disorders such as dysphagia, dysmotility, gastroesophageal reflux, and constipation.[26] Any GI disorder should be treated nutritionally, medically, and surgically (see the section on dysmotility in this chapter). If feeding by mouth is stressful for the child and takes longer than 3 hours a day, tube feeding should be considered.[25,26]

New recommendations suggest that gastrostomy-tube placement should be considered before signs and symptoms of undernutrition develop.[27] Once a child with neurologic impairment exhibits poor weight gain or growth or micronutrient deficiencies, tube placement becomes more critical.[25,26] Feeding via gastrostomy tube significantly improves growth, nutritional status, and quality of life.[35-37]

The selection of an enteral formula should be individualized and based on the patient's GI symptoms. Usually, polymeric or peptide-based, age-appropriate formulas are well tolerated. Blenderized tube feeding improves GI symptoms.[38] If a low volume of formula is being given (less than the recommended Dietary Reference Intakes), a protein supplement and vitamin and mineral supplement are essential. Vitamin D supplementation at 800 to 1,000 International Units daily is recommended with chronic antiseizure medication use. Consider calcium supplementation with long-term antireflux medication use. The practitioner should always consider fluid adequacy.

Dysmotility

Motility disorders are becoming more recognized in children. These disorders can cause considerable abdominal pain, which can lead to decreased nutritional intake. Some of the motility disorders are difficult to diagnose, resulting in a delay in therapies. If symptoms become chronic, patients may be unable to consume an adequate diet and become malnourished. Two important motility disorders in children are gastroparesis and chronic intestinal pseudo-obstruction. The former is much more common than the latter.

Clinical Presentation and Diagnosis

Gastroparesis

Gastroparesis is characterized by the delayed emptying of gastric contents, usually solid foods, without evidence of mechanical obstruction; it leads to nausea, early satiety, vomiting, and abdominal pain. Gastroparesis can be chronic or transient, depending on the cause. It can occur temporarily after anesthesia, infection, or use of certain medications. The disorder is commonly seen in premature infants and may not resolve as the infant grows and matures. It can be more of a chronic condition in patients with an underlying neuromuscular disorder, poorly controlled diabetes mellitus, postsurgical interventions (such as fundoplication and vagotomy), and connective tissue disorders. It is common in patients with significant cardiovascular disease due to poor perfusion, which can also be transient. Some cases are idiopathic.[39] Gastroparesis is typically diagnosed clinically. Gastric emptying scintigraphy can be beneficial; however, there are no standard values described in the pediatric population. For more complex cases that do not improve with therapy, antroduodenal manometry may be needed.

Chronic Intestinal Pseudo-Obstruction

Chronic intestinal pseudo-obstruction is a rare disorder that results from impairment of GI peristalsis and contractions, which leads to symptoms that mimic a mechanical obstruction. It can occur along any segment of the GI tract. Symptoms can range from nausea, vomiting, anorexia, or early satiety to constipation, abdominal pain, and abdominal distention, depending on which area of the intestinal tract is affected. Given the nonspecific symptoms, it is difficult to diagnose, and diagnosis is often delayed. Because of this, patients often do not receive adequate nutrition or the correct medical therapy, which leads to a higher morbidity and mortality rate among these patients.[40]

Treatment and Nutrition Management

Nutrition Intervention

A nutrition assessment of any pediatric patient includes monitoring anthropometric measurements for growth and a nutrition focused physical examination.[41] The assessment of nutritional intake is critical in children with dysmotility because the severity of symptoms (eg, vomiting, gastroesophageal reflux, and constipation) can adversely affect nutrient intake and absorption.[42]

Because patients with dysmotility may have exacerbated symptoms or poor nutrient absorption (or both), the nutrition intervention will vary from person to person. If absorption is adequate, these patients are encouraged to eat smaller, more frequent meals that are lower in fiber and fat.[42] Thorough chewing of solids should be encouraged (as age and developmentally appropriate). Typically, the gastric emptying of liquids is preserved, so patients should be encouraged to consume liquids that are high in protein (eg, supplemental shakes) and increase their liquid consumption as the day progresses and fullness worsens.[39,42] When possible, enteral therapy should always be the first choice. If the patient cannot consume enough kilocalories because of their symptoms, a nasoenteric tube should be considered. If tube feedings are needed for longer than 8 weeks, surgically placed tubes are recommended. Where the tube terminates is determined by the severity of symptoms. Gastric feedings are preferred and allow for larger feeding volumes, but risk of aspiration is increased with this method.[42] Cyclic feedings, with a short break between feedings, can be used when feeding into the stomach. Postpyloric feedings, while decreasing the risk of aspiration, limit the volume of feedings, and feedings must be given over a longer period of time, either continuously or overnight.[42] Many cases of dysmotility are transient and only require a short-term intervention. In the most severe cases, patients may require parenteral nutrition.[40]

Medical Management

The goal of pharmacologic management is to promote intestinal motility and decrease the risk of small intestinal bacterial overgrowth (SIBO). The area of the GI tract affected will determine the most appropriate medication to use, as the site of action varies. For patients with upper GI involvement, medications such as erythromycin, metoclopramide, and domperidone are effective. Pyridostigmine and prucalopride have been shown to be more beneficial in patients with lower GI involvement. However, not all of these medications are approved in the pediatric population.[39,40]

Other medications are used to treat complications and symptoms from dysmotility, such as SIBO. A variety of antibiotic regimens are used to treat SIBO, and there are no established guidelines. Antibiotics are typically given in a 1- to 2-week rotation and can include amoxicillin-clavulanate, metronidazole, rifaximin, and ciprofloxacin. One of the most common concerns of patients with dysmotility is abdominal pain. The typical medications for functional abdominal pain, such as tricyclic antidepressants and serotonin-norepinephrine reuptake inhibitors, can help the patient with abdominal pain; but they should be given at low doses and titrated up slowly in an effort to decrease some of the side effects of these medications, such as constipation.[40]

Surgical Management

Some patients with dysmotility can benefit from surgical intervention. For some, intermittent decompression with nasogastric tubes is beneficial, and patients may opt for gastrostomy. If only a small section of the intestinal tract is impaired, surgical removal may be an option to alleviate symptoms. More severe cases may require diverting ostomies for relief.

Constipation

Clinical Presentation and Diagnosis

Constipation is the most common symptom treated by pediatricians and pediatric gastroenterologists. It is characterized by infrequent bowel movements or hard, painful bowel movements, or both.[43] Some underlying disorders can lead to constipation, including Hirschsprung disease, CF, hypothyroidism, and sometimes celiac disease. If there are red flags for an underlying medical condition, further investigation is required. This may include a contrast enema, rectal biopsy, laboratory tests, a sweat chloride test, or colonic or anorectal manometry. However, for the majority of cases, there is no underlying medical disease that explains the constipation. Functional constipation is diagnosed clinically.

Treatment and Nutrition Management

Nutrition Intervention

Limited evidence exists to support the effectiveness of nutrition interventions for constipation, but dietitians usually encourage a balanced diet of whole grains, fruits, and vegetables to provide fiber.[42,43] If tube-fed, the child can be given a formula with soluble fiber. Children with constipation should consume an adequate amount of fluid, and fluid intake should be increased as needed. Fruit juices may be helpful, but should not replace whole fruit.[42] Daily juice intake should be limited because juice is limited in nutrients but calorie-dense.

Medical Management

Osmotic laxatives are usually the first line of therapy in children with functional constipation. Typically, for small infants, lactulose is the medication of choice. It is a good option for infants because it is highly concentrated and can be given in a small volume. The most commonly used medication in children is polyethylene glycol, which comes in a powder formulation and can be mixed with any clear liquid. It is typically well tolerated. For some patients, the stool's consistency and the inability to evacuate the bowel may be the issue. These patients will also benefit from a stimulant laxative, such as senna or bisacodyl.[43] Patients with pelvic floor dysfunction benefit from pelvic floor rehabilitation and behavioral therapy.

Complications

Chronic constipation can lead to multiple complications, including anal fissures, rectal prolapse, and, rarely, hemorrhoids in the pediatric population. Fecal impaction with encopresis is another complication frequently seen in the pediatric population. This can be traumatizing as well as socially problematic for school-age children. Poorly controlled constipation can lead to hospitalizations for manual disimpaction or nasogastric tube osmotic solution stool cleanouts.

Summary

CF is a complex disease affecting many organ systems. A multidisciplinary approach can provide patients with optimal care and decrease the number of physician visits. An early diagnosis leads to overall improved survival. Maintaining close follow-up that includes a nutrition assessment at each visit is vital to treating patients with this disease.

Food-induced immune-mediated GI disorders present in different ways and in different age groups. It is essential to obtain a thorough diet history when evaluating these patients. Overall, these disorders improve once the offending food agent is removed from the diet. Working closely with an experienced RDN helps practitioners to provide the best therapeutic plans for each individual patient.

The inborn errors of metabolism are a set of rare disorders resulting from genetic defects that result in the disruption of a cell's normal biochemical pathways. These diseases should be investigated when a patient's GI symptoms are not attributable to one of the more common causes.[20] Currently, the majority of these disorders are treated with dietary management. The general approach is to eliminate or reduce the intake of the substrates that result in toxicity. Some patients may require therapies that bypass or supply substances normally produced by the body's metabolic pathways.

Because each child with a neurologic impairment is unique, the nutrition plan must be tailored to the individual patient's needs. A multidisciplinary team should closely monitor the child's nutritional status and adjust the plan as needed.[23]

Patients with dysmotility are at high risk of developing malnutrition. Diagnosing the disorder early is critical to starting appropriate therapy and preventing malnutrition. For patients with secondary dysmotility from other chronic diseases, therapy should be targeted toward the primary disease.

For patients with chronic constipation, the goal of therapy is to have soft, regular bowel movements. With dietary changes, pharmacologic therapy, or both, constipation can be resolved or managed. When constipation is adequately managed, the quality of life of both the pediatric patient and the caregiver improves.

References

1. Goetz D, Ren CL. Review of cystic fibrosis. *Pediatr Ann.* 2019;48(4):e154-e161.
2. Sullivan JS, Mascarenhas MR. Nutrition: Prevention and management of nutritional failure in Cystic Fibrosis. *J Cyst Fibros.* 2017;16 Suppl 2:S87-S93.
3. Altman K, McDonald CM, Michel SH, Maguiness K. Nutrition in cystic fibrosis: From the past to the present and into the future. *Pediatr Pulmonol.* 2019;54 Suppl 3:S56-S73.
4. Freeman AJ, Sellers ZM, Mazariegos G, et al. A multidisciplinary approach to pretransplant and posttransplant management of cystic fibrosis-associated liver disease. *Liver Transpl.* 2019;25(4):640-657.
5. Mousan G, Kamat D. Cow's milk protein allergy. *Clin Pediatr (Phila).* 2016;55(11):1054-1063.
6. Ahn KM, Han YS, Nam SY, Park HY, Shin MY, Lee SI. Prevalence of soy protein hypersensitivity in cow's milk protein-sensitive children in Korea. *J Korean Med Sci.* 2003;18(4):473-477.
7. Kattan JD, Cocco RR, Järvinen KM. Milk and soy allergy. *Pediatr Clin North Am.* 2011;58(2):407-426.
8. Klemola T, Vanto T, Juntunen-Backman K, Kalimo K, Korpela R, Varjonen E. Allergy to soy formula and to extensively hydrolyzed whey formula in infants with cow's milk allergy: a prospective, randomized study with a follow-up to the age of 2 years. *J Pediatr.* 2002;140:219-224.
9. Dupont C, Chouraqui JP, Linglart A, et al. Nutritional management of cow's milk allergy in children: An update. *Arch Pédiatr.* 2018;25(3):236-243.
10. Cherian S, Varshney P. Food protein-induced enterocolitis syndrome (FPIES): review of recent guidelines. *Curr Allergy Asthma Rep.* 2018;18(4):28.
11. Nowak-Wegrzyn A, Berin MC, Mehr S. Food protein-induced enterocolitis syndrome. *J Allergy Clin Immunol Pract.* 2020;8(1):24-35.

12. Nowak-Wegrzyn A, Jarocka-Cyrta E, Moschione Castro A. Food protein-induced enterocolitis syndrome. *J Investig Allergol Clin Immunol.* 2017;27(1):1-18.

13. Vinit C, Dieme A, Courbage S, et al. Eosinophilic esophagitis: Pathophysiology, diagnosis, and management. *Arch Pédiatr.* 2019;26(3):182-190.

14. Ferreira CT, Vieira MC, Furuta GT, Barros F, Chehade M. Eosinophilic esophagitis-Where are we today? *J Pediatr (Rio J).* 2019;95(3):275-281.

15. Gomez-Aldana A, Jaramillo-Santos M, Delgado A, Jaramillo C, Luquez-Mindiola A. Eosinophilic esophagitis: Current concepts in diagnosis and treatment. *World J Gastroenterol.* 2019;25(32):4598-4613.

16. Groetch M, Venter C, Skypala I, et al. Dietary therapy and nutrition management of eosinophilic esophagitis: a work group report of the American Academy of Allergy, Asthma, and Immunology. *J Allergy Clin Immunol Pract.* 2017;5(2):312-324.e329.

17. Straumann A, Katzka DA. Diagnosis and treatment of eosinophilic esophagitis. *Gastroentero.* 2018;154(2):346-359.

18. Gambello MJ, Li H. Current strategies for the treatment of inborn errors of metabolism. *J Genet Genomics.* 2018;45(2):61-70.

19. Vernon HJ. Inborn errors of metabolism: advances in diagnosis and therapy. *JAMA Pediatr.* 2015;169(8):778-782.

20. Guerrero RB, Kloke KM, Salazar D. Inborn errors of metabolism and the gastrointestinal tract. *Gastroenterol Clin North Am.* 2019;48(2):183-198.

21. Valle DL, Antonarakis S, Ballabio A, Beaudet AL, Mitchell GA. Eds. *The Online Metabolic and Molecular Bases of Inherited Disease.* McGraw Hill; 2019. Accessed December 14, 2021. https://ommbid .mhmedical.com/content.aspx?bookid=2709

22. Blackburn PR, Gass JM, Vairo FP, et al. Maple syrup urine disease: mechanisms and management. *App Clin Genet.* 2017;10:57-66.

23. Evans M, Truby H, Boneh A. The relationship between dietary intake, growth, and body composition in inborn errors of intermediary protein metabolism. *J Pediatr.* 2017;188:163-172.

24. van Calcar S. Nutrition management of maple syrup urine disease. In: Bernstein LER, Fran; Helm, Joanna R. *Nutrition Management of Inherited Metabolic Disorders.* Springer International Publishing Switzerland; 2015:173-183.

25. Penagini F, Mameli C, Fabiano V, Brunetti D, Dilillo D, Zuccotti GV. Dietary intakes and nutritional issues in neurologically impaired children. *Nutrients.* 2015;7(11):9400-9415.

26. Romano C, Dipasquale V, Gottrand F, Sullivan PB. Gastrointestinal and nutritional issues in children with neurological disability. *Dev Med Child Neurol.* 2018;60(9):892-896.

27. Romano C, van Wynckel M, Hulst J, et al. European Society for Paediatric Gastroenterology, Hepatology and Nutrition guidelines for the evaluation and treatment of gastrointestinal and nutritional complications in children with neurological impairment. *J Pediatr Gastroenterol Nutr.* 2017;65(2):242-264.

28. Araújo LA, Silva LR. Anthropometric assessment of patients with cerebral palsy: which curves are more appropriate? *J Pediatr (Rio J).* 2013;89(3):307-314.

29. Bell KL, Benfer KA, Ware RS, et al. Development and validation of a screening tool for feeding/swallowing difficulties and undernutrition in children with cerebral palsy. *Dev Med Child Neurol.* 2019;61(10):1175-1181.

30. Minocha P, Sitaraman S, Choudhary A, Yadav R. Subjective global nutritional assessment: a reliable screening tool for nutritional assessment in cerebral palsy children. *Indian J Pediatr.* 2018;85(1):15-19.

31. Bebars GM, Afifi MF, Mahrous DM, Okaily NE, Mounir SM, Mohammed EA. Assessment of some micronutrients serum levels in children with severe acute malnutrition with and without cerebral palsy- A follow up case control study. *Clin Nutr Exp.* 2019;23:34-43.

32. Teagarden DL, Meador KJ, Loring DW. Low vitamin D levels are common in patients with epilepsy. *Epilepsy Res.* 2014;108(8):1352-1356.

33. Dura-Trave T, Gallinas-Victoriano F, Malumbres-Chacon M, Moreno-Gonzalez P, Aguilera-Albesa S, Yoldi-Petri ME. Vitamin D deficiency in children with epilepsy taking valproate and levetiracetam as monotherapy. *Epilepsy Res.* 2018;139:80-84.

34. Green Corkins K. Nutrition-focused physical examination in pediatric patients. *Nutr Clin Pract.* 2015;30(2):203-209.

35. Smith SW, Camfield C, Camfield P. Living with cerebral palsy and tube feeding: a population-based follow-up study. *J Pediatr.* 1999;135(3):307-310.

36. Dipasquale V, Catena MA, Cardile S, Romano C. Standard polymeric formula tube feeding in neurologically impaired children: a five-year retrospective study. *Nutrients.* 2018;10(6):684. doi:10.3390/nu10060684

37. Suh CR, Kim W, Eun BL, Shim JO. Percutaneous endoscopic gastrostomy and nutritional interventions by the pediatric nutritional support team improve the nutritional status of neurologically impaired children. *J Clin Med.* 2020;9(10).

38. Bobo E. Reemergence of blenderized tube feedings: exploring the evidence. *Nutr Clin Pract.* 2016;31(6):730-735: 3295. doi:10.3390/jcm9103295

39. Camilleri M, Chedid V, Ford AC, et al. Gastroparesis. *Nat Rev Dis Primers.* 2018;4(1):41.

40. Di Nardo G, Di Lorenzo C, Lauro A, et al. Chronic intestinal pseudo-obstruction in children and adults: diagnosis and therapeutic options. *Neurogastroenterol Motil.* 2017;29(1):e12945.

41. Green Corkins K, Teague EE. Pediatric nutrition assessment: anthropometrics to zinc. *Nutr Clin Pract.* 2017;32(1):40-51.

42. Krasaelap A, Kovacic K, Goday PS. Nutrition management in pediatric gastrointestinal motility disorders. *Nutr Clin Pract.* 2020;35(2):265-272.

43. Tabbers MM, DiLorenzo C, Berger MY, et al. Evaluation and treatment of functional constipation in infants and children: evidence-based recommendations from ESPGHAN and NASPGHAN. *J Pediatr Gastroenterol Nutr.* 2014;58(2):258-274.

Gastrointestinal Oncology

Mary J. Marian, DCN, RDN, CSO, FAND, FASPEN

KEY POINTS

- Cancer is expected to become the leading cause of death in the United States, and many malignancies are thought to be preventable.
- Gastrointestinal cancers, including cancers of the esophagus, stomach, small bowel, large bowel, rectum, liver, gallbladder, and pancreas, account for approximately 20% of all newly diagnosed cancers annually.
- Nutrition screening identifies patients with cancer who are at high risk for nutritional deterioration or who are malnourished. Medical nutrition therapy plays an essential role in maintaining or improving the nutritional status of cancer survivors.

Introduction

The incidence of new cancers in the United States is more than 1.9 million cases annually (excluding basal and squamous cell skin cancers), with cancer accounting for one in every four deaths.[1] When deaths are aggregated by age, cancer surpasses heart disease as the leading cause of death for individuals younger than 85 years.[2] The American Cancer Society estimates that approximately 17 million adults in the United States have a history of a cancer diagnosis and that the overall costs related to cancer diagnoses will reach approximately $245 billion per year by the year 2030.[3,4] Gastrointestinal (GI) cancers, including cancers of the esophagus, stomach, small bowel, large bowel, rectum, liver, gallbladder, and pancreas, account for approximately 20% of all newly diagnosed cancers annually (see Table 10.1).[5]

Approximately one-third of cancer deaths are related to excess body fat, sedentary lifestyle, and poor diet, all of which are largely modifiable contributors.[6] Chronic inflammation is thought to play a key role in carcinogenesis, although scientists do not know the precise mechanisms.[6] Increased cell proliferation and oxidative stress resulting in dysplasia

TABLE 10.1 Gastrointestinal Cancers in US Adults[5]

Cancer type	New diagnoses per year[a]	Estimated deaths per year	Comments
Esophageal	19,260	15,530	Adenocarcinoma rates are increasing.
Gastric	26,560	11,180	More common in people aged more than 70 years.
Small bowel	11,390	2,100	Median age at diagnosis is 67 years.
Colorectal	149,500	52,980[b]	Third most common cancer, but incidence is decreasing.
Pancreatic	60,430	48,220	Incidence is stable in men and increasing in women; early detection can be difficult.
Hepatocellular and intrahepatic bile duct	42,230	30,230	

[a] Based on 2021 estimates.
[b] Deaths from rectal cancer and deaths from colon cancer are typically combined as colorectal cancer mortality statistics.

are key aspects of inflammation that are thought to contribute to carcinogenesis. Increased amounts of reactive oxygen and nitrogen species and DNA damage due to oxidative stress are also thought to be key contributors.[6] Box 10.1 presents factors associated with increased risk and protective factors for the development of GI cancers.[7-12]

BOX 10.1

Factors Associated With Risk for Gastrointestinal Cancers[7-12]

Mouth (oral)

Increased risk	Consumption of alcohol
Decreased risk	Consumption of nonstarchy vegetables, fruits, carotenoids

Esophageal

Increased risk	Abdominal fatness
	Consumption of alcohol and smoked foods
	Longstanding gastroesophageal reflux disease
Decreased risk	Consumption of nonstarchy cruciferous vegetables, vitamin C, carotenoids

Gastric

Increased risk	Consumption of salt and salted foods
	Smoking
	Helicobacter pylori infection
Decreased risk	Consumption of nonstarchy allium vegetables, vitamin C, whole grains, carotenoids, green tea

Large bowel

Increased risk	Consumption of red meat, processed meats, alcohol
	Body fatness
	Adult-attained height
Decreased risk	Consumption of fruits, vegetables, high-fiber foods, garlic, calcium
	Physical activity

Liver

Increased risk	Consumption of aflatoxins and alcohol
	Body fatness
Decreased risk	Consumption of fruits

Pancreas

Increased risk	Consumption of red meat
	Body fatness
	Smoking
	Chronic pancreatitis, diabetes, family history of pancreatic cancer
Decreased risk	Consumption of fruits, carotenoids, high-folate foods
	Physical activity

Gastrointestinal Cancer Prevention

The role that lifestyle and diet play in cancer risk is becoming increasingly clear, and it is now estimated that 42% of cancers are preventable.[6] Observational and epidemiologic studies reflect substantial differences in cancer rates among countries. Migration patterns exhibit the importance of environmental influences, as the incidence of cancer increases among populations that migrate from developing countries to more westernized societies.[13] Tobacco and alcohol use have also been found to play an important role in the development of many GI cancers. (See Box 10.1 for diet and lifestyle factors associated with GI cancer risk.[7-12])

Carcinogenesis is a multistep process with three critical steps: initiation, promotion, and progression. Chemoprevention involves preventing, suppressing, or reversing a premalignancy so it does not progress into cancerous cells. Epidemiologic evidence provides support that natural dietary bioactive compounds can modify this response.[14] A number of studies have shown that individuals in the lower quartiles for intake of fruits and vegetables have about twice the risk for cancers when compared with individuals in the upper quartiles.[6,13,14] Although the nutrient profile varies among these foodstuffs, plant foods are typically rich sources of many natural substances associated with a reduced risk for cancers: fiber, vitamins, minerals, flavonoids, sulforaphane, resveratrol, and organosulfur compounds. Food sources rich in chemopreventive phytochemicals include cruciferous vegetables, carrots, celery, tomatoes, peppers, flaxseed, grapes, soybeans, parsley, garlic, onions, turmeric, and ginger.[14]

The chemopreventive benefits that may be provided by specific phytonutrients are reviewed in Box 10.2; possible effects include the following[14]:

- antioxidant and anti-inflammatory effects
- induction of phase II enzymes and anti–cell growth signaling pathways
- induction of cellular defense systems resulting in apoptosis, cell cycle arrest, or both
- insulin-sensitizing effects that increase adiponectin levels or enhance adiponectin signaling

---

BOX 10.2

Phytochemicals and Gastrointestinal Cancer Prevention[14]

Allylic sulfides

Food sources Garlic, onion, shallots, chives, leeks

Clinical significance Anticancer activity; may decrease risk for colon and stomach cancers; decreases lipid peroxidation

α-Linoleic acid

Food sources Flaxseed, soy, walnuts

Clinical significance

Reduces inflammation; may protect against breast cancer; enhances immunity

Anthocyanins

Food sources Blackberries, blueberries, strawberries, other berries

Clinical significance Antioxidants; inhibit β-hydroxy-β-methylglutaryl-CoA reductase

Box continues

BOX 10.2 (CONTINUED)

Ascorbic acid

Food sources Green and yellow vegetables; fruits

Clinical significance Antioxidant

β-carotene

Food sources Green and yellow fruits and vegetables

Clinical significance Reduces risk for lung and breast cancers; enhances immunity (in older adults)

Capsaicin

Food sources Chili peppers

Clinical significance Antioxidant; reduces risk for colon, gastric, and rectal cancers

Catechin (flavonoid): theaflavins, thearubigins

Food sources Green and black tea, berries

Clinical significance Reduces risk for gastric cancer; antioxidant; increases immune function

Coumarin

Food sources Parsley, carrots, citrus

Clinical significance Reduces cancer risk

Curcumin (plant phenol)

Food sources Turmeric, curry, cumin

Clinical significance Anti-inflammatory properties; reduces risk for skin cancer

Cynarin

Food sources Artichokes

Clinical significance Decreases cholesterol levels

Ellagic acid (polyphenol)

Food sources Wine, grapes, currants, nuts (pecans), berries (strawberries, blackberries, raspberries), seeds

Clinical significance Reduces cancer risk

Flavonoids, polyphenolic acids, and other phenolic compounds (caffeic acid, ferulic acids, sesame, vanillin)

Food sources Parsley, carrots, citrus fruits, broccoli, cabbage, cucumbers, squash, yams, tomatoes, eggplant, peppers, soy products, berries, potatoes, broad beans, pea pods, colored onions, radishes, horseradish, tea, onions, apples, red wine, grape juice

Clinical significance Extend activity of vitamin C; act as antioxidants; anticarcinogenic activity

Box continues

BOX 10.2 (CONTINUED)

Genistein (isoflavone)

Food sources	Soybeans
Clinical significance	Reduces risk for hormone-dependent cancers

Indoles

Food sources	Cabbage, broccoli, brussels sprouts, spinach, watercress, cauliflower, turnips, kohlrabi, kale, rutabagas, horseradish, mustard greens
Clinical significance	Reduce risk for hormone-related cancers; may "inactivate" estrogen

Isoflavones and saponins

Food sources	Soybeans and soybean products
Clinical significance	Decrease risk for certain cancers

Isothiocyanates, such as sulforaphane (released during chewing of cruciferous vegetables)

Food sources	Cabbage, cauliflower, broccoli and broccoli sprouts, brussels sprouts, mustard greens, horseradish, radish
Clinical significance	Reduce risk for tobacco-induced tumors; stimulate glutathione S-transferase activity

Lignans (phytoestrogen)

Food sources	High-fiber foods, especially seeds; flax
Clinical significance	Reduce cancer risk (colon); bind to estrogen receptor sites and may reduce risk for estrogen-stimulated breast cancer

Lignin

Food sources	Soybean products, flaxseed
Clinical significance	May reduce risk for certain types of cancers, including breast and prostate

d-Limonene

Food sources	Citrus, citrus oils
Clinical significance	Antioxidant; reduces cancer risk

Lycopene (carotenoid)

Food sources	Tomato sauce, ketchup, red grapefruit, guava, dried apricots, watermelon
Clinical significance	Antioxidant; reduces risk for prostate cancer; may reduce cardiovascular disease

Box continues

BOX 10.2 (CONTINUED)

Monoterpenes

Food sources Parsley, carrots, celery, broccoli, cabbage, cauliflower, cucumbers, squash, yams, tomatoes, eggplant, peppers, mint, basil, caraway seed oil

Clinical significance Anticancer activity

Organosulfur compounds (allylic acid)

Food sources Garlic, onion, watercress, cruciferous vegetables, leeks

Clinical significance Decrease lipid peroxidation; reduce risk of gastric cancer

Phenolic acid

Food sources Cruciferous vegetables, eggplant, peppers, tomatoes, celery, parsley, soy, licorice root, flaxseed, citrus, whole grains, berries

Clinical significance Inhibits cancer through inhibition of nitrosamine formation; reduces risk for lung and skin cancers

Plant sterols

Food sources Broccoli, cabbage, cucumbers, squash, yams, tomatoes, eggplant, peppers, soy products, whole grains

Clinical significance May decrease risk for colon, rectal, stomach, lung, and breast cancers; decrease cardiovascular disease

Polyacetylene

Food sources Parsley, carrots, celery

Clinical significance Decreases risk for tobacco-induced tumors; alters prostaglandin formation

Retinol

Food sources Green and yellow vegetables, fruits

Clinical significance Potentially decreases risk for certain cancers

Selenium

Food sources Seafood, garlic

Clinical significance Antioxidant

Tocopherol (vitamin E)

Food sources Nuts, wheat germ, oils

Clinical significance Antioxidant

Nutritional Implications of Gastrointestinal Cancer and Cancer Therapies

Available anticancer therapies for GI cancers include surgery, chemotherapy, radiation, immunotherapy, and targeted therapy. Both the disease itself and treatment-related toxicities can contribute to deteriorations in nutritional status, including substantial weight loss and malnutrition. In fact, malnutrition is often the ultimate cause of death in patients with cancer.[6,13]

Weight Loss and Cancer Cachexia

The prevalence of weight loss among patients with cancer seems to be influenced by the type of tumor and stage of cancer. For example, 30% to 85% individuals with GI cancers have significant weight loss. Breast cancer, lymphomas, leukemias, and sarcomas are associated with the lowest incidence of weight loss.[15]

The following factors may be associated with weight loss:

- decreased nutritional intake
- acute metabolic stress and increased nutrient demands associated with surgery, radiotherapy, or chemotherapy
- an increase in nutrient demands resulting from the systemic effect of the tumor, which competes with the host for nutrients, resulting in metabolic derangements leading to anorexia, increased basal metabolic rate, and abnormal metabolism of nutrients (cachexia)[15]
- tumor phenotype or host genotype (although weight loss is not universal in all patients with similar tumor types)[16]

The wasting syndrome known as cancer anorexia-cachexia syndrome (CACS) is a major cause of malnutrition.[6,13,15] CACS is defined as a multifactorial syndrome characterized by a continual loss of skeletal muscle mass (fat loss may or may not occur) due to inadequate intake of energy and protein orchestrated by alterations in metabolism that lead to reductions in oral intake, impairments in functional status, and a poorer tolerance to treatment.[13] A weight loss of more than 5%, or a weight loss of more than 2% in individuals already showing depletion according to current body weight and height (BMI <20) or skeletal muscle mass (sarcopenia), are the agreed-upon criterion for a diagnosis of CACS.[13]

In addition to profound losses in weight and lean body mass, CACS is often characterized by the following:

- anorexia, early satiety, dysgeusia, nausea, constipation, fatigue, anemia, and edema
- other inflammatory conditions, such as cardiac failure, rheumatoid arthritis, and chronic obstructive pulmonary disease

Moreover, cachexia is estimated to be the primary cause of death in up to 33% of patients with cancer.[15,16] Weight loss before a cancer diagnosis is an important prognosticator of morbidity and mortality. A review of cancer-associated cachexia found that a weight loss of as little as 6% in patients predicted their response to therapy, influenced their overall survival rate, and correlated with their performance status and quality of life, all of which decreased concurrently with weight.[16] Malnutrition is underdiagnosed in the oncology population and, if not detected and treated, can lead to cancer cachexia.

Cancer cachexia is not a homogeneous syndrome, but experts agree that it presents with different stages, from precachexia to refractory cachexia. Patients are more likely to respond to nutrition interventions in the early stages, whereas severely malnourished patients with cancer typically do not respond to nutrition interventions when experiencing refractory cachexia.[15-17]

Mechanisms of Cancer Anorexia-Cachexia Syndrome

CACS is a multifactorial proinflammatory syndrome that has profound effects on dietary intake, body composition, functional status, tolerance to treatment, and mortality. The syndrome is poorly understood. Although the precise mechanisms involved are not clear, research has definitively shown that tumor-induced cytokines—tumor necrosis factor α, interleukin-1, interleukin-6 (which is a family of cytokines), and interferon-γ—play a role in promoting alterations in energy balance, appetite, gluconeogenesis, and lipolysis.[15-17] Alterations in proteostasis, reflecting the enhancement of proteolysis with simultaneous decreases in protein synthesis, are also involved; however, protein synthesis can be activated with the provision of nutrition. Other mediators may play a role in promoting CACS through various pathways, leading to reductions in lean body mass but also adversely affecting the central nervous system and both white and brown adipose tissue; these include transforming growth factor γ, activin A, myostatin, and proteolysis-inducing factor (PIF; a glycoprotein).[16]

Treatments for Cancer Cachexia

Curing the cancer is the most effective way to treat cancer cachexia, although a cure is not always possible in the advanced stages of cancer. Increasing nutrient intake would seem to be a logical way to reverse weight loss and promote nutritional repletion; however, this strategy is not always successful.[17]

Investigations have revealed that a multimodal approach targeting the various mechanisms associated with inflammation, anorexia, and cachectic mediators or signaling pathways is likely to be more effective than the use of single agents.[15,17] Pharmacologic agents (eg, megestrol acetate, a synthetic progestin) are used to stimulate appetite. Megestrol acetate, when compared to placebo in one study, led to improvements in weight and intake, although this benefit disappeared when megestrol acetate was compared with other drugs, such as dronabinol and dexamethasone.[18]

Eicosapentaenoic acid (EPA) is an omega-3 fatty acid that has been evaluated for its ability to attenuate weight loss. EPA's benefits are thought to be related to its ability to inhibit the activation of nuclear factor κB by PIF through preventing signaling pathways upstream—potentially by inhibiting the release of arachidonic acid from phospholipids.[19] EPA also seems to downregulate zinc-α2-glycoprotein expression by interfering with glucocorticoid signaling, which may, in turn, preserve adipose tissue.[19] The results of clinical studies investigating the benefits of EPA regarding weight loss have been mixed, and the strength of the evidence is limited by poor adherence, poor study design, and short study duration.[20-22] Well-designed placebo-controlled trials are needed to continue investigating the anticachetic activity of EPA. Further information about EPA is provided later in this chapter, in the section on selected nutrition interventions for patients with cancer.

β-Hydroxy-β-methylbutyrate (HMB) has been shown to downregulate PIF-induced muscle protein degradation by reducing the expression and activity of the ubiquitin-proteasome pathway.[23] In placebo-controlled clinical trials, HMB, together with L-glutamine and L-arginine, resulted in increased body weight and lean tissue mass, with no changes in fat mass in study participants with advanced cancers; however, conversely, in another study no benefits were found with HMB supplementation, reflecting the need for further investigation.[23,24]

Malnutrition Related to Antineoplastic Treatments

Antineoplastic therapies, including surgery, chemotherapy, and radiation, are known contributors to malnutrition (see Box 10.3 on page 156). Surgically induced malnutrition results from a reduced GI absorptive capacity for nutrients or from postoperatively increased metabolic demands for tissue repair in the face of inadequate nutritional intake.

As outlined in Box 10.4, chemotherapy can result in a number of treatment-related side effects, and radiation therapy also promotes deterioration in nutritional status when the radiotherapy field involves regions associated with the mechanics of eating or nutrient absorption. Treatment-related toxicities should be aggressively managed to prevent or reduce the likelihood of malnutrition associated with these therapies. Box 10.4 provides nutrition intervention strategies for combating these treatment-related issues.[25,26]

BOX 10.3

Anticancer Modalities That Affect Nutritional Status

Treatment modality	Potential adverse effects
Cytotoxic chemotherapy	Nausea, vomiting, anorexia, diarrhea, myelosuppression, fatigue, mucositis, dysgeusia, renal or hepatic side effects, peripheral neuropathies
Immunotherapy	Nausea, vomiting, diarrhea, fatigue, severe colitis (rare), diabetes mellitus
Radiation to the oropharyngeal region	Anorexia, dysphagia, mucositis, odynophagia, early satiety, fatigue
Radiation to the thorax region	Esophagitis, dysphagia, nausea, anorexia, fatigue, odynophagia
Radiation to the abdominal or pelvic region	Nausea, vomiting, diarrhea, abdominal cramping, abdominal bloating and gas, lactose intolerance, malabsorption, chronic colitis, enteritis
Surgery	Reduced surface area for digestion or absorption, increased nutrient needs, delayed wound healing, chyle leak, dumping syndrome, diarrhea, abdominal bloating and gas, gastroparesis, lactose intolerance, fluid and electrolyte imbalance
Targeted therapies	Weight loss, increased loss of skeletal muscle

BOX 10.4

Strategies for the Management of Treatment-Related Nutrition Impact Symptoms[25,26]

Anorexia

Cause	Pain, depression, cytokine oncological therapies
Recommendation	Small, frequent, nutrient-dense meals; no fluids with meals; no low-energy filler foods; increased physical activity; appetite stimulants

Constipation

Cause	Antineoplastic therapies, pain medication
Recommendation	Adequate hydration; high-fiber diet; fiber supplements; laxatives and stool softeners; physical activity

Box continues

BOX 10.4 (CONTINUED)

Diarrhea

Cause   Antineoplastic therapies

Recommendation   Low-fat, lactose-free diet; increased soluble fiber and reduced insoluble fiber; no spicy foods; no caffeine or alcohol; increased fluid intake; probiotics; antidiarrheal medications

Dysgeusia

Cause   Antineoplastic therapies

Recommendation   Strong-flavored foods (spicy, tart); zinc supplements; avoidance of metallic eating utensils

Dysphagia

Cause   Tumor burden, antineoplastic therapies

Recommendation   Thickened, moist, soft, blenderized, ground, and pureed foods; enteral nutrition support when risk of aspiration is too great for oral intake

Early satiety

Cause   Tumor burden, antineoplastic therapies

Recommendation   Small, frequent, nutrient-dense meals; no fluids with meals; low-fat and low-fiber meals and foods

Fatigue

Cause   Tumor burden, antineoplastic therapies, anemia, dehydration, chronic pain, medications, stress, depression, poor nutrition, poor sleep

Recommendation   Small, frequent, nutrient-dense meals; physical activity; assistance with meal planning, shopping, and preparation; stress management; depression treatment; better sleep hygiene; adequate hydration

Nausea and vomiting

Cause   Antineoplastic therapies, malignant gastroparesis

Recommendation   Small, frequent, low-fat and low-fiber meals; no spicy foods or caffeine; no eating for 1-2 h before treatment; ginger supplements; antiemetics; hypnosis; acupuncture; music therapy

Stomatitis and mucositis

Cause   Antineoplastic therapies

Recommendation   Soft, nonirritating, nutrient-dense foods; liquids and nutritional supplements; "magic mouthwash"; viscous lidocaine swishes; lemon glycerin swabs; analgesics; no extremely hot or cold foods

Weight gain

Cause   Antineoplastic therapies, edema, steroids

Recommendation   No excess energy intake; increased physical activity; fluid status assessment

Box continues

BOX 10.4 (CONTINUED)

Weight loss

Cause	Tumor burden, cachexia, antineoplastic therapies
Recommendation	Small, frequent, nutrient-dense meals and snacks; liquid or powder nutritional supplements; appetite stimulants; omega-3 fatty acids

Xerostomia

Cause	Tumor burden, antineoplastic therapies
Recommendation	Drinking or swallowing of small amounts of food at one time; sipping water or other fluid after each bite; sweet or tart foods; soft or pureed foods; sucking on hard candies; artificial saliva; acupuncture

Nutrition Screening, Assessment, and Intervention for Cancer

Ideally, a nutrition screening and surveillance program should be in place in all types of oncology settings. However, most patients with cancer are likely to receive therapy in an outpatient setting, where nutrition screening and intervention protocols are less likely to be implemented than in acute care. Both the Malnutrition Screening Tool and the Patient-Generated Subjective Global Assessment (PG-SGA), which has been adapted from the Subjective Global Assessment tool (SGA), have been validated for use in patients with cancer.[15] Patients identified with malnutrition or who are at high risk for becoming malnourished should receive a comprehensive nutrition assessment. Currently, there is no consensus on the ideal nutrition assessment tool, but the PG-SGA has been specifically validated for patients with cancer. Additional tools include the original, validated SGA (see Chapter 1) and the Academy of Nutrition and Dietetics and American Society for Parenteral and Enteral Nutrition (ASPEN) criteria for detecting malnutrition (not validated).[28-30]

The use of nutrition protocols or algorithms for nutrition referral can lead to optimized nutrition care. Patients with new cancer diagnoses may have a variety of symptoms and nutrition problems, including the following[15]:

- abdominal fullness (present in 60% of patients with new diagnoses)
- constipation (present in 58%)
- taste changes (present in 46%)
- mouth dryness (present in 40%)
- nausea (present in 39%)
- vomiting (present in 27% prior to initiation of oncologic treatment)

Attention to weight loss at early points in time can successfully prevent the deterioration of weight, body composition, and performance status. CACS should be suspected when an involuntary weight loss of 5% within 6 months is detected, especially when muscle wasting is manifested, as cachexia contributes to poorer prognosis and weight stabilization has been shown to improve survival in patients with GI cancers.[28,31] However, the significance of weight loss varies based on the percentage of weight lost and BMI, with a grading system developed and validated that correlates with probable survival.[28]

Patients identified to be at nutritional risk should receive a comprehensive nutrition assessment, which evaluates the following:

- anthropometric measurements (including weight-for-height, weight history, BMI, and waist-to-hip ratio)
- nutrition history

- nutrition focused physical examination findings that can indicate potential nutritional deficiencies
- laboratory data (eg, electrolytes; data related to renal function; glucose; serum albumin and prealbumin [as a reflection of inflammation]; and hemoglobin and hematocrit together with mean corpuscular volume or mean corpuscular hemoglobin concentration)
- performance status (using scales such as the Karnofsky scale to reflect level of functional impairment) and quality of life

After the assessment, an individualized nutrition plan that includes goals for clinical outcomes should be developed. Strategies for how to meet the patient's nutritional requirements, as well as strategies to combat treatment-related toxicities, should be reviewed with the patient with cancer. Nutrition care plans should consider the intent of treatment (palliative vs curative) and the patient's or caregiver's wishes. Reassessment should also occur at regular intervals. Nutrition outcome goals can include the following:

- maintaining or improving nutritional status
- avoiding or improving treatment-related toxicities
- avoiding nutrition-related interruptions in treatment
- decreasing morbidity related to disease or treatment
- maintaining or improving functional ability
- maintaining or improving quality of life

As noted previously, nutrition management strategies for patients struggling to consume adequate oral intake or facing other short-term and long-term issues, such as diarrhea, xerostomia, or mucositis, are described in Box 10.4.

Nutrition Requirements of Patients With Cancer

Adequate intake of energy, protein, and micronutrients can improve nutritional status for most patients with cancer.[27,28] The nutrition principles outlined by the American Cancer Society's guidelines on diet, nutrition, and cancer prevention should be used for the basis of a healthy diet for all patients with cancer, including those who are well nourished, during and after treatment.[25,26]

Energy

The impact of cancer on energy needs is inconsistent. Resting energy expenditure may be unchanged, increased, or decreased in comparison to predicted needs.[28] The European Society for Clinical Nutrition and Metabolism (ESPEN) consensus guidelines recommend 25 to 30 kcal/kg of body weight per day depending on the individual's functional status when resting energy expenditure cannot be measured directly.[28] However, ESPEN states that these recommendations are less accurate for individuals who are underweight.

In a 2008 study, the energy needs of weight-losing, nonambulatory patients with GI tumors were found to range from 24 to 28 kcal/kg/d.[31] More recently, another study noted that patients with newly diagnosed colorectal cancers (with primarily stage II and stage III cancers) needed on average approximately 30 kcal/kg/d, although energy needs varied widely from 20 to 49 kcal/kg/d due to differences in BMI (most study participants were either overweight or obese) and body composition.[32]

Protein

Protein metabolism is altered with cancer, and protein needs typically increase with treatment because of the stress and cellular damage that commonly occur with therapies, particularly radiation. In general, the protein requirement for patients with cancer is thought to be a minimum of 1 g/kg of body weight per day with a target goal range of 1.2 to 2 g/kg/d, particularly in inactive patients and patients with systematic inflammation.[28] However, protein intake in patients with chronic kidney disease should not exceed 1.5 g/kg/d; and in those with acute kidney disease, it should not exceed 1.2 g/kg/d.[33]

Micronutrients

Individuals with cancer may be at risk for micronutrient deficiencies because of poor nutrient intake, increased nutrient requirements, and/or increased nutrient losses. Specific guidelines are not available; however, the Tolerable Upper Intake Levels of the Dietary Reference Intakes should not be exceeded unless some objective data indicate a need for a greater intake to facilitate repletion.

Selected Nutrition Interventions for Patients With Cancer

Immune-Enhancing Formulas

The efficacy of using immune-enhancing formulas (containing arginine, omega-3 fatty acids, and nucleotides) vs standard formulas preoperatively and perioperatively, in terms of their impact on clinical outcomes in patients with cancer, has been examined. A 2020 meta-analysis and systematic review found that malnourished patients with cancer who received immune-enhancing formulations (25–30 kcal/kg/d) for 5 to 7 days preoperatively experienced fewer infections and wound complications, as well as decreased length of hospital stay, although there was no difference in all-cause mortality.[34]

Clinical practice guidelines recommend the perioperative use of immune-enhancing formulations for patients undergoing elective surgeries (including surgeries for cancer) and for critically ill patients to achieve favorable clinical outcomes.[35,36] However, further study is warranted before the use of these formulas can be recommended on a more global basis for all patients with cancer.

Oral Nutritional Supplements

The strategies for maintaining adequate oral intake depend on the challenges experienced by the individual patient (see Box 10.4). Studies have shown that the aggressive management of nutrition impact symptoms not only improves or maintains nutritional status but also enhances quality of life and social interactions, although mortality is not affected.[25,26,28,37] The use of commercially prepared oral nutritional supplements (ONS) can result in increased weight gain and reduced incidence of postoperative complications in patients undergoing surgery; it can also help avoid unnecessary delays in treatment for patients with GI cancers.[37,38] Conversely, a 2018 meta-analysis reported that use of ONS did not improve body weight in patients undergoing concurrent chemotherapy and radiation; this was determined through subgroup analysis, which was required because of considerable heterogeneity among the studies.[39] The investigators theorized this was likely due to insufficient energy intake, as the study participants did not reach their recommended energy goals (actual intakes of 1,700–2,000 kcal/d vs goals of 2,100–2,800 kcal/d), reflecting poor adherence to recommendations. However, they noted that ONS enriched with protein and omega-3 fatty acids helped to prevent CACS and increase body weight and muscle mass when gaps in energy and protein intake were minimized during chemotherapy. Data are scarce regarding the impact of ONS on preventing treatment-related toxicities or delays in treatment; further research is needed, as most studies done thus far lack adequate sample size, homogeneous populations, and adequate length of follow-up.

Nutrition Support

Nutrition support should be considered when oral nutritional intake is insufficient to maintain nutritional status or is contraindicated.[28,35,36] See Chapter 19, 20, and 22 for more on nutrition support, including home nutrition support. When to start nutrition support in patients with cancer depends on their prognosis and nutritional status, the potential benefits of treatment, and the wishes of the individual patient or the patient's caregivers. Nutrition support should be considered for patients with an expected survival of months or years, tumors obstructing the GI tract, severe mucositis and dysphagia, and ongoing weight loss.[28,35] If a patient is not expected to survive more than a few weeks, noninvasive interventions that promote comfort should be considered.[28]

Enteral Nutrition

Weight loss and decreases in lean body mass can lead to poorer quality of life, treatment toxicity, delays in treatment, and increased morbidity and mortality. Therefore, ESPEN recommends that patients presenting with weight loss and malnutrition who are receiving antineoplastic therapies and are unlikely to consume adequate nutrition for more than 2 weeks be considered as candidates for nutrition support.[28] An analysis of data from a longitudinal study noted that a "window of anabolic potential" exists, as patients with advanced cancer who are within 90 days of death are unlikely to benefit from nutrition interventions that halt or reverse CACS.[40]

Enteral nutrition (EN) should be considered for patients who are unable to consume adequate oral nutrition, if the GI tract can be safely used. When specialized nutrition support is warranted and the GI tract is functional and accessible, EN is clearly preferred over parenteral nutrition (PN) because EN is associated with fewer complications.[28] EN in various GI oncology populations has resulted in fewer chemotherapy-related hematological issues, improved weight, fewer unplanned hospitalizations, a greater chance of completing prescribed chemotherapy, and in some studies, improved survival.[41-44]

Parenteral Nutrition

The ASPEN and ESPEN clinical guidelines for nutrition support during adult anticancer treatment support the perioperative use of PN for severely malnourished patients with cancer.[28,35,36] PN for patients receiving chemotherapy with or without radiation can result in increased weight and body fat mass, correction of vitamin and mineral deficiencies, improved hydration, and, possibly, improved survival.[28] Clinical practice guidelines suggest that PN should not be routinely used in all patients.[28,35,36] For ethical reasons, no prospective, randomized controlled trials have been done to examine the benefits of PN in patients with cancer.[35] In summary:

- PN should not be routinely administered to patients with cancer who are undergoing chemotherapy, radiation, or surgery.[28,35,36]
- PN should be considered only in patients who are moderately to severely malnourished and unable to tolerate EN or oral diet for at least 1 week.
- PN should be initiated if the duration of therapy will be more than 7 days.[36]
- Perioperative PN may be indicated for moderately to severely malnourished patients in whom surgery may safely be delayed 7 to 14 days and when EN is not possible.[36]
- PN is recommended for individuals with severe mucositis, ileus, or intractable vomiting following hematopoietic stem cell transplantation.[28]

Nutrition Support in Alternative-Care Sites and Home Care

Nutrition support, especially EN, is widely used in long-term-care and alternative-care sites.[28] Clinical practice guidelines for the provision of home nutrition support stress the importance of conducting the following before making decisions about home nutrition support[28,44]:

- an in-depth nutrition assessment;
- an assessment of the patient's home environment;
- an evaluation the patient's medical suitability for EN or PN; education level; religious, culture and ethical background; and rehabilitative potential and expected survival; and
- a close evaluation of reimbursement sources.

PN or EN should be terminated when the patient no longer benefits from the therapy or the burden exceeds the benefit.[28,35] There is no benefit to nutrition support during the last few weeks of life, and predicting how long a patient will survive is difficult; thus, the decision to initiate nutrition support or not should be based on clinical judgment, patient and caregiver wishes, and the risks and benefits that may be conveyed by the nutrition support. However, PN may prolong survival in patients with cancer (primarily those with intestinal obstruction and hypophagia) compared with no support.[44-46] For more information on home EN and PN, see Chapter 22.

Nutrition and Specific Gastrointestinal Cancers

Head and Neck Cancer

Malnutrition plays a key role in the morbidity of patients with head and neck cancer who are undergoing surgery, chemotherapy, or radiotherapy; many patients with head and neck cancer receive concurrent chemoradiotherapy, which has been found to promote better survival.[47] However, profound side effects (eg, severe mucositis, dysphagia, xerostomia, early satiety, and constipation) are nutrition impact symptoms commonly associated with treatment that can promote further nutritional deterioration.[47-49] Weight loss before a diagnosis of head and neck cancer is common and is associated with poorer survival.[47-49] Following diagnosis, an additional 10% of pretherapy body weight may be lost during radiotherapy or combined-modality treatment.[49] A weight loss of more than 20% during chemoradiotherapy has been associated with poor survival.[49]

Individualized nutrition counseling effectively increases dietary intake, maintains or improves nutritional and functional status, and improves the quality of life in patients undergoing radiotherapy for a variety of head and neck cancers; however, because of the detrimental side effects of treatment, percutaneous endoscopic gastrostomy tubes are often placed prophylactically.[47-49] Even with a feeding tube in place, however, most patients will continue to lose weight during treatment, as they are unable to achieve their nutrition goals related to energy and protein needs.[49] Barriers to adequate EN include severe nausea, early satiety, and lack of motivation, among others.[49]

Estimates of the percentage of patients who must depend on EN support for 6 to 12 months after surgical, radiotherapy, or chemotherapy interventions (or a combination of these modalities) because of chronic dysphagia and xerostomia vary from 6% to 64%.[47-49] At long-term follow-up (≥1 year) after chemoradiation, patients without recurrence of cancer typically have at least some oral intake, but more than 10% still require supplemental enteral support because of chronic dysphagia.[50]

Esophageal Cancer

Although esophageal cancer is relatively uncommon compared to other types of cancer (approximately 18,440 new cases in the United States in 2020), the incidence of adenocarcinoma of the esophagus is increasing, with the tumors being located primarily in the distal esophagus.[1] Unfortunately, the prognosis for individuals with esophageal cancer is poor, with a 5-year survival rate of approximately 20%.[51]

Esophageal cancer affects males more than females, and White people are at increased risk compared with other racial groups.[52] Risk factors for esophageal cancer include the following:

- tobacco and alcohol use
- obesity
- Barrett esophagus (which is associated with persistent gastric acid reflux)
- diet
- sedentary lifestyle

Dietary factors that may increase risk include the following[7]:

- ingestion of very hot foods and beverages
- diets low in fruits and vegetables
- diets high in processed meat

To effectively treat esophageal cancer, patients typically undergo neoadjuvant therapy followed by an esophagectomy.[53] Patients with esophageal cancer should be screened for malnutrition and reassessed at established interval as an estimated 79% of patients with esophageal cancer experience malnutrition.[53]

Esophageal obstruction, dysphagia, anorexia, thick oral secretions, and the side effects of treatment modalities (such as severe mucositis and vomiting) often affect nutritional status in this patient population.[53-57] Progressive dysphagia resulting in weight loss affects more than 75% of patients before esophageal cancer is diagnosed, and continued weight loss is common once antineoplastic therapies are initiated.[56] Early signs of esophageal cancer can also include complaints of food "sticking" in the throat, retrosternal discomfort, or a burning sensation. Esophageal stents may be placed to "open up the esophagus" and facilitate the passage of food and liquids. Soft foods and foods that can be moistened (eg, sauces, gravies, butter) are recommended. Foods are that crumbly, dry, or hard may be more difficult for patients to swallow. Nutritional supplements can also help to increase energy and protein intakes.

Patients with esophageal cancer often require EN because of the frequency of severe dysphagia or luminal obstruction; a jejunostomy tube is commonly placed. Clinical practice guidelines recommend the use of perioperative nutrition support for moderately to severely malnourished patients, including patients with esophageal cancer, if it can be administered for 7 to 14 days preoperatively.[28,35] Moreover, some studies have found that when consumed preoperatively, either orally or through a feeding tube, immune-enhancing formulations (vs a standard diet) containing a combination of arginine, omega-3 fatty acids, glutamine, antioxidants, and nucleotides are associated with positive outcomes, such as enhanced immune function, fewer infectious complications, and shorter length of hospital stay.[58,59] Conversely, other studies have reported no benefits to consuming an immune-enhancing formulation preoperatively.[60]

Studies examining whether perioperative use of immune-enhancing formulas provides benefits have had mixed results.[61-63] Many of these studies failed to distinguish whether enrolled study participants were malnourished or not. Additionally, determining the optimal timing for using such formulations requires further exploration in well-designed, prospective, randomized clinical trials.

Gastric Cancer

Gastric cancer (also called stomach cancer) is the 15th most commonly diagnosed cancer in the United States. More than 27,000 cases of gastric cancer are diagnosed annually, and approximately 11,000 deaths are caused each year by this type of cancer.[1] Incidence in the United States is relatively low, but gastric cancer is the third leading cause of cancer deaths worldwide, with particularly high incidence rates in Asia and South America.[64] Individuals older than 65 years are the most likely to receive a diagnosis of gastric cancer, and the overall survival rate in the United States is about 31%. The most common type of gastric cancer (>90% of cases) is adenocarcinoma.[64]

Risk factors for gastric cancer include[64]:

- genetic factors (Asian descent),
- obesity,
- environmental factors (smoking), and
- dietary factors (including high intake of salted or smoked foods; N-nitroso compounds, processed and red meats, or alcoholic beverages; and low intake of fruits and vegetables)

Chronic superficial gastritis and gastric atrophy are thought to play a role in the progression to gastric cancer.[64] Chronic gastritis caused by chronic *Helicobacter pylori* infection and pernicious anemia results in chronic atrophic gastritis and intestinal metaplasia.[65]

As with esophageal cancer, gastroesophageal reflux disease (GERD) has been associated with an increased risk for gastric cancer.[64,66] GERD-related stomach cancer is becoming more common than *H pylori*–related disease.

Gastric resection is associated with an increased risk for morbidity, depending on the disease state and type of resection needed.[67-69] The presence and type of disease dictates whether a small portion of the stomach must be removed vs a total gastrectomy. Whether a Billroth I operation (anastomosis of the esophagus or the remaining stomach to the duodenum) or a Billroth II operation (anastomosis of the esophagus or remaining stomach to the jejunum) is done, the patient's ability to consume adequate oral nutrition postoperatively is affected.

After gastric surgery, dumping syndrome is common, especially when the pylorus is removed or bypassed. Dumping syndrome occurs when the food passes through the GI tract quickly without being substantially absorbed. Symptoms of dumping syndrome include abdominal cramping, diarrhea, sweating, nausea, dizziness, and tachycardia.[70] Symptoms usually appear within 2 to 3 hours after eating.

Dietary modifications to help combat these symptoms include the following:

- eating small, frequent, bland, low-fat meals
- avoiding spicy foods, alcohol, and sugar and sweets
- avoiding very hot or cold foods
- limiting fluids to 4 oz during meals and instead drinking liquids 30 to 45 minutes before and after eating

Some nutrients, vitamins, and minerals may be poorly absorbed because of anatomical alterations or intestinal bacterial overgrowth (or both), leading to subsequent deficiencies in iron, vitamin D, folate, and vitamin B12.[71] Reportedly, up to 77% of patients have small intestinal bacterial overgrowth following total gastrectomy procedures.[72] To avoid or correct nutrient deficiencies, patients may need to take liquid or chewable multivitamin and multimineral supplements that contain iron and vitamin B12 (taken sublingually or as an intramuscular injection).

Small Intestine Cancers

Small intestine cancers, also called small bowel cancers, are extremely rare (slightly more than 11,000 cases diagnosed annually).[1,73] The most common type diagnosed is adenocarcinoma. Other types include sarcoma, carcinoid tumors, and lymphoma, which together account for between 1% and 2% of all GI cancers.[73] The 5-year survival rate for small intestine cancer varies between 20% (for resectable adenocarcinomas) and 50% (for leiomyosarcoma tumors).[73]

The treatment modalities for the other types of GI cancers previously discussed are also used for the treatment of small bowel cancers. Surgery is the most common treatment, when resection of the tumor is possible. See Chapter 17 for more on GI surgeries.

Pancreatic Cancer

Pancreatic cancer is the fourth leading cause of cancer-related deaths in the United States, Canada, and Western Europe.[1] In the United States, approximately 57,600 cases are diagnosed annually, and roughly 47,000 people die from it each year.[1] Pancreatic cancer is rare in individuals younger than 45 years of age; however, rates increase sharply thereafter, with males affected more often than females. Compared with other racial groups, Black people are at increased risk.[74,75] Risk factors for pancreatic cancer also include the following[74-76]:

- a first-degree relative with a history of the disease (5% to 10% of pancreatic cancers are thought to occur in individuals with a first-degree relative who has had pancreatic cancer)
- smoking
- hereditary chronic pancreatitis and other inherited cancer-susceptibility syndromes
- obesity
- diabetes mellitus, alterations in glucose metabolism, and insulin resistance
- tall height
- lower levels of physical activity

Some, but not all, studies have found that an increased risk for pancreatic cancer is associated with consumption of a Western-style diet that is high in fat or meat (or both). Although coffee consumption has not been associated with an increased risk for pancreatic cancer, as was previously thought, lifetime alcohol exposure has been noted to increase the risk.[77-78] Lastly, the potential association between serum vitamin D levels and pancreatic cancer risk has been evaluated in case-control studies.[79,80] However, more research is needed before public health recommendations about vitamin D and pancreatic cancer risk can be made.

The most common treatment options for pancreatic cancer are chemotherapy and radiation; approximately 20% of patients undergo surgery.[81] Tumor resection with curative intent is possible in only 10% to 15% of patients, with many patients facing limited therapeutic options and a poor prognosis.[81-83]

At the time of diagnosis, many patients with pancreatic cancer present with substantial weight loss. Such weight loss is associated with impairments in functional status and worse outcomes; as many as 80% of patients with advanced pancreatic cancer die of cancer cachexia.[82] Reduced intake is caused by a number of factors, including nausea, pain, anxiety, depression, and gastric outlet obstruction.[81] Palliative management strategies include gastric bypass or placement of a small bowel stent. Malabsorption and altered glucose tolerance further complicate nutritional status.

Malabsorption should be suspected in the face of continued weight loss and the presence of abdominal symptoms (eg, bloating, abdominal pain, greasy stools). Pancreatic enzymes should be prescribed when malabsorption is diagnosed. Enzymes are typically dosed according to lipase content.[84-86] See Chapter 8 for more information on the use of pancreatic enzymes.

Malabsorption also typically leads to vitamin and mineral deficiencies. Absorption of vitamins A, D, E, and K is dependent on fat absorption; vitamin B12 absorption relies on the presence of protease enzymes. Iron, calcium, vitamin B12, and vitamin D deficiencies can occur when proton pump inhibitors are prescribed. Whipple procedures can result in deficiencies of calcium, zinc, and iron.[81,84] Guidelines for providing vitamin and mineral supplements to patients with pancreatic cancer are lacking. Supplementation needs are likely to vary depending on the severity of malabsorption.

A multivitamin supplement with the fat-soluble vitamins provided as water-soluble components is recommended. The use of omega-3 fatty acid supplements has been investigated in this patient population with mixed results.[87,88] More recently, a randomized, controlled, double-blind trial found that omega-3 fatty acids, supplemented either as marine phospholipids or as a fish oil supplement combined with medium-chain triglycerides, led to a stabilization of body weight at a low dose of 300 mg/d of omega-3 fatty acids for 6 weeks in study participants with pancreatic cancer.[88]

Large Bowel Cancers

The most common type of large bowel cancer is colon cancer, which is the third most common type of cancer worldwide and the second most common cause of cancer deaths in the United States.[1] Although, in general, colon cancer incidence continues to decline in the United States thanks to effective screening measures, the incidence has been increasing among US adults under the age of 50 years.[89] Genetic factors may play a role in the development of colon cancer, although colon cancer is more common in Westernized countries than in developing countries, and it is thought to be strongly influenced by lifestyle factors.[89] Commonly cited risk factors include[89,90]:

- family history, particularly of familial adenomatous polyposis and hereditary non-polyposis colon cancer,
- personal or family history of breast, ovarian, or endometrial cancers,
- presence of adenomatous polyps,
- inflammatory bowel disease (chronic ulcerative colitis or Crohn's disease),
- cholecystectomy,
- obesity,
- systemic inflammation,
- diabetes and insulin resistance,
- advanced age (colon cancer is rare before 40 years of age but more recently has been increasing in those under 40),
- sedentary lifestyle, and
- smoking.

In addition, the consumption of red and processed meats, consumption of alcoholic drinks, body fatness, abdominal fatness, and a tall adult-attained height are reportedly strong risk factors for colorectal cancer (CRC), whereas the consumption of fiber, whole grains, calcium, vitamin D, and dairy products, as well as being physically active, are associated with a reduced risk.[9,89,90]

A meta-analysis reported that greater consumption of foods with proinflammatory potential, as measured by the Dietary Inflammatory Index for food, may increase the risk for CRC.[90] A higher adherence to the Mediterranean diet has been reported to decrease the risk for CRC, as well as for other malignancies.[91,92]

Additionally, individuals can decrease their risk by increasing their physical activity, and also by increasing their consumption of milk, cheese, and calcium. Additionally, calcium supplementation ranging from 200 to 1,000 mg/d may reduce risk. Six of eight cohort studies showed consistent inverse relationships between calcium supplement use and CRC.[9] Lastly, the evidence that vitamin D decreases the risk for colorectal cancers is limited but suggests that consuming foods high in vitamin D or using a vitamin D supplement decreases the risk for colon cancer.[9,89] However, serum and plasma vitamin D levels have not been correlated with risk.[9]

Treatment for CRC includes the traditional adjuvant and neoadjuvant oncological therapies—namely, surgery, chemotherapy, and radiation. Prehabilitation therapies, such as exercise, nutrition, and psychological therapies, following neoadjuvant treatments can improve cardiorespiratory parameters and may reduce postoperative complications.[93]

The recommendations for the use of nutrition support for patients with CRC are the same as for patients with other cancers. As outlined by the ESPEN clinical practice guidelines for patients with cancer, the recommendations for nutrition in the CRC population include the following[28]:

- Avoid long periods of preoperative fasting.
- Begin oral feeding as early as possible after surgery.
- Start nutrition support early, as determined by nutritional risk.
- Reduce factors that exacerbate stress-related catabolism and impairment of the GI tract.

A randomized controlled trial compared individualized nutrition counseling with the use of ONS and the consumption of a typical Western-style diet. When adjusted for tumor stage, nutritional deterioration was substantially greater in the patients who consumed a Western-style diet, and deterioration was the least severe in patients who received individualized counseling.[94] Moreover, the median survival in the nutrition counseling group was 7.3 years, compared with 6.5 years for the ONS group and 4.9 years for the group consuming the Western-style diet ($P < .01$). Study participants who took ONS and those who ate a Western-style diet also experienced more late radiotherapy toxicity than those in the nutrition counseling group. This illustrates the value of one-on-one nutrition education in comparison to solely using ONS.

Summary

Cancer is expected to become the leading cause of death in the United States, and many malignancies are thought to be preventable. Multiple lifestyle factors, including tobacco and alcohol use, an unhealthy diet, excess body weight, and lack of regular physical activity, have been identified as risk factors. Basic lifestyle changes can, therefore, have a major impact on modifying one's risk.

Medical nutrition therapy plays an essential role in maintaining or improving the nutritional status of patients with cancer. Nutrition screening identifies patients at high risk for nutritional deterioration or who are experiencing malnutrition. Many anticancer therapies are associated with treatment-related toxicities that have a profound impact on a patient's nutritional status. Such treatment-related toxicities should be aggressively managed to maintain or improve the patient's nutritional status and quality of life. Following the completion of antineoplastic treatment, cancer survivors should receive a survivorship plan that focuses on reducing the risks for recurrence or maintaining nutritional status and quality of life while living with cancer. For additional information on medical nutrition therapy for patients with cancer, readers are encouraged to review the Academy of Nutrition and Dietetics Oncology (2013) Evidence-Based Nutrition Practice Guideline and the book *Oncology Nutrition for Clinical Practice* (2021).[95,96]

References

1. American Cancer Society. *Cancer Facts and Figures 2021*. American Cancer Society; 2021. Accessed January 4, 2022. www.cancer.org/content/dam/cancer -org/research/cancer-facts-and-statistics/annual-cancer-facts-and-figures /2021/cancer-facts-and-figures-2021.pdf

2. American Cancer Society medical and editorial content team. Lifetime risk of developing or dying from cancer. American Cancer Society. Last updated January 13, 2020. Accessed January 4, 2022. www.cancer.org/cancer/cancer-basics /lifetime-probability-of-developing-or-dying-from-cancer.html

3. Simon S. Population of US cancer survivors grows to nearly 17 million. American Cancer Society. June 11, 2019. Accessed January 4, 2022. www.cancer.org/latest -news/population-of-us-cancer-survivors-grows-to-nearly-17-million.html

4. Cancer care costs in the United States are projected to exceed $245 billion by 2030. News release. American Association for Cancer Research. June 10, 2020. Accessed July 20, 2020. www.aacr.org/about-the-aacr/newsroom/news-releases /cancer-care-costs-in-the-united-states-are-projected-to-exceed-245-billion -by-2030

5. Cancer Statistics Center, American Cancer Society. Accessed January 4, 2022. https://cancerstatisticscenter.cancer.org/?_ga=2.13704383.967077499 .1598308468-1020226238.1594496459#!

6. Islami F, Sauer AG, Miller KD, et al. Proportion and number of cancer cases and deaths attributable to potentially modifiable risk factors in the United States. *CA Cancer J Clin*. 2018;68(1):31-54. doi:10.3322/caac.21440

7. Continuous Update Project: mouth, pharynx, larynx cancers. American Institute for Cancer Research. Last updated January 9, 2020. Accessed January 4, 2022. www.aicr.org/research/the-continuous-update-project/mouth-pharynx-larynx -cancers

8. Continuous Update Project: esophageal cancer. American Institute for Cancer Research. Last updated January 9, 2020. Accessed January 4, 2022. www.aicr.org /research/the-continuous-update-project/esophageal-cancer

9. Continuous Update Project: stomach cancer. American Institute for Cancer Research. Last updated January 9, 2020. Accessed January 4, 2022. www.aicr.org /research/the-continuous-update-project/stomach-cancer

10. Continuous Update Project: colorectal cancer. American Institute for Cancer Research. Last updated January 9, 2020. Accessed January 4, 2022. www.aicr.org /research/the-continuous-update-project/colorectal-cancer

11. Continuous Update Project: liver cancer. American Institute for Cancer Research. Last updated January 9, 2020. Accessed January 4, 2022. www.aicr.org/research /the-continuous-update-project/liver-cancer

12. Continuous Update Project: pancreatic cancer. American Institute for Cancer Research. Last updated January 9, 2020. Accessed January 4, 2022. www.aicr.org /research/the-continuous-update-project/pancreatic-cancer

13. Fearon K, Strasser F, Amlar S, et al. Definitions and classifications of cancer cachexia: an international consensus. *Lancet Oncol*. 2011;12(5):489-495. doi:10 .1016/S1470-2045(10)70218-7

14. Nosrati N, Bakovic M, Paliyath G. Molecular mechanisms and pathways as targets for cancer prevention and progression with dietary compounds. *Int J Mol Sci*. 2017;18(10):2050. doi:10.3390/ijms18102050

15. Zhang X, Edwards BJ. Malnutrition in older adults with cancer. *Curr Oncol Rep. 2019;*21(9):80. doi:10.1007/s11912-019-0829-8

16. Biswas AK, Acharyya S. Cancer-associated cachexia: a systemic consequence of cancer progression. *Annu Rev Cancer Biol*. 2020;4:391-411. doi:10.1146/annurev -cancerbio-030419-033642

17. Marceca GP, Londhe P, Calore F. Management of cancer cachexia: attempting to develop new pharmacological agents for new effective therapeutic options. *Front Oncol*. 2020;10:298. doi:10.3389/fonc.2020.00298

18. Ruiz GV, Lopez-Briz E, Carbonell SR, et al. Megestrol acetate for treatment of anorexia-cachexia syndrome. *Cochrane Database Syst Rev*. 2013;(3):CD004310.

19. Freitas RDS, Campos MM. Protective effects of omega-3 fatty acids in cancer- related complications. *Nutrients*. 2019;11(5):945. doi:10.3390/nu11050945

20. Chagas TR, Borges DS, de Oliveira PF, et al. Oral fish oil positively influences nutritional-inflammatory risk in patients with haematological malignancies during chemotherapy with an impact on long-term survival: a randomised clinical trial. *J Hum Nutr Diet.* 2017;30(6):681-692. doi:10.1111/jhn.12471

21. Abe K, Uwagawa T, Haruki K, et al. Effects of ω-3 fatty acid supplementation in patients with bile duct or pancreatic cancer undergoing chemotherapy. *Anticancer Res.* 2018;38(4):2369-2375. doi:10.21873/anticanres.12485

22. Bruera E, Strasser F, Palmer JL, et al. Effect of fish oil on appetite and other symptoms in patients with advanced cancer and anorexia/cachexia: a double-blind, placebo-controlled study. *J Clin Oncol.* 2003;21(1):129-134. doi:10.1200/JCO.2003.01.101

23. May PE, Barber A, D'Olimpio JT, Hourihane A, Abumrad NN. Reversal of cancer-related wasting using oral supplementation with a combination of beta-hydroxy-beta-methylbutyrate, arginine, and glutamine. *Am. J. Surg.* 2002;183:471-479. doi:10.1016/S0002-9610(02)00823-1

24. Berk L, James J, Schwartz A, et al. A randomized, double-blind, placebo-controlled trial of a b-hydroxy-b-methylbutyrate, glutamine, and arginine mixture for the treatment of cancer cachexia (RTOG 0122). *Support Care Cancer.* 2008;16(10):1179-1188. doi:10.1007/s00520-008-0403-7

25. Rock CL, Doyle C, Demark-Wahnefried W. Nutrition and physical activity guidelines for cancer survivors. *CA Cancer J Clin.* 2012;62(4):243-274. doi:10.3322/caac.21142

26. American Cancer Society medical and editorial content team. Nutrition for People with Cancer. American Cancer Society. Last updated June 9, 2020. Accessed January 4, 2022. www.cancer.org/content/dam/CRC/PDF/Public/6711.00.pdf

27. Muscaritoli M, Lucia S, Farcomeni A, et al. Prevalence of malnutrition in patients at first medical oncology visit: the PreMiO study. *Oncotarget.* 2017;8(45):79884-79896. doi:10.18632/oncotarget.20168

28. Arends J, Bachmann P, Baracos V, et al. ESPEN guidelines on nutrition in cancer patients. *Clin Nutr.* 2017;36(1):11-48. doi:10.1016/j.clnu.2016.07.015

29. Jager-Wittenaar H, Ottery FD. Assessing nutritional status in cancer: role of the Patient-Generated Subjective Global Assessment. *Curr Opin Clin Nutr Metabolic Care.* 2017;20(5):322-329. doi:10.1097/MCO.0000000000000389

30. White JV, Guenter P, Jensen G, et al. Consensus statement: Academy of Nutrition and Dietetics and American Society for Parenteral and Enteral Nutrition: characteristics recommended for the identification and documentation of adult malnutrition (undernutrition). *JPEN J Parenter Enteral Nutr.* 2012;36(3):275-283. doi:10.1177/0148607112440285

31. Bencini L, Di Leo A, Pozzessere D, Bozzetti F. Total energy expenditure in patients with advanced solid tumours: a preliminary report. *Nutr Ther Met.* 2008;26:45-47.

32. Purcell SA, Elliott SA, Walter PJ, et al. Total energy expenditure in patients with colorectal cancer: associations with body composition, physical activity, and energy recommendations. *Am J Clin Nutr.* 2019;110(2):367-376. doi:10.1093/ajcn/nqz112

33. Cano N, Fiaccadori E, Tesinsky P, et al. ESPEN guidelines on enteral nutrition: adult renal failure. *Clin Nutr.* 2006;25(2):295-310. doi:10.1016/j.clnu.2006.01.023

34. Yu K, Zheng X, Wang G, et al. Immunonutrition vs standard nutrition for cancer patients: a systematic review and meta-analysis (part 1). *JPEN J Parenter Enteral Nutr.* 2020;44(5):742-767. doi:10.1002/jpen.1736

35. Taylor BE, McClave SA, Martindale RG, et al. Guidelines for the provision and assessment of nutrition support therapy in the adult critically ill patient: Society of Critical Care Medicine (SCCM) and American Society for Parenteral and Enteral Nutrition (A.S.P.E.N.). *Crit Care Med.* 2016;44(2):390-438. doi:10.1097/CCM.0000000000001525

36. Weimann A, Braga M, Carli F, et al. ESPEN guideline: clinical nutrition in surgery. *Clin Nutr.* 2017;36(3):623-650. doi:10.1016/j.clnu.2017.02.013

37. Cereda E, Cappello S, Colombo S, et al. Nutritional counseling with or without systematic use of oral nutritional supplements in head and neck cancer patients undergoing radiotherapy. *Radiother Oncol.* 2018;26:81-88. doi:10.1016/j.radonc.2017.10.015

38. Kim SH, Lee SM, Jeung HC, et al. The effect of nutrition intervention with oral nutritional supplements on pancreatic and bile duct cancer patients undergoing chemotherapy. *Nutrients.* 2019;11(5):1145. doi:10.3390/nu11051145

39. de van der Schueren MAE, Laviano A, Blanchard H, et al. Systematic review and meta-analysis of the evidence for oral nutritional intervention on nutritional and clinical outcomes during chemo(radio)therapy: current evidence and guidance for design of future trials. *Ann Oncol.* 2018;29(5):1141-1153. doi:10.1093/annonch/mdy114

40. Prado CM, Sawyer MG, Ghosh S, et al. Central tenet of cancer cachexia therapy: do patients with advance cancer have exploitable anabolic potential? *Am J Clin Nutr.* 2013;98:1012-1019. doi:10.3945/ajcn.113.06022

41. Miyata H, Yano M, Yasuda T. et al. Randomized study of clinical effect of enteral nutrition support during neoadjuvant chemotherapy on chemotherapy-related toxicity in patients with esophageal cancer. *Clin Nutr.* 2012;31:330-336. doi:10.1016/j.clnu.2011.11.002

42. De Waele E, Mattens S, Honore PM, Spapen H, De Greve J, Pen JJ. Nutrition therapy in cachectic cancer patients: the Tight Caloric Control (TiCaCo) pilot trial. *Appetite.* 2015;91:298-301. doi:10.1016/j.appet.2015.04.049

43. Gavazzi C, Colatruglio S, Valoriani F, et al. Impact of home enteral nutrition in malnourished patients with upper gastrointestinal cancer: a multicentre randomised clinical trial. *Eur J Cancer.* 2016;64:107-112. doi:10.1016/j.ejca.2016.05.032

44. Bischoff SC, Austin P, Boeykens K, et al. ESPEN guideline on home enteral nutrition. *Clin Nutr.* 2020;39(1):5-22. doi:10.1016/j.clnu.2019.04.022

45. Theilla M, Cohen J, Kagan I, Attal-Singer J, Lev S, Singer P. Home parenteral nutrition for advanced cancer patients: contributes to survival? *Nutrition.* 2018;54:197-200. doi:10.1016/j.nut.2017.03.005

46. Bozzetti F, Santarpia L, Pironi L, et al. The prognosis of incurable cachectic cancer patients on home parenteral nutrition: a multi-centre observational study with prospective follow-up of 414 patients. *Ann Oncol.* 2014;25:487-493. doi:10.1093/annonc/mdt549

47. Della Valle S, Colatruglio S, La Vela V, Tagliabue E, Mariani L, Gavazzi C. Nutritional intervention in head and neck cancer patients during chemo-radiotherapy. *Nutrition.* 2018;51:95-97. doi:10.1016/j.nut.2017.12.012

48. Yanni A, Dequanter D, Lechien JR, et al. Malnutrition in head and neck cancer patients: impacts and indications of a prophylactic percutaneous endoscopic gastrostomy. *Eur Ann Otorhinolaryngol Head Neck Dis.* 2019;136(3):S27-S33. doi:10.1016/j.anorl.2019.01.001

49. Orell H, Schwab U, Saarilahti K, Österlund P, Ravasco P, Mäkitie A. Nutritional counseling for head and neck cancer patients undergoing (chemo) radiotherapy-a prospective randomized trial. *Front Nutr.* 2019;6:22. doi:10.3389/fnut.2019.00022

50. Sachdev S, Refaat T, Bacchus ID, Sathiaseelan V, Mittal BB. Age most significant predictor of requiring enteral feeding in head-and-neck cancer patients. *Radiat Oncol.* 2015;10:93. doi:10.1186/213014-015-0408-6

51. Esophagus. Cancer Statistics Center, American Cancer Society. Accessed August 31, 2020. https://cancerstatisticscenter.cancer.org/#!/cancer-site/Esophagus

52. PDQ Adult Treatment Editorial Board. Esophageal cancer treatment (adult) (PDQ)—health professional version. National Cancer Institute. Updated July 31, 2020. Accessed August 31, 2020. www.cancer.gov/types/esophageal/hp/esophageal-treatment-pdq

53. Jordan T, Mastnak DM, Palamar N, Kozjek NR. Nutritional therapy for patients with esophageal cancer. *Nutr Cancer.* 2017;70(1):23-29. doi:10.1080/01635581.2017.1374417

54. Garth AK, Newsome CM, Simmance N, Crowe TC. Nutritional status, nutrition practices and postoperative complications in patients with gastrointestinal cancer. *J Hum Nutr Diet.* 2010;23(4):393. doi:10.1111/j.1365-277X.2010.01058.x

55. D'Journo XB, Ouattara M, Loundou A, et al. Prognostic impact of weight loss in 1-year survivors after transthoracic esophagectomy for cancer. *Dis Esophagus.* 2012;25(6):527-534. doi:10.1111/j.1442-2050.2011.01282

56. Deans DA, Tan BH, Wigmore SJ, Ross JA, de Beaux AC, Paterson-Brown S, Fearon KC. The influence of systemic inflammation, dietary intake and stage of disease on rate of weight loss in patients with gastro-oesophageal cancer. *Br J Cancer.* 2009;100(1):63-69. doi:10.1038/sj.bjc.6604828

57. Huddy JR, Huddy FMS, Markar SR, Tucker O. Nutritional optimization during neoadjuvant therapy prior to surgical resection of esophageal cancer—a narrative review. *Dis Esophagus.* 2018;31(1):1-11. doi:10.1093/dote/dox110. Erratum in: *Dis Esophagus.* 2018;31(4).

58. Fukuda T, Seto K, Yamada K, et al. Can immune-enhancing nutrients reduce postoperative complications in patients undergoing esophageal surgery? *Dis Esophagus.* 2008;21:708-711. doi:10.1111/j.1442-2050.2008.00861x

59. Kubota K, Kuroda J, Yoshida M, et al. Preoperative oral supplementation support in patients with esophageal cancer. *J Nutr Health Aging.* 2014;18(4):437-440. doi:10.1007/s12603-014-0018-2

60. Aiko S, Kumano I, Yamanaka N, et al. Effects of an immune-enhanced diet containing antioxidants in esophageal cancer surgery following neoadjuvant therapy. *Dis Esophagus.* 2012;25:137-145. doi:10.1111/j.1442-2050.2011.01221.x

61. Sakurai Y, Masui T, Yoshida I, et al. Randomized clinical trial of the effects of preoperative use of immune-enhancing enteral formula on metabolic and immunological status in patients undergoing esophagectomy. *World J Surg.* 2007;31:2150-2157. doi:10.1007/s00268-007-9170-8

62. Ryan AM, Reynolds JV, Healy L, et al. Enteral nutrition enriched with eicosapentaenoic acid (EPA) preserves lean body mass following esophageal cancer surgery: results of a double-blinded randomized controlled trial. *Ann Surg.* 2009;249:355-363. doi:10.1097/SLA.0b013e31819a4789

63. Healy LA, Ryan A, Doyle SL, et al. Does prolonged enteral feeding with supplemental omega-3 fatty acids impact on recovery post-esophagectomy: results of a randomized double-blind trial. *Ann Surg.* 2017;266:720-728. doi:10.1097/SLA.0000000000002390

64. Rawla P, Barsouk A. Epidemiology of gastric cancer: global trends, risk factors and prevention. *Prz Gastroenterol.* 2019;14(1):26-38. doi:10.5114/pg.2018.80001

65. Wroblewski LE, Peek RM Jr, Wilson KT. *Helicobacter pylori* and gastric cancer: factors that modulate disease risk. *Clin Microbiol Rev.* 2010;23(4):713-739. doi:10.1128/CMR.00011-10

66. Fujiya K, Kawamura T, Omae K Makuuchi R, Irino T, Tokunaga M, Tanizawa Y, Bando E, Terashima. Impact of malnutrition after gastrectomy for gastric cancer on long-term survival. *Ann Surg Oncol.* 2018;25(4):974-983. doi:10.1245/s10434-018-6342-8

67. Liu X, Qiu H, Kong P, Zhou Z, Sun X. Gastric cancer, nutritional status, and outcome. *Onco Targets Ther.* 2017;10:2107-2114. doi:10.2147/OTT.S132432

68. Yoon SH, Kye BH, Kim HJ, Jun KH, Cho HM, Chin HM. Risk of malnutrition after gastrointestinal cancer surgery: a propensity score matched retrospective cohort study. *Surg Metab Nutr.* 2018;9(1):16-25. doi:10.18858/smn.2018.9.1.16

69. Rosania R, Chiapponi C, Malfertheiner P, Venerito M. Nutrition in patients with gastric cancer: an update. *Gastrointest Tumors*. 2016;2(4):178-187. doi:10.1159 /000445188

70. Scarpellini E, Arts J, Karamanolis G, et al. International consensus on the diagnosis and management of dumping syndrome. *Nat Rev Endocrinol*. 2020;16:448-466. doi:10.1038/s41574-020-0357-5

71. Veeralakshmanan P, Tham JC, Wright A, et al. Nutritional deficiency post esophageal and gastric cancer surgery: a quality improvement study. *Ann Med Surg (Lond)*. 2020;56:19-22. doi:10.1016/j.amsu.2020 .05.032

72. Paik C, Choi M, Lim C, Park J, Chung W, Lee K. The role of small intestinal bacterial overgrowth in postgastrectomy patients. *Neuro Gastroenterol Motil*. 2011;23(5):191-196. doi:10.1111/j.1365-2982.2011 .01686.x

73. Cancer stat facts: small intestine cancer. Surveillance, Epidemiology, and End Results Program, National Cancer Institute. Accessed August 14, 2020. https:/ /seer.cancer.gov/statfacts/html/smint.html

74. Xu M, Jung X, Hines OJ, Eibl G, Chen Y. Obesity and pancreatic cancer: overview of epidemiology and potential prevention by weight loss. *Pancreas*. 2018;47(2):158-162. doi:10.1097/MMPA .00000000000000974

75. American Cancer Society medical and editorial content team. Pancreatic cancer risk factors. American Cancer Society. Last updated June 9, 2020. Accessed August 14, 2020. www.cancer.org/cancer/pancreatic-cancer /causes-risks-prevention/risk-factors.html

76. De Souza A, Irfan K, Masud F, Saif MW. Diabetes type 2 and pancreatic cancer: a history unfolding. *JOP*. 2016;17(2):144-148.

77. Lu PY, Shan SS, Chen XJ, Zhang XY. Dietary patterns and pancreatic cancer risk: a meta-analysis. *Nutrients*. 2017;9(1)38. doi:10.3390/nu9010038

78. Naudin S, Li K, Jaouen T, et al. Lifetime and baseline alcohol intakes and risk of pancreatic cancer in the European Prospective Investigation into Cancer and Nutrition study. *Int J Cancer*. 2018;143(4):801-812. doi:10.1002/ijc.31367

79. Waterhouse M, Risch HA, Bosetti C, et al. Vitamin D and pancreatic cancer: a pooled analysis from the Pancreatic Cancer Case-Control Consortium. *Ann Oncol*. 2015;26(8):1776-1783. doi:10.1093/annonc/mdv236

80. Duijnhoven FJB, Jenab M, Hveem K, et al. Circulating concentrations of vitamin D in relation to pancreatic cancer risk in European populations. *Int J Cancer*. 2018;142(6):1189-1201. doi:10.1002/ijc.31146

81. Gilliland TM, Villafane-Ferriol N, Shah KP, et al. Nutritional and metabolic derangements in pancreatic cancer and pancreatic resection. *Nutrients*. 2017;9(3):243. doi:10.3390/nu9030243

82. Mueller TC, Burmeister MA, Bachmann J, Martignoni ME. Cachexia and pancreatic cancer: are there treatment options? *World J Gastroenterol*. 2014;20(28):9361–9373. doi:10.3748/wjg.v20.i28.9361

83. Mitchell T, Clarke L, Goldberg A, Bishop KS. Pancreatic cancer cachexia: the role of nutritional interventions. *Healthcare* (Basel). 2019;7(3):89. doi:10.3390 /healthcare7030089

84. Nemer L, Krishna SG, Shah ZK, et al. Predictors of pancreatic cancer-associated weight loss and nutritional interventions. *Pancreas*. 2017;46(9):1152-1157. doi:10.1097/MPA.0000000000000898

85. Saito T, Hirano K, Isayama H, et al. The role of pancreatic enzyme replacement therapy in unresectable pancreatic cancer: a prospective cohort study. *Pancreas*. 2017;46(30):341-346. doi:10.1097 /MPA.0000000000000767

86. Roberts KJ, Bannister CA, Schrem H. Enzyme replacement improves survival among patients with pancreatic cancer: results of a population based study. *Pancreatology*. 2019;19(1):114-121. doi:10.1016/j.pan .2018.10.010

87. Colomer R, Moreno-Nogueira JM, García-Luna PP, et al. N-3 fatty acids, cancer and cachexia: a systematic review of the literature. *Br J Nutr*. 2007;97(5):823-831. doi:10.1017/S000711450765795X

88. Werner K, Küllenberg de Gaudry D, Taylor LA, et al. Dietary supplementation with n-3-fatty acids in patients with pancreatic cancer and cachexia: marine phospholipids versus fish oil—a randomized controlled double-blind trial. *Lipids Health Dis*. 2017;16:104. doi:10.1186/s12944-017-0495-5

89. Thanikachalam K, Khan G. Colorectal cancer and nutrition. *Nutrients*. 2019;11(1):164. doi:10.3390 /nu11010164

90. Shivappa N, Godos J, Hebert JR, et al. Dietary Inflammatory Index and colorectal cancer risk—a meta-analysis. *Nutrients*. 2017;9:1043. doi:10.3390 /nu9091043

91. Schwingshackl L, Schwedhelm C, Galbete C, Hoffmann G. Adherence to Mediterranean diet and risk of cancer: an updated systematic review and meta-analysis. *Nutrients*. 2017;9(10):1063. doi:10.3390/nu9101063

92. Mentella MC, Scaldaferri F, Ricci C, Gasbarrini A, Miggiano GAD. Cancer and Mediterranean diet: a review. *Nutrients*. 2019;11(9):2059. doi:10.3390/ nu11092059

93. Barberan-Garcia A, Ubré M, Roca J, et al. Personalized prehabilitation in high-risk patients undergoing elective major abdominal surgery: a randomized blinded controlled trial. *Ann Surg*. 2018;267(1):50-56. doi:10.1097/SLA.0000000000002293

94. Ravasco P, Monteiro-Grillo I, Camillo M. Individualized nutrition intervention is of major benefit to colorectal cancer patients: long-term follow-up of a randomized controlled trial of a nutritional therapy. *Am J Clin Nutr*. 2012;96:1346-1353. doi:10.3945/ajcn.111.018838

95. Academy of Nutrition and Dietetics. Oncology (ONC) guideline (2013). Evidence Analysis Library. Accessed August 27, 2021. www.andeal.org/topic.cfm?menu =5291&cat=5066

96. Voss A, Williams V, eds. *Oncology Nutrition for Clinical Practice*. 2nd ed. Academy of Nutrition and Dietetics; 2021.

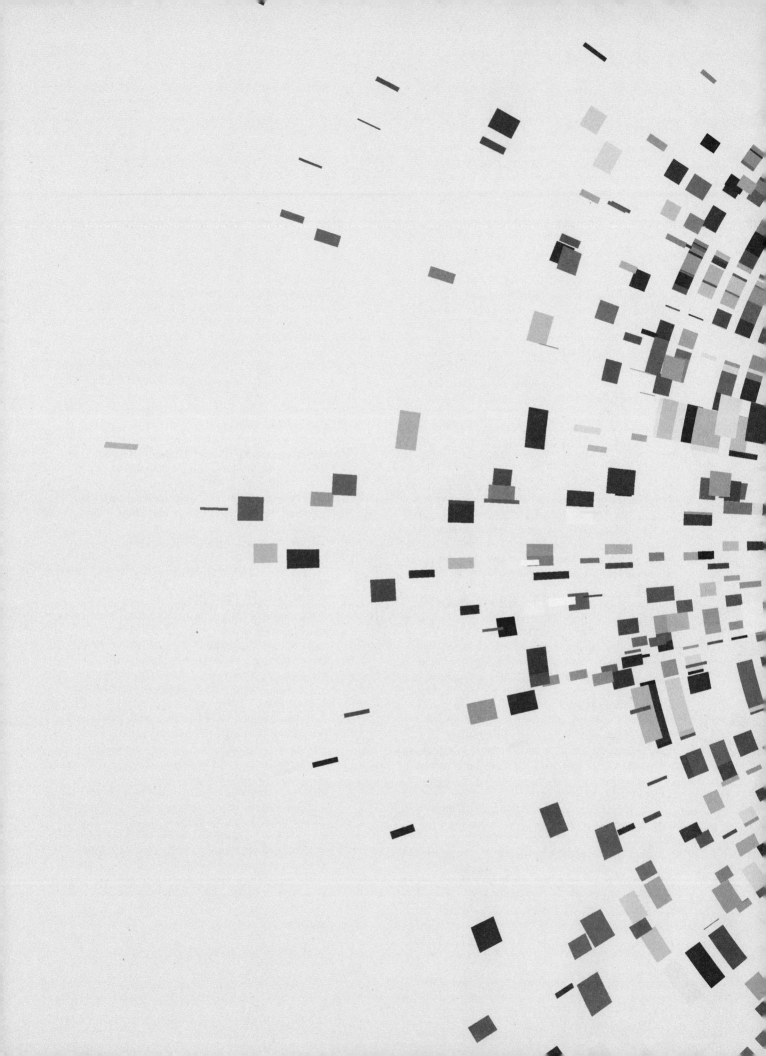

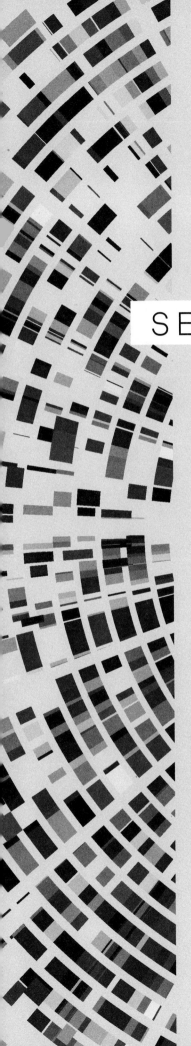

Nutrition and Gastrointestinal-Related Systemic Disorders

Medical Treatment of Obesity

Lawrence J. Cheskin, MD, FACP, FTOS
Tammy L. Wagner, PhD, RDN

KEY POINTS

- Successful weight loss will often lessen the risk for gastrointestinal disorders and reduce symptoms and progression for those who already suffer from gastrointestinal and liver disorders associated with weight gain and obesity.
- Losing weight and maintaining weight loss require interventions that target changing lifestyle behaviors to decrease energy intake and increase energy expenditure.
- The intensity and frequency of treatment visits for weight control are important predictors of outcome success.

Introduction

Obesity is highly prevalent worldwide and is a growing medical and public health problem in the United States. Obesity in adults is defined as a BMI of 30 or higher and is a condition of excess body fat.[1,2] According to the National Center for Health Statistics, more than 42% of adults in the United States suffer from obesity, and more than 9% suffer from severe obesity (BMI ≥40).[2] Obesity has been shown to be associated with many chronic diseases, including heart disease,[3] hypertension, type 2 diabetes mellitus, and end-stage renal disease.[4] It is also associated with other serious health risks including, notably, such gastrointestinal (GI) disorders as gastroesophageal reflux disease, nonalcoholic fatty liver disease, and Barrett esophagus.[5]

In fact, the increased prevalence of GI conditions in the United States may in part be related to the increased prevalence of obesity. It is important to recognize the role of a high BMI (and particularly increased *abdominal* adiposity) in the development of GI morbidity. For this reason, measurement of waist circumference is recommended in patients presenting with GI complaints or abnormal liver function test results. Studies have shown that obesity can be associated with other types of GI disorders, including esophageal adenocarcinoma, erosive gastritis, gastric cancer, gallstones, colon polyps, hepatocellular carcinoma, acute pancreatitis, and pancreatic cancer.[6-10] Changes in GI motility, which can have a substantial impact on appetite and satiety, may also be associated with obesity.[11,12]

This chapter focuses on specific interventions for managing obesity. The ultimate goal of these interventions is for the patient to not only lose weight but also maintain a healthy weight. In addition to its many other potential benefits, achieving successful weight loss and maintenance can often lessen the risk for developing GI disorders, as well as reduce disease symptoms and progression in those who already suffer from GI and liver disorders associated with weight gain and obesity. Chapter 18 addresses surgical interventions for the treatment of obesity.

Pathogenesis of Obesity and Related Gastrointestinal Disorders

The GI tract produces gut hormones that influence appetite, aiding in the efficient absorption of nutrients and thus energy intake. Changes in bile acids, the gut microbiome, and metabolic products of nutrient digestion can all affect metabolic factors that are associated with obesity. Obesity also has medical effects on digestive diseases; for example, it increases the levels of circulating free fatty acids and alters adipocytokines. The physiological effects of obesity may also contribute to esophageal disease and may trigger various GI symptoms, such as heartburn. For this reason, two important goals of treating patients with concurrent obesity and GI disorders are weight loss and maintenance of a healthy weight.

At a basic level, obesity occurs only when more energy is consumed than is burned, and the excess energy is stored as body fat. Obesity can be caused by a medical condition, such as hypothyroidism, but this is more often claimed than demonstrated. The vast majority of cases of obesity are related to eating an unhealthful diet characterized by excess energy intake, coupled with relative inactivity. Many Americans' diets are too high in energy content as a result of a large intake of energy-dense foods and high-energy beverages. Inactivity, or sedentary lifestyle, is also prevalent in the United States.

Losing weight and maintaining weight loss require interventions that target changing lifestyle behaviors to decrease energy intake and increase energy expenditure. The overall aim is to improve the patient's health as weight is reduced through improved diet and increased physical activity. This, in combination with supportive behavioral therapy, tends to improve outcomes. Thus, a multidisciplinary treatment approach that includes education from experts in nutrition, exercise, and behavior modification is the best way to help individuals maintain weight loss and achieve lasting success.

Management Strategies for Weight Loss and Weight Stabilization

The essential strategies for maintaining a lifelong healthy weight are to eat the appropriate amounts and types of food (appropriate energy intake) and to exercise and move more each day (appropriate energy expenditure). When energy intake exceeds energy expenditure, weight gain occurs. When energy expenditure is greater than energy intake, weight loss occurs. To sustain weight loss over time, interventions that target lifestyle behaviors that decrease energy intake are necessary, preferably in concert with improvements in diet quality and increases in energy expenditure. These interventions will allow weight maintenance once a person returns to a healthy weight. Thus, the features most likely to lead to successful weight loss include a moderate reduction in energy intake, an increase in energy expenditure, and behavioral strategies to enact the necessary changes in diet and physical activity.

The concept of small changes in diet and physical activity behaviors is worth highlighting. Many individuals pursue aggressive, rapid changes, and although this does result in greater initial weight loss in some people, many regain a large amount of weight after the initial loss. Small changes in dietary and exercise behaviors can promote more sustainable weight management and help prevent weight regain.

Decrease Energy Intake

Unless a patient has an unusually low resting metabolic rate that has been documented via indirect calorimetry, the prescribed dietary intake should be no lower than 1,000 kcal/d in females and no lower than 1,200 kcal/d in males, to achieve a goal weight loss of 0.5 to 2 lb (0.2 to 0.9 kg) per week. Helpful behavioral strategies for patients who are trying to lose weight include keeping a food diary, logging physical activity, and journaling. Portion control is also important, and educating patients as to what is considered a normal portion for each food group is helpful. Patients should also be advised to increase their daily intake of nutrient-dense foods and decrease their portion sizes of energy-dense foods. Additional dietary strategies are detailed in a later section of the chapter.

Increase Energy Expenditure

Physical activity is also important for weight loss and weight maintenance, to the extent that it contributes to a negative energy balance. An initial goal of 30 minutes of moderate exercise a day is recommended, with a gradual increase to 60 minutes on most days. The *Physical Activity Guidelines for Americans* recommend at least 150 minutes of moderate-to-vigorous physical activity per week for weight control.[13] Even longer durations of physical activity may be needed for weight loss and maintenance, and up to 300 minutes of moderate-to-vigorous physical activity weekly is recommended for improvements in health outcomes. The guidelines also recommend moving more during the day and sitting less. A reduction in sedentary behavior (defined as sitting or reclining activities with very low energy expenditure) is also associated with improvements in weight and cardiometabolic heath because either a reallocation of sedentary time to light activity increases energy expenditure, or a reduction in food consumption often associated with sedentary time (eg, snacking while watching television) decreases energy intake.[14] Although some interventions have been shown to decrease sedentary time, particularly the use of sit-stand workstations, their effects on long-term weight management are not clear.[15] It is clear, however, that behavioral weight management programs that include both diet and exercise interventions result in greater long-term weight loss (at 12-18 months) compared with exercise-only programs.[16]

Behavioral Strategies

Behavioral strategies can help patients make lifestyle changes and maintain weight loss over the long term. Although making and sustaining lifestyle changes can be difficult, it is important to emphasize to patients that the results are worth the effort. Cognitive behavioral therapy (CBT), which helps people change how they think about themselves, how they act, and how they cope with the circumstances that influence their actions, is an effective behavioral paradigm for weight control.[17] Patients should be advised to focus on attainable, specific changes and maintain these over the long term. Effective CBT strategies for weight loss and lifestyle behavior change include goal setting, self-monitoring, having a positive attitude, and reinforcement through feedback.

Setting both short-term and long-term goals is helpful. Specific, measurable, attainable, realistic, and timely goals (sometimes collectively referred to as SMART goals) are a great way to incorporate measurable and meaningful changes that can be monitored to measure progress. The more specific and realistic the goals are, the better the chances are for success.

Self-monitoring, through food diaries, physical activity logs, and journaling, can help patients both track their progress and develop a greater awareness of what is working and what is not. The more the patient records, the easier it is for the patient and the care team to identify any barriers to weight loss and develop a plan to address these issues.

Establishing a supportive and positive attitude sets an individual up for early success, and success breeds more success, which builds patients' confidence in their ability to achieve their original goals. Lastly, outside feedback can help keep a patient's expectations ambitious but realistic. For example, having a personal accountability partner to check in with daily can provide the necessary support and help sustain motivation.

Patients should be reminded that adopting a healthier lifestyle is not about making short-term changes to the way they eat or temporarily adjusting exercise routines; lifestyle changes take a sustained effort over time.

Popular Dietary Interventions for Obesity

Energy-Restricted Diets

Although energy-restricted diets vary greatly in the magnitude and source of energy restriction and in the level of structure required, both the low-calorie diet and the very low-calorie diet (VLCD) have been mainstays of treatment for obesity since the 1970s. Low-calorie diets typically range from 1,200 to 1,600 kcal/d and impose structure through the use of meal plans, which specify food choices and portion sizes. Meal replacements, such as bars and shakes, may help improve diet adherence, as they have a fixed, prespecified energy content and limit other food choices. A partial meal-replacement diet is more effective for short-term weight loss than a low-calorie diet with conventional foods,[18] and two daily meal replacements are more effective than one in patients with overweight or obesity and type 2 diabetes mellitus.[19]

A medically supervised VLCD provides fewer than 800 kcal/d and is appropriate for patients who are severely obese (BMI ≥40) or for patients who are obese (BMI ≥30) and have serious medical conditions related to their obesity.[20] A VLCD may consist of whole foods, commercially available meal replacements or liquids, or a combination of the two. Patients being considered for a VLCD should undergo a comprehensive medical evaluation and have regular (weekly or biweekly) visits for medical supervision while on the VLCD. With full adherence, weight loss averages 2.4 to 4 lb (1.1 to 1.8 kg) per week, depending on the person's initial body mass (more rapid weight loss typically occurs with more severe obesity) and physical activity level. In a meta-analysis of studies in adults with class III obesity (BMI ≥40), VLCDs that involved the use of liquid meal-replacement products for at least 6 weeks resulted in a clinically relevant weight loss (which ranged from 10.2% to 28% of initial body weight).[20]

Intermittent fasting regimens (also called semifasting regimens) allow for fasting and nonfasting cycles over a given period and may work by improving patient adherence better than other energy-restricted diets. Alternate-day fasting is one such regimen; it involves a partial fasting day, during which the person consumes a diet similar to a VLCD, followed by a normal feeding day, when foods and beverages are consumed ad libitum. Alternate-day fasting is associated with better diet adherence, greater reduction of fat mass, and greater preservation of lean body mass than VLCDs.[20]

Macronutrient-Focused Diets

Macronutrient-based dietary changes focus on one target macronutrient (carbohydrate, fat, or protein), although changes in the dietary intake of one macronutrient will result in changes in the intake of other macronutrients. In 2005, the Institute of Medicine (now the National Academy of Medicine) established the acceptable distribution ranges for macronutrients based on percentage of total energy intake (protein, 10%–35%; fat, 20%–35%; and carbohydrate, 45%–65%) by considering the epidemiological evidence, which suggested that consumption within these ranges is associated with a reduction in the risk of chronic diseases.[21] Although macronutrient-focused diets involve intakes that often fall outside of these ranges, as a short-term approach, they are typically safe.

Many studies have been conducted to determine the optimal macronutrient distribution for a weight-loss diet. A 2005 data analysis found that, among the more than 4,000 adults enrolled in the National Weight Control Registry—a database that tracks individuals who have been successful at long-term weight loss and maintenance, which today includes more than 10,000 participants—the most common strategy for achieving weight control was to follow a low-calorie, low-fat diet,[22] yet recently the popularity of low-fat diets has declined in favor of low-carbohydrate diets.

Low-carbohydrate dieting was first popularized by Robert Atkins, MD, in the 1970s and is usually defined as a carbohydrate intake of less than 20 g/d, without restriction of energy or other macronutrients. Once a desired weight loss is achieved, carbohydrate intake is somewhat liberalized to 50 g/d. A 2006 meta-analysis of five randomized controlled trials compared low-carbohydrate diets to low-fat diets and found that low-carbohydrate diets were more effective for weight loss, initially, than low-fat diets. Low-fat diets were found to lead to a greater decrease in total cholesterol and low-density lipoprotein cholesterol compared to low-carbohydrate diets, whereas the low-carbohydrate diets reduced blood triglycerides and increased high-density lipoprotein cholesterol levels more than the low-fat, low-calorie diets.[23]

An increasingly popular diet that uses a more extreme restriction of carbohydrates to induce serum and urinary ketones is the ketogenic diet—a low-carbohydrate, high-protein, and typically also high fat diet. A 2013 meta-analysis comparing randomized controlled trials of the ketogenic diet vs a low-fat diet found significantly greater weight loss with the ketogenic diet for up to 24 months. However, a significant increase in low-density lipoprotein cholesterol was also observed,[24] though the clinical importance of this increase is not known. It has been noted that dropout rates for ketogenic diets range from 13% to 84% across studies.[25] In addition to their use for weight control, ketogenic diets may play a promising role in epilepsy treatment.[26]

The positive weight-loss outcomes associated with low-carbohydrate diets may be attributable, in part, to their typically high protein content. A high-protein diet is defined as one in which at least 20% of energy intake comes from protein, with no restriction in fat or carbohydrates.[27] A 2012 meta-analysis that included 24 randomized controlled trials comparing isocaloric high-protein vs low-protein diets found that the high-protein diets resulted not only in greater weight loss but also in greater loss of fat mass. Weight loss may be enhanced by the increased satiety and resting energy expenditure that accompany a higher protein intake.[28] Yet patients following high-protein diets, like those following ketogenic diets, suffer from a gradual decline in adherence and eventually regain weight; adherence to daily energy restriction declines as well. Many high-protein diets involve the use of portion-controlled liquid and solid meal replacements. In one study of patients with obesity and the metabolic syndrome, participants who consumed two high-protein meal replacements daily lost more body weight and more fat mass than those who ate a diet with conventional levels of protein.[29]

Pattern-Based Diets

Long-term weight loss and attendant metabolic and cardiovascular disease control may require more permanent alterations in diet and lifestyle than what short-term diets provide. Pattern-based diets focus on the overall diet by offering recommendations for the types of foods to consume rather than the amounts of energy or macronutrients to consume. The *2020-2025 Dietary Guidelines for Americans* (DGA) provide recommendations on a high-nutrient-density eating pattern, which is associated with weight maintenance and a reduction in chronic disease risk.[30] The DGA is a resource for health professionals and policymakers, particularly those working on the design and implementation of food assistance programs, but it can also be used by the public to make healthier food choices for those aged 2 years and older.

The Dietary Approaches to Stop Hypertension (DASH) diet was developed to reduce hypertension among individuals with moderate to high blood pressure.[31-33] The diet is high in fruits, vegetables, fat-free or low-fat dairy products, whole grains, lean meats, nuts, legumes, and seeds, and is low in sweets, added sugars, and red meat. The consumption of dietary sodium is reduced to 2,300 mg/d (standard DASH) or 1,500 mg/d (low-sodium DASH), the latter being in line with American Heart Association recommendations.[34] The original DASH diet does not stipulate daily energy restrictions; however, the addition of exercise and weight loss to the DASH diet results in even larger reductions in blood pressure compared to DASH alone.[35]

The traditional Mediterranean diet is based on the dietary pattern observed in Mediterranean regions of the world (particularly Greece and Italy) during the 1960s. It focused on plant-based foods, including fruits, vegetables, grains, nuts, and seeds; minimally processed foods; olive oil as the main fat source; dairy, fish, and poultry consumed moderately; very limited red meat consumption; and the frequent but moderate intake of red wine.[36] Early studies found that the Mediterranean diet resulted in similar energy deficits to a low-fat diet but had more favorable effects on glycemic markers (glucose, insulin), and it had a high adherence rate (85% at 2 years).[37] More recently, the PREDIMED (Prevención con Dieta Mediterránea) multicenter, randomized controlled trial was conducted among individuals at high risk for cardiovascular disease in Spain to test two modified versions of the Mediterranean diet (one supplemented with extra-virgin olive oil and the other with nuts) against just advice on adhering to a low-fat diet. PREDIMED demonstrated that both of the supplemented Mediterranean diets led to decreases in diastolic blood pressure as well as to improvements in other cardiovascular end points, and more so than a low-fat diet.[38] These improvements in cardiovascular end points are frequently of about the same magnitude as effects observed with statin therapy, though further studies are needed in this area.[39] Much of the benefits associated with the Mediterranean diet are thought to be due to the high intake of unsaturated fat and antioxidants that is characteristic of the diet.

Overall, vegetable-based dietary patterns that involve substituting plant-based protein foods for animal proteins have become increasing popular and widespread. Both the DGA and the Academy of Nutrition and Dietetics highlight the benefits of plant-based dietary patterns, while acknowledging the need for appropriate planning to ensure that vegetarian and vegan diets are nutritionally adequate.[30,40] Such diets include legumes, nuts, grains, and, in ovolacto-vegetarian diets, dairy products and eggs. However, in vegan diets, all animal-derived products are avoided, limiting some of these options. In observational studies, vegetarians generally had lower body weight, lower blood pressure, less diabetes, and fewer other health issues than people who consumed foods from animal sources, as well as less weight gain.[41,42] Evidence from clinical trials supports that vegetarian diets, and vegan diets in particular, reduce body weight.[43] However, the long-term effects of vegetarian diets and their effects on weight maintenance remain unclear, as most studies reviewed have had less than 1 year of follow-up.[44]

Medical Management of Obesity

Most comprehensive lifestyle intervention programs combine an energy restriction (not lower than 500 kcal/d) with a physical activity prescription of at least 150 minutes of moderate-to-vigorous physical activity per week and structured behavioral change strategies. These programs are designed to achieve weight loss of at least 1 lb (0.45 kg) per week. A multidisciplinary team is desirable to support patients in achieving the maximal benefit from the program. The team should ideally include the following: a primary physician or nurse practitioner with expertise in the medical complications of obesity and obesity pharmacotherapy, a dietitian, an exercise specialist, and a counselor for behavior change. This combination of expertise can best provide a comprehensive, in-depth, personalized weight-loss program by incorporating the most effective interventions from each discipline. Such a personalized weight-loss program can be complemented by consultations with a pharmacist, case manager, and specialty physicians, such as a bariatric surgeon, psychiatrist, and gastroenterologist, or other specialists if specific comorbidities are present (eg, a podiatrist, cardiologist, nephrologist, or endocrinologist). Weight-management programs such as the ones used in the Look AHEAD clinical trial are comprehensive interventions with proven success.[45] Look AHEAD used CBT to assist with changing eating and activity behaviors. Typical CBT strategies, some of which have already been mentioned, include self-monitoring, goal setting, problem-solving and preplanning, stimulus control, and relapse prevention. Intensive lifestyle interventions are best implemented with the assistance of a multidisciplinary team, using patient-centered care, and evidence-based and protocol-driven treatment choices.[46] Well-informed providers are essential to the effective management of a chronic condition like obesity.

Intensity and Delivery of Interventions for Obesity

The intensity and frequency of treatment visits for weight control are important predictors of outcome success. Guidelines suggest that one or two face-to-face treatment sessions per month for at least 6 months results in a weight loss of 4.4 to 8.8 lb (2 to 4 kg) over 6 to 12 months, and a high-intensity intervention (>14 sessions in 6 months) yields greater weight loss than a low-to-moderate–intensity intervention.[47] There is probably some limit to the benefit of increasing the intensity of interventions, however, because "diet fatigue" may occur with very prolonged or very taxing intervention schemes. A break from intensive interventions of modest duration may be useful in resetting engagement. Interventions can be delivered with the use of technology to decrease costs, increase reach, and possibly decrease attrition, but may produce less weight loss than face-to-face interventions. Smartphone-based delivery may have benefits over computer-based delivery, as interventions can be more frequently delivered (or even "ever-present"), interactive, and more readily incorporate tailored messaging.[48] The efficacy of smartphone delivery compared with other methods is not yet clear.

Pharmacotherapy for Obesity

Whether or not to use medications that are designed to assist in weight loss is a decision best made in concert with the patient. Typical weight loss achieved with and without pharmacotherapy is summarized in Box 11.1. Specific agents currently available are described in Table 11.1. Assuming the patient is receptive and there are no contraindications for the specific agent or agents being considered, it is usually appropriate to strongly consider adding such an agent when it becomes clear that weight loss has halted for the patient or that excessive hunger is interfering with dietary or behavioral adherence. Appetite-suppressing drugs are not a cure-all, but they can reinvigorate a weight-loss trajectory that has begun to falter in appropriate candidates; however, practitioners should monitor their patients for adverse side effects or lack of efficacy in the individual patient.

BOX 11.1

Overview of Approaches to Weight Loss With and Without Pharmacotherapy

Lifestyle changes (diet, exercise, behavior modification)

Criteria for use	BMI ≥25
Typical weight loss achieved	3% to 10%

Lifestyle changes with pharmacotherapy[a]

Criteria for use	BMI ≥27 with comorbidity *or* BMI ≥30
Typical weight loss achieved	4% to 12%

[a] See list of pharmacotherapy agents in Table 11.1

TABLE 11.1 Approved Pharmacotherapy for Obesity[a,49]

Generic name	Trade name	DEA schedule	Mechanism of appetite suppression	Dosage	Estimated % weight loss[b]
Phentermine HCl	Various	IV	Noradrenergic agonist	15 mg or 37.5 mg PO, qd	5.1% at 28 wk (15 mg, qd)
Orlistat	Xenical, Alli	None	Lipase inhibitor	120 mg PO, tid, with meals	3.1% at 1 y
Phentermine and topiramate ER	Qysmia	IV	Adrenergic agonist (phentermine); neurostabilizer (topiramate)	Dose escalation (gradual and individualized): 3.75 mg phentermine and 23 mg topiramate (3.75 mg/23 mg) PO, qd 7.5 mg/46 mg PO, qd 11.25 mg/69 mg PO, qd 15 mg/92 mg PO, qd	6.6% at 1 y (7.5 mg/46 mg, qd)
Naltrexone SR and bupropion SR	Contrave	None	Opioid receptor antagonist (naltrexone); norepinephrine and dopamine reuptake inhibitor (bupropion)	Dose escalation: Wk 1: 8 mg naltrexone and 90 mg bupropion (8 mg/90 mg) PO, qd, in AM Wk 2: 8 mg/90 mg PO, bid Wk 3: 16 mg/180 mg PO in am and 8mg/90 mg PO in PM Wk 4: 16 mg/180 mg PO, bid	4.8% at 56 wk (16 mg/180 mg, bid)
Liraglutide	Saxenda	None	Glucagon-like peptide-1 analogue	Dose escalation: Wk 1: 0.6 mg SC, qd Wk 2: 1.2 mg SC, qd Wk 3: 1.8 mg SC, qd Wk 4: 2.4 mg SC, qd Wk 5: 3 mg SC, qd	5.4% at 56 wk (3 mg, qd)

bid = twice a day | DEA, US Drug Enforcement Administration | ER = extended-release | IV = intravenous | PO = by mouth | qd = every day | SC = subcutaneous | SR = sustained release | tid = three times daily
[a] Approved by the US Food and Drug Administration
[b] Medications compared with placebo; intent-to-treat data

Summary

The management of obesity through medical means has been challenging for both patients and providers. Nonetheless, there have been steady advances in treatment options and the understanding of mechanisms and paths of treatment. Tailoring of the diet and other treatment components by a knowledgeable and caring provider can have a positive effect on outcomes for patients.

References

1. National Heart, Lung, and Blood Institute. *Managing Overweight and Obesity in Adults: Systematic Evidence Review From the Obesity Expert Panel, 2013*. National Heart, Lung, and Blood Institute; 2013. Accessed January 5, 2022. www.nhlbi.nih.gov/health-topics/managing-overweight-obesity-in-adults

2. Hales C, Carroll M, Fryar C, Ogden C. Prevalence of obesity and severe obesity among adults: United States, 2017-2018. NCHS Data Brief, no. 360. National Center for Health Statistics; 2020.

3. Li TY, Rana JS, Manson JE, et al. Obesity as compared with physical activity in predicting risk of coronary heart disease in women. *Circulation.* 2006;113(4):499-506.

4. Hsu CY, McCulloch CE, Iribarren C, Darbinian J, Go AS. Body mass index and risk for end-stage renal disease. *Ann Intern Med.* 2006;144(1):21-28.

5. Kopelman PG. Obesity as a medical problem. *Nature.* 2000;404(6778):635-643.

6. Nam SY. Obesity-related digestive diseases and their pathophysiology. *Gut Liver.* 2017;11(3):323-334.

7. Fujihara S, Mori H, Kobara H, et al. Metabolic syndrome, obesity and gastrointestinal cancer. *Gastroenterol Res Pract.* 2012;2012:483623. doi:10.1155/2012/483623

8. Nam SY, Choi IJ, Ryu KH, Park BJ, Kim HB, Nam BH. Abdominal visceral adipose tissue volume is associated with increased risk of erosive esophagitis in men and women. *Gastroenterology.* 2010;139:1902-1911.

9. Nam SY, Kim BC, Han KS, et al. Abdominal visceral adipose tissue predicts risk of colorectal adenoma in both sexes. *Clin Gastroentrol Hepatol.* 2010;8:443-450.

10. Colicchio P, Tarantino G, del Genio F, et al. Non-alcoholic fatty liver disease in young adult severely obese non-diabetic patients in South Italy. *Ann Nutr Metab.* 2005;49:289-295.

11. Mushref MA, Srinivasan S. Effect of high fat-diet and obesity in gastrointestinal motility. *Ann Transl Med.* 2013;1(2):14. doi:10.3978/j.issn.2305-5839.2012.11.01

12. Xing J, Chen JD. Alterations of gastrointestinal motility in obesity. *Obes Res.* 2004;12:1723-1732.

13. US Department of Health and Human Services. *Physical Activity Guidelines for Americans*. 2nd ed. US Department of Health and Human Services; 2019. Accessed January 15, 2022. https://health.gov/our-work/nutrition-physical-activity/physical-activity-guidelines/current-guidelines

14. Dunstan DW, Howard B, Healy GN, Owen N. Too much sitting—a health hazard. *Diabetes Res Clin Pract.* 2012;97(3):368-376. doi:10.1016/j.diabres.2012.05.020

15. Chau JY, Daley M, Dunn S, et al. The effectiveness of sit-stand workstations for changing office workers' sitting time: results from the Stand@Work randomized controlled trial pilot. *Int J Behav Nutr Phys Act.* 2014;11:127. doi:10.1186/s12966-014-0127-7

16. Johns DJ, Hartmann-Boyce J, Jebb SA, Aveyard P; Behavioural Weight Management Review Group. Diet or exercise interventions vs combined behavioral weight management programs: a systematic review and meta-analysis of direct comparisons. *J Acad Nutr Diet.* 2014;114(10):1557-1568. doi:10.1016/j.jand.2014.07.005

17. Cooper Z, Fairburn CG, Hawker DM. *Cognitive-Behavioral Treatment of Obesity: A Clinician's Guide*. Guilford Press; 2003.

18. Heymsfield SB, van Mierlo CAJ, van der Knaap HCM, Heo M, Frier HI. Weight management using a meal replacement strategy: meta and pooling analysis from six studies. *Int J Obes Relat Metab Disord.* 2003;27(5):537-549. doi:10.1038/sj.ijo.0802258

19. Leader NJ, Ryan L, Molyneaux L, Yue DK. How best to use partial meal replacement in managing overweight or obese patients with poorly controlled type 2 diabetes. *Obes.* 2013;21(2):251-253. doi:10.1002/oby.20057

20. Tsai AG, Wadden TA. The evolution of very-low-calorie diets: an update and meta-analysis. *Obes.* 2006;14(8):1283-1293. doi:10.1038/oby.2006.146

21. Institute of Medicine. *Dietary Reference Intakes for Energy, Carbohydrate, Fiber, Fat, Fatty Acids, Cholesterol, Protein, and Amino Acids*. National Academies Press; 2005. doi:10.17226/10490

22. Wing RR, Phelan S. Long-term weight loss maintenance. *Am J Clin Nutr.* 2005;82(1 suppl):222S-225S. doi:10.1093/ajcn/82.1.222S

23. Nordmann AJ, Nordmann A, Briel M, et al. Effects of low-carbohydrate vs low-fat diets on weight loss and cardiovascular risk factors: a meta-analysis of randomized controlled trials. *Arch Intern Med.* 2006;166(3):285-293. doi:10.1001/archinte.166.3.285

24. Bueno NB, de Melo ISV, de Oliveira SL, da Rocha Ataide T. Very-low-carbohydrate ketogenic diet v. low-fat diet for long-term weight loss: a meta-analysis of randomised controlled trials. *Br J Nutr.* 2013;110(7):1178-1187. doi:10.1017/S0007114513000548

25. Mansoor N, Vinknes KJ, Veierød MB, Retterstøl K. Effects of low-carbohydrate diets v. low-fat diets on body weight and cardiovascular risk factors: a meta-analysis of randomised controlled trials. *Br J Nutr.* 2016;115(3):466-479. doi:10.1017/S0007114515004699

26. Martin K, Jackson CF, Levy RG, Cooper PN. Ketogenic diet and other dietary treatments for epilepsy. *Cochrane Database Syst Rev.* 2016;(2):CD001903. doi:10.1002/14651858.CD001903.pub3

27. Westerterp-Plantenga MS, Lemmens SG, Westerterp KR. Dietary protein—its role in satiety, energetics, weight loss and health. *Br J Nutr.* 2012;108(suppl 2):S105-112. doi:10.1017/S0007114512002589

28. Wycherley TP, Moran LJ, Clifton PM, Noakes M, Brinkworth GD. Effects of energy-restricted high-protein, low-fat compared with standard-protein, low-fat diets: a meta-analysis of randomized controlled trials. *Am J Clin Nutr.* 2012;96(6):1281-1298. doi:10.3945/ajcn.112.044321

29. Flechtner-Mors M, Boehm BO, Wittmann R, Thoma U, Ditschuneit HH. Enhanced weight loss with protein-enriched meal replacements in subjects with the metabolic syndrome. *Diabetes Metab Res Rev.* 2010;26(5):393-405. doi:10.1002/dmrr.1097

30. US Department of Health and Human Services, US Department of Agriculture. *2020-2025 Dietary Guidelines for Americans.* 9th ed. US Department of Health and Human Services and US Department of Agriculture; 2020. Accessed January 15, 2022. www.dietaryguidelines.gov/resources/2020-2025-dietary-guidelines-online-materials

31. Appel LJ, Moore TJ, Obarzanek E, et al. A clinical trial of the effects of dietary patterns on blood pressure. DASH Collaborative Research Group. *N Engl J Med.* 1997;336(16):1117-1124. doi:10.1056/NEJM199704173361601

32. Sacks FM, Obarzanek E, Windhauser MM, et al. Rationale and design of the Dietary Approaches to Stop Hypertension trial (DASH): a multicenter controlled-feeding study of dietary patterns to lower blood pressure. *Ann Epidemiol.* 1995;5(2):108-118. doi:10.1016/1047-2797(94)00055-x

33. Epstein DE, Sherwood A, Smith PJ, et al. Determinants and consequences of adherence to the dietary approaches to stop hypertension diet in African-American and white adults with high blood pressure: results from the ENCORE trial. *J Acad Nutr Diet.* 2012;112(11):1763-1773. doi:10.1016/j.jand.2012.07.007

34. Arnett DK, Blumenthal RS, Albert MA, et al. 2019 ACC/AHA guideline on the primary prevention of cardiovascular disease: executive summary: a report of the American College of Cardiology/American Heart Association Task Force on Clinical Practice Guidelines. *J Am Coll Cardiol.* 2019;74(10):1376-1414. doi:10.1016/j.jacc.2019.03.009

35. Blumenthal JA, Babyak MA, Hinderliter A, et al. Effects of the DASH diet alone and in combination with exercise and weight loss on blood pressure and cardiovascular biomarkers in men and women with high blood pressure: the ENCORE study. *Arch Intern Med.* 2010;170(2):126-135. doi:10.1001/archinternmed.2009.470

36. Willett WC, Sacks F, Trichopoulou A, et al. Mediterranean diet pyramid: a cultural model for healthy eating. *Am J Clin Nutr.* 1995;61(6 suppl):1402S-1406S. doi:10.1093/ajcn/61.6.1402S

37. Shai I, Schwarzfuchs D, Henkin y, et al. Weight loss with a low-carbohydrate, Mediterranean, or low-fat diet. *N Engl J Med.* 2008;359(3):229-241. doi:10.1056/NEJMoa0708681

38. Toledo E, Hu FB, Estruch R, et al. Effect of the Mediterranean diet on blood pressure in the PREDIMED trial: results from a randomized controlled trial. *BMC Med.* 2013;11:207. doi:10.1186/1741-7015-11-207

39. Ros E, Martínez-González MA, Estruch R, et al. Mediterranean diet and cardiovascular health: teachings of the PREDIMED study. *Adv Nutr.* 2014;5(3):330S-336S. doi:10.3945/an.113.005389

40. Melina V, Craig W, Levin S. Position of the Academy of Nutrition and Dietetics: vegetarian diets. *J Acad Nutr Diet.* 2016;116(12):1970-1980. doi:10.1016/j.jand.2016.09.025

41. Orlich MJ, Fraser GE. Vegetarian diets in the Adventist Health Study 2: a review of initial published findings. *Am J Clin Nutr.* 2014;100(suppl 1):353S-358S. doi:10.3945/ajcn.113.071233

42. Rosell M, Appleby P, Spencer E, Key T. Weight gain over 5 years in 21,966 meat-eating, fish-eating, vegetarian, and vegan men and women in EPIC-Oxford. *Int J Obes.* 2006;30(9):1389-1396. doi:10.1038/sj.ijo.0803305

43. Barnard ND, Levin SM, yokoyama y. A systematic review and meta-analysis of changes in body weight in clinical trials of vegetarian diets. *J Acad Nutr Diet.* 2015;115(6):954-969. doi:10.1016/j.jand.2014.11.016

44. Huang R-Y, Huang C-C, Hu FB, Chavarro JE. Vegetarian diets and weight reduction: a meta-analysis of randomized controlled trials. *J Gen Intern Med.* 2016;(1):109-116. doi:10.1007/s11606-015-3390-7

45. Look AHEAD Research Group; Wing RR. Long-term effects of lifestyle intervention on weight and cardiovascular outcomes in individuals with type 2 diabetes mellitus: four-year results of the Look AHEAD trial. *Arch Internal Med.* 2010;170(17):1566-1575. doi:10.1001/archinternmed.2010.334

46. Foster D, Sanchez-Collins S, Cheskin LJ. Multidisciplinary team-based obesity treatment in patients with diabetes: current practices and the state of the science. *Diabetes Spectr*. 2017;30(4):244-249. doi:10.2337/ds17-0045

47. Academy of Nutrition and Dietetics. Adult weight management (AWM) systematic review (2020-21). Evidence Analysis Library website. Accessed January 28, 2022. www.andeal.org/topic.cfm?menu=5276&cat=6108

48. Lin M, Mahmooth Z, Dedhia N, et al. Tailored, interactive text messages for enhancing weight loss among African American adults: the TRIMM randomized controlled trial. *Am J Med*. 2015;128(8):896-904. doi:10.1016/j.amjmed.2015.03.013

49. Prescribers' Digital Reference. Accessed January 15, 2022. www.pdr.net

CHAPTER

12

Eating Disorders

Jennifer Leah Goetz, MD
Angela S. Guarda, MD

KEY POINTS

- Eating disorders are relatively common—at least one in 20 individuals in the United States has a clinically significant eating disorder. These serious psychiatric conditions come with a variety of associated gastrointestinal and nutritional complications.

- Gastrointestinal and nutritional complications can be a consequence of prolonged starvation, engagement in purging behaviors, or the refeeding process itself, which should occur under appropriate medical supervision and guidance.

- Recognizing the signs and symptoms of eating disorders, as well as the common gastrointestinal and nutritional complications, is critical.

Introduction

Eating disorders are serious psychiatric conditions that have a variety of associated gastrointestinal (GI) and nutritional complications.[1] The two most well-recognized eating disorders, anorexia nervosa (AN) and bulimia nervosa (BN), are characterized by a drive for thinness, body image dissatisfaction, feelings of shame and embarrassment, and frequent denial of the seriousness of the illness. As a result, individuals with eating disorders are often ambivalent toward treatment. They may preferentially present to nonpsychiatric medical providers with GI or other somatic concerns that are a consequence of their disordered eating and weight-control behaviors but without disclosing their diagnosis. Binge eating disorder is also commonly associated with body dissatisfaction, and affected individuals are often overweight. Individuals with binge eating disorder may seek help with weight loss from registered dietitian nutritionists (RDN) in an attempt to improve their body image concerns.

The *Diagnostic and Statistical Manual of Mental Disorders*, 5th Edition (*DSM-5*), recognizes six eating disorders: AN, BN, binge eating disorder (BED), avoidant/restrictive food intake disorder (ARFID), other specified feeding or eating disorder (OSFED), and unspecified feeding or eating disorder (UFED). This chapter focuses primarily on AN and BN, as these are the most studied. The severity of eating disorders can be categorized by either the degree of weight loss or the frequency of engagement in compensatory behaviors, when present (see Table 12.1 on page 186).[2]

Eating disorders are relatively common, and experts estimate that at least one in 20 individuals in the United States has a clinically significant eating disorder. According to a 2020 publication by Deloitte Access Economics, 9% of the US population, or 28.8 million Americans, will have an eating disorder in their lifetime.[3]

Recognizing the signs and symptoms of eating disorders, as well as the common GI and nutritional complications arising from starvation or purging behaviors or as a consequence of renourishment, is critical for the practicing gastroenterologist and allied health specialists. A strong alliance between primary providers and behavioral health specialists is an important factor in successful treatment.

This chapter reviews (1) clinical criteria for identifying eating disorders; (2) pathological mechanisms underlying their development; (3) GI and nutritional complications attributable to starvation, purging behavior, and refeeding; and (4) empirically based treatment modalities.

TABLE 12.1 Eating Disorder Severity[2]

Severity[a]	Anorexia nervosa[b]	Bulimia nervosa	Binge eating disorder
Mild	BMI ≥17.00	1-3 episodes a week of inappropriate compensatory behavior[c]	1-3 binge eating episodes a week
Moderate	BMI = 16.00-16.99	4-7 episodes a week of inappropriate compensatory behavior[c]	4-7 binge eating episodes a week
Severe	BMI = 15.00-15.99	8-13 episodes a week of inappropriate compensatory behavior[c]	8-13 binge eating episodes a week
Extreme	BMI <15.00	14 or more episodes a week of inappropriate compensatory behavior[c]	14 or more binge eating episodes a week

[a] Severity of diagnosis may be increased based on clinical judgment of other factors, including symptoms or functional disability.
[b] BMI ranges are based on World Health Organization categories for thinness in adults. Use corresponding BMI percentiles for children and adolescents.
[c] Typical incidence

Diagnostic Categories of Eating Disorders

Anorexia Nervosa

There are two subtypes of AN: a predominantly restricting subtype, characterized by extreme restriction of energy intake as the primary means of weight control; and a binge-purge subtype, which involves regular bingeing or purging behaviors (self-induced vomiting and the misuse of laxatives, diuretics, or enemas) as means of weight control. Transitioning from the restricting subtype to the binge-purge subtype over time is common.[4,5] Compulsive exercise is also common and occurs in up to 80% of patients with AN.[6]

BMI can be a useful indicator of the degree or severity of weight loss in AN. A cutoff BMI of less than 18.5 is most commonly used as the general threshold for underweight status. Although there is no absolute BMI or weight cutoff criteria for making the diagnosis, BMI can be a helpful marker when looking at weight trajectories over time.

A shift in dietary preferences to low-energy-density foods and restriction of food variety are typical presenting features. As affected individuals lose weight, their preoccupation with food, weight, and body shape increases, as does anxiety and resistance to straying from self-imposed food rules and exercise regimens. Patients may offer seemingly rational explanations for their food choices based on personal ethical or environmental values (eg, vegetarianism, a preference for organic foods, health concerns, food intolerances) that do not, however, explain their state of malnourishment. Anxiety about behavior change—especially about eating more foods with higher energy density, decreasing exercise, or making an effort to gain weight—is often prominent and can lead to a number of problematic behaviors that interfere with treatment. Some of these include denial of illness and treatment avoidance, a preference for treatments that emphasize talk therapies rather than behavior change, and a focus on relieving the symptoms of complications that arise from the disordered eating and weight-control behaviors (including symptoms of GI complications)—all at the expense of treating the underlying eating disorder. See Box 12.1 for a summary of diagnostic criteria for AN.[2]

Bulimia Nervosa

Binge eating is a hallmark behavior of BN (as well as of BED) and is defined in the *DSM-5* as "eating more than most people would eat in a discrete period of time"; patients often consume several thousand kilocalories in a 1- to 2-hour time period. Bingeing is usually a secretive behavior associated with feelings of shame and embarrassment. In BN, binge eating is followed by a compensatory behavior to prevent weight gain. Purging by vomiting is the most common of these compensatory behaviors. Many people with BN report that

BOX 12.1

Diagnostic Criteria for Anorexia Nervosa[2]

The patient restricts oral intake, leading to significantly low body weight (in the context of the patient's age, sex, development, and physical health).

The patient has a fear of gaining weight or becoming fat, or exhibits persistent behaviors that interfere with weight gain despite low weight.

The patient has a body weight or body shape disturbance and does not recognize the seriousness of low weight.

purging alleviates both the physical discomfort associated with the binge and the fear of weight gain. In some individuals, purging and the associated sense of relief becomes the goal of the binge itself. In patients who are underweight and meet the criteria for AN, and who engage in either bingeing or purging behaviors, the diagnosis is AN–binge/purge, a subtype of AN. Weight status (underweight vs normal or above normal) can help distinguish AN–binge/purge from BN. See Box 12.2 for a summary of diagnostic criteria for BN.[2]

BOX 12.2

Diagnostic Criteria for Bulimia Nervosa[2]

The patient has repeated episodes of binge eating.

The patient engages in repeated compensatory activities to prevent weight gain, including self-induced vomiting; misuse of laxatives, diuretics, or other medications; fasting; and excessive exercise.

The behaviors occur, on average, at least once a week for 3 months.

The patient's self-worth is excessively influenced by weight and body shape.

The behaviors do not occur primarily during episodes of anorexia nervosa.

Binge Eating Disorder

A diagnosis of BED places the patient at increased risk of lifetime and current obesity.[7] Unlike in BN, individuals with BED do not regularly engage in compensatory behaviors. Triggers for binge eating in both BN and BED can include negative affect, interpersonal stressors, dietary restraint, environmental cues, and boredom. Although binge eating may serve to alleviate negative feelings in the short term, increased dysphoria and negative self-evaluation often result from the behavioral pattern. See Box 12.3 for a summary of diagnostic criteria for BED.[2]

BOX 12.3

Diagnostic Criteria for Binge Eating Disorder[2]

The patient has repeated episodes of binge eating.

The binge eating episodes are associated with at least three of the following:

- eating more rapidly than normal
- eating until uncomfortably full
- eating large amounts of food when not feeling hungry
- eating alone due to feeling embarrassed by the amount one is eating
- feeling disgusted, depressed, or guilty after eating

The patient experiences excessive distress regarding binge eating.

The binge eating occurs, on average, at least once a week for 3 months.

The binge eating is not associated with the repeated use of compensatory behavior (as in bulimia nervosa) and does not occur exclusively during the course of bulimia nervosa or anorexia nervosa.

Avoidant/Restrictive Food Intake Disorder

ARFID is a relatively new diagnosis and was added to the *DSM-5* to describe individuals who engage in restrictive eating behaviors that result in malnutrition and functional impairment but who do not exhibit associated concerns about body weight and shape, as is typical in AN, BN, or BED. See Box 12.4 for a summary of diagnostic criteria for ARFID.[2]

BOX 12.4

Diagnostic Criteria for Avoidant/ Restrictive Food Intake Disorder[2]

The patient lacks interest in eating or food, or avoids eating based on sensory characteristics of food or concerns about aversive consequences of eating, as evidenced by a persistent failure to meet nutrition or energy needs (or both) and leading to one or more of the following:

- significant weight loss or failure to gain weight; or faltering growth in children
- significant nutritional deficiency
- dependence on enteral feeding or oral nutritional supplements
- significant interference with psychosocial functioning

The disturbance is not better explained by lack of available food or an associated culturally sanctioned practice.

The eating disturbance does not occur exclusively during the course of anorexia nervosa or bulimia nervosa, and there is no evidence of a disturbance in the way in which body weight or shape is experienced.

The eating disorder is not attributable to another medical condition or mental disorder. If the eating disturbance occurs in the context of another condition or disorder, the severity of the eating disturbance exceeds that associated with the condition and warrants additional clinical attention.

Patients with ARFID are a heterogeneous group of individuals from across the weight spectrum. There are limited data available to date on the presentation, prevalence, pathogenesis, or clinical course of the disorder, though more data are available for the pediatric population than the adult population. Three preliminary subtypes have been described: (1) a subtype characterized by a lifelong low appetitive drive and low weight; (2) a subtype characterized by concerns about food texture and sensitivities (typical of patients with autism spectrum disorders); and (3) a subtype in which food restriction (of either quantity or type of foods consumed) is rooted in anxiety over the possible consequences of eating (eg, fear of choking, nausea or vomiting, abdominal pain, bloating).[5] In a retrospective study of patients from a tertiary care center who underwent neurogastroenterology examination, ARFID symptoms were found to be most frequently related to fear of GI symptoms. Patients with any of these subtype characteristics should be evaluated for symptoms of ARFID, especially when dietary interventions are considered.[8] Evidence suggests that the subtypes are not mutually exclusive and that many individuals with ARFID are of mixed subtype.

Other Specified Feeding or Eating Disorder, and Unspecified Feeding or Eating Disorder

The *DSM-5* includes two additional catchall categories of eating disorders—OSFED (see Box 12.5) and UFED. UFED is a preliminary diagnosis that can be used when there is insufficient information to characterize the type of eating disorder, as, for example, in emergency situations or initial consultations, when inadequate information is available. OSFED is diagnosed in individuals who present with symptoms of an eating disorder that result in substantial functional impairment but who do not meet the full criteria for AN, BN, BED, or ARFID. Atypical anorexia is one example of OSFED. This category includes patients who present with all the symptoms of AN, including substantial weight loss, restricted food intake, and overvaluation of body weight and shape but who lost weight from an above average weight and are still within the normal or above-normal range for height. Despite not being underweight by BMI, people with atypical anorexia and extreme eating behaviors, including frequent purging or fasting and rapid weight loss, can be medically unstable and present with substantial functional impairment.

Pathogenesis of Eating Disorders

The etiology of eating disorders is multifactorial and includes predisposing, precipitating, and perpetuating factors. Although eating disorders used to be thought of as sociocultural conditions arising from the pressure to be thin, it is increasingly clear that they are biologically based and arise from a combination of genetic and environmental factors. Predisposing factors for the development of an eating disorder include genetic vulnerabilities, temperamental features, and individual personality traits. There is a significant genetic predisposition to eating disorders, especially for AN, with elevated rates of concordance in monozygotic compared to dizygotic twins, and a sevenfold risk for an eating disorder in first- and second-degree relatives of an affected proband.[9] A recent large, genome-wide association study identified eight key chromosomal loci associated with AN. Additionally, genetic correlations found positive associations with psychiatric conditions and negative associations with metabolic characteristics associated with obesity, including glycemic, lipid, and anthropometric profiles.[10] As with substance use disorders, it is likely that a higher genetic diathesis is associated with greater chronicity and severity of illness. Personality traits associated with AN and BN include perfectionism, neuroticism, sensitivity to criticism, and obsessional traits, all of which are heritable and common in first-degree relatives of affected individuals.[11]

In genetically vulnerable individuals, a number of precipitating factors are thought to trigger the onset of an eating disorder. As eating disorders occur most typically during adolescence and young adulthood, and for AN and BN the preponderance of cases are in females, hormonal changes related to puberty may play a role in onset. Additional factors linked to the onset of illness include dieting and exercise behaviors, life stressors, and trauma. As the disorder progresses, physiological consequences of starvation and of binge-purge behaviors lead to disturbances in homeostatic hunger and satiety signaling, in fear conditioning and habit formation, and in brain reward circuitry. These changes are increasingly believed to underlie maintenance of the disorder and contribute to its self-sustaining, or feed-forward, nature.[12] Over time, as a disorder becomes chronic, these secondary sustaining factors are thought to maintain the behavioral cycle of the eating disorder, despite the increasing cost to the individual. The behavioral model of eating disorders has important implications for treatment that will be discussed in the section on treatment later in the chapter.

Comorbidity

Psychiatric comorbidities are common in patients with eating disorders, especially mood disorders, anxiety disorders, obsessive compulsive disorder, personality disorders, and substance use disorders.[13] Anxiety disorders are the most common comorbid psychiatric condition and often precede the onset of the eating disorder. It can be challenging to distinguish whether concurrent psychopathology is due to a comorbid psychiatric disorder or simply a consequence of binge-purge behavior or malnutrition (or both), because mood, cognition, and behavior are all affected by the starved state and by the physiological consequences of disordered eating. Indeed, starvation can result in a syndrome of depression that is identical to major depressive disorder but which resolves rapidly with renourishment. In severe BN and BED, demoralization and shame, as well as disruption in the sleep-wake cycle and poor concentration, can similarly amplify depressive symptomatology in the acutely ill state. A personal or family history of a premorbid psychiatric condition may help clarify whether symptoms are due to a co-occurring psychiatric illness. Suicide rates are elevated in patients with eating disorders, especially those with AN complicated by alcohol use disorder.[14] Prompt and early recognition and treatment of coexisting conditions is essential to recovery. Medical conditions having elevated comorbidity with eating disorders include type 1 diabetes mellitus (T1DM). When co-occurring with an eating disorder, T1DM is of serious concern because patients may underdose their insulin as a way to purge energy intake, and this can result in higher risks for diabetic ketoacidosis and end-organ complications of T1DM. Some autoimmune conditions, including inflammatory bowel disease and celiac disease, may also have an increased prevalence in patients with eating disorders and may complicate disease course and management.[15]

Comorbid medical conditions associated with BED include those associated with being overweight—cardiovascular disease, type 2 diabetes mellitus, gallbladder disease, arthritis, and infertility. In addition, comorbid mood disorders, particularly major depressive disorder, are common in BED, though they are not related directly to malnutrition as is often the case in AN-associated mood disorders. Up to 32% of patients with BED have depression, according to the National Comorbidity Survey Replication study.[16]

Epidemiology: Prevalence Estimates

Body dissatisfaction is extremely common in the general population and is associated with the development of disordered eating (doesn't meet criteria for an eating disorder but there is significant disruption in eating behaviors) and eating disorders. A national sample of more than 36,000 US adults from the 2012–2013 National Epidemiological Survey on Alcohol and Related Conditions found that lifetime prevalence estimates for AN, BN, and BED were 0.8% to 0.9%, 0.28% to 1.5%, and 0.85% to 1.9%, respectively.[7,17] The prevalence of ARFID is undetermined but is estimated to be 3% to 5% in children, with males potentially having a higher risk than females for this disorder.[18] In an Australian-based population study, the 3-month prevalence of ARFID in those over 15 years of age was 0.3% in 2014 and 0.3% in 2015.[3] OSFED and UFED are new diagnoses in the *DSM-5*, and epidemiological data is lacking. OSFED is estimated to be the most common eating disorder, with a lifetime prevalence of 3.82% among females and 1.61% among males.[2]

Mortality rates for patients who have ever been hospitalized for AN are five times higher than those for the general population when matched for sex and age, with peak deaths occurring in young adulthood, between the ages of 25 and 34 years, according to one large study published in 2016.[19] Mortality in this population is related to the consequences of prolonged starvation, malnutrition, and suicide.[20] AN has the highest mortality rate of any psychiatric conditions other than opioid use disorder and is additionally associated with high morbidity and burden of illness.[3]

Clinical Presentation and Diagnosis of Eating Disorders

Patients who present with clinical suspicion of an eating disorder should undergo a thorough evaluation that includes a history, physical examination, and laboratory work-up. Medical complications are best thought of as secondary either to the severity of starvation or the severity of bingeing and purging behaviors. Patients who are both starved and engaging in binge-purge behaviors are, therefore, at the highest risk. Importantly, this risk can be high even in individuals presenting at a normal or above-normal weight who do not purge but who have lost weight rapidly (ie, in atypical AN).

Individuals may present with anxiety, depression, or somatic discomfort as a result of medical complications, including GI complications. The latter may include a variety of symptoms, such as choking, nausea, vomiting, heartburn, pain with eating, bloating, constipation, and diarrhea. Many patients will, therefore, present to gastroenterologists with primary GI concerns. Refer to Box 12.6 for information to gather from the patient during a clinical evaluation for a possible eating disorder.

BOX 12.6

Clinical Evaluation for Diagnosing Eating Disorders

Highest and lowest body weight (Ask: "What is the most and least you have weighed at your current height?"), or growth charts for children and adolescents

Desired body weight (Ask: "What weight would you be most comfortable at?")

Any rapid, substantial, recent weight changes (Ask: "Has your weight changed in the past year? By how much?")

Frequency of self-weighing (daily, weekly, monthly, or less often)

Meal patterns (typical breakfast, lunch, and dinner; variety of foods consumed; snacking or grazing habits; skipped meals; preference for low-energy-density foods)

Number and frequency of binge eating episodes and self-induced vomiting episodes; amount and frequency of use of laxatives, diuretics, and diet pills; amount of time spent exercising (current and lifetime maximum frequency per day, week, or month, for all of these behaviors)

Excessive preoccupation with food, weight, or body image

Menstrual status (oligomenorrhea or amenorrhea)

Any passive death wishes, suicidal thoughts, suicide attempts, or self-injurious behaviors

Current and lifetime mood, anxiety, impulse control, substance use disorders

Psychosocial functioning

Family history of eating disorders and associated psychopathology (anxiety, mood, or substance use disorders)

Physical Examination

The key elements of a complete physical examination in patients suspected of having an eating disorder are weight and height, orthostatic vital signs, temperature, skin condition, oropharyngeal examination, abdominal examination, and neurologic examination. In addition, potential signs to watch for include bitemporal wasting, lanugo hair, hair loss, parotid gland enlargement, poor dentition, and scarring or calluses on the dorsum of the hand (resulting from use of fingers to induce vomiting).

Laboratory Assessment

When considering laboratory evaluation to aid in the diagnosis of an eating disorder, testing should be guided by the patient's presenting symptoms and physical findings (see Box 12.7).

BOX 12.7

Laboratory Tests for Diagnosis of Eating Disorders

Complete blood count and differential: to rule out anemia, leukopenia, thrombocytopenia

Comprehensive metabolic panel (blood urea nitrogen/creatinine ratio, liver function tests, albumin, calcium, phosphate, magnesium): to identify electrolyte abnormalities, third spacing, or organ dysfunction in patients who have lost a substantial amount of weight or are purging, or both

Amylase and lipase levels: to assess for recent purging (especially if suspicion is high but the patient denies purging behaviors) and pancreatitis

Thyroid function tests (thyrotropin [thyroid-stimulating hormone], triiodothyronine and thyroxine): to identify alternative causes of weight loss or euthyroid sick syndrome, a common consequence of malnutrition

Hormone levels: luteinizing hormone, follicle-stimulating hormone, estrogen, and testosterone, all of which are typically suppressed in the starved state

Vitamin D level: to assess for deficiency often seen in eating disorders, and resulting effects on bone mineral density

Urinalysis: to assess specific gravity; may be low in "water loading" in order to artificially inflate weight

Dual-energy x-ray absorptiometry scan: to assess for bone loss or osteoporosis in patients restricting intake for longer than 6 months

Electrocardiogram: to assess for abnormal cardiac rhythm, including bradycardia or prolonged QT interval corrected for heart rate

---

Complications of Eating Disorders

Starvation induces protein and fat catabolism that leads to loss of cellular volume and atrophy of the heart, brain, liver, intestines, kidneys, and muscles. The primary risk factors for developing medical complications in AN are the degree and speed of weight loss, the severity of purging behaviors, and the chronicity of the illness.

Nutrition-Related Deficiencies and Complications

The macronutrient and micronutrient intakes of individuals with eating disorders vary; however, those with restrictive eating behavior tend to avoid foods containing more than trace amounts of fats and often have a very stereotyped and restricted food repertoire.

Although most malnutrition is due to low energy intake, certain micronutrient deficiencies are also seen. Some people restrict meats and dairy without substituting appropriate vegetarian alternatives, which leads to deficiencies mainly in the B vitamins.[21] Excessive intake of one food can result in hypervitaminosis (eg, carotenemia and orange skin pigmentation from excess vitamin A intake) or poisoning (eg, mercury toxicity from excess tuna intake).

The true extent of a patient's nutrient deficiencies may not become apparent until the patient has entered the refeeding stage of treatment, as increased energy intake leads to improved cellular metabolism, tissue repair, and cell turnover, all of which increases nutrient utilization and may deplete already-low nutrient stores. In studies of diet history and recall, the reliability of which is limited, females with AN were found to be at elevated risk for deficiencies in the following nutrients: zinc, calcium, vitamin D, folate, vitamin B12, magnesium, and copper.[22] A more recent study found that nearly 50% of patients with AN had at least one micronutrient deficiency before starting treatment.[23]

Electrolyte Disturbances

Electrolyte deficiencies are the most acutely dangerous micronutrient deficiencies and commonly result from purging behaviors (self-induced vomiting, laxative and diuretic abuse). Hypokalemia is commonly associated with frequent purging and is a major cause of cardiac arrythmia and sudden death. Oral repletion is preferable in most cases, and addressing the underlying causative behavior is critical to decreasing ongoing risk. Chronic vomiting may result in hypochloremic metabolic alkalosis, whereas chronic laxative abuse can cause a metabolic acidosis, hypomagnesemia or hypermagnesemia, and hypophosphatemia or hyperphosphatemia and may result in acute renal impairment.

Hyponatremia occurs for a variety of reasons, the most common of which is associated with hypovolemia and low serum tonicity. This may be due to extrarenal or renal sodium loss from purging behaviors (including vomiting, diarrhea, or diuretic abuse) or severe fluid restriction and hypovolemia in patients in extremely malnourished and fluid-restricted states. The decrease in circulating vascular volume causes the release of antidiuretic hormone, which leads to reabsorption of water by the kidneys. Hyponatremia is most dangerous when it presents rapidly (over course of a few hours) or with very significant drops in serum sodium level (below 120–125 mEq/L).[2] Care should be taken when repleting sodium intravenously; repletion should happen slowly to avoid central pontine myelinolysis.[24] Hypoglycemia related to fasting behavior and starvation is associated with tachycardia, sweating, anxiety, irritability, and feeling faint, lightheaded, or shaky.

Vitamin and Mineral Deficiencies

Vitamin D

Vitamin D deficiency (<30 ng/mL) is common in patients with limited dairy intake and low sunshine exposure. Low bone mineral density, defined as a z score under 2 standard deviations, in AN is multifactorial in origin; it is attributable to low levels of estrogen, vitamin D, and calcium, and elevated cortisol levels. The severity of malnutrition, long duration of illness, and amenorrhea are risk factors for bone loss and osteoporosis, with the risk of fracture in this population being seven times that of the general population.[25] Weight gain sufficient to produce menses is important in preventing continued bone loss.[26] Recommended supplementation is with 50,000 International Units (IU) of vitamin D3 weekly for 8 weeks in patients with vitamin D levels below 30 ng/mL, followed by a maintenance dose of 1,000 to 2,000 IU per day thereafter, unless the patient is getting adequate amounts of vitamin D from fortified foods and a general multivitamin.

Thiamin

Thiamin is found in many foods, though patients who restrict carbohydrates may have inadequate intake. Patients with both a restrictive eating disorder and an alcohol use disorder are at particularly high risk for thiamin deficiency because alcohol interferes with thiamin absorption. Patients with an eating disorder who have undergone bariatric surgery are also at increased risk for thiamin deficiency, which can result in Wernicke encephalopathy (ocular abnormalities, ataxia, confused state, hypothermia, coma) or Korsakoff syndrome (retrograde and anterograde amnesia, confabulation). A deficiency of thiamin can also cause or worsen psychiatric symptoms, including depression and cognitive impairment, so supplementation is recommended for patients with history of inadequate intake, though the appropriate dose, frequency, and duration are not universally agreed upon (recommendations range from 100 to 500 mg once to three times daily).

Folate and Vitamin B12

Patients with eating disorders may be deficient in both folate and vitamin B12. Symptoms of a deficiency of either of these include fatigue, lack of energy, paresthesia, oral ulcers, muscle weakness, visual disturbances, depression, confusion, memory difficulties, and macrocytic anemia. It is especially important to check for these symptoms in patients with eating disorders who consume large quantities of alcohol or have undergone bariatric surgery, for they are at particularly high risk for deficiencies. An elevated plasma concentration of total homocysteine is a more sensitive indicator of folate deficiency. Supplementation with 400 mcg folate daily is recommended by the Centers for Disease Control and Prevention for all people of childbearing age. Vitamin B12 deficiency is diagnosed at serum levels below 200 pg/mL and is also indicated by elevated levels of methylmalonic acid and total homocysteine. Deficiency is treated with 1 mg cyanocobalamin per month, though depending on the severity of deficiency, this may be supplemented with 500 mcg daily.

Calcium

Inadequate calcium intake is fairly common among patients with eating disorders, though this may not be reflected in their serum calcium levels because calcium is released from bone in order to maintain serum levels in the stable or normal range. A food log or dietary intake history can help identify inadequate calcium intake. For patients at risk for osteoporosis or bone loss, supplementation with 1,500 mg elemental calcium per day, divided over two to three doses and taken with meals, is recommended.

Iron

Patients with eating disorders who are vegetarians or vegan often have insufficient iron in their diets and may ingest foods that inhibit iron absorption, such as coffee and tea, in greater amounts. Symptoms of iron deficiency include fatigue, weakness, and inability to stay warm, all of which mimic symptoms of general energy malnutrition. The best indicator of long-term iron stores is serum ferritin; repletion is a long-term process and may continue even after oral intake is normalized.

Zinc

Zinc is crucial for proper functioning of GI and neuroendocrine systems. Zinc is released from catabolic tissues—so in the initial stage of weight loss, serum levels may not accurately reflect zinc status; supplementation may be helpful even for patients whose levels are slightly low or whose dietary intake is inadequate. Caution should be taken, however, because zinc can inhibit copper absorption. Zinc deficiency is common in patients who restrict their meat consumption and exercise heavily, and it can cause symptoms such as weight loss, changes in taste or smell, loss of appetite, dermatitis, amenorrhea, and depression.[27]

Gastrointestinal-Related Complications

GI complications in patients with eating disorders are the norm rather than the exception and can include both structural and functional symptoms. Co-occurring GI disease, including inflammatory bowel disease or celiac disease, may also be present in a minority of patients with eating disorders. The majority of patients with eating disorders do not seek behavioral health treatment but may seek out gastroenterologists and allied health care providers to request symptomatic treatment of the GI complications of their disorder. These patients may present a diagnostic challenge. Most GI complications of eating disorders will reverse with the normalization of eating behavior and do not require—and generally do not respond to—symptomatic treatment alone (ie, with pharmaceutical agents). Gastroenterologists and RDNs should be familiar with the common GI concerns of patients with eating disorders, know how to elicit a diagnosis, recognize typical signs and symptoms, and refer patients for early psychiatric intervention.

Functional Gastrointestinal Disorders

Functional GI disorders related to GI dysmotility are present in the vast majority of patients with eating disorders. In fact, up to 97% of patients admitted to a specialty program for treatment of eating disorders meet the criteria for one or more functional GI disorders.[28] The most common symptoms include heartburn, abdominal pain, bloating, and constipation. Improvement of GI symptoms can be expected with treatment of the underlying behavioral disorder, normalization of eating cessation weight-control behaviors, and reversal of the starved state.

GI motility is typically delayed in starvation and disrupted in patients with binge-purge behaviors.[29,30] Patients with frequent self-induced vomiting may ruminate and regurgitate food after meals and have a diminished or absent gag reflex.

Starvation or purging behavior can result in delayed gastric emptying and gastroparesis in both AN and BN and in presenting complaints of both early satiety and fullness.[31] Although metoclopramide and erythromycin can be prescribed to shorten gastric emptying time, the safest and most efficacious therapy for gastroparesis in eating disorders is nutritional rehabilitation and interruption of the restrict-binge-purge cycle. A very rare but life-threatening complication of extreme bingeing occasionally seen in severely underweight individuals with AN is acute gastric dilatation with risk of gastric perforation. Acute gastric dilatation can usually be managed conservatively with nasogastric tube insertion for decompression but may require emergency surgical intervention.

Starvation in AN is also associated with delayed whole gut transit times, and constipation is a common concern.[31] Treatment of constipation in eating disorders is important because rectal distention may reflexively inhibit gastric emptying time, further complicating eating with feelings of fullness and associated discomfort.[29] Nonstimulant laxatives are recommended (ie, psyllium and polyethylene glycol 3350) on an as-needed or standing basis, depending on the degree and severity of constipation.

Laxative abuse involves the use of large quantities of stimulant laxatives or enemas, or both, to relieve symptoms of constipation and to lose weight. Although weight loss from laxative abuse is almost entirely due to fluid loss in the colon rather than small intestinal malabsorption, patients often use purging with laxatives as a way to suppress their appetite and fast, as laxative abuse comes with associated nausea. Frequent and excessive laxative use depletes potassium and can lead to muscle weakness, acute renal insufficiency, and cardiac arrhythmia. Hypermagnesemia can occur with magnesium-containing laxatives and can lead to weakness. Laxative abuse can result in secondary hyperaldosteronemia in response to chronic dehydration—and acute cessation of laxatives can precipitate severe water and sodium retention with anasarca and potential cardiac and pulmonary fluid overload. In general, the prescribed use of laxatives for constipation in eating disorders should be limited. We recommend restricting prescribed laxatives to fiber laxatives, osmotic agents, and stool softeners and avoiding stimulant laxatives. Nutritional rehabilitation and meal-based behavioral treatment is effective in relieving constipation in most individuals within weeks. Pelvic dyssynergy is a commonly overlooked contributing condition that can impede colonic transit and should be considered in females with difficult-to-manage constipation. Straining upon defecation is a classic symptom of pelvic dyssynergy, and first-line treatment is biofeedback.[4]

Laxative abuse can cause mucosal damage from castor oil, and anthracene derivative-containing products can lead to melanosis coli.

Structural Gastrointestinal Disorders

Oral Manifestations   Oral manifestations of eating disorders include enamel erosion of the lingual surface of the teeth, dental caries, and periodontal disease from chronic acid exposure caused by repeated emesis or severe regurgitation and rumination behaviors. Additionally, gingivitis, periodontitis, and cheilosis—all relatively uncommon in children, adolescents, and young adults—should raise suspicion for an underlying eating disorder. In extreme AN, protein-energy malnutrition can cause immune compromise and result in oral candidiasis. Repetitive vomiting is frequently associated with sialadenosis (parotid gland enlargement), which may lead some patients with BN or the binge-purge subtype of AN to seek care out of cosmetic concerns. Serum salivary amylase is usually elevated and normalizes gradually, along with the sialadenosis, within weeks to months of purging cessation. Providers should be aware of these oral pathologies, ask patients about disordered eating and weight-control practices when detected, and refer patients to dental providers when indicated.

Esophageal Lesions   Esophageal damage from self-induced vomiting and regurgitation is common in patients with eating disorders and can range from mild esophagitis to dysplasia (Barrett esophagus), esophageal erosions, Mallory-Weiss tears and hematemesis, or, in extreme cases, esophageal rupture (Boerhaave syndrome). Patients present with severe chest pain, painful swallowing, tachypnea, and pneumomediastinum, and they generally require surgical intervention and have significant mortality.[31] There have been rare reports of oropharyngeal dysphagia with aspiration in severely malnourished patients with AN, and it is thought to be secondary to oropharyngeal muscle wasting.[30] Endoscopy should be considered in patients with chronic purging behaviors who present with moderate or severe upper GI symptoms; however, esophageal manometry is not recommended unless emesis does not appear to be consistent with self-induced vomiting.[31]

Pancreatic and Hepatic Manifestations   Acute pancreatitis has been reported in patients with AN. Potential mechanisms include malnutrition-related microlithiasis, ischemia, and structural damage. Benign and asymptomatic moderate elevations in amylase and lipase may occur during the refeeding process. Serum salivary amylase is often elevated in patients who purge by vomiting and may be distinguished from pancreatic amylase with a fractionated amylase test. Serum lipase and pancreatic isoamylase are more sensitive and specific indicators of pancreatitis.

Liver injury can also occur in patients with AN and BN. In malnourished individuals, liver injury is most commonly an asymptomatic transaminitis and rarely progresses to hepatic failure. Starvation-induced autophagy and glycogen hepatocyte depletion may be involved in cell death, leading to transaminitis, which is typically moderate but may transiently worsen with refeeding before normalizing with nutritional rehabilitation.

Intestinal Manifestations Superior mesenteric artery (SMA) syndrome is a rare complication of AN that is caused by severe malnutrition as a result of loss of the fatty tissue surrounding the SMA. It leads to intestinal obstruction and can cause postprandial nausea and epigastric abdominal pain secondary to extrinsic compression of the third part of the duodenum by the aorta posteriorly and the superior mesenteric artery anteriorly. Treatment of SMA syndrome involves nutritional rehabilitation and weight gain to restore the fat pad that cushions the artery.[32]

Necrotizing colitis is a rare complication from severe malnutrition in AN and may occur even with cautious refeeding. It is thought to be caused by starvation-induced intestinal hypoperfusion with hypoxic-ischemic bowel injury, intestinal dysmotility, and compromised intestinal mucosal integrity.

Cathartic colon, characterized by abnormal peristalsis due to continuous usage of stimulant laxatives, has rarely been reported.

Rectal and Pelvic Floor Manifestations Pelvic floor dysfunction may be present in patients with AN. In one study, 40% of patients with AN had pelvic floor dysfunction and after a 4-week refeeding program did not show any improvements in pelvic function, suggesting potential structural damage.[33] This correlation has been hypothesized to be related to protracted evacuation efforts, laxative abuse, excessive exercise, and repeated forced vomiting that induce a rise in intra-abdominal pressure, which causes structural damage of the pelvic floor musculature, as well as atrophy and rhabdomyolysis secondary to malnutrition.

There appears to be a relationship between BN, the binge-purge subtype of AN, and rectal prolapse whereby the process of vomiting involves strong contractions of the diaphragm downward with abdominal musculature to expel stomach contents. This repetitive intra-abdominal pressure, along with preexisting pelvic floor weakness, misuse of laxatives, manual self-disimpaction, and overexercise, has been hypothesized as the rationale for the relationship between the eating disorders and rectal prolapse.[34,35]

Other Medical Complications

Eating disorders can affect all organ systems, and a comprehensive overview is beyond the scope of this chapter. Box 12.8 on pages 198 and 199 outlines some of the more important complications observed in this patient population.

The mainstay of treatment for medical complications includes nutritional rehabilitation and cessation of binge-purge behaviors, as most common complications can be expected to resolve with appropriate treatment and cessation of disordered eating and weight-control behaviors.

Treatment of Eating Disorders

The most accepted treatment for eating disorders involves a multidisciplinary team approach. Essential members of the team include a psychiatrist, an internist or pediatrician, an RDN (with experience in treating eating disorders), and a mental health professional (PhD, PsyD, or LICSW). Expertise in managing eating disorders and familiarity with the basic, empirically supported nutritional and behavioral interventions for eating disorders are more important factors, however, than the specific disciplines involved. Patients who consult a gastroenterologist or RDN may be reluctant to seek care from a mental health provider with specialty training in eating disorders because they are concerned about the stigma associated with mental illness. It is, therefore, important for clinicians to be aware of both the signs and symptoms of eating disorders and the basic first-line interventions that are useful in the treatment of eating disorders. In a team approach, it is crucial for the team to work collaboratively with the patient and encourage referral for psychiatric treatment when indicated; and comanagement and communication between the gastroenterologist, RDN, and psychiatric provider should be prioritized. Involving family and loved ones is often helpful for obtaining collateral information and supporting treatment recommendations.

Weight gain is an essential component of a successful outcome in the patient who is severely underweight and malnourished, and weight restoration can correct many of the physiologic consequences of an eating disorder. Adolescent AN responds most favorably to family-based treatment, an outpatient behavioral intervention involving parental support for weight gain.[36] Most adolescents with a short duration of illness respond favorably to this intervention; if medically unstable, however, they may require a short inpatient hospitalization for medical stabilization and energy-intake advancement, but most of the refeeding can be done in outpatient family-based treatment, thereafter. A substantial proportion of adults with short duration of illness or no prior treatments can also respond favorably to outpatient-based refeeding interventions. These interventions commonly employ nutrition education as well as cognitive behavioral and motivational interviewing psychotherapeutic interventions.

BOX 12.8

Medical Complications of Eating Disorders

Cardiac

Starvation-related complications

Cardiac arrhythmias, conduction abnormalities, cardiomyopathy or myocardial atrophy, bradycardia, mitral valve prolapse, pericardial effusion, bradycardia, hypotension

Purging-related complications

Cardiac arrhythmias, conduction abnormalities, cardiomegaly (ipecac toxicity), bradycardia

Pulmonary

Purging-related complications

Aspiration pneumonia, pneumothorax, subcutaneous emphysema, rib fractures

Metabolic

Starvation-related complications

Hypoglycemia, hypophosphatemia, hyperlipidemia, osteoporosis, euthyroid sick syndrome

Purging-related complications

Hypoglycemia, hypokalemia, hypochloremia, metabolic alkalosis, hyperlipidemia, hyperamylasemia

Gastrointestinal

Starvation-related complications

Early satiety, gastroparesis, delayed gastrointestinal transit time, bloating, abdominal pain, constipation

Box continues

BOX 12.8 (CONTINUED)

Purging-related complications

Dental enamel erosion, Mallory-Weiss tears, Boerhaave syndrome, gastroesophageal reflux disease, ileus, pancreatitis, transaminitis

Immunologic

Starvation-related complications

Leukopenia, anemia, thrombocytopenia

Renal

Starvation-related complications

Hyperaldosteronemia, hypokalemia, elevated serum creatinine, renal disease

Purging-related complications

Hyperaldosteronemia

Neurological

Starvation-related complications

Irritability, confusion, brain atrophy, Wernicke encephalopathy, Korsakoff syndrome

Reproductive

Starvation-related complications

Amenorrhea or oligomenorrhea, infertility

Purging-related complications

Amenorrhea or oligomenorrhea, infertility

Integument

Starvation-related complications

Lanugo

Nutritional Rehabilitation

A program of nutritional rehabilitation should be established for all patients with AN who are underweight. There are no consensus guidelines as to best practices for nutritional rehabilitation. We present here an outline of recommendations used by our practice.

The goal weight range for adolescents should be established using the patient's growth curve. For adolescents who have historically fallen between the 25th and 50th percentile BMI, the goal weight range is calculated by carrying out their weight trajectory. For those who have historically fallen below the 25th percentile, the 25th percentile should be used as a goal weight. For those who have historically fallen above the 50th percentile, the 50th percentile should be used as the target weight range. For adults, a BMI of 20.5 to 21 is generally sufficient to trigger menses in those with female biology and can be used to estimate goal weight range.[5] For patients who are not underweight at presentation, the initial goals should be weight maintenance and normalization of eating and weight-control behaviors. Attempts to lose weight should not be the focus of care, as restrictive eating is likely to exacerbate binging behavior.

Patients should be prescribed three regular meals a day with sufficient variety and inclusive of all nutrient groups. Whenever possible, restrictive specialty diets (vegan, vegetarian, gluten-free, lactose-free) should be discouraged in favor of broadening the food repertoire and focusing on balanced meals. In the case of gluten-free diets, a biopsy showing histological changes of celiac disease is recommended before initiating a restrictive gluten-free diet.

Behavioral monitoring is one of the most effective tools for helping patients change their behavior and for identifying maladaptive eating and weight-control patterns. Patients should be instructed to keep a food log of all meals and foods consumed to be reviewed during treatment sessions. The food log should include any bingeing or purging episodes or skipped meals. Because calorie-counting is often part of an individual's eating disorder, use of an exchange-based system is preferable in order to balance macronutrient intake and teach portioning (protein, carbohydrate, fat, dairy, vegetable, and fruit exchanges).

Intake usually begins at 30 to 40 kcal per kilogram of body weight per day (1,200–2,000 kcal/d), depending on medical status. Energy intake can be advanced by 500 kcal every 2 to 3 days. Target energy intake should be 3,500 to 4,000 kcal/d for patients who are underweight and require a weight gain diet, and 2,000 to 2,500 kcal/d for patients whose treatment goal is weight maintenance. Patients with extreme AN whose BMI is less than 14 or 60% of ideal body weight and patients with frequent purging behaviors should be assessed for medical stability for outpatient care. If laboratory values and vital signs are stable, outpatients with very low BMIs should start refeeding at 1,200 kcal/d on a lower-salt diet to minimize risks of refeeding syndrome, including edema and hypophosphatemia, and the diet should be advanced gradually over 10 to 14 days. For outpatients whose BMI is 14 to 21, energy intake should start at 1,500 kcal/d and can advance 500 kcal/d weekly until 3,500 kcal/d is reached. Energy intake above 2,500 kcal/d should be administered as high-energy liquid supplements. These can then be discontinued once the target weight is reached and can be presented as temporary "medicine" while focusing on standard portioning of food in meals. Some patients may require up to 4,000 kcal/d if they are unable to gain sufficient weight on 3,500 kcal/d. Once a patient reaches the appropriate goal weight range, energy intake is lowered gradually to maintain weight in a healthy range.

Exercise may be incorporated into the patient's daily routine cautiously in a gradual, stepwise fashion; this is contingent on continued weight gain in those who are underweight. In general, exercise recommendations should be made on an individual basis and be consistent with the needs of the patient, taking into account relevant aspects of the patient's illness, such as a history of excessive exercise.

For those that are unable to eat and are severely medically compromised as a result, short-term nasogastric tube feeding has been used to initiate weight restoration and nutritional rehabilitation. This modality should be employed only if medically necessary and for the shortest time possible, so as to facilitate the restoration of regular eating patterns.[37]

Recommended rates of weight gain for patients with AN have historically been 2 to 3 lb (0.9 to 1.4 kg) per week for inpatients and 0.5 to 1 lb (0.2 to 0.5 kg) per week for outpatients because of concerns about the risk of refeeding syndrome. More recent research has challenged this standard as too slow and suggests that target weight gain rates should be closer to 4 lb (1.8 kg) per week. The rationale is that this faster rate of gain is safe in closely monitored settings (inpatient) and that the risk of hypophosphatemia and refeeding syndrome appears more closely related to the patient's BMI at the time of admission than to the rate of weight gain itself.[38]

Complications of Refeeding

Although weight gain is the cornerstone of treatment for patients with AN, serious and potentially fatal complications can arise when refeeding is administered too rapidly or aggressively. Termed *refeeding syndrome*, this constellation of fluid and electrolyte imbalances can result in clinical complications that include peripheral and central edema, congestive heart failure, cardiac arrhythmias, pulmonary edema, and death. The hallmark feature of this syndrome is hypophosphatemia, though it can also include alterations in sodium and fluid balance; changes in glucose, protein, and fat metabolism; thiamin deficiency; hypokalemia; and hypomagnesemia.[39] During starvation, the body changes from using carbohydrates to using protein and fat stores for energy, the basal metabolic rate decreases to preserve muscle breakdown, and intracellular minerals are depleted (though serum levels often remain normal). During refeeding, the intake of glucose leads to increased insulin and decreased secretion of glucagon. Insulin stimulates glycogen, fat, and protein synthesis via cellular uptake of glucose, magnesium, phosphate, and water, with concurrent decreases in the plasma concentration of these elements, which are often already depleted from malnutrition. Thiamin is a cofactor for carbohydrate metabolism, and as refeeding progresses, the demand for thiamin increases; thus thiamin is typically supplemented, even when laboratory values are within normal range, in anticipation of increased demand. For these reasons, careful attention must be paid to the refeeding process, with prompt repletion of electrolyte imbalances, ideally under supervised inpatient conditions in the case of patients who are severely malnourished.

Medical and Psychiatric Interventions

Pharmacotherapy

Pharmacotherapy for AN has been largely disappointing, with few trials demonstrating efficacy and mostly for comorbid depressive and obsessive-compulsive disorders. The antipsychotic olanzapine has been shown to have modest effects on weight gain; however, studies of other agents have often been underpowered to detect differences.[40] Behavioral refeeding remains the treatment of choice for AN.[41] Pharmacotherapy for BN has been more successful than that for AN, and antidepressant drugs have been the most widely studied. A number of trials have shown a reduction in binge eating and vomiting in patients treated with fluoxetine at higher doses (60 mg).[42]

Pharmacotherapy for BED has been more encouraging than that for the other eating disorders; however, psychotherapy—including cognitive behavioral therapy (CBT) and interpersonal therapy approaches—remains more efficacious for BED. Several medications have been studied, including the selective serotonin reuptake inhibitors, antiepileptics (topiramate and zonisamide) and stimulants (lisdexamfetamine). In 2015, following an expedited review, lisdexamfetamine became the first medication approved by the US Food and Drug Administration for the treatment of BED. Though it has shown efficacy in reducing the number of binge eating episodes at dosages of 50 and 70 mg/d, early studies were limited by the exclusion of patients with comorbid psychiatric conditions, making generalizability difficult.[43] Furthermore long-term efficacy is limited, and there is risk of abuse and dependence with use of stimulant medications.

Behavioral Interventions

Behavioral interventions are among the most effective treatment modalities and are components of a wide variety of evidence-based treatment approaches, including CBT, dialectical behavioral therapy, and family-based treatment for eating disorders. These modalities may be provided by various members of the treatment team, including therapists, psychiatrists, internists or pediatricians, and RDNs, depending on their level of experience and expertise in treating eating disorders. Behavior change is inherent to each of these therapeutic modalities as a core and necessary component of treatment. Key behavioral techniques employed across treatment modalities include normalizing eating patterns, identifying triggers and coping strategies, enhancing cognitive flexibility, and managing negative emotions. Recently, interest has grown in the application of "exposure and response prevention" techniques to manage anxiety over food and body image and to counter avoidant and safety behaviors that may reinforce eating-disorder cognitions—including beliefs about weight gain and the value of body checking and body comparisons, enhancement of self-esteem, and reduction in beliefs around the value of perfectionism. Behavioral-skills training includes meal planning and parent behavioral training (of adolescent patients).[44]

Cognitive Behavioral Therapy
The most studied form of treatment to date for eating disorders has been CBT, which emphasizes the relationship of thoughts and feelings to behaviors and helps patients learn to recognize and manage the emotional and cognitive triggers associated with disordered eating.[45] The CBT model for the treatment of eating disorders emphasizes the important role played by cognitive and behavioral factors in contributing to and maintaining the eating disorder and its associated pathology. Cognitive factors include attitudes about weight and body shape and their control. Behavioral factors include dietary restriction, binge eating, and purging. CBT has been shown to be more efficacious than both inactive (wait list or treatment as usual) and active psychotherapeutic treatment modalities for both BN and BED. It has been shown to reduce behavioral and cognitive symptoms of the disorders, including binge and purge frequency, with improvements in core behavioral symptoms sustained at follow-up, suggesting an enduring effect of CBT beyond the end of treatment.[46] RDNs are uniquely poised to help patients with various food-related exposures, including food challenges, grocery shopping, and dining out, all of which may be part of this treatment modality.

Dialectical Behavior Therapy
Dialectical behavioral therapy can complement the core CBT-based treatment with sessions that focus on mindfulness, distress tolerance, emotional regulation, and interpersonal effectiveness. It was first designed to treat borderline personality disorder and can be especially useful when this comorbidity is present.

Dialectical behavior therapy appears promising in individuals with eating disorders, especially those in whom affective regulation and impulsivity have been especially problematic; it has also shown promise in AN, for emotional and behavioral overcontrol.[47]

Family-Based Treatment
Also known as the Maudsley method, family-based treatment is highly effective for children and adolescents with AN and has been shown to be superior to other forms of therapy in this age group. This type of therapy involves parental control and supervision of meals, with a gradual return of control to the child or adolescent as their weight stabilizes with associated exploration of normative developmental tasks.[48]

Monitoring and Follow-Up of Eating Disorders

Individuals with eating disorders can receive care in a variety of settings, including outpatient, inpatient, residential, or partial hospitalization programs, depending on their medical stability, severity and frequency of symptoms, psychiatric comorbidity, patient safety, psychosocial supports, and response to current and prior treatments.[9] A majority of individuals are cared for in the outpatient setting by a multidisciplinary treatment team that may include a gastroenterologist and an RDN.

Levels of Care

Inpatient care is for patients who are acutely medically or psychiatrically unstable or unable to make progress in the outpatient setting. Once stabilized, patients may benefit from a variety of step-down programs (eg, partial hospitalization or intensive outpatient evening programs) before returning to the care of their outpatient providers.

Inpatient care is generally indicated for patients whose weight is less than 85% of their ideal body weight (<75% in adolescents) and who have abnormal vital signs (bradycardia, hypotension, abnormal electrolytes) or abnormal electrocardiogram results (prolonged QTc). Other reasons for hospital admission include dehydration, syncope, seizures, and severe eating disorder symptomatology (eg, uncontrollable bingeing and purging or acute food refusal). Comorbid psychiatric conditions requiring psychiatric hospitalization may also influence the need for admission (eg, severe depression, suicidal ideation), or inpatient care may be indicated when outpatient treatment has failed (ie, poor weight gain, failure to decrease frequency of binge-purge episodes).[49,50]

Monitoring in the outpatient setting depends on the individual's specific symptoms and behaviors and should include regular weight checks and monitoring of orthostatic vital signs and electrolytes in individuals with binge-purge behaviors (see Box 12.9).

BOX 12.9

Suggested Outpatient Medical and Nutritional Interventions for Patients With Eating Disorders

Weighing

Underweight	Weekly at appointments
Normal or above-normal weight	Monthly

Energy prescription

Underweight	BMI of 14 through 20: start at 1,500 kcal/d
Normal or above-normal weight	2,000 kcal/d

Energy-intake advancement (of sufficient variety across all food groups)

Underweight	BMI of less than 14: increase to 1,500 kcal/d after 1 week
	BMI of 14 to 21: increase in increments of 500 kcal/d weekly until at 3,500 kcal/d; once 2,500 kcal/d is reached, calories above this amount should be from oral nutrition supplements or equivalent shakes.
Normal or above-normal weight	Maintenance at 2,000 kcal/d; may adjust depending on whether patient gains or loses weight

Box continues

BOX 12.9 (CONTINUED)

Laboratory tests (baseline)

Underweight	Complete blood count, comprehensive metabolic panel, calcium, magnesium, phosphate, thiamin, thyrotropin (thyroid-stimulating hormone), vitamin D, electrocardiogram
Normal or above-normal weight	Complete blood count, comprehensive metabolic panel, calcium, magnesium, phosphate, thiamin, thyrotropin (thyroid-stimulating hormone), human chorionic gonadotropin, vitamin D, electrocardiogram

Electrolyte supplementation

Underweight	Weekly if purging daily
Normal or above-normal weight	Weekly if purging daily

Summary

Eating disorders are a complex group of behavioral disorders. GI symptoms are common in this population, and patients often present to the gastroenterologist with a variety of somatic concerns arising from their disordered eating or weight-control behaviors. Gastroenterologists and RDNs are uniquely qualified to identify eating disorders at an early stage and to help direct patients to the appropriate care and treatment. The latter is especially important, as these are treatable conditions yet about 50% of affected individuals do not seek specialty care from an eating disorder treatment provider.

GI and nutritional complications of eating disorders can be a consequence of prolonged starvation, engagement in purging behaviors, or the refeeding process itself, which should take place under appropriate medical supervision and guidance.

Patients are treated for eating disorders in both inpatient and outpatient settings, and treatment typically involves a multidisciplinary team. Although weight stabilization and control of bingeing and purging are necessary, they are not sufficient for recovery. Often, the greatest barrier to treatment is the denial that accompanies these disorders. With a team approach, there is hope and evidence that full recovery is attainable.

References

1. Bern E, Woods ER, Rodriguez L. Gastrointestinal manifestations of eating disorders. *J Pediatr Gastroenterol Nutr.* 2016;63(5):e77-e85. doi:10.1097/MPG.0000000000001394
2. American Psychiatric Association. *Diagnostic and Statistical Manual of Mental Disorders: DSM-5.* 5th ed. American Psychiatric Association; 2013. doi:10.1176/appi.books.9780890425596
3. Deloitte Access Economics. *The Social and Economic Cost of Eating Disorders in the United States of America: A Report for the Strategic Training Initiative for the Prevention of Eating Disorders and the Academy for Eating Disorders.* June 2020. Accessed February 12, 2022. www.hsph.harvard.edu/striped/report-economic-costs-of-eating-disorders
4. Pearson CM, Miller J, Ackard DM, et al. Stability and change in patterns of eating disorder symptoms from adolescence to young adulthood. *Int J Eat Disord.* 2017;50(7):748-757. doi:10.1002/eat.22692
5. Norris ML, Spettigue W, Hammond NG, et al. Building evidence for the use of descriptive subtypes in youth with avoidant restrictive food intake disorder. *Int J Eat Disord.* 2018;51(2):170-173. doi:10.1002/eat.22814

6. Hebebrand J, Exner C, Hebebrand K, et al. Hyperactivity in patients with anorexia nervosa and in semistarved rats: evidence for a pivotal role of hypoleptinemia. *Physiol Behav.* 2003;79(1):25-37. doi:10.1016/s0031-9384(03)00102-1

7. Udo T, Grilo CM. Prevalence and correlates of DSM-5 eating disorders in nationally representative sample of United States adults. *Biol Psychiatry.* 2018;84(5):345-354. doi:10.1016/j.biopsych.2018.03.014

8. Murray HB, Bailey AP, Keshishian AC, et al. Prevalence and characteristics of avoidant/restrictive food intake disorder in adult neurogastroenterology patients. *Clin Gastroenterol Hepatol.* 2020;18(9):1995-2002.e1. doi:10.1016/j.cgh.2019.10.030

9. Lilenfeld LR, Kaye WH, Greeno CG, et al. A controlled family study of anorexia nervosa and bulimia nervosa: psychiatric disorders in first-degree relatives and effects of proband comorbidity. *Arch Gen Psychiatry.* 1998;55(7):603-610. doi:10.1001/archpsyc.55.7.603

10. Watson HJ, Yilmaz Z, Thornton LM, et al. Genome-wide association study identifies eight risk loci and implicates metabo-psychiatric origins for anorexia nervosa. *Nat Genet.* 2019;51(8):1207-1214. doi:10.1038/s41588-019-0439-2

11. Woodside DB, Bulik CM, Halmi KA, et al. Personality, perfectionism, and attitudes toward eating in parents of individuals with eating disorders. *Int J Eat Disord.* 2002;31(3):290-299. doi:10.1002/eat.10032

12. Steinglass JE, Walsh BT. Neurobiological model of the persistence of anorexia nervosa. *J Eat Disord.* 2016;4(1):19. doi:10.1186/s40337-016-0106-2

13. Ulfvebrand S, Birgegård A, Norring C, Högdahl L, von Hausswolff-Juhlin Y. Psychiatric comorbidity in women and men with eating disorders results from a large clinical database. *Psychiatry Res.* 2015;230(2):294-299. doi:10.1016/j.psychres.2015.09.008

14. Papadopoulos FC, Ekbom A, Brandt L, Ekselius L. Excess mortality, causes of death and prognostic factors in anorexia nervosa. *Br J Psychiatry.* 2009;194(1):10-17. doi:10.1192/bjp.bp.108.054742

15. Mascolo M, Geer B, Feuerstein J, Mehler PS. Gastrointestinal comorbidities which complicate the treatment of anorexia nervosa. *Eat Disord.* 2016;25(2):122-133. doi:10.1080/10640266.2016.1255108

16. Hudson JI, Hiripi E, Pope HG, Kessler RC. The prevalence and correlates of eating disorders in the National Comorbidity Survey Replication. *Biol Psychiatry.* 2007;61(3):348-358. doi:10.1016/j.biopsych.2006.03.040

17. Smink FRE, van Hoeken D, Hoek HW. Epidemiology of eating disorders: incidence, prevalence and mortality rates. *Curr Psychiatry Rep.* 2012;14(4):406-414. doi:10.1007/s11920-012-0282-y

18. Norris ML, Spettigue WJ, Katzman DK. Update on eating disorders: current perspectives on avoidant/restrictive food intake disorder in children and youth. *Neuropsychiatr Dis Treat.* 2016;12:213-218. doi:10.2147/NDT.S82538

19. Fichter MM, Quadflieg N. Mortality in eating disorders—results of a large prospective clinical longitudinal study. *Int J Eat Disord.* 2016;49(4):391-401. doi:10.1002/eat.22501

20. Chesney E, Goodwin GM, Fazel S. Risks of all-cause and suicide mortality in mental disorders: a meta-review. *World Psychiatry.* 2014;13(2):153-160. doi:10.1002/wps.20128

21. Hanachi M, Dicembre M, Rives-Lange C, et al. Micronutrients deficiencies in 374 severely malnourished anorexia nervosa inpatients. *Nutrients.* 2019;11(4):792. doi:10.3390/nu11040792

22. Hadigan CM, Anderson EJ, Miller KK, et al. Assessment of macronutrient and micronutrient intake in women with anorexia nervosa. *Int J Eat Disord.* 2000;28(3):284-292. doi:10.1002/1098-108X(200011)28:33.0.CO;2-G

23. Achamrah N, Coëffier M, Rimbert A, et al. Micronutrient status in 153 patients with anorexia nervosa. *Nutrients.* 2017;9(3):225. doi:10.3390/nu9030225

24. George JC, Zafar W, Bucaloiu ID, Chang AR. Risk factors and outcomes of rapid correction of severe hyponatremia. *Clin J Am Soc Nephrol.* 2018;13(7):984-992. doi:10.2215/cjn.13061117

25. Misra M. Long-term skeletal effects of eating disorders with onset in adolescence. *Ann N Y Acad Sci.* 2008;1135(1):212-218. doi:10.1196/annals.1429.002

26. Gosseaume C, Dicembre M, Bemer P, Melchior J, Hanachi M. Somatic complications and nutritional management of anorexia nervosa. *Clin Nutr Exp.* 2019;28:2-10. doi:10.1016/j.yclnex.2019.09.001

27. Setnick J. Micronutrient deficiencies and supplementation in anorexia and bulimia nervosa. *Nutr Clin Pract.* 2010;25(2):137-142. doi:10.1177/0884533610361478

28. Boyd C, Abraham S, Kellow J. Appearance and disappearance of functional gastrointestinal disorders in patients with eating disorders. *Neurogastroenterol Motil.* 2010;22(12):1279-1283. doi:10.1111/j.1365-2982.2010.01576.x

29. Benini L, Todesco T, Dalle Grave R, Deiorio F, Salandini L, Vantini I. Gastric emptying in patients with restricting and binge purging subtypes of anorexia nervosa. *Am J Gastroenterol.* 2004;99(8):1448-1454. doi:10.1111/j.1572-0241.2004.30246.x

30. Holmes SRM, Gudridge TA, Gaudiani JL, Mehler PS. Dysphagia in severe anorexia nervosa and potential therapeutic intervention: a case series. *Ann Otol Rhinol Laryngol.* 2012;121(7):449-456. doi:10.1177/000348941212100705

31. Bern EM, Woods ER, Rodriguez L. Gastrointestinal manifestations of eating disorders. *J Pediatr Gastroenterol Nutr.* 2016;63(5):e77-e85. doi:10.1097/MPG.0000000000001394

32. Watters A, Gibson D, Dee E, Mascolo M, Mehler PS. Superior mesenteric artery syndrome in severe anorexia nervosa: a case series. *Clin Case Rep.* 2019;8(1):185-189. doi:10.1002/ccr3.2577

33. Giuseppe C, Gabrio B, Antonella M, et al. Anorectal dysfunction in constipated women with anorexia nervosa. *Mayo Clin Proc.* 2000;75(10):1015-1019. doi:10.4065/75.10.1015

34. Santonicola A, Gagliardi M, Guarino MPL, Siniscalchi M, Ciacci C, Iovino P. Eating disorders and gastrointestinal diseases. *Nutrients.* 2019;11(12):3038. doi:10.3390/nu11123038

35. Mitchell N, Norris ML. Rectal prolapse associated with anorexia nervosa: a case report and review of the literature. *J Eat Disord.* 2013;1(1):39. doi:10.1186/2050-2974-1-39

36. LE Grange D. The Maudsley family-based treatment for adolescent anorexia nervosa. *World Psychiatry.* 2005;4(3):142-146.

37. Rizzo SM, Douglas JW, Lawrence JC. Enteral nutrition via nasogastric tube for refeeding patients with anorexia nervosa: a systematic review. *Nutr Clin Pract.* 2019;34(3):359-370. doi:10.1002/ncp.10187

38. Redgrave GW, Coughlin JW, Schreyer CC, et al. Refeeding and weight restoration outcomes in anorexia nervosa: challenging current guidelines. *Int J Eat Disord.* 2015;48(7):866-873. doi:10.1002/eat.22390

39. Mehanna HM, Moledina J, Travis J. Refeeding syndrome: what it is, and how to prevent and treat it. *BMJ.* 2008;336(7659):1495-1498. doi:10.1136/bmj.a301

40. Attia E, Steinglass JE, Walsh BT, et al. Olanzapine versus placebo in outpatient adults with anorexia nervosa: a randomized clinical trial. *Am J Psychiatry.* 2019;176(6):449-456. doi:10.1176/appi.ajp.2018.18101125

41. Yager J, Devlin MJ, Halmi KA, et al. Guideline watch: practice guideline for the treatment of patients with eating disorders, 2nd edition. *Focus.* 2005;3(4):546-551. doi:10.1176/foc.3.4.546

42. Fluoxetine Bulimia Nervosa Collaborative Study Group. Fluoxetine in the treatment of bulimia nervosa: a multicenter, placebo-controlled, double-blind trial. *Arch Gen Psychiatry.* 1992;49(2):139-147. doi:10.1001/archpsyc.1992.01820020059008

43. McElroy SL, Hudson JI, Mitchell JE, et al. Efficacy and safety of lisdexamfetamine for treatment of adults with moderate to severe binge-eating disorder: a randomized clinical trial. *JAMA Psychiatry.* 2015;72(3):235-246. doi:10.1001/jamapsychiatry.2014.2162

44. Waller G, Raykos B. Behavioral interventions in the treatment of eating disorders. *Psychiatr Clin North Am.* 2019;42(2):181-191. doi:10.1016/j.psc.2019.01.002

45. Whittal ML, Agras WS, Gould RA. Bulimia nervosa: a meta-analysis of psychosocial and pharmacological treatments. *Behav Ther.* 1999;30(1):117-135. doi:10.1016/S0005-7894(99)80049-5

46. Linardon J, Wade TD, de la Piedad Garcia X, Brennan L. The efficacy of cognitive-behavioral therapy for eating disorders: a systematic review and meta-analysis. *J Consult Clin Psychol.* 2017;85(11):1080-1094. doi:10.1037/ccp0000245

47. Chen EY, Segal K, Weissman J, et al. Adapting dialectical behavior therapy for outpatient adult anorexia nervosa—a pilot study. *Int J Eat Disord.* 2015;48(1):123-132. doi:10.1002/eat.22360

48. Lock J, Le Grange D, Agras WS, Moye A, Bryson SW, Jo B. Randomized clinical trial comparing family-based treatment to adolescent focused individual therapy for adolescents with anorexia nervosa. *Arch Gen Psychiatry.* 2010;67(10):1025-1032. doi:10.1001/archgenpsychiatry.2010.128

49. Yager J, Devlin MJ, Katherine A, et al. *Practice Guideline for the Treatment of Patients With Eating Disorders.* 3rd ed. American Psychiatric Association; 2010. Accessed February 15, 2022. www.psychiatryonline.org/pb/assets/raw/sitewide/practice_guidelines/guidelines/eatingdisorders.pdf

50. Society for Adolescent Health and Medicine, Golden NH, Katzman DK, et al. Position paper of the society for adolescent health and medicine: medical management of restrictive eating disorders in adolescents and young adults. *J Adolesc Health.* 2015;56(1):121-125. doi:10.1016/j.jadohealth.2014.10.259

Food Allergies and Food Intolerances

Maeson L. Zietowski
John Leung, MD
Jaclyn Quinlan, MPH, RD, LDN

KEY POINTS

- Food allergies and food intolerances are common phenomena, and a growing body of evidence suggests that the prevalence of these conditions is increasing. Food allergies represent an adverse, reproducible effect stemming from a humoral or cellular immune response upon exposure to a select food; if left unmanaged, they can become life-threatening.
- Food allergies and food intolerances encompass a diverse set of conditions and reactions. Given the potential for life-threating reactions associated with immunoglobulin E–mediated food allergies, it is important to distinguish them from other adverse food reactions.
- Patients with food allergies or food intolerances are often unable to manage their dietary needs alone and, therefore, require nutrition counseling to improve both their quality of life and overall health.

Introduction

Food allergies and food intolerances are common phenomena, and a growing body of evidence suggests that the prevalence of these conditions is increasing.[1] Food allergies represent an adverse, reproducible effect stemming from a humoral or cellular immune response (immune-mediated) upon exposure to a select food. These reactions can become life-threatening if left unmanaged. Food intolerances, on the other hand, are less severe in nature and are not rooted in immunological responses.[2] It is essential to understand the differences between food allergies and food intolerances because the management of these conditions and their associated risks hinges on proper differentiation. This chapter highlights the differences in prevalence, associated risk, and management of food allergies and food intolerances.

Prevalence of Food Allergies

An accurate prevalence for food allergies is difficult to ascertain, as food allergies vary greatly in their severity, triggers, and presentation.[1] However, evidence supports that true food allergies affect up to 5% of adults and 8% of children. Rates as high as 10% have been documented in infants.[3,4] These figures are supported by the reported increase in hospitalizations, ambulatory care visits, and outpatient visits for food allergies over the past 20 years in pediatric patients.[1] Notably, self-reported rates of food allergies are consistently higher, with data suggesting that about 19% of US adults believe they have a true food allergy and may be adding unnecessary constraints to their diets as a result.[5]

Overall, in the United States, the most commonly identified food allergies are to the proteins in eggs, milk, peanuts, tree nuts, wheat, fish, crustacean shellfish, and soy. Sesame allergy has been increasingly documented in North America, and as a result it was named the ninth major food allergen in 2021.[6,7] The most common food allergies differ in adult vs pediatric populations. Peanuts, tree nuts, and fin fish are the most common food allergies in adults.[5,8] In children, milk, eggs, and peanuts are the three most common triggers.[8] Studies have shown that 80% to 95% of children outgrow their milk allergy by age 5 years, and 80% of children outgrow egg allergies by age 16 years.[9] In comparison, a variety of studies have demonstrated that only a small percentage of children with a peanut allergy develop tolerance in adulthood, with data suggesting anywhere from 3% to 20% tolerance in adults after a previous peanut reaction.[10]

Clinical Presentation of Immunoglobulin E—Mediated Food Allergies

Immunoglobulin E (IgE)–mediated food allergies have a wide variety of clinical presentations that can involve multiple systems (skin, respiratory, cardiovascular, and gastrointestinal) and range from mild to severe, including anaphylaxis. It is important to understand the various manifestations of food allergies to ensure their proper diagnosis and subsequent treatment. The most common food-allergy reactions involve skin and mucosal tissue and include conditions such as urticaria and angioedema. These symptoms have been shown to occur in up to 92% of anaphylactic episodes.[10]

Chronic urticaria (lasting more than 6 weeks) is rarely caused by a food allergy. In cases of acute urticaria, symptoms typically appear within minutes to up to 2 hours following ingestion of the offending food and are commonly associated with angioedema. Acute urticaria caused by an IgE-mediated food allergy is reproducible with reexposure to the allergen.[11] It is important to recognize symptoms, as angioedema can also involve the upper airways and necessitate urgent medical attention.[10]

The relationship between atopic dermatitis and food allergy is not yet completely understood. Management of atopic dermatitis should begin with optimal skin care as a first-line therapy. Food allergy testing is indicated when immediate-type allergic reactions are a concern. An elimination diet is only prescribed when the patient has been formally diagnosed with a food allergy and the patient or patient's guardians have been educated by a physician and registered dietitian nutritionist (RDN).[12,13] Children with atopic dermatitis are at greater risk of food allergy, so removing foods that are tolerated may do more harm than good. Families should be informed of the limited benefits and possible harms of an elimination diet, such as loss of tolerance to previously tolerated foods, and increased risk of serious allergic reactions, including anaphylaxis.[13,14] Although a few studies have demonstrated that dietary restriction of trigger foods can improve atopic dermatitis symptoms, elimination diets for this condition are controversial because of the limited evidence and aforementioned health risks.[15-17]

The most serious reaction caused by a food allergy is anaphylaxis. Anaphylaxis occurs rapidly and can be fatal if left untreated. A suspected food allergy is the leading reason for emergency room visits in which the patient presents with anaphylaxis, constituting more than 50% of reported anaphylaxis cases in emergency rooms.[18] The major organ systems affected in an anaphylactic reaction include the skin and mucosal tissue, cardiovascular system, gastrointestinal (GI) system, and upper and lower respiratory systems. GI symptoms including vomiting, nausea, and abdominal pain occur in up to 45% of anaphylactic episodes and typically come about within minutes to a few hours after food ingestion.[10,19] Exceptions to this time frame (eg, as in alpha-gal syndrome) are discussed later in this section.

The majority of anaphylactic episodes are not fatal, even without emergency intervention, but proper treatment is crucial to avoid preventable consequences.[20] Most cases of fatality due to anaphylaxis are correlated with delayed administration of epinephrine. Epinephrine administration is the most effective way to halt anaphylaxis.[21,22]

The current criteria for identifying and defining an anaphylactic episode are shown in Box 13.1. These criteria were published in 2006 by the National Institute of Allergy and Infectious Diseases (NIAID) and the Food Allergy and Anaphylaxis Network (FAAN; now Food Allergy Research and Education or FARE) to aid in the diagnosis of anaphylaxis in emergency departments.[18] They should serve as a guideline for identifying cases of possible anaphylaxis in patients after they have experienced a suspected reaction. However, the final diagnosis and treatment must be left to a qualified physician. Patients with suspected food allergy reactions should be referred to an allergist for further evaluation.

BOX 13.1

Diagnostic Criteria for
Anaphylaxis[18]

Patient must meet one of the following criteria for anaphylaxis:

- Acute onset (minutes to hours) with symptoms involving the skin and/or mucosal tissue *and* the presence of respiratory symptoms and/or attenuated blood pressure and/or indications of end-organ dysfunction
- At least two of the following rapidly occurring symptoms after allergen exposure:
  - involvement of the skin or mucosal tissue
  - respiratory system involvement
  - gastrointestinal system involvement
  - lowered blood pressure
- Lowered blood pressure directly resulting from allergen exposure

The NIAID/FAAN guidelines were reevaluated in recent years after the World Allergy Organization (WAO) proposed slightly modified diagnostic criteria for anaphylaxis in 2019.[23] The 2019 proposal differed by adding categories for patients exposed to probable triggers who present with symptoms of respiratory compromise with bronchospasm or laryngeal involvement, as well as a category for patients with severe GI symptoms after exposure to nonfood allergens.[23] The 2006 NIAID/FAAN criteria were shown to have a 95% sensitivity with a 71% specificity; therefore, 9f5% of anaphylaxis cases meet the 2006 NIAID/FAAN criteria.[23,24] In 2021, the American Academy of Allergy, Asthma, and Immunology suggested that the 2019 WAO proposed criteria should also be useful in emergency departments, as the criteria are very similar to the 2006 version.[25] The 2006 criteria are presented in Box 13.1 for reference, as they are widely used and accepted as the standard.

There are some uncommon food-allergy reactions that fall outside of the normal scope and do not present with the typical symptoms. These include food-dependent exercise-induced anaphylaxis and alpha-gal syndrome. Food-dependent exercise-induced anaphylaxis is an anaphylactic reaction that occurs during or shortly after exercise if a food trigger is ingested in the 2 to 4 hours before exercise. The anaphylactic episode is caused by the combination of the ingestion of the food to which the person is sensitized and the exercise.[26] In alpha-gal syndrome, patients develop a sensitivity to the carbohydrate galactose-f-1,3-galactose, which is found in mammalian meat such as beef, lamb, and pork. This can occur after a lone star tick (*Amblyomma americanum*) bite that induces the production of IgE antibodies against galactose-α-1,3-galactose, which causes a delayed (3–7 hours) immunological response after meat ingestion.[27] This condition is distinct in that symptoms occur several hours after food ingestion, as opposed to the near-immediate reaction typical of IgE-mediated food allergies.[28]

Two other conditions that may mimic an IgE-mediated allergic reaction are scombroid poisoning and ciguatera poisoning. In scombroid poisoning, symptoms occur rapidly after eating scombroid fish (eg, tuna, bonito, mackerel) and include diarrhea, flushing, and rashes. These symptoms are caused by contaminated fish that have accumulated toxic levels of histamine during processing. Although the symptoms can be mistaken for anaphylaxis, this is not an IgE-mediated food allergy and is typically treated with an H_1 antihistamine.[29] The symptoms of ciguatera poisoning include vomiting, diarrhea, and abdominal pain. This condition is caused by the ingestion of fish contaminated with toxins such as ciguatoxin, saitotoxin, and scaritoxin. Symptoms can resolve on their own within 48 hours, or mannitol may be given.[30] By obtaining a detailed history of the incident, a physician should be able to differentiate a true IgE-mediated food allergy from these conditions.

Finally, it is important to distinguish between oral allergy syndrome (also called pollen-food allergy syndrome) and a systemic IgE-mediated food allergy. Oral allergy syndrome may be the most common food allergy in adult populations.[31] Symptoms occur after the ingestion of raw fruits and vegetables in patients with an existing tree pollen allergy (eg, birch, ragweed, grass). Proteins in some raw fruits and vegetables trigger cross-reactivity with the pollen allergy and cause localized symptoms, such as oral pruritus and swelling in the mouth, lips, and throat immediately after eating. Generally, patients with oral allergy syndrome do not experience symptoms when the trigger foods are cooked, as the majority of the responsible proteins are heat-labile and can, therefore, be tolerated when canned or cooked.[31] Symptoms remain localized to the oropharynx and resolve after a few minutes. It is very rare for a patient with oral allergy syndrome to experience a systemic reaction.[32]

Diagnosing Immunoglobulin E–Mediated Food Allergies

The patient history is the cornerstone of food allergy diagnosis. A detailed clinical history should include questions about the potential food trigger, the onset and duration of the reaction, previous encounters with the trigger, and associated symptoms at each encounter. Many patients may require a referral to an allergist, who may conduct additional testing, such as skin testing, in vitro assays, or, in some cases, an oral food challenge to confirm the diagnosis. Using both quantitative and qualitative methods, the specialist can then contextualize the results to determine the appropriate course of treatment.[10] Other tests that have not been validated for food allergy diagnosis are kinesiology, electrodermal testing, hair analysis, intradermal or sublingual provocation-neutralization tests, flow cytometry food tests, and mediator release testing.[33,34] Box 13.2 compares and contrasts the available types of food allergy testing.[35] Skin testing or skin prick testing (SPT) and IgE antibody testing are the most commonly used methods to support an IgE-mediated food allergy diagnosis. Skin tests and IgE antibody tests must be interpreted within the context of the patient's history, however, as there are benefits and limitations to these methods, and a positive test result does not necessarily indicate a pathological response to a food antigen.[36] Both SPT and IgE antibody testing have similar test performance, as evidenced by their high sensitivity (>90%) but modest specificity. This indicates that they are most suited for ruling out food allergies because there is a greater possibility of a false positive than a false negative.[37] Many patients may believe that a positive result is equivalent to a food allergy, but this is often not the case because of the high false-positive rate of these tests.[38]

As previously mentioned, a detailed clinical history that includes the food trigger, symptoms, frequency, onset, and duration of the reaction is the best diagnostic tool; tests

---

BOX 13.2

Available Food Allergy Testing[35]

Recommended

Oral food challenge

Oral challenge with escalating allergen dose until response seen

Pros	Double-blind study is gold standard
Cons	Expensive, inconvenient, potential for severe allergic reaction

Box continues

BOX 13.2 (CONTINUED)

Skin prick test

Allergen introduced subcutaneously; detects presence of allergen-specific immunoglobulin E (sIgE) bound to subcutaneous mast cells

Pros	High sensitivity, high negative predictive value
Cons	Low positive predictive value, low specificity

Allergen-specific IgE

Fluorescent enzyme labeled antibody assay measuring sIgE

Pros	Absolute sIgE levels may correlate directly with likelihood of clinical reaction
Cons	More expensive, results from different assays not necessarily comparable

Patch testing

Allergen-containing chambers lined on adhesive tape strips applied to intact skin and reaction checked 48 to 72 hours later

Pros	May be useful for evaluation for triggers for eosinophilic esophagitis (EoE), but not food allergy in EoE
Cons	Used primarily in research settings, variable sensitivity and specificity

Elimination diet

Elimination of six foods: eggs, soy, cow's milk, wheat, seafood, peanut or tree nuts

Pros	Can be therapeutic and diagnostic in EoE
Cons	Can lead to nutritional deficiency with long-term use

Not recommended

Intradermal tests

Intradermal injection of food allergen

Pros	Higher sensitivity than skin test for immunoglobulin E (IgE)–mediated food allergy
Cons	Not performed due to higher risk of systemic adverse effects (ie, anaphylaxis)

Total serum IgE

Detects IgE

Pros	Not applicable
Cons	Insufficient sensitivity and specificity

Unvalidated

Allergen-specific immunoglobulin G (IgG)

Detects IgG, which is marker of exposure (and also tolerance) to food

Pros	Not applicable
Cons	High false-positive rate, may not be elevated in patients with true IgE-mediated allergy

such as SPTs should be used in conjunction with the patient's history and the judgment of the clinician to determine if the patient is at high or low risk for a food allergy. If there is a low suspicion for food allergy, the physician can definitively rule out an IgE-mediated food allergy through a formal oral food challenge.

In clinical practice, oral food challenges can be done in a single-blind or open fashion and should be carried out in a monitored setting by an experienced, board-certified allergist, given the risk of a serious allergic reaction. Typically, a small dose of the suspected trigger food is consumed by the patient, followed by an increasingly larger dose every 15 to 30 minutes, until the patient either develops symptoms, thereby confirming a food allergy, or consumes the desired quantity of food (typically a meal-size portion), thereby ruling out the food allergy. Oral food challenges can cause anxiety for patients and their families. For this reason, and because of other psychosocial facets of these challenges, they should only be performed when the probability of a reaction is low and the test is needed to confirm a diagnosis or confirm tolerance to an existing allergy. After an oral food challenge rules out a food allergy, the reintroduction of previously avoided food items can substantially increase the quality of life for some patients.

Management of Immunoglobulin E–Mediated Food Allergies

Management of an IgE-mediated food allergy can be divided into initial and long-term management. In initial management, the first step is to identify anaphylaxis. If anaphylaxis is identified, the first-line treatment is an epinephrine autoinjector, with dosing determined by patient weight: 0.1 mg for infants less than 10 kg (22 lb); 0.15 mg for patients weighing between 10 kg and 25 kg (55 lb); or 0.3 mg for patients weighing 25 kg or more. If a 0.1 mg autoinjector is not accessible, the 0.15 mg autoinjector should be given to infants.[10,18] Intramuscular epinephrine should be administered immediately upon anaphylaxis identification, given that delayed administration has been associated with increased fatalities.[10,18] In the event that the patient is nonresponsive to the first dose of epinephrine, repeat injections may be given.

After epinephrine has been administered, antihistamines or glucocorticoids (or both) can be used as a second-line therapy for symptomatic relief.[10] Following the acute event, the patient should be discharged with a prescription for an epinephrine autoinjector and referred to an allergist for further management. An allergist will confirm or rule out a food allergy diagnosis and then educate the patient on how and when to properly self-administer an epinephrine autoinjector.

Once a diagnosis has been established, the allergy is managed over the long term through avoidance, education, and emergency epinephrine prescriptions.[39] The patient should work with an allergist to determine an appropriate emergency action plan and should carry the prescribed medications.[40]

For long-term management, patients should be referred to an RDN who can provide strategies for preventing food allergy reactions and ensure that patients meet their weight and nutrition goals. Preventive strategies can include, but are not limited to, accurate label reading, ingredient substitutions, and avoiding cross-contamination in food preparation. Patients may find it difficult to navigate this aspect of management without counsel. It should be noted that under the Food Allergen Labeling Consumer Protection Act of 2004, food manufacturers are required to list on their Nutrition Facts labels any ingredients that contain protein from a major food allergen. Until 2021, the eight major allergens were milk, eggs, fish, crustacean shellfish, tree nuts, peanuts, wheat, and soybeans. The definition of a major food allergen was expanded to include sesame as a ninth major allergen when the Food Allergy Safety, Treatment, Education, and Research Act of 2021 was signed into law. However, changes in labeling for sesame-containing products are not required to be initiated until January 1, 2023.[6] Care must be taken, therefore, to ensure that patients with sesame allergies are able to identify sesame-containing foods, as "sesame" may not be fully disclosed as an ingredient on the product label. For example, some foods may not list "sesame" as an ingredient but instead list "sesamol," "sim sim," "benne," or some other term.[41] These words all mean sesame or sesame seed, but they may not be known to patients. Additionally, patients with allergies outside of the major food allergens require further counseling on how to avoid triggers in their daily lives because Nutrition Facts labels are not required to list ingredients by their simplest name.[42]

A dietary consultation is especially important for infants and children at certain developmental stages given that infants and children with food allergies have been shown to have insufficient nutrient levels.[43] Many of the major allergens contain important macronutrient and micronutrient components that are essential for adequate growth and development, and the traditional substitutes may fall short. If, for example, an infant is allergic to cow's milk, the RDN must work closely with the supervising physician to ensure that the infant's nutritional needs are met.[43] As children get older, RDNs can continue to assist in finding suitable replacements for allergens so that their patients can still enjoy foods that they would like to eat while meeting their nutritional needs. In addition, RDNs should encourage their patients, or their patients' caregivers, to carry the necessary prescribed medications with them at all times in case of accidental allergen ingestion.

In recent years, oral immunotherapy (OIT) has also been proposed as a treatment option for food allergies.[44] OIT induces tolerance to a food trigger by introducing escalated doses of the trigger food over time until the patient reaches a desired maintenance dose, which is then ingested daily. The goal is to protect the patient from severe allergic reaction on accidental exposure. This process should be individualized according to the patient's allergy severity and timeline. Given that this is an individualized process and relatively new, there is great variability among both the volume of maintenance doses and the duration of regular maintenance dose ingestion.[45] In early 2020, the US Food and Drug Administration approved a peanut allergen OIT powder (brand name Palforzia) to be used by Risk Evaluation and Mitigation Strategy–certified clinicians in health care settings to treat children aged 4 years and older who are allergic to peanuts.[46]

Despite its efficacy, there is concern about the safety of OIT. Data show an increased risk of reactions during OIT, and evidence suggests that patients undergoing OIT are more likely to develop anaphylactic reactions during this treatment.[47] In the short term, the patient may be at higher risk for reactions; however, in the long term, OIT has been shown to increase patient quality of life, as it provides security against accidental exposure.[48,49] The decision tree for suspected food allergies and possible treatment options is shown in Figure 13.1.

FIGURE 13.1 Decision tree for food allergy treatment

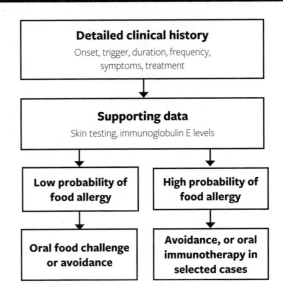

Non–Immunoglobulin E-Mediated Disorders

Food Protein–Induced Enterocolitis Syndrome

A variety of adverse reactions to food are not IgE-mediated. One of these is food protein–induced enterocolitis syndrome (FPIES). The specific mechanisms underlying FPIES are largely unknown; however, the leading theory proposes that alterations in food-specific T cells generate a systemic response.[50] FPIES is typically diagnosed in early infancy, and patients present with repeated projectile vomiting that is often associated with diarrhea. Patients can also exhibit dehydration, lethargy, intermittent vomiting, weight loss, and failure to thrive.[38] In the United States, the most common trigger foods are cow's milk and soy, but there is evidence that certain solid foods including poultry, rice, cereal, and oats (among others) may also cause a reaction in patients with FPIES.[51,52] In FPIES that is triggered by solid foods, symptoms usually start at around 4 to 7 months of age, when the solid foods are first introduced.[53,54]

FPIES can be classified into acute and chronic phases. The differences between the two phases, as well as the similarity to other GI disorders such as inflammatory bowel disease, make FPIES difficult to diagnosis. Acute FPIES occurs when a triggering food is ingested infrequently, introduced for the first time, or removed and then reintroduced. In this phase, symptoms such as repeated vomiting and diarrhea begin more immediately, usually 1 to 3 hours after ingestion and last up to several hours before subsiding. Other symptoms can include shock, pallor, hypertonia, and hypothermia, making some cases of acute FPIES severe.[55] In contrast, in chronic FPIES, the triggering food is regularly ingested and the infant presents with more intermittent, but chronic symptoms (diarrhea, weight loss, vomiting). Over time, the infant can develop hypoproteinemia, hypoalbuminemia, and poor weight gain. Typically, chronic FPIES is caused by the regular feeding of cow's milk or a soy-based formula, but symptoms can also be triggered by solid foods, depending on the frequency of ingestion.[56]

Diagnosis is made primarily by thorough examination of the patient's clinical history and improvement with elimination of the trigger food. It is also possible to proceed with an oral food challenge if the diagnosis or trigger foods are not clear, but there is evidence that about 15% to 20% of FPIES reactions result in shock, so appropriate caution must be taken and resources must be available during oral food challenges.[51] The decision to proceed with an oral challenge must be left to an experienced allergist in a monitored setting, as reactions can be severe. An FPIES diagnosis can generally be made by history alone.

After diagnosis, the suspected allergen should be eliminated from the diet, and an emergency treatment plan should be discussed with the physician. For infants with soy or cow's milk triggers, experts recommended switching the infant to a casein hydrolysate–based formula. It is also possible, but less likely, that the infant will require an amino acid–based formula. If the infant is breastfed, the breastfeeding mother should be instructed to avoid any consumption of soy and cow's milk. After eliminating these triggers, infants generally show improvement within 3 to 10 days.[52] The majority of infants outgrow this sensitivity, but a subsequent, supervised oral food challenge is needed to determine if the trigger food can safely be reintroduced.[57] Given that FPIES reactions can be very severe, it may be necessary to place an intravenous access prior to the oral food challenge. This decision and the timeline for reintroduction should be left to the discretion of the supervising physician.

When introducing new foods to an infant with FPIES, the family should not delay introducing solid foods beyond 6 months of age. Evidence shows that if the child can tolerate a food in one food group, there is greater likelihood of tolerance to other foods in same group. The order and timing of introducing food groups should be adjusted at the physician's discretion and under supervision, depending on the severity of the previous FPIES reaction. The current recommendations for food introduction in patients with FPIES are based on a single medical center's published experience, so it is important that the patient consult a physician with expertise in FPIES for an appropriate and personalized treatment plan. Also, infants with a cow's milk or soy FPIES trigger are more likely to react to a solid food as well, with the most common solid food trigger being rice or oats. In general, food introduction should begin with low-risk vegetables (eg, broccoli, cauliflower, and turnips) followed by low-risk fruits (eg, watermelon, peaches, and plums) before moving on to meats, grains, and nuts. Examples of higher-risk foods include green peas, bananas, oat cereals, rice, eggs, and fish.[52]

As in the traditional management of food allergies, after eliminating an FPIES trigger, the family should seek counsel from an RDN to determine how to meet the infant's nutritional needs. The RDN should monitor the patient's weight and height regularly during this process, and special care should be taken to expose the patient to a variety of textures and flavors via food preparation, even if the diet is restrictive in order to prevent unwanted feeding behaviors.[52]

Food Protein–Induced Allergic Proctocolitis

Food protein–induced allergic proctocolitis (FPIAP) is generally self-limiting and benign. The major symptom is noticeable blood in the stool of an otherwise healthy baby. This condition manifests in the first few months of infancy (up to 6 months) and occurs mostly in those who are breastfed, with up to 60% of cases occurring in breastfed infants.[58] It can be triggered by the mother's ingestion of cow's milk or soy or by the infant's ingestion of milk or soy proteins in formula. Corn and egg triggers have also been documented, although they are much less common.[58] FPIAP bleeding presents as soft, mucoid stool with blood mixed throughout.[58,59] In order to diagnosis FPIAP, other causes of rectal bleeding, such as fissures and infection, must be ruled out. Also, the infant will typically respond to dietary restrictions and show marked or complete resolution of symptoms within 72 hours. Generally, a casein hydrolysate formula is used until symptoms resolve, and then the allergen must be removed from the mother's diet or the infant's formula. In general, the food is eliminated for at least 6 months before attempted reintroduction. Research suggests that negative skin test results for the allergen or allergens may also help to guide the timeline of reintroduction. The specific timing of allergen reintroduction should be informed by an experienced and qualified allergist. The majority of children with FPIAP regain tolerance to their allergen by 3 years of age.[58,60]

Eosinophilic Gastrointestinal Disorders

Eosinophilic GI disorders include multiple inflammatory diseases defined by an increased eosinophilic infiltration of the GI tract and are diagnosed via endoscopic biopsies of mucosal tissue. The disorders are then classified based on the site of infiltration, such as the esophagus, stomach, small bowel, or colon.[61]

Of all the disorders, eosinophilic esophagitis (EoE) is the most studied. EoE is diagnosed when a patient presents with symptoms of esophageal dysfunction and esophageal biopsies show 15 or more eosinophils per high-power field, with no other cause for the esophageal symptoms or eosinophilia in the esophagus.[62] Symptoms range in scope and severity and can present differently in pediatric vs adult populations. The symptoms in children are commonly vomiting, abdominal pain, heartburn, and failure to thrive; the symptoms in adults are typically dysphagia, heartburn, and impaction.[62,63] In the adult EoE population, dysphagia is the most common symptom reported in more than 60% of patients.[62-64]

Studies have also found links between atopic conditions and EoE.[64,65] Experts estimate that 26% to 86% of adults with EoE and 42% to 93% of children with EoE have atopic conditions (allergic rhinitis, food allergy, asthma, dermatitis).[66] There is also some evidence to support a mild increase in risk of EoE if a family history of EoE is identified.[67,68] EoE prevalence and incidence have been increasing over the past few decades, with estimates putting the prevalence between 0.03% and 0.05%.[68,69]

Following a diagnosis of EoE, the options for first-line therapy include a food elimination diet, swallowed topical corticosteroids, or proton pump inhibitors. Patients who want to avoid the potential side effects of topical steroids or proton pump inhibitors may be more likely to choose an elimination diet. The three commonly used elimination diets for EoE treatment are an empirical elimination diet, an allergy testing–guided elimination diet, and an elemental (amino acid–based) elimination diet.

Although an elemental diet has the highest efficacy, approaching about 90% efficacy in multiple studies, difficulties with long-term compliance and higher costs make it a less desirable choice.[70-72] Following this dietary approach, patients can only ingest amino acid–based formula, which is not palatable, making this diet especially difficult for children, adolescents, and adults.[71] Allergy testing–guided elimination diets gained popularity in the last decade but have largely been replaced by empirical elimination diets. There are limited data comparing the efficacy of empirical and allergy testing–guided diets, but experts in the field are moving away from those guided by allergy testing because their efficacy is generally lower and associated costs are higher.[73] With empirical elimination diets, the patient eliminates the most common trigger foods for EoE, ranging from one to six different foods; however, there is no consensus on how many foods should be eliminated in the first step. It depends on the patient's dietary preferences, medical expertise of health professionals providing care, and underlying dietary restrictions dictated by other medical conditions. The most common trigger for EoE in adults and children is cow's milk; about 66% of patients are triggered by this allergen. Wheat, eggs, soy, fish, shellfish, peanuts, and tree nuts are other common triggers.[74]

After histological and symptomatic remission is achieved with a multiple-food elimination diet, specific trigger food groups are then identified by serial reintroduction of each food group, followed by histological and symptom assessment to confirm the absence of eosinophilic infiltration. On the other hand, if a patient starts with a single-food elimination diet and does not achieve remission, one can choose to expand the elimination diet to include other common food triggers. Symptoms do not necessarily correlate with disease severity, so histological evaluation with esophageal biopsies is usually required every 4 to 6 weeks following food reintroduction.[72] Overall, empirical food elimination diets have been shown to have an efficacy of about 55% to 85%.[75-78]

It is critical that patients meet with an RDN for nutrition counseling during this time because they may be unable to comply with the constraints of an elimination diet without counseling, especially if they regularly eat one of the eliminated foods. RDNs should also consider factors including patient preferences, dietary goals, and other restrictions (eg, current IgE-mediated food allergies). It is helpful to provide palatable replacement options for eliminated foods. For example, if a patient must eliminate all milk products, oat milk may be a good substitute for cow's milk. RDNs should also educate patients about "hidden" sources of trigger foods (eg, sauces) and food preparation technique. The overall goal is to create a maintainable and tolerable diet for the patient that adheres to the restrictions of the food elimination diet.

Food Intolerances

A food intolerance is an adverse reaction to a food trigger, but it is nonimmunologic in nature.[2] Food intolerances include conditions such as carbohydrate intolerance, reactions to monosodium glutamate and other chemicals, and reflux. The focus here will be on carbohydrate intolerance (particularly FODMAP intolerance), as it is one of the most common adverse food reactions encountered in clinical practice.

The prevalence of food intolerances is estimated to be as high as 20%, which is much higher than the prevalence of IgE-mediated food allergies.[2,3] One of the most common food intolerances is an adverse effect from consumption of the type of carbohydrates known as FODMAPs (fermentable oligosaccharides, disaccharides, monosaccharides, and polyols). There are five main FODMAPs: fructose, lactose, polyols, fructan, and galacto-oligosaccharides.[2] Symptoms of FODMAP intolerance vary and may present as bloating, abdominal discomfort, bowel movement irregularity, and flatulence. Most patients with irritable bowel syndrome may actually be suffering from food intolerance, as evidenced by substantial symptom relief in patients with this syndrome after following a low-FODMAP diet.[79] The cause of these symptoms stems from an osmotic effect in the small intestine from FODMAPs that are not absorbed.[80] This is paired with increased gas production from bacteria in the colon as the carbohydrate is fermented.[80,81] See Chapter 5 for additional discussion of the low-FODMAP diet for treatment of irritable bowel syndrome.

The first-line therapy for suspected FODMAP intolerance includes a low-FODMAP diet, which has been proven to reduce symptoms by anywhere from 50% to 80%.[2,82,83] While following this diet, patients should consult an RDN to ensure that they are receiving proper nutrition and are complying with the diet, especially given that the low-FODMAP diet is very restrictive.[83] FODMAP sugars (eg, fructose, lactose, and fructan) are reintroduced one by one to identify which sugar or sugars are causing the symptoms. Once the offending substance is identified, the patient should be instructed to avoid excess consumption of that substance for long-term management of the intolerance.[84] Also, it is advisable for the patient to work with an RDN to establish a sustainable, long-term diet that avoids the trigger food and is based on patient preference and nutritional needs. This process can be supported and guided with hydrogen breath testing. Physicians can identify specific FODMAP intolerances with serial hydrogen breath tests using a variety of substrates, such as lactose, glucose, fructose, sucrose, and sorbitol.[85]

To ensure the accuracy of hydrogen breath testing, small intestinal bacterial overgrowth must first be ruled out using a glucose substrate.[85] The current consensus for breath testing details the appropriate preparation, indications, dosing, and interpretation of test results for use in diagnosing carbohydrate intolerance; however, large knowledge gaps remain with regard to optimal timing, pediatric dosing, and differences in baseline hydrogen level.[85]

Summary

Food allergies and food intolerances encompass an extraordinarily diverse set of conditions and reactions. Given the potential for life-threating reactions associated with IgE-mediated food allergies, it is important to distinguish IgE-mediated food allergies from other adverse food reactions. Collaboration between a physician specializing in allergies or gastroenterology and an RDN is essential for the accurate and safe treatment of patients with these diet-related conditions. Patients with food allergies or food intolerances are often unable to manage their dietary needs alone and require nutrition counseling to improve both their quality of life and overall health. Patients with food-related disorders carry the lifelong burden of managing their dietary restrictions; therefore, the role of the RDN is not only to provide patient education and critical skills, such how to read Nutrition Facts labels, but also to work within the lifestyle and preferences of the patient to find agreeable and sustainable dietary substitutions. The scientific field of food allergy and intolerance is constantly evolving, as new information is brought to light. Given their position as health care providers, RDNs must be in constant pursuit of new knowledge as they seek to better serve their patients.

References

1. Sicherer SH, Sampson HA. Food allergy: a review and update on epidemiology, pathogenesis, diagnosis, prevention, and management. *J Allergy Clin Immunol.* 2018;141(1):41-58. doi:10.1016/j.jaci.2017.11.003

2. Tuck CJ, Biesiekierski JR, Schmid-Grendelmeier P, Pohl D. Food Intolerances. *Nutrients.* 2019;11(7). doi:10.3390/nu11071684

3. Lomer MCE. Review article: the aetiology, diagnosis, mechanisms and clinical evidence for food intolerance. *Aliment Pharmacol Ther.* 2015;41(3):262-275. doi:10.1111/apt.13041

4. Osborne NJ, Koplin JJ, Martin PE, et al. Prevalence of challenge-proven IgE-mediated food allergy using population-based sampling and predetermined challenge criteria in infants. *J Allergy Clin Immunol.* 2011;127(3):668-676.e2. doi:10.1016/j.jaci.2011.01.039

5. Gupta RS, Warren CM, Smith BM, et al. Prevalence and severity of food allergies among US adults. *JAMA Netw Open.* 2019;2(1):e185630. doi:10.1001/jamanetworkopen.2018.5630

6. FASTER Act of 2021, S 578, 117th Cong (2021). Accessed May 25, 2021. www.congress.gov/bill/117th-congress/senate-bill/578

7. Protudjer JLP, Abrams EM. Sesame: the new priority allergen? *JAMA Netw Open.* 2019;2(8):e199149. doi:10.1001/jamanetworkopen.2019.9149

8. Sampson HA. Update on food allergy. *J Allergy Clin Immunol.* 2004;113(5):805-819. doi:10.1016/j.jaci.2004.03.014

9. Radlović N, Leković Z, Radlović V, Simić D, Ristić D, Vuletić B. Food allergy in children. *Srp Arh Celok Lek.* 2016;144(1-2):99-103. doi:10.2298/sarh1602099r

10. Anvari S, Miller J, Yeh C-Y, Davis CM. IgE-mediated food allergy. *Clin Rev Allergy Immunol.* 2019;57(2):244-260. doi:10.1007/s12016-018-8710-3

11. Abrams EM, Sicherer SH. Diagnosis and management of food allergy. *CMAJ Can Med Assoc J.* 2016;188(15):1087-1093. doi:10.1503/cmaj.160124

12. Lim NR, Lohman ME, Lio PA. The role of elimination diets in atopic dermatitis—a comprehensive review. *Pediatr Dermatol.* 2017;34(5):516-527. doi:10.1111/pde.13244

13. Eigenmann PA, Beyer K, Lack G, et al. Are avoidance diets still warranted in children with atopic dermatitis? *Pediatr Allergy Immunol.* 2020;31(1):19-26. doi:10.1111/pai.13104

14. Chang A, Robison R, Cai M, Singh AM. Natural history of food-triggered atopic dermatitis and development of immediate reactions in children. *J Allergy Clin Immunol Pract.* 2016;4(2):229-236.e1. doi:10.1016/j.jaip.2015.08.006

15. Juto P, Engberg S, Winberg J. Treatment of infantile atopic dermatitis with a strict elimination diet. *Clin Allergy.* 1978;8(5):493-500. doi:10.1111/j.1365-2222.1978.tb01502.x

16. Kjaer HF, Eller E, Høst A, Andersen KE, Bindslev-Jensen C. The prevalence of allergic diseases in an unselected group of 6-year-old children: the DARC birth cohort study. *Pediatr Allergy Immunol.* 2008;19(8):737-745. doi:10.1111/j.1399-3038.2008.00733.x

17. Bath-Hextall F, Delamere FM, Williams HC. Dietary exclusions for established atopic eczema. *Cochrane Database Syst Rev.* 2008;(1):CD005203. doi:10.1002/14651858.CD005203.pub2

18. Shaker MS, Wallace DV, Golden DBK, et al. Anaphylaxis—a 2020 practice parameter update, systematic review, and Grading of Recommendations, Assessment, Development and Evaluation (GRADE) analysis. *J Allergy Clin Immunol.* 2020;145(4):1082-1123. doi:10.1016/j.jaci.2020.01.017

19. Grabenhenrich LB, Dölle S, Moneret-Vautrin A, et al. Anaphylaxis in children and adolescents: the European Anaphylaxis Registry. *J Allergy Clin Immunol.* 2016;137(4):1128-1137.e1. doi:10.1016/j.jaci.2015.11.015

20. Turner PJ, Jerschow E, Umasunthar T, Lin R, Campbell DE, Boyle RJ. Fatal anaphylaxis: mortality rate and risk factors. *J Allergy Clin Immunol Pract.* 2017;5(5):1169-1178. doi:10.1016/j.jaip.2017.06.031

21. Grabenhenrich LB, Dölle S, Ruëff F, et al. Epinephrine in severe allergic reactions: the European Anaphylaxis Register. *J Allergy Clin Immunol Pract.* 2018;6(6):1898-1906.e1. doi:10.1016/j.jaip.2018.02.026

22. Prince BT, Mikhail I, Stukus DR. Underuse of epinephrine for the treatment of anaphylaxis: missed opportunities. *J Asthma Allergy.* 2018;11:143-151. doi:10.2147/JAA.S159400

23. Turner PJ, Worm M, Ansotegui IJ, et al. Time to revisit the definition and clinical criteria for anaphylaxis? *World Allergy Organ J.* 2019;12(10):100066. doi:10.1016/j.waojou.2019.100066

24. Loprinzi Brauer CE, Motosue MS, Li JT, et al. Prospective validation of the NIAID/FAAN criteria for emergency department diagnosis of anaphylaxis. *J Allergy Clin Immunol Pract.* 2016;4(6):1220-1226. doi:10.1016/j.jaip.2016.06.003

25. Ade J, Jeffery M, Hagan J, et al. Validation of the revised National Institute of Allergy and Infectious Disease[s]/Food Allergy and Anaphylaxis Network diagnostic criteria in emergency department patients. *J Allergy Clin Immunol.* 2021;147(2):AB240. doi:10.1016/j.jaci.2020.12.021

26. Giannetti MP. Exercise-induced anaphylaxis: literature review and recent updates. *Curr Allergy Asthma Rep.* 2018;18(12):72. doi:10.1007/s11882-018-0830-6

27. Commins SP, James HR, Stevens W, et al. Delayed clinical and ex vivo response to mammalian meat in patients with IgE to galactose-alpha-1,3-galactose. *J Allergy Clin Immunol.* 2014;134(1):108-115.e11. doi:10.1016/j.jaci.2014.01.024

28. Crispell G, Commins SP, Archer-Hartman SA, et al. Discovery of alpha-gal-containing antigens in North American tick species believed to induce red meat allergy. *Front Immunol.* 2019;10:1056. doi:10.3389/fimmu.2019.01056

29. Ridolo E, Martignago I, Senna G, Ricci G. Scombroid syndrome: it seems to be fish allergy but … it isn't. *Curr Opin Allergy Clin Immunol.* 2016;16(5):516-521. doi:10.1097/ACI.0000000000000297

30. Friedman MA, Fernandez M, Backer LC, et al. An updated review of ciguatera fish poisoning: clinical, epidemiological, environmental, and public health management. *Mar Drugs.* 2017;15(3). doi:10.3390/md15030072

31. Kashyap RR, Kashyap RS. Oral allergy syndrome: an update for stomatologists. *J Allergy (Cairo).* 2015;2015:543928. doi:10.1155/2015/543928

32. Muluk NB, Cingi C. Oral allergy syndrome. *Am J Rhinol Allergy.* 2018;32(1):27-30. doi:10.2500/ajra.2018.32.4489

33. Mullin GE, Swift KM, Lipski L, Turnbull LK, Rampertab SD. Testing for food reactions: the good, the bad, and the ugly. *Nutr Clin Pract.* 2010;25(2):192-198. doi:10.1177/0884533610362696

34. Kelso JM. Unproven diagnostic tests for adverse reactions to foods. *J Allergy Clin Immunol Pract.* 2018;6(2):362-365. doi:10.1016/j.jaip.2017.08.021

35. Onyimba F, Crowe SE, Johnson S, Leung J. Food allergies and intolerances: a clinical approach to the diagnosis and management of adverse reactions to food. *Clin Gastroenterol Hepatol.* 2021;19(11):2230-2240.e1. doi:10.1016/j.cgh.2021.01.025

36. Gocki J, Bartuzi Z. Role of immunoglobulin G antibodies in diagnosis of food allergy. *Postepy Dermatol Alergol.* 2016;33(4):253-256. doi:10.5114/ada.2016.61600

37. Chafen JJS, Newberry SJ, Riedl MA, et al. Diagnosing and managing common food allergies: a systematic review. *JAMA.* 2010;303(18):1848-1856. doi:10.1001/jama.2010.582

38. Food allergy: a practice parameter update—2014. *J Allergy Clin Immunol.* 2014;134(5):1016-1025.e43. doi:10.1016/j.jaci.2014.05.013

39. Leung J, Dadlani A, Crowe S. Food allergies, food intolerances, and carbohydrate malabsorption. In: Lacy B, DiBaise J, Pimentel M, Ford A, eds. *Essential Medical Disorders of the Stomach and Small Intestine.* Springer, Cham; 2019:437-457. doi:10.1007/978-3-030-01117-8_21

40. Food Allergy and Anaphylaxis Emergency Care Plan. Food Allergy Research and Education. Accessed April 9, 2021. www.foodallergy.org/living-food-allergies/food-allergy-essentials/food-allergy-anaphylaxis-emergency-care-plan

41. Sesame allergy. Food Allergy Research and Education. Accessed April 12, 2021. www.foodallergy.org/living-food-allergies/food-allergy-essentials/common-allergens/sesame

42. Food Allergen Labeling and Consumer Protection Act of 2004 questions and answers. *FDA.* December 12, 2005. Updated July 18, 2006. Accessed January 31, 2021. www.fda.gov/food/food-allergensgluten-free-guidance-documents-regulatory-information/food-allergen-labeling-and-consumer-protection-act-2004-questions-and-answers

43. Hobbs CB, Skinner AC, Burks AW, Vickery BP. Food allergies affect growth in children. *J Allergy Clin Immunol Pract.* 2015;3(1):133-134.e1. doi:10.1016/j.jaip.2014.11.004

44. Brotons-Canto A, Martín-Arbella N, Gamazo C, Irache JM. New pharmaceutical approaches for the treatment of food allergies. *Expert Opin Drug Deliv.* 2018;15(7):675-686. doi:10.1080/17425247.2016.1247805

45. Keet CA, Seopaul S, Knorr S, Narisety S, Skripak J, Wood RA. Long-term follow-up of oral immunotherapy for cow's milk allergy. *J Allergy Clin Immunol.* 2013;132(3):737-739.e6. doi:10.1016/j.jaci.2013.05.006

46. Hise K, Rabin RL. Oral immunotherapy for food allergy—a US regulatory perspective. *Curr Allergy Asthma Rep.* 2020;20(12):77. doi:10.1007/s11882-020-00973-x

47. Abbasi J. Weighing the risks and rewards of peanut oral immunotherapy. *JAMA.* 2019;322(7):596-598. doi:10.1001/jama.2019.9142

48. Mori F, Barni S, Liccioli G, Novembre E. Oral immunotherapy (OIT): a personalized medicine. *Medicina (Kaunas).* 2019;55(10):684. doi:10.3390/medicina55100684

49. Sánchez-García S, Cipriani F, Ricci G. Food allergy in childhood: phenotypes, prevention and treatment. *Pediatr Allergy Immunol.* 2015;26(8):711-720. doi:10.1111/pai.12514

50. Goswami R, Blazquez AB, Kosoy R, Rahman A, Nowak-Węgrzyn A, Berin MC. Systemic innate immune activation in food protein-induced enterocolitis syndrome. *J Allergy Clin Immunol*. 2017;139(6):1885-1896.e9. doi:10.1016/j.jaci.2016.12.971

51. Cherian S, Varshney P. Food protein-induced enterocolitis syndrome (FPIES): review of recent guidelines. *Curr Allergy Asthma Rep*. 2018;18(4):28. doi:10.1007/s11882-018-0767-9

52. Nowak-Węgrzyn A, Chehade M, Groetch ME, et al. International consensus guidelines for the diagnosis and management of food protein-induced enterocolitis syndrome: executive summary—workgroup report of the Adverse Reactions to Foods Committee, American Academy of Allergy, Asthma, and Immunology. *J Allergy Clin Immunol*. 2017;139(4):1111-1126.e4. doi:10.1016/j.jaci.2016.12.966

53. Mehr S, Kakakios A, Frith K, Kemp AS. Food protein-induced enterocolitis syndrome: 16-year experience. *Pediatrics*. 2009;123(3):e459-e464. doi:10.1542/peds.2008-2029

54. Nowak-Wegrzyn A, Sampson HA, Wood RA, Sicherer SH. Food protein-induced enterocolitis syndrome caused by solid food proteins. *Pediatrics*. 2003;111(4):829-835. doi:10.1542/peds.111.4.829

55. Vazquez-Ortiz M, Argiz L, Machinena A, et al. Diagnostic criteria for acute FPIES: what are we missing? *J Allergy Clin Immunol Pract*. 2020;8(5):1717-1720.e2. doi:10.1016/j.jaip.2019.11.034

56. Baker MG, Nowak-Wegrzyn A. Diagnosis and management of chronic FPIES. In: Brown-Whitehorn TF, Cianferoni A, eds. *Food Protein Induced Enterocolitis (FPIES): Diagnosis and Management*. Springer International Publishing; 2019:77-89. doi:10.1007/978-3-030-21229-2_6

57. Agyemang A, Nowak-Wegrzyn A. Food protein-induced enterocolitis syndrome: a comprehensive review. *Clin Rev Allergy Immunol*. 2019;57(2):261-271. doi:10.1007/s12016-018-8722-z

58. Nowak-Węgrzyn A. Food protein-induced enterocolitis syndrome and allergic proctocolitis. *Allergy Asthma Proc*. 2015;36(3):172-184. doi:10.2500/aap.2015.36.3811

59. Cetinkaya PG, Ocak M, Sahiner UM, Sekerel BE, Soyer O. Food protein-induced allergic proctocolitis may have distinct phenotypes. *Ann Allergy Asthma Immunol*. 2021;126(1):75-82. doi:10.1016/j.anai.2020.08.021

60. Mennini M, Fiocchi AG, Cafarotti A, et al. Food protein-induced allergic proctocolitis in infants: literature review and proposal of a management protocol. *World Allergy Organ J*. 2020;13(10):100471. doi:10.1016/j.waojou.2020.100471

61. Collins MH, Capocelli K, Yang G-Y. Eosinophilic gastrointestinal disorders pathology. *Front Med (Lausanne)*. 2018;4:261. doi:10.3389/fmed.2017.00261

62. Dellon ES, Liacouras CA, Molina-Infante J, et al. Updated international consensus diagnostic criteria for eosinophilic esophagitis: proceedings of the AGREE conference. *Gastroenterology*. 2018;155(4):1022-1033.e10. doi:10.1053/j.gastro.2018.07.009

63. Reed CC, Dellon ES. Eosinophilic esophagitis. *Med Clin North Am*. 2019;103(1):29-42. doi:10.1016/j.mcna.2018.08.009

64. Dellon ES, Kim HP, Sperry SLW, Rybnicek DA, Woosley JT, Shaheen NJ. A phenotypic analysis shows that eosinophilic esophagitis is a progressive fibrostenotic disease. *Gastrointest Endosc*. 2014;79(4):577-585.e4. doi:10.1016/j.gie.2013.10.027

65. Williamson P, Aceves S. Allergies and eosinophilic esophagitis—current updates for the pediatric gastroenterologist. *Curr Gastroenterol Rep*. 2019;21(11):56. doi:10.1007/s11894-019-0729-y

66. Ishihara S, Kinoshita Y, Schoepfer A. Eosinophilic esophagitis, eosinophilic gastroenteritis, and eosinophilic colitis: common mechanisms and differences between East and West. *Inflamm Intest Dis*. 2016;1(2):63-69. doi:10.1159/000445131

67. Gonsalves NP, Aceves SS. Diagnosis and treatment of eosinophilic esophagitis. *J Allergy Clin Immunol*. 2020;145(1):1-7. doi:10.1016/j.jaci.2019.11.011

68. Gomez Torrijos E, Gonzalez-Mendiola R, Alvarado M, et al. Eosinophilic esophagitis: review and update. *Front Med (Lausanne)*. 2018;5:247. doi:10.3389/fmed.2018.00247

69. Navarro P, Arias Á, Arias-González L, Laserna-Mendieta EJ, Ruiz-Ponce M, Lucendo AJ. Systematic review with meta-analysis: the growing incidence and prevalence of eosinophilic oesophagitis in children and adults in population-based studies. *Aliment Pharmacol Ther*. 2019;49(9):1116-1125. doi:10.1111/apt.15231

70. Simon D, Straumann A, Schoepfer AM, Simon H-U. Current concepts in eosinophilic esophagitis. *Allergo J Int*. 2017;26(7):258-266. doi:10.1007/s40629-017-0037-8

71. Warners MJ, Vlieg-Boerstra BJ, Verheij J, et al. Elemental diet decreases inflammation and improves symptoms in adult eosinophilic oesophagitis patients. *Aliment Pharmacol Ther*. 2017;45(6):777-787. doi:10.1111/apt.13953

72. Lucendo AJ, Molina-Infante J, Arias Á, et al. Guidelines on eosinophilic esophagitis: evidence-based statements and recommendations for diagnosis and management in children and adults. *United Eur Gastroenterol J*. 2017;5(3):335-358. doi:10.1177/2050640616689525

73. Anyane-Yeboa A, Wang W, Kavitt RT. The role of allergy testing in eosinophilic esophagitis. *Gastroenterol Hepatol (N Y)*. 2018;14(8):463-469.

74. Spergel J, Aceves SS. Allergic components of eosinophilic esophagitis. *J Allergy Clin Immunol*. 2018;142(1):1-8. doi:10.1016/j.jaci.2018.05.001

75. Molina-Infante J, Arias Á, Alcedo J, et al. Step-up empiric elimination diet for pediatric and adult eosinophilic esophagitis: the 2-4-6 study. *J Allergy Clin Immunol*. 2018;141(4):1365-1372. doi:10.1016/j.jaci.2017.08.038

76. Lucendo AJ, Molina-Infante J. Dietary therapy for eosinophilic esophagitis: chances and limitations in the clinical practice. *Expert Rev Gastroenterol Hepatol*. 2020;14(10):941-952. doi:10.1080/17474124.2020.1791084

77. Cotton CC, Eluri S, Wolf WA, Dellon ES. Six-food elimination diet and topical steroids are effective for eosinophilic esophagitis: a meta-regression. *Dig Dis Sci.* 2017;62(9):2408-2420. doi:10.1007/s10620-017-4642-7

78. Kagalwalla AF, Sentongo TA, Ritz S, et al. Effect of six-food elimination diet on clinical and histologic outcomes in eosinophilic esophagitis. *Clin Gastroenterol Hepatol.* 2006;4(9):1097-1102. doi:10.1016/j.cgh.2006.05.026

79. Varjú P, Farkas N, Hegyi P, et al. Low fermentable oligosaccharides, disaccharides, monosaccharides and polyols (FODMAP) diet improves symptoms in adults suffering from irritable bowel syndrome (IBS) compared to standard IBS diet: a meta-analysis of clinical studies. *PLoS ONE.* 2017;12(8):e0182942. doi:10.1371/journal.pone.0182942

80. Major G, Pritchard S, Murray K, et al. Colon hypersensitivity to distension, rather than excessive gas production, produces carbohydrate-related symptoms in individuals with irritable bowel syndrome. *Gastroenterology.* 2017;152(1):124-133.e2. doi:10.1053/j.gastro.2016.09.062

81. Ong DK, Mitchell SB, Barrett JS, et al. Manipulation of dietary short chain carbohydrates alters the pattern of gas production and genesis of symptoms in irritable bowel syndrome. *J Gastroenterol Hepatol.* 2010;25(8):1366-1373. doi:10.1111/j.1440-1746.2010.06370.x

82. Harvie RM, Chisholm AW, Bisanz JE, et al. Long-term irritable bowel syndrome symptom control with reintroduction of selected FODMAPs. *World J Gastroenterol.* 2017;23(25):4632-4643. doi:10.3748/wjg.v23.i25.4632

83. Staudacher HM, Kurien M, Whelan K. Nutritional implications of dietary interventions for managing gastrointestinal disorders. *Curr Opin Gastroenterol.* 2018;34(2):105-111. doi:10.1097/MOG.0000000000000421

84. Whelan K, Martin LD, Staudacher HM, Lomer MCE. The low FODMAP diet in the management of irritable bowel syndrome: an evidence-based review of FODMAP restriction, reintroduction and personalisation in clinical practice. *J Hum Nutr Diet.* 2018;31(2):239-255. doi:10.1111/jhn.12530

85. Rezaie A, Buresi M, Lembo A, et al. Hydrogen and methane-based breath testing in gastrointestinal disorders: the North American consensus. *Am J Gastroenterol.* 2017;112(5):775-784. doi:10.1038/ajg.2017.46

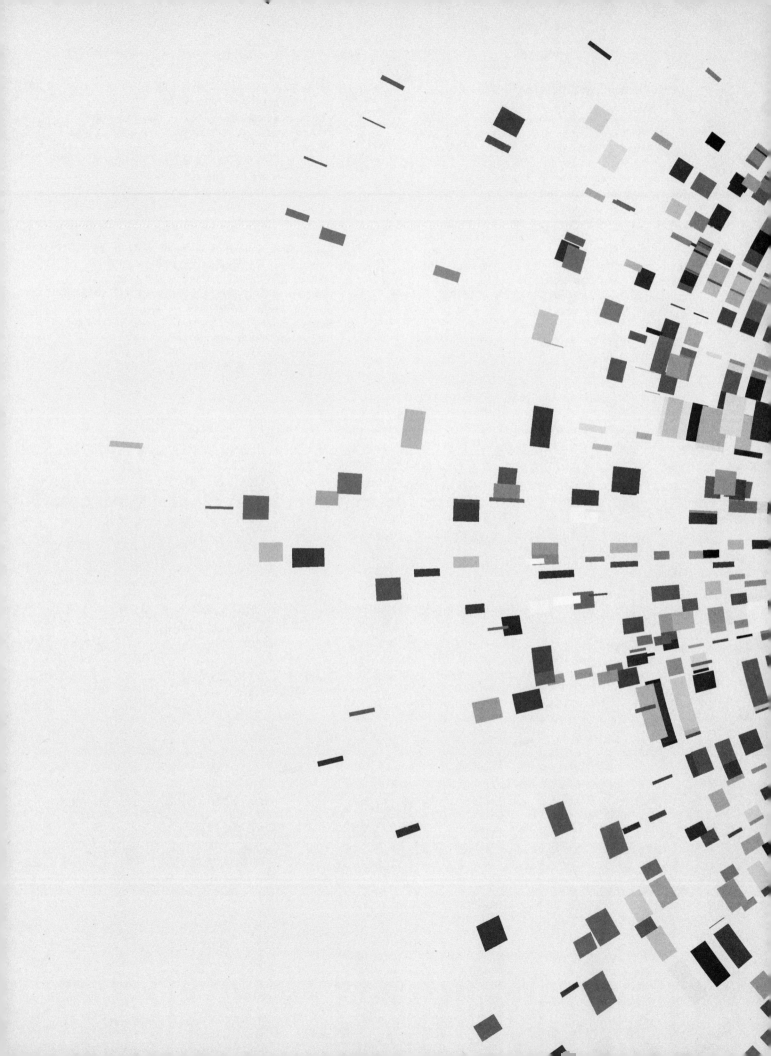

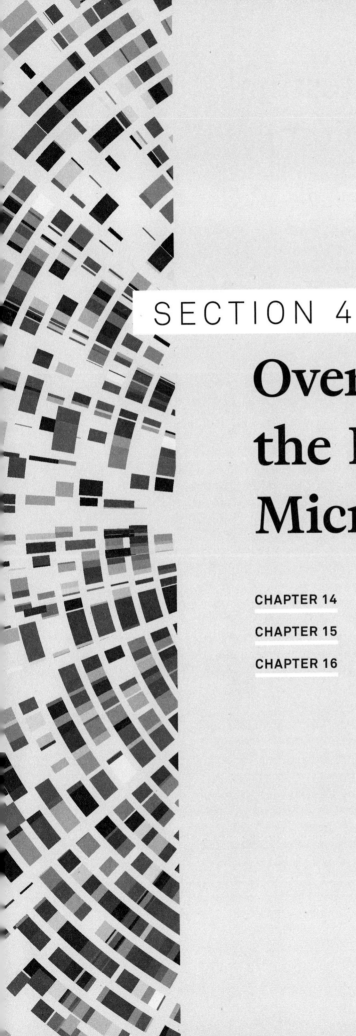

Overview of the Intestinal Microbiome

14

The Intestinal Microbiome

Riley L. Hughes, PhD
Hannah D. Holscher, PhD, RD

KEY POINTS

- The gastrointestinal microbiota is a collection of microorganisms, including bacteria, archaea, viruses, and eukaryotes (including fungi), that inhabit the human gastrointestinal tract.
- Many microorganisms in the gut microbiota are either commensal or mutualistic, providing functions for the human host, including nutrient metabolism, training of host immunity, endocrine and neurological signaling, and xenobiotic metabolism.
- Diet affects the gut microbiota and changes in microbial composition and function have been connected with health outcomes.

Introduction

Research has increasingly revealed the crucial role of the gastrointestinal (GI) microbiome in mediating the effects of diet on human health.[1] Thus, nutrition and dietetics practitioners must understand the GI microbiome to provide appropriate dietary guidance. This chapter introduces the GI microbiome: what it is, what it does, the effects of diet on it, and its effects on human health. See Chapters 15 and 16 for more detailed information specific to prebiotics and probiotics, respectively.

Overview of the Gastrointestinal Microbiome

The GI microbiota is a collection of microorganisms, including bacteria, archaea, viruses, and eukaryotes (including fungi), that inhabit the human GI tract.[1] Bacteria generally make up the majority of the GI microbiota (>90%). Interestingly, these bacteria equal or outnumber the human cells in our body and the number of microbial genes present in the microbiome outnumber the genes in the human genome by at least 100 to one.[2] Many microorganisms in the gut microbiota are commensal or mutualistic, providing functions for the human host, including nutrient metabolism, training of host immunity, endocrine and neurological signaling, and xenobiotic metabolism.[1]

Though the terms *microbiota* and *microbiome* are often used interchangeably, they represent two different concepts. *Microbiota* refers to the collection of microorganisms contained in a particular environment (eg, within the gut); *microbiome*, on the other hand, refers to the collection of microbial *genomes* present in that environment (see Box 14.1). To determine a microbiome, gene sequencing is used to characterize the microbes present and their genetic capabilities. Furthermore, different aspects of the microbiome can be characterized, including composition, function, diversity, richness, abundance of keystone species, and dysbiosis (see Box 14.1). *Composition* refers to what microbes are present. *Function* refers to what microbes have the functional capacity to do. Specifically, metagenomic sequencing allows for determining the genes present in the environment that could enable an action. For example, the presence of butyryl–coenzyme A in the genome suggests the microorganisms can convert two molecules of acetate to butyrate.[3] However, to assess actual functions of the intestinal microbiome, other measures, such as metabolomics, must be employed. There are different levels of taxonomic classification that can be used to identify microorganisms,

BOX 14.1

The Intestinal Microbiome: Key Terms and Definitions

Microbiome vs microbiota: Microbiome refers to the collection of microbial genomes within a particular environment, whereas microbiota refers only to the collection of microorganisms within that environment. The gene sequencing method used determines the level of characterization: 16S ribosomal RNA gene sequencing (also called amplicon sequencing) allows for characterization of the microbiota composition, whereas metagenomic (or whole genome) sequencing—that is, sequencing all of the DNA present—enables characterization of the microbiome.

Commensal and mutualistic vs pathogenic: Both commensal and mutualistic microorganisms can coexist with their host organisms. In commensal relationships, one organism benefits and the other is unaffected; in mutualistic relationships, both organisms (ie, both the microbe and the host) benefit. Pathogenic microbes, on the other hand, may cause infection or disease in their hosts and actively attempt to invade the host, triggering an immune response and inflammation. Pathobionts are microbes that can coexist with the host in the absence of overt disease but may drive disease development under certain circumstances.

Composition vs function: Composition refers to what microbes are present; function refers to what functional genes of microbes are present.

Richness vs diversity: Richness refers to the number of species found in the community. Diversity refers to how many species are present and how evenly distributed their numbers are. There are multiple methods used to measure each of these, such as α-diversity (Shannon, Simpson, Faith PD), β-diversity (weighted and unweighted UniFrac, Bray-Curtis, Jaccard), and richness (Chao1, ACE).

Abundance: Abundance is the amount of a specific microbe present in a community. It can be measured in absolute numbers (counts) and relative numbers (percentages), the latter of which is more common.

Keystone species: A keystone species is a microbial taxon that is crucial for a specific function and whose removal would cause a loss of function and potentially a dramatic shift in an ecosystem.

Enterotype grouping: Enterotype grouping is the classification of individual microbial communities into compositional categories based on the dominance of particular taxa.

Dysbiosis: Dysbiosis is a state of dysregulated (abnormal) microbiota composition. The concept is not well defined and is often used when comparing the gut microbiota of individuals with and without disease (eg, obesity, diabetes, colon cancer, irritable bowel disease).

ranging from the broad (ie, phylum) to the specific (ie, species) (Figure 14.1 on page 226). Microbial taxa that share more specific taxonomic classification levels are more closely related and are more likely to share similar functional characteristics.

Other ways of characterizing the community are richness (ie, how many taxa are present), diversity (ie, how many taxa are present and how evenly they are distributed), and enterotype grouping.[4-6] Diversity is of two types, α-diversity and β-diversity; the former refers to species differences *within* a community and the latter to differences *between* communities. Some correlational research has revealed that greater GI microbiota diversity is associated with superior health outcomes, such as reduced adiposity, insulin resistance, and dyslipidemia. However, other studies reveal that greater diversity caused by long colonic transit time is associated with increased risk factors for colorectal cancer.[7] Furthermore, in infants, being breastfed is associated with less GI microbiota diversity than being

FIGURE 14.1 Taxonomy

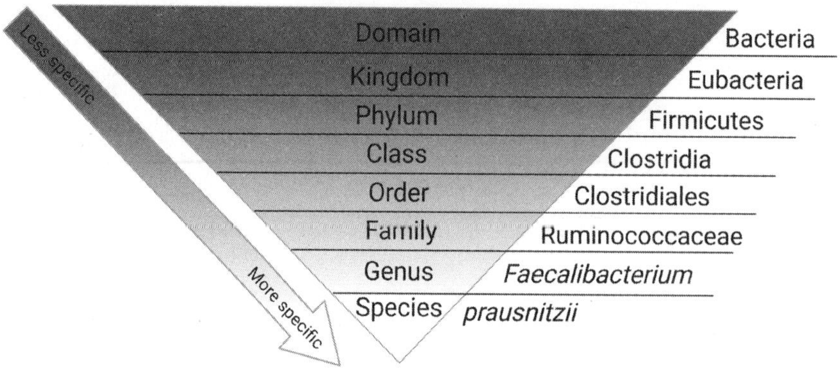

Microbes can be identified at different levels of taxonomic classification. The taxonomy is shown for the taxon *Faecalibacterium prausnitzii*.

formula-fed.[8] Importantly, few randomized controlled trials have demonstrated causality between diversity and health measures, with the exception of research on *Clostridioides difficile* (previously known as *Clostridium difficile*). *C difficile* infection is characterized by a loss of microbe diversity, usually due to aggressive antibiotic treatments, which results in a bloom of *C difficile* and subsequently life-threatening diarrhea.[9] For this reason, findings based on associations should be interpreted with care.

Enterotype grouping based on microbiota characteristics, such as having a greater abundance of *Prevotella* species relative to *Bacteroides* species, may be important in determining an individual's response (eg, weight loss, metabolic improvement) to fiber intake.[10] However, enterotype distinctions may exist along a gradient or spectrum rather than in distinct groups as initially thought.[11] Also, associations may be driven by individual taxa within these taxonomic groups. For instance, in one study, the protective association between adherence to the Mediterranean diet and cardiometabolic disease risk was significantly greater among individuals with a lower abundance of *Prevotella copri*.[12] Sometimes, certain microbes, when present at specific amounts, are important in facilitating a metabolic process or disease state; these keystone species may be specifically targeted to facilitate a health outcome when present in an efficacious amount. For example, *Ruminococcus bromii* was designated a keystone species in the degradation of resistant starch.[13]

Ultimately, there is no consensus on what constitutes a "healthy" GI microbiome. More research is needed to determine normal levels of variation within healthy people across populations and the contextual relevance and function of certain microbes under different circumstances. Indeed, rather than a binary "good" or "bad," the GI microbiota should be viewed as a spectrum, with the emergence of the disease being dependent on varying levels of disease-associated or health-associated taxa.[14] Certain conditions have been associated with an abnormal microbiota composition (ie, dysbiosis), which can be characterized either by the presence of specific pathogenic microbes or by broader measures, such as the loss of richness or diversity.[1,15]

How the Gastrointestinal Microbiome Is Measured

Stool is the most commonly used sample for GI microbiota and microbiome studies; however, biopsies and ostomy (eg, ileostomy) sampling are also used. Following extraction of the DNA from the sample, target regions of the DNA are amplified using primers to allow for the microbiota characterization. The 16S ribosomal RNA (rRNA) gene, which is approximately 1,500 base pairs long and includes nine variable regions (V1-V9), is unique to bacteria and archaea. Thus, one or multiple regions of the 16S rRNA gene (eg, V1-V4) can be amplified and then sequenced to allow for taxonomic identification of bacteria and archaea. For fungi, primers are designed for an intertranscribed region of the genome (eg, V1-V4) to allow taxonomic classification. For characterization of the microbiome, segments of the entire microbial genome are sequenced. This type of metagenomic sequencing, or whole genome sequencing, allows for taxonomic classification of microorganisms (eg, bacteria, archaea, and fungi) and their functional potential. Both 16S rRNA gene sequencing and metagenomic sequencing rely on reference databases to match the sequence data to interpretable information, including taxa and functional genes.[16]

To understand what the microbes are doing at the time of measurement, RNA gene expression, proteins, and metabolites can be measured using metatranscriptomics, metaproteomics, and metabolomics, respectively. Metatranscriptomics and metaproteomics study RNA gene expression and proteins, respectively, from microbial communities, whereas metabolomics studies the collection of small molecules (ie, metabolites) within a sample.[17] Multimodal approaches that combine these different "omic" approaches allow for an integrated and comprehensive view of the complexity of the microbiome and its interaction with the human host.

How the Gastrointestinal Microbiome Develops

The initial colonization of the infant microbiota may begin in utero but primarily occurs during the birthing process.[18,19] Delivery method (vaginal delivery or cesarean section) affects the establishment of the microbial community, after which breastfeeding and subsequent introduction to solid foods continues to shape the developmental trajectory of the GI microbiota.[18,20] The infant GI microbiota has low diversity and contains a relatively large proportion of *Bifidobacterium* spp, which thrive on human milk oligosaccharides; the introduction of solid foods, as well as environmental exposure, leads to the maturation and diversification of this community toward a more adultlike pattern over the first few years of life.[21,22] Research is limited on the GI microbiota of children and adolescents, but evidence suggests that there may be compositional and functional differences between the GI microbiomes of children and adults that reflect the need to support ongoing development in children.[23]

Among healthy adults, although the GI microbiota experiences stochastic changes from day to day, an individual's microbiota composition remains relatively stable, and interindividual variability is much greater than intraindividual variability.[24,25] Whereas genetics may play a minor role in the GI microbiome, lifestyle factors including diet, medication and antibiotic use, exercise, and environment exert a strong influence on the composition and function of the GI microbiome and contribute to much of the observed interindividual variability.[26]

The interindividual variability in GI microbiota composition increases with age. Still, it continues to be influenced by factors such as residence (eg, community, day hospital, rehabilitation, long-term residential care), medications, and diet.[27,28] Decreased intestinal motility, resulting in longer transit times, and poor dentition play a role in altered nutrient intake and turnover, thus affecting the physical and nutritional environment for the GI microbiota.[21] The GI microbiota of elderly individuals is correlated with age-related declines in health, presenting a potential therapeutic opportunity.[29]

Gastrointestinal Microbiome Functioning

The GI microbiome provides many necessary and beneficial functions to the host (see Box 14.2 on page 228).[6,15,30-39] Within the GI tract, the microbiome aids in the metabolism of dietary components, resulting in the production of vitamins and bioactive metabolites, such as short-chain fatty acids (SCFAs), that can influence the local GI environment or be absorbed into the systemic circulation.[30] Commensal and mutualistic microbes in the GI tract also influence epithelial barrier integrity and immune system defenses to promote the

BOX 14.2

Functions of the Gastrointestinal Microbiome[6,15,30-39]

Metabolism: The gastrointestinal (GI) microbiome metabolizes nondigested dietary components, including certain dietary fibers, and produces short-chain fatty acids (SCFAs). SCFAs serve as energy substrates (particularly by colonocytes), substrates for gluconeogenesis, histone deacetylase inhibitors, and signaling molecules. SCFAs influence inflammation and enteroendocrine (eg, insulin) signaling.[30] Microbes also metabolize protein and micronutrients, such as polyphenols, to produce bioactive compounds. The GI microbiome also synthesizes vitamins, including vitamin K and B vitamins, that may be used by the host and other resident microbes.[35] The GI microbiome may also produce metabolites that can be harmful at high concentrations, such as phenols, indoles, and ammonia.[30]

Immunity: Gut microbes and their metabolites affect the innate immune system via two types of signals: microbial cell components and metabolites.[15,31] These interactions are critical during infancy for priming immune cell development and affect the development of immune-related diseases (eg, allergies, asthma, inflammatory bowel disease).[36] The gut microbiota also influences the adaptive immune system via induction of secretory IgA and immune cell differentiation. The intestinal mucosa and epithelial cell layers prevent the invasion of bacteria via physical barrier function and pattern recognition. The integrity of the intestinal epithelium is enhanced by microbial metabolites, such as butyrate and tryptophan.[15] Commensal microbes may also protect against pathogenic colonization via competitive exclusion, production of antimicrobial peptides and secretory immunoglobulin A, and pH reduction due to SCFA production.[15,36,37]

Systemic gut axes: The GI microbiome interacts and communicates with extraintestinal systems, including the brain, skeletal muscle, bone, kidney, and liver.[6,32-34,38] Production of metabolites, including SCFAs and neurotransmitters, influences the production of cytokines (ie, substances secreted by immune system cells), allowing the GI microbiome to communicate with the brain via immune and endocrine pathways and to influence neurochemistry and behavior.[38] The GI microbiome is connected to muscle and bone health, potentially via SCFA production, which increases fuel availability and glycogen storage in muscle, increases calcium absorption, and reduces inflammation to aid bone health.[6,39] The GI microbiome affects the liver via the biliary tract, portal vein, and systemic mediators to regulate bile acid synthesis and hepatic glucose and lipid metabolism, affecting the risk for liver diseases, such as nonalcoholic fatty liver disease.[33] Altered microbiota composition, bile acid metabolism, SCFA production, and excessive production of uremic toxins by the GI microbiome have been implicated in the progression of various kidney diseases.[34] Inherent in all of these connections is the potential to develop microbiome-targeted therapies to manage disease symptoms and promote health.

development of the immune system, as well as prevent local and systemic inflammation, the establishment of opportunistic pathogens, and the development of autoimmune diseases such as inflammatory bowel disease (IBD).[31] Pathobionts may also contribute to the development and maturation of the immune system in immunocompetent hosts, though they may also drive the development of autoimmunity and disease under certain conditions.[40]

There are also various routes, or axes, by which intestinal microbes communicate with other parts of the body, including the brain, skeletal muscle, bone, kidney, and liver, all of which ultimately influence health and disease risk.[6,32-34,41] As an example, the bidirectional communication between the gut and the brain (the gut-brain axis) may affect mood and behavior and the development of neurologic pathologies.[41] Gut microbes can communicate with the brain via the vagus nerve, SCFAs, cytokines, and tryptophan-derived neurotransmitters.

FIGURE 14.2 Microbial metabolites in health and disease

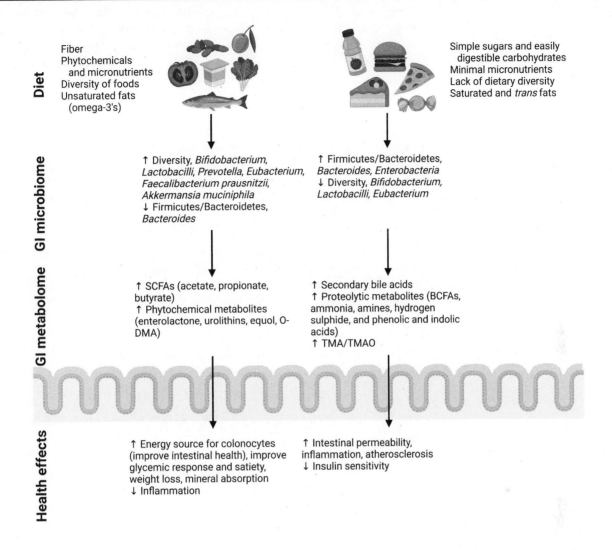

BCFA = branched-chain fatty acid | GI = gastrointestinal | O-DMA = O-desmethylangolensin | SCFA = short-chain fatty acid | TMA = trimethylamine | TMAO = trimethylamine-*N*-oxide. Created with BioRender.com

Microbial metabolites may also exert their effects indirectly via immune regulation, enteric nervous system activation, or epigenetic modulation (eg, histone deacetylation).[41,42] Dysregulation of the gut-brain axis, such as with stress and activation of the hypothalamic-pituitary-adrenal axis, may then disrupt the GI microbiome and luminal environment, leading to inflammation, dysbiosis, and potential development of neurologic pathologies (eg, depression, Parkinson disease, Alzheimer disease).[41,43]

Microbial Metabolites

One of the main ways the GI microbiome communicates with and affects health is through the production of metabolites.[7] Dietary nutrients modulate the GI microbiota and metabolome, contributing to the effects of diet on human health (see Figure 14.2). Furthermore, metabolites from the primary fermentation of dietary components can stimulate the growth of other microbes in the community in a process called cross-feeding, which means that substrate metabolism affects the GI microbiota beyond those taxa that directly utilize the substrate.[44]

SCFAs (eg, acetate, propionate, and butyrate) serve various functions. They act as energy sources for colonocytes, reduce the body's glycemic response and increase satiety, promote weight loss, enhance mineral absorption, reduce systemic inflammation, and improve intestinal health.[7,45,46] Between 90% and 95% of SCFAs are absorbed in the gut or used by microbes; however, small amounts of SCFAs are absorbed into the systemic circulation and influence pathways such as glucose homeostasis, lipid metabolism, appetite regulation, and immune function.[44,45,47] Excessive or abnormal production of SCFAs has been linked to obesity and type 2 diabetes mellitus (T2DM), potentially because of the increased energy harvest, suggesting that there may be an optimal concentration of SCFAs.[7,48]

Although some proteolytic fermentation products have negative effects on health, this is not universally true and is likely dependent on the amino acid composition of the protein, the type and concentration of metabolites, and concurrent fiber intake.[49] Similarly, the effects of the interaction between the GI microbiome and the host's lipid metabolism on health depend on the amount and type of fat, which differentially affects the production of secondary bile acids and SCFAs by the GI microbiome.[7,48] Increases in secondary bile acids and decreases in SCFAs resulting from high intakes of fat and saturated fat have been associated with negative health outcomes, such as inflammation, intestinal permeability, and glucose and lipid homeostasis.[7,50] In contrast, polyunsaturated fats, particularly omega-3 fatty acids, maintain SCFA levels and have been associated with positive effects on these health outcomes.[50,51] Additional metabolites (eg, trimethylamine [TMA] and trimethylamine-N-oxide [TMAO] produced from dietary carnitine, choline, and phosphatidylcholine) may also affect health outcomes. Thus, microbial metabolites form the basis for host-microbial communication and act as a bridge that connects diet-induced alterations in the GI microbiota and human health implications.

Microbial Diversity, Dysbiosis, and Diet-Related Chronic Disease

Although they are not stand-alone indicators of a health-associated microbiota, diversity and richness of gut microorganisms have been associated with measures of health in adults.[1,7] High levels of diversity and richness have been linked to lower adiposity, insulin resistance, and dyslipidemia.[7] Conversely, a low degree of diversity is regularly observed in people with IBD, type 1 diabetes mellitus (T1DM) and T2DM, obesity, celiac disease, atopic eczema, psoriatic arthritis, and arterial stiffness compared with healthy individuals.[52] However, measures of diversity and richness may be confounded by long colonic transit time, which is a risk factor for colorectal cancer and Parkinson disease and increases protein fermentation but is also associated with higher microbial richness.[7] Also, increasing single sources of dietary fibers, as is done in intervention studies, can reduce microbial diversity by enriching specific bacteria capable of metabolizing the provided fiber.[52] Therefore, though diversity indicates that the GI microbiota is potentially more robust against environmental changes, diversity alone does not indicate a "healthy gut." Furthermore, there is increasing interest in dysbiosis, which is poorly defined but commonly reported in disease states such as obesity, T1DM and T2DM, colon cancer, and irritable bowel disease.

Digestion, Absorption, and Physiology of the Gastrointestinal Tract

To understand the influence of diet on the GI microbiome, it is important to understand the luminal environment's effects on the microbial community. This includes pH, oxygen concentrations, transit time, secretion of immune factors, and nutrient availability as a function of digestion or absorption (or both) of macronutrients and micronutrients.[53,54] These factors lead to regional variations in the microbial communities throughout the GI tract. Some gut microbes reside in the small intestine, where they help the body utilize simple carbohydrates, but most microbes reside in the large intestine, where they ferment

FIGURE 14.3 Digestion

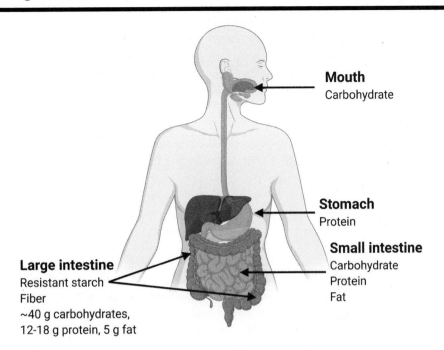

Mouth
Carbohydrate

Stomach
Protein

Small intestine
Carbohydrate
Protein
Fat

Large intestine
Resistant starch
Fiber
~40 g carbohydrates,
12-18 g protein, 5 g fat

Digestion and absorption occur primarily in the small intestine, but a portion of ingested nutrients make it down to the large intestine, where they interact with the GI microbiota. The macronutrient gram amounts shown are per day. Created with BioRender.com

undigested nutrients.[54,55] Many of these factors, including pH, transit time, and nutrient availability, are influenced by dietary intake, digestion and absorption of nutrients, and the subsequent fermentation of remaining nutrients by gut microbes in the large intestine.

The small intestine is the most active site of digestion and absorption.[56] The *bioaccessibility* of a nutrient or compound is defined as the proportion of that nutrient or compound that is released from a complex food matrix during digestion and is, thus, made available for absorption.[57] Depending on the volume and composition of nutrient intake, however, some nutrients escape digestion and absorption and reach the large intestine (see Figure 14.3).

Approximately 40 g dietary carbohydrates, 12 to 18 g protein, and 5 g fat escape digestion and make it to the large intestine each day, where the microbiota then metabolize these macronutrients.[58] Low-digestible or nondigestible carbohydrates, including dietary fibers, are resistant to digestion by host enzymes and are a preferred fuel source for microbes. The proportion of residual dietary protein in the large intestine (roughly 10% of protein intake) depends on the amount and type of protein consumed.[58] Although most dietary fat is absorbed in the small intestine, the food matrix, bile acid secretion, and microbial metabolism of bile acids affect fatty acid malabsorption and the presence of fatty acids in the colon.[58] Also, though the microbiota can synthesize some vitamins, dietary micronutrients ingested by the host, including vitamins, minerals, and polyphenols, also modulate the composition and function of the GI microbiome, with implications for pathogen inhibition and production of bioactive metabolites that influence host health.[59]

The GI microbiota can metabolize unabsorbed nutrients that make it to the large intestine. Metabolites found in stool provide a functional readout of gut microbial activity, but because microbial metabolites are also absorbed into the circulation, host-microbe interactions are also reflected in blood and urine and can be used to predict dietary intake.[7] The preferred fuel source for many bacteria within the intestines is dietary fiber, which is metabolized into SCFAs: acetate, propionate, butyrate, lactate, and succinate.[7,60] However, depending on the availability of fiber in the large intestine, pH, and transit time, there is a trade-off between saccharolytic (carbohydrate) and proteolytic (protein) metabolism, with low fiber and high protein intake, high pH, and long transit times resulting in increased proteolytic fermentation.[7,60] Protein fermentation can also result in the production of SCFAs, primarily propionate, and generates various other bioactive metabolites, such as branched-chain fatty acids (BCFAs; isovalerate, valerate, and isobutyrate), ammonia, amines, hydrogen sulfide, and phenolic and indolic acids.[7] Though the mechanism is poorly understood, the GI microbiome also modifies dietary fatty acids and influences the host's lipid metabolism, possibly via modulation of the bile acid pool or production of SCFAs.[50] Besides the production of metabolites from the fermentation of macronutrients, an extremely diverse array of metabolites are produced from phytonutrients, such as polyphenols, that have the potential to affect host health. Indeed, the bioactive metabolites produced from the microbial metabolism of polyphenols often have greater bioavailability and biological activity than their dietary precursors.[61] Thus, fermentation by the GI microbiome represents an additional step in the human digestive process and is an important means by which dietary components are modified and interact with the host.

The Effect of Diet on the Gastrointestinal Microbiome

Diet affects the GI microbiome because it is the main source of substrates for microbial metabolism.[58] Specific dietary components (eg, certain fibers that are not digested) become fuel for the GI microbiota, promoting the growth of certain taxa that possess the metabolic capacity to hydrolyze the glycosidic bonds linking monosaccharides together that are resistant to digestion by human alimentary enzymes. Nutrients are not typically consumed in isolation, however, but in the form of whole foods, which are complex mixtures of these different nutrients (ie, the food matrix) that have been shown to influence the GI microbiota.[62-65] To further add to the complexity, habitual dietary patterns, such as the Western-style diet and the Mediterranean diet, and short-term diet patterns involving extreme changes can affect the GI microbiome composition and function.[66-70]

Effects of Specific Dietary Components

Fiber

Dietary fiber is defined by the US Food and Drug Administration (FDA) as "non-digestible soluble and insoluble carbohydrates (with three or more monomeric units) and lignin that are intrinsic and intact in plants; isolated or synthetic non-digestible carbohydrates (with three or more monomeric units) determined by FDA to have physiological effects that are beneficial to human health."[71] Dietary fibers that are intrinsic and intact are found in plant foods, including whole grains, vegetables, fruits, nuts, and legumes. Epidemiological studies consistently suggest the benefits of dietary fiber intake from plant foods on obesity, cardiovascular disease, cancer, and T1DM and T2DM.[72] Synthetic, isolated, or extracted fibers, such as inulin and resistant starch type 2, are also added to a range of processed foods, including cereals, bars, baked goods, and ice creams. Clinical trials often use isolated fibers in supplement form to elucidate specific effects; however, the properties and bioaccessibility of the fiber may differ when consumed in whole foods and in combination with other dietary components.[72] Ultimately, in order to be listed on a Nutrition Facts label as dietary fiber, isolated and synthetic fibers must, through their consumption, contribute a physiological benefit to human health.[71]

Human digestive enzymes cannot digest most dietary fibers because of their inability to access or degrade the linkages between carbohydrate molecules; thus, fibers are allowed to pass into the large intestine, where they are used as a fuel source for the GI microbiota.[44] Fibers may be broadly divided into resistant starches and nonstarch polysaccharides (eg, pectin, β glucan, inulin-type fructans, galacto-oligosaccharides, pectin, cellulose, hemicellulose, gums, and psyllium), the latter of which are the main components of plant cell walls.[72] Resistant starches are divided into four categories: physically inaccessible starches (RS1), native starch granules (RS2), retrograde starches (RS3), and chemically modified food starches (RS4). In addition to RS4, other chemically synthesized carbohydrate compounds approved as dietary fibers by the FDA include dextrin, polydextrose, and hydroxypropylmethylcellulose.[73] Chemical composition, food matrix interactions, physicochemical properties (ie, fermentability, solubility, viscosity), and processing and cooking all influence the functional properties of fibers and, thus, their effects on the GI microbiome.[44,72] And although some bacteria, such as those of the genus *Bacteroides*, can make use of a wide array of fibers, increasing in response to the intake of a broad range of fiber types, other bacteria can only utilize one or a few different types. This functional diversity adds to the complex interaction between dietary fibers and the GI microbiome and provides a basis for variability in response to fiber intake based on fiber type and amount, host genetics, and the unique microbiota composition of the individual, such as the presence of bacteria able to ferment the fiber or fibers of interest.[44]

Prebiotics, Probiotics, Synbiotics, and Fermented Foods

Probiotics, prebiotics, and synbiotics provide health benefits by affecting the GI microbiome. Probiotics are "live microorganisms that, when administered in adequate amounts, confer a health benefit on the host," and prebiotics are "substrates that [are] selectively utilized by host microorganisms conferring a health benefit."[74,75] Synbiotics are "a mixture comprising live microorganisms and substrate(s) selectively utilized by host microorganisms that confers a health benefit on the host."[76] Commonly used and accepted probiotics include *Bifidobacterium* (*adolescentis, animalis, bifidum, breve,* and *longum*), *Lactobacillus* (*acidophilus, casei, fermentum, gasseri, johnsonii, paracasei, plantarum, rhamnosus, salivarius*), and *Streptococcus thermophilus*.[75] Among the most researched and commonly used prebiotics are fructooligosaccharides, galactooligosaccharides, and inulin, though other nondigestible oligosaccharides and plant polyphenols may also be considered prebiotics or candidate prebiotics.[74] A synbiotic may be a combination of a probiotic and a prebiotic (complementary synbiotic) or may consist of individual components that do not necessarily need to meet the criteria for probiotics and prebiotics but act synergistically when coadministered (synergistic synbiotic).[76] Fundamental to these definitions are the concepts of "selective" and "beneficial." Bacterial functions are species-dependent and often strain-dependent, requiring probiotics, prebiotics, and synbiotics to be specific and selective to elicit the desired beneficial health effects.[75]

Live cultures associated with fermented foods are excluded from the probiotic framework.[75,77] Fermented foods and beverages such as yogurt, kefir, kimchi, sauerkraut, and kombucha are "made through desired microbial growth and enzymatic conversions of food components."[77] To qualify as a probiotic fermented food, evidence of a strain-specific benefit from an intervention study, with confirmation of safety and sufficient quantity of the strain in the final product, is needed. Though all fermented foods require live cultures, not all fermented foods contain probiotics because they contain undefined microbial consortia, at variable levels, chosen for their performance characteristics rather than demonstrated health effects. The health benefits of fermented foods may be attributable to the improved nutritional value of the raw ingredients (eg, phytate detoxification, reduced sugar, increased bioavailability of polyphenols), the biosynthesis of bioactive compounds (eg, vitamin biosynthesis, bioactive peptides, conjugated linoleic acid), the modification of the GI microbiota, or the development and modification of the immune system.[77] Aside from studies of yogurt and other cultured dairy products (eg, kefir, cultured milk), there are too few studies within each fermented food category to establish consistent effects of each type on the GI microbiota and subsequent health benefits.[77,78] However, consumption of fermented foods may modify the GI microbiota and metabolites.[75,78,79] Compared to nonconsumers, consumers of fermented foods have a higher abundance of bacteria derived from the ingested fermented foods, such as *Lactobacillus* spp, *Prevotella* spp, and *Bacteroides* spp, and have higher fecal concentrations of conjugated linoleic acid.[77,79]

Sugars and Sweeteners

On average, Americans consume in excess of 100 g added sugar per person per day, which is four times the recommended maximum daily intake. The sharp increase in added-sugar consumption is thought to contribute to the concurrent rise in metabolic syndrome, obesity, T2DM, and cardiovascular disease, among other disorders. Increasingly, evidence suggests that the detrimental effects of excessive sugar consumption are partially mediated via the GI microbiome by altering the pool of available carbohydrates and shaping the community structure and function. Sucrose, glucose, fructose, and high-fructose corn syrup are the most-consumed sugars in the United States, but we have also seen a rise in the consumption of sugar alcohols and low-energy or no-energy sweeteners. Most of these sugars are digested and absorbed in the small intestine. However, sugar alcohols and some sweeteners (eg, sucralose) are poorly absorbed and make it to the large intestine in greater quantities. Overconsumption may promote greater malabsorption and overflow into the large intestine.[80] A food's glucose and fructose load and fructose-to-glucose ratio also influence absorption efficiency and, therefore, differentially affect gut microbial fermentation, and in some individuals, GI intolerance. For instance, a food with a higher fructose-to-glucose ratio increases malabsorption in the small intestine and leads to greater fermentation and gas production in the large intestine.[81]

Excess intake of refined sugar decreases bacterial diversity and *Lactobacillus* species while increasing bacteria classes Clostridia, Proteobacteria, and Bacilli.[82] In animal models, refined-sugar intake also alters the metabolite pool; it causes a decrease in fecal butyrate and propionate concentrations and an increase in both cecal and circulating serum levels of lipopolysaccharide, a proinflammatory bacterial product, indicating an increase in metabolic endotoxemia.[80,82] These effects on the GI microbiota and their metabolites may occur via both direct (eg, substrate utilization, toxicity) and indirect mechanisms (eg, reduced mucus thickness, impaired barrier integrity).[80]

Although an increase in refined-sugar intake and decrease in fiber intake are known to have detrimental effects on the GI microbiome and metabolic health, less is known about the relative effects of low-energy or no-energy sweeteners on the GI microbiome and consequent health outcomes.[80,83,84] Common low- or no-energy sweeteners include acesulfame potassium (acesulfame K), advantame, aspartame, monk fruit extract, neotame, saccharin, sucralose, and steviol glycosides (eg, rebaudioside A).[85] Low- or no-energy sweeteners vary in their digestion, absorption, metabolism, and excretion, which means that their effects on the GI microbiota also vary.[80,84] Consumption of these sweeteners in amounts relevant to humans, and within the acceptable daily intake (ADI), seem to have little effect on the GI microbiota.[83] Indeed, studies of the effects of several of the most commonly consumed low- or no-energy sweeteners (aspartame, cyclamate, neotame, and saccharin) in doses within the ADI have demonstrated inconclusive results.[86-89] Although several other studies have been conducted in humans, many have important confounding factors, such as lack of dietary control.[83] Ultimately, the variability in findings, lack of control for confounding factors including habitual dietary intake, and evidence of effects in animal models warrant further investigation into the effects of low- or no-energy sweeteners on the GI microbiota and the subsequent effects on metabolic health.[86]

Health practitioners should encourage patients to keep their intake of added refined sugars to a minimum and to increase their intake of food sources that also contain fiber and beneficial phytochemicals (eg, fruit). There is limited evidence at this time to support avoidance of low- or no-energy sweeteners for the sake of the GI microbiome.

Phytochemicals

Phytochemicals are bioactive plant compounds that are found in abundance in fruits, vegetables, nuts, grains, and seeds. Common phytochemicals found in these food sources include dietary fiber, flavonoids, isoflavonoids, carotenoids, and glucosinolates, among others.[51,90] Herbs and spices are also a source of phytochemicals, particularly phenolic compounds; among the herbs and spices with high levels of these compounds are turmeric (which contains curcumin, demethoxycurcumin, and bisdemethoxycurcumin), star anise (which contains quercetin derivatives, kaempferol derivatives, and isorhamnetin derivatives), ginger (which contains gingerols and shogaols), and cinnamon (which contains procyanidins, cinnamic acid, kaempferitrin, cinnamaldehyde, and 2-hydroxycinnamaldehyde).[91]

Phytochemical compounds, at specific amounts, can have a range of physiologic effects, including antioxidant, antiestrogenic, anti-inflammatory and immunomodulatory, cardioprotective, and anticarcinogenic effects.[51,91] However, food sources of these components often contain lower concentrations than are used in research studies and, therefore, may not have the same effects. Additionally, the absorption, bioavailability, and effects of phytochemicals often depend on their conversion by the GI microbiota into bioactive metabolites.[46,51,92] For example, the production of metabolites equol and O-desmethylangolensin from soy isoflavones and enterodiol, respectively, and enterolactone from plant lignans have been associated with anticarcinogenic effects, and the production of urolithin metabolites from ellagitannin (present in nuts and berries) is associated with anti-inflammatory effects and decreased risk for cardiovascular disease.[93,94] The ability to metabolize phytochemicals and produce these bioactive compounds, therefore, depends on the GI microbiota composition and the presence of taxa involved in these pathways.[59,93,94] This may lead to interindividual variability in exposure to bioactive metabolites from dietary intake, and thus variability in health effects. Unfortunately, many animal studies use pharmacologic-level doses or metabolic forms that do not reflect dietary intake in humans, limiting the physiological relevance of these studies.[95]

Phytochemicals and their metabolites also influence the GI microbiota composition, exerting prebiotic-like effects by stimulating the growth of commensal bacteria, such as *Bifidobacterium*, *Lactobacillus*, *Faecalibacterium prausnitzii*, and *Roseburia*.[51,59,92] Thus, the bidirectional interaction between the GI microbiota and dietary phytochemicals has the potential to influence health outcomes related to phytochemical intake.

Micronutrients

Micronutrients, including vitamins, minerals, and trace elements, are essential for human health and may interact with the GI microbiota under circumstances of both excess (eg, supplements) and deficiency.[59] Vitamins A, C, D, and E modulate the abundance of *Bifidobacterium* and *Lactobacillus* species, suggesting beneficial effects on the GI microbiota.[59] Additionally, gut bacteria can synthesize vitamin K and B vitamins, which the host and other resident microbes may then utilize.[35]

The GI microbiome may also influence the absorption of minerals from dietary intake.[96,97] For instance, prebiotic (eg, soluble corn fiber, galacto-oligosaccharides, fructans) or probiotic (eg, *L acidophilus*, *L rhamnosus*, *L bulgaricus*, *B breve*, *B lactis*, *B longum*, *S thermophilus*) supplementation in humans increases calcium absorption with concurrent, correlated alterations in the GI microbiota composition.[97-103] Conversely, mineral intake also influences the GI microbiota composition. Excess iron supplementation in infants increases pathogenic microbes and contributes to intestinal inflammation, but iron deficiency also causes decreases in commensal microorganisms, such as *Roseburia*, *Bacteroides*, and *Eubacterium rectale*.[96,97] The effects of micronutrient supplementation are likely dependent on the micronutrient status of the host, with oversupplementation having potentially adverse effects on the GI microbiota and health.[59]

Fat

The amount and type of fat consumed influence the GI microbiota.[50,58,59,69,104] Though most fatty acids are absorbed in the small intestine, some fat does reach the large intestine and interacts with the GI microbiota.[50,58] High-fat diets (30%–70% of energy from fat) increase the ratio of Firmicutes to Bacteroidetes in the gut and decrease diversity, richness, *Bifidobacterium*, and SCFAs in mice.[50] However, interventional studies in humans are few, and effects at the genus level are variable and may be due more to differences in fatty acid composition or compensatory changes in fermentable carbohydrate intake than fat intake, per se.[50,58] Observational and cross sectional studies in humans show decreased diversity, richness, *F prausnitzii*, and *Akkermansia muciniphila* and increased Firmicutes, *Bacteroides*, and *Clostridium* with high fat intake, changes that are associated with obesity and impaired glucose tolerance in humans.[104] The effects of a low-fat or high-fat diet may also depend on the health status of the individual, as people without a diagnosis of metabolic disease show little effect of a high fat intake on the GI microbiota.[59]

The type of dietary fat is also important in determining the effects on the GI microbiota. Intake of saturated fat reduces *Bifidobacterium*, *Roseburia*, and *Lactobacillus* and increases *Blautia* and *Bacteroides*—changes that are associated with increases in obesogenic traits in humans.[104,105] However, the effects of dairy-derived saturated fat on the GI microbiota are unclear and warrant further investigation, given the positive associations between dairy intake and health.[106,107] Conversely, unsaturated fats from olive, flax, and fish oil increase the abundance of Bacteroidaceae, *Bifidobacterium*, *Lactobacillus*, and *A muciniphila*.[50,59,69] However, though monounsaturated fat decreases richness, polyunsaturated fat shows either a null or positive effect on microbial richness and diversity in clinical trials.[50,59,69] More specifically, omega 3 and omega-6 polyunsaturated fats may have differential effects on the GI microbiome, with omega-3 fatty acids having bifidogenic and anti-inflammatory effects compared to omega-6 fatty acids.[50] Unfortunately, there is little research on the effects of dietary intake of SCFAs, plant sterols, or conjugated linoleic acid on the GI microbiota.[50] When assessing study results, health practitioners should be aware of confounding factors, such as the amount and type of carbohydrate and protein sources in the diet that may independently affect the GI microbiota.

Protein

The amount and type of protein in the diet affect the GI microbiome composition and function.[49,58,59,69] Increased protein decreases microbial richness, butyrate, and butyrate-producing taxa, as well as the abundance of *Bifidobacterium*.[49] These changes are accompanied by increased concentrations of proteolytic metabolites, including BCFAs, ammonia, amines, hydrogen sulfide, and phenolic and indolic acids.[7] Many of these protein-derived metabolites have been associated with detrimental effects in animal models and humans, including impaired barrier function, inflammation, and insulin resistance. However, indole metabolites have been found to have beneficial effects, suggesting that the ultimate health effects of protein fermentation are likely dependent on the balance of metabolites and the absorption and detoxification of potentially harmful metabolites.[7,49] Like the impact of high-fat intake, the potentially detrimental effects of high-protein intake on the GI microbiome and production of proteolytic metabolites may be due to decreases in carbohydrate intake and may be mitigated by increasing carbohydrate, fiber, and prebiotic consumption.[7,49,58]

Research into the effect of different protein types on the GI microbiota has centered on the impact of animal-based vs plant-based proteins. In animal models, meat-based proteins have been shown to increase the abundance of *Lactobacillus* while decreasing butyrate and SCFA-producing bacteria, compared to nonmeat proteins. Taking meat proteins and plant proteins as opposite ends of a spectrum, dairy proteins (whey and casein) seem to have intermediate effects between meat- and plant-based proteins on mouse microbiota.

However, these studies have been conducted almost exclusively in animal models, and well-controlled clinical studies are lacking.[108]

In addition to differences in amino acid profiles, animal- and plant-based proteins also differ in fat and carbohydrate content and profiles, as well as in the presence of other bioactive compounds, thus complicating interpretations of whole-food interventions. For instance, meat and eggs are rich in carnitine, choline, and phosphatidylcholine, which are metabolized by the GI microbiota to TMA, which is then converted to TMAO in the liver by an enzyme called flavin-containing monooxygenase 3 (FMO3).[68] Some research has shown that TMAO is a proatherogenic compound and, owing to the presence of its dietary precursors in foods such as red meat, is an indicator of an unhealthy dietary pattern.[109] However, the associations between TMAO and disease do not indicate a causative role but may be confounded by or dependent on the effects of kidney function, the GI microbiome, and FMO3 genotype.[1,109-111] Additionally, fish is rich in preformed TMAO and has the greatest impact on circulating TMAO concentrations; however, fish intake is associated with decreased risk of cardiovascular disease, whereas habitual intake of red meat and acute feeding of phosphatidylcholine are not associated with increased circulating TMAO.[1,109-112] There is also evidence that the amount of choline in the diet and its relationship with TMAO concentrations is related to the food form, with consumption of eggs resulting in lower circulating concentrations compared to a similar dose of choline within a supplement.[113] Ultimately, this suggests that TMAO is not an indicator of an unhealthy dietary pattern and is not increased by lipid-soluble choline, which is the predominant form of choline in foods such as eggs. Overall, the conflicting reports on TMAO limit its utility as a gut microbiota–derived marker of diet quality or health. As both fat and fermentable-carbohydrate intake are greater determinants of GI microbiota composition than protein amount or type, practitioners should focus on the overall composition and combination of macronutrients in the diet rather than on a single component.[105,108,114]

Effects of Specific Foods

In addition to the diversity of foods, consumption of individual foods affects the GI microbiota composition. A broad overview of foods and their effects on the GI microbiota and metabolites is provided in Box 14.3 (see page 238).[62-65,115] Whole plant foods (eg, nuts, fruits, vegetables, grains) are sources of dietary fibers and phytochemicals that contribute to effects on the GI microbiota.[44] The diversity of chemical compositions and physicochemical properties of fibers and phytochemicals in different foods leads to variability in their specific effects on the GI microbiota.[44,116]

Nuts

Nuts contain numerous nutrients that may influence the GI microbiome, including fiber, unsaturated fatty acids, and polyphenols.[117] Also, the structure of cell walls in whole, unprocessed nuts decreases the bioaccessibility of these nutrients, allowing them to resist digestion and absorption in the upper GI tract and, therefore, have a greater chance of interacting with the GI microbiota in the colon.[57] Nuts may increase bacterial diversity, though results have not been consistent.[62,63,118] Some experts suggest that nuts may have a prebiotic effects on the GI microbiota. However, a 2020 meta-analysis of studies investigating the effect of nuts on the GI microbiota showed that nut consumption did not increase *Bifidobacterium* or α-diversity, though there was a high degree of variability between studies due to differences in nut type, nut amount, and study duration.[117] Nut consumption did increase *Clostridium*, *Dialister*, *Lachnospira*, and *Roseburia* and decreased *Parabacteroides*.[116,117] *Clostridium*, *Lachnospira*, and *Roseburia* produce butyrate, an SCFA that is crucial for intestinal health and has been associated with beneficial metabolic effects. Furthermore, *Roseburia* has been negatively associated with fecal secondary bile acid concentrations, which have been associated

BOX 14.3

Overview of Effects of Foods on the Gut Microbiota and Metabolites[62-65,115]

	Gut microbiome	Metabolites
Nuts	↑[a] *Clostridium, Dialister, Lachnospira, Roseburia* ↓[b] *Parabacteroides*	↑ Short-chain fatty acids (SCFAs), urolithins, phenolic acids ↓ Secondary bile acids
Fruits	↑ Diversity with increased diversity of plant foods consumed ↑ Firmicutes (*Faecalibacterium*, Ruminococcaceae, Clostridiales)	↑ SCFAs, polyphenol metabolites (eg, urolithins)
Vegetables	↑ Diversity with increased diversity of plant foods consumed ↓ Firmicutes:Bacteroidetes ratio	↑ SCFAs, polyphenol metabolites (eg, enterolactone)
Grains	↑ Diversity, *Bifidobacterium, Clostridium,* Ruminococcaceae, *Lachnospira, Akkermansia, Roseburia, Lactobacillus*	↑ SCFAs, enterolactone
Legumes	↔[c] Diversity ↑ *Bifidobacterium, Lactobacillus*	↑ SCFAs
Dairy	↑ *Bifidobacterium, Lactobacillus*	↑ SCFAs, hippurate, malonate ↓ Trimethylamine-*N*-oxide, choline
Fermented foods	↑ *Lactobacillus, Prevotella, Bacteroides*	↑ Conjugated linoleic acid

[a] ↑ = increase
[b] ↓ = decrease
[c] ↔ = increase or decrease

with diseases such as IBD, metabolic syndrome, and cancer.[117] Therefore, the GI microbiome may contribute to the established health benefits of nuts.

Fruits and Vegetables

Fruits and vegetables contain dietary fiber, an abundance of vitamins and minerals, and a wide array of phytochemicals, such as flavonoids, isoflavonoids, lignins, stilbenoids, tannins, and polyphenols. Yet, though many studies have investigated the effects of supplementation of isolated plant compounds on the GI microbiome, there are few well-controlled interventions with whole plant foods. Additionally, most studies provide few details on the clinical relevance of observed changes in the microbiota. Furthermore, interindividual variability in the microbial response to these interventions is often observed, suggesting that an individual's baseline microbiota composition or habitual dietary intake may influence the effect or trajectory of the microbial community in response to the intervention.[116] Although intake of specific types or increased amounts of fruits and vegetables has been associated with increased GI microbiota diversity in some cases, these interventions generally do not increase diversity. As discussed, this may be more dependent on the diversity of plant foods rather than on a specific type or increased amount.[65,116,119]

The consumption of certain plant foods, however, does influence the abundance of specific taxa. For instance, broccoli, which is rich in dietary fiber and glucosinolates, decreased the Firmicutes:Bacteroidetes ratio by enriching *Bacteroides*.[64] The classification of vegetables, such as cruciferous or apiaceous vegetables, based on fiber and phytochemical content may be a useful way to categorize the effects of different vegetable foods. For example, adding cruciferous vegetables to a low-phytochemical, low-fiber diet resulted in increases in *Eubacterium*, *Alistipes*, *Eggerthella*, and *Phascolarctobacterium*, bacteria involved in the production of SCFAs and other bioactive metabolites such as enterolignans.[120-123] Classifying fruits and vegetables by the type of fiber they contain may also be useful. Intake of vegetables high in inulin-type fructans (an established prebiotic fiber), including artichokes, leeks, salsify, and onions, increases *Bifidobacterium*.[124] These strategies of classification may help alleviate the need to individually test the effects of different vegetables. However, other factors such as cooking method, host genotype (eg, glutathione *S*-transferase), gut transit time, and BMI that influence or have been associated with the metabolism of fiber or phytochemical components must also be taken into account.[64,120]

In addition to having unique fiber and phytochemical content compared to vegetables, many fruits also contain a higher concentration of sugars (eg, fructose and glucose) that can influence fermentation by the GI microbiota.[81] As the ratio of fructose to glucose alters the absorption of fructose in the small intestine, this may contribute to differential effects of fruits with different ratios of these sugars. For instance, the higher fructose-to-glucose ratio in apple juice vs white grape juice resulted in malabsorption and greater fermentation in the large intestine in humans in one randomized controlled trial.[81] Consumption of whole apples, rather than juice, has the addition of fiber (eg, pectin) and increases *Bifidobacterium* and *Lactobacillus*, as well as acetate concentrations.[125] Another study on apple intake, however, found no effect on the GI microbiota, highlighting the need for more studies on the effects of whole-food plant intake to clarify the effects of different foods.[126] Owing to their fatty acid composition and fiber content, avocados increase the concentration of stearic acid and palmitic acid, acetate, α-diversity, *Faecalibacterium*, *Lachnospira*, and *Alistipes*, while decreasing the concentrations of cholic acid and chenodeoxycholic acid (bile acids).[65] For all these reasons, the fiber, phytochemical, and sugar composition of various fruits will differentially affect the impact of fruit on the GI microbiota.

Grains and Legumes

Grains and legumes are predominant food sources for much of the world, with wheat being especially predominant in Western populations.[127] Much like the research on fruits and vegetables, most research into the effects of grains and legumes on the GI microbiota has focused on isolated fibers rather than intact cereal grains and pulses because of the complexity of fiber molecules and food matrices (eg, fatty acids, protein, vitamins, minerals, phytochemicals).[127] Though the effects of individual types of whole-grain cereals on the GI microbiota vary, the intake of mixed whole grains increases bacterial diversity, *Bifidobacterium*, *Clostridium*, Ruminococcaceae, and *Lachnospira*.[127-129] Conversely, reducing fiber intake by replacing whole grains with refined grains decreases Bacteroidetes, *Roseburia*, *Eubacterium*, and *Bifidobacterium*, as well as fecal SCFAs, particularly butyrate.[127] These changes may contribute to the benefits of consuming whole grains on health outcomes, such as liver fat, inflammation, and postprandial glucose and insulin.[128,129] Yet the high interindividual variability in responses may again be due to baseline microbiota composition and habitual dietary intake, particularly baseline fiber intake.[127,129] For instance, people with a habitually low fiber intake or low baseline microbiota diversity were determined, in a systematic review of relevant studies, to be more responsive to increases in whole grain and fiber intake, which suggests that these individuals may benefit more from an increase in whole-grain intake.[127] The literature on the effects of legumes on the GI microbiota is sparse, and results are inconsistent; but studies suggest that eating legumes does not increase GI microbial diversity.[130]

Animal and in vitro studies indicate that some pulses, such as chickpeas and mung beans, may increase the abundance of *Bifidobacterium*, *Lactobacillus*, and SCFAs,[131] but these results have not been replicated in humans.

Dairy

Dairy foods are sources of protein, calcium, and other essential nutrients, such as magnesium, potassium, phosphorus, zinc, and B vitamins.[107] Though there are some conflicting data on the health benefits of dairy, particularly high-fat dairy foods, meta-analyses reveal that dairy intake, including the consumption of high-fat dairy and fermented dairy products, has beneficial effects on cardiovascular disease risk, T2DM, and weight management.[132-136] The multitudinous dairy products, including milks of varying fat content and fortified with vitamins and minerals, fermented milk products (eg, cheese, yogurt, kefir), and dairy derivatives (eg, casein, whey) exhibit distinct nutrient profiles that may differentially determine their GI effects.[107] These effects may be mediated in part by the GI microbiome, as milk components—including lactose, protein, and fat—affect the GI microbiota composition.

Differences in lactose digestion and absorption affect the quantity of lactose that reaches the large intestine.[137] Lactose maldigestion results in lactose fermentation by the GI microbiota. In some people, greater increases in *Bifidobacterium* and gas production can cause GI distress, which is subsequently classified as lactose intolerance.[137,138] Fermented dairy products, such as yogurt and kefir, have lower lactose content due to lactose metabolism by microbes during the fermentation process (ie, the food production process), which allows for improved tolerance of these dairy products. However, lactose fermentation in the gut also increases *Bifidobacterium* and *Lactobacillus*, which are commensal bacteria.[137] Indeed, different dairy types, including milk, yogurt, and kefir, increase the abundance of *Bifidobacterium* and *Lactobacillus*, though these effects are not observed with the consumption of casein or whey derivatives.[107] The increase in these commensal bacteria via dairy intake or probiotic supplementation may help overcome or lessen the symptoms of lactose intolerance.[139] Because of the lack of clinical studies investigating the effects of different dairy types and components on the GI microbiome, it is unclear whether factors such as fat content may influence the effects of dairy on the GI microbiome and subsequent health outcomes. In sum, the consumption of dairy foods, but not isolated derivatives such as whey and casein, may beneficially modulate the GI microbiome while providing a dense source of nutrition.

Dietary Diversity

Dietary diversity is important for ensuring adequate intake of nutrients and microbial diversity in the GI tract. The diversity of foods, particularly plant foods, rather than traditional nutrient profiles (eg, macronutrients or micronutrients) or dietary categories (eg, vegan, vegetarian, omnivore) was shown to be the primary determinant of GI microbiota diversity and composition.[24,119,140] The American Gut Project, a collaborative research effort that includes samples from thousands of individuals, reported that people who consumed more than 30 types of plants per week and those who ate more fruits and vegetables had greater fecal bacterial diversity, greater abundance of SCFA-producing bacteria (eg, *F prausnitzii* and *Oscillospira*), and differing metabolite profiles, particularly higher levels of conjugated linoleic acid, compared to individuals who ate fewer than 10 types of plants.[119] Daily sampling of a small subset of individuals in a longitudinal study showed that GI microbiota profiles were more strongly correlated to foods than nutrient profiles, though food-microbe correlations were highly personalized. This study also reported that dietary diversity, rather than dietary stability (ie, eating the same foods consistently from day to day), was positively correlated with the stability of microbiota composition over time.[24] Though dietary diversity was not correlated with microbiota diversity in this small, longitudinal study, the resilience of the GI microbiota to perturbations and alterations in substrate availability is characteristic of a diverse ecosystem.[140] In sum, a greater diversity of plant foods, especially those with higher fiber and prebiotic content, may be important drivers of gut microbial diversity and composition.

Dietary Patterns

Although individual nutrients and foods may have specific effects on the GI microbiota, the totality of foods and nutrients consumed ultimately determines the overall composition and function of the gut microbial community (see Box 14.4).[66-70]

BOX 14.4

Effects of Common Dietary Patterns on Gut Microbiota and Metabolites[66-70]

	Effects on gut microbiome	Effects on metabolites
Western-style diet	↓[a] Richness, diversity, *Bifidobacterium, Lactobacillus, Eubacterium*	↓ Short-chain fatty acids (SCFAs), polyphenol metabolites
	↑[b] Firmicutes:Bacteroidetes ratio, *Bacteroides*, enterobacteria	↑ Trimethylamine-*N*-oxide, secondary bile acids, proteolytic metabolites
Mediterranean diet	↑ Richness, diversity, *Prevotella, Bifidobacterium, Faecalibacterium, Akkermansia*	↑ SCFAs, polyphenol metabolites
	↓ Firmicutes:Bacteroidetes ratio, *Bacteroides*	
Vegan or vegetarian diet	↑ Richness, Bacteroidetes	↑ Polyphenol metabolites
		↓ Bile acids, proteolytic metabolites
		↔[c] SCFAs
Ketogenic diet	↓ *Bifidobacterium, Lactobacillus*, Firmicutes:Bacteroidetes ratio	↔ Bile acids, SCFAs
	↑ *Fusobacteria, Escherichia*	↑ Hydrogen sulfide, lactate
Low-FODMAP[d] diet	↓ *Bifidobacterium, Lactobacillus*	↔/↓ SCFAs
		↓ Hydrogen, histamine
Gluten-free diet	↓ *Bifidobacterium, Lactobacillus, Roseburia, Ruminococcus bromii, Faecalibacterium prausnitzii*	↔ SCFAs
	↑ *Enterobacteriaceae, Escherichia coli*	

[a] ↓ = decrease
[b] ↑ = increase
[c] ↔ = increase or decrease
[d] FODMAP = fermentable oligosaccharides, disaccharides, monosaccharides, and polyols

---

Western-Style Diet

The Western-style diet is characterized by high intakes of animal protein; fat, particularly saturated and *trans* fats; sugar; and processed foods, as well as a low intake of fiber. Consequently, the high digestibility (ie, degradation and absorption in the small intestine) of this dietary pattern alters the amount and profile of substrates that reach the GI microbiota. This dietary pattern is often used in diet-microbiome studies to investigate the connection between high-fat and high-sugar consumption, the GI microbiome, and health outcomes such as obesity, T2DM, and cardiovascular disease. The Western-style diet has been associated with lower diversity and richness of bacteria and a lower abundance of *Bifidobacterium*, *Lactobacillus*, and *Eubacterium* and a higher abundance of *Bacteroides* and enterobacteria.[68,69] Diversity and richness, although not standalone indicators of a healthy microbiota, are generally associated with health in adults.[1] Likewise, *Bifidobacterium*, *Lactobacillus*, and *Eubacterium* contribute to beneficial health outcomes, such as immune modulation and butyrate production. The Western-style diet has also been associated with a higher ratio of Firmicutes:Bacteroidetes, which is a characteristic of the GI microbiota in individuals with obesity.[69] However, there is a lack of consistency between the Firmicutes:Bacteroidetes ratio and BMI; a meta-analysis of studies investigating the link between obesity and the GI microbiota found no statistically significant relationship between the ratio or individual abundances of these microbes and BMI.[141]

Mediterranean Diet

The Mediterranean diet is characterized by a high intake of fruits and vegetables, legumes, whole grains, nuts, seeds, and aromatic herbs, with extra-virgin olive oil as the main source of fat.[68] The Mediterranean diet is not a low-fat diet, as the total fat consumption is high (roughly 40% total energy intake), but extra-virgin olive oil is high in monounsaturated fat, so the ratio of monounsaturated to saturated fat is high (≥ 2).[142] Consuming a Mediterranean diet has been associated with a higher diversity of bacteria and higher abundance of *Prevotella*, *Bifidobacterium*, *Faecalibacterium*, and *Akkermansia*, and a lower Firmicutes:Bacteroidetes ratio and abundance of *Bacteroides*, compared to a Western-style diet.[68] The higher fiber and polyphenol content of the Mediterranean diet provides substrates for these enriched taxa and results in the production of microbial-derived metabolites, such as SCFAs and bioactive polyphenol metabolites (including urolithins, enterodiol, and enterolactone) that contribute to the anti-inflammatory and cardioprotective qualities of this dietary pattern.[7,68] Compared to the high saturated-fat intake typical of the Western-style diet, the fatty acid profile of the Mediterranean diet, which is high in polyunsaturated omega-3 fatty acids from fish and monounsaturated fat from olive oil, differentially modulates the composition and function of the GI microbiome.[50,59,68] Therefore, a Mediterranean diet may promote a GI microbiota composition and metabolite profile that contributes to beneficial health effects.

Vegetarian and Vegan Diets

A vegetarian diet restricts the intake of meat-based products and focuses primarily on plant-based foods. A vegan diet restricts the intake of all animal-based products and focuses exclusively on plant-based foods. Well-planned vegetarian and vegan diets may have beneficial health effects for the prevention and treatment of cardiovascular disease, T2DM, cancer, and obesity.[143] Studies have attempted to determine whether these dietary patterns induce changes to the GI microbiota that may contribute to their health benefits.[66,143-145] Indeed, different enterotype groupings have been associated with a high-carbohydrate, vegetarian diet (*Prevotella*) vs a high-protein diet rich in animal products (*Bacteroides*).[66] However, the taxonomic differences between omnivores and vegetarians and vegans are marginal, though some differences such as higher richness and abundance of Bacteroidetes in vegetarians and vegans have been reported.[119,143,144] The similarity in GI microbiota composition between omnivores, vegetarians, and vegans may reflect the common intake of nutrients (despite differences in food sources) or indicate the importance of different dietary classifications, such as dietary plant diversity.[119,143] Despite the lack of taxonomic differences, differences in metabolites between the omnivore, vegetarian, and vegan diet groups have been reported, including higher plasma concentrations of polyphenol metabolites and lower plasma concentrations of bile acids and proteolytic metabolites among vegans and vegetarians.[7,144] There are no differences in fecal SCFA concentrations between these diet groups, though the concentrations were correlated with intake of fruits, vegetables, and legumes, suggesting that plant intake, regardless of dietary group, is the main determinant of SCFA production.[119,144,146]

Ketogenic Diet

The ketogenic diet is characterized by a high fat intake (70%–90% of energy) and a very low carbohydrate intake (5%–10% of energy, or <50 g/d), with adequate protein (10%–20% of energy), though variations of the original diet have developed that vary in energy restriction and fat source.[147,148] Originally designed to treat epilepsy in children, the ketogenic diet has been popularized as a rebuttal to the low-fat approach to achieving weight loss.[148] Its effects on the GI microbiome, however, remain unclear, as studies are often confounded by other energetic or macronutrient intake changes. The limitation of carbohydrates, including nondigestible carbohydrates that are a preferred substrate for the GI microbiota, can alter the microbial community composition and function. In a clinical study conducted in 17 adults with overweight or class I obesity and without diabetes, consumption of a ketogenic diet decreased the abundances of *Bifidobacterium* and *Lactobacillus* and increased the abundances of Fusobacteria and *Escherichia*. The effects of a ketogenic diet were distinct from those of a high-fat diet, though, in that the ketogenic diet reversed the increase in the Firmicutes:Bacteroidetes ratio that was observed on a high-fat diet. The distinction between the effects of a high-fat diet and a ketogenic diet on the GI microbiota was due to ketone production, which inhibited bifidobacterial growth. These changes in the GI microbiota in response to a ketogenic diet may help mediate its neurological and immunomodulatory effects; however, the short- and long-term effects of these changes on GI and metabolic health are unclear.[149]

Low-FODMAP Diet

Recent dietary trends have also focused on a more targeted restriction of carbohydrates based on their FODMAP content—that is, on the amount of fermentable oligosaccharides, disaccharides, monosaccharides, and polyols (FODMAPs) they contain. Certain individuals experience GI discomfort, bloating, and diarrhea in response to eating FODMAPs because of GI conditions, including irritable bowel syndrome, IBD, or a sensitivity to these dietary components (see Chapters 3, 5, and 13). Some of these symptoms are due to the fermentation of carbohydrates by the GI microbiota, creating gas in the intestinal tract, and other symptoms are due to the osmotic activity of these compounds, drawing water into the intestinal tract.[150] Regardless, a low-FODMAP diet—less than 3 g oligosaccharides per day and less than 1 g polyols per day—effectively manages symptoms and decreases gas (eg, hydrogen) production.[151] A low-FODMAP diet decreases the abundance of *Bifidobacterium* and *Lactobacillus* in both healthy and diseased individuals.[150] Low-FODMAP diets may also decrease SCFAs, though study results are mixed because of differences in study design and SCFA quantification methods.[152]

A study in people with functional GI disorders showed that, compared to a low-FODMAP diet, low-dose prebiotic (β-galacto-oligosaccharide) supplementation in combination with a Mediterranean diet had similar beneficial effects on alleviating symptoms of GI discomfort while increasing the abundance of *Bifidobacterium*. The prebiotic group also experienced more lasting symptom relief following cessation of the diet compared to the low-FODMAP group. Though more research is needed to establish this as a reliable strategy, this approach may be a viable alternative to dietary restriction in individuals with functional GI disorders.[153]

The low-FODMAP diet consists of a restrictive phase, in which all FODMAP foods are eliminated, and a reintroduction phase, in which foods are systematically reintroduced to determine what foods may be consumed without triggering symptoms. Most studies only report results at the end of the restrictive period, without considering the less-stringent and prolonged reintroduction and maintenance phases, precluding the determination of long-term effects.[150] For these reasons, the reintroduction of FODMAP foods and the consumption of nonrestricted sources of dietary fiber, such as gluten-free grains and legumes (eg, brown rice, quinoa, lentils) and low-FODMAP fruits and vegetables (eg, broccoli, berries, tomatoes), may help restore the abundance of *Bifidobacterium* and *Lactobacillus* while also maintaining alleviation of symptoms.[154]

Gluten-Free Diet

Celiac disease and nonceliac gluten or wheat sensitivity cause various GI and extra-intestinal symptoms as a result of increased GI permeability and inflammation in response to gluten ingestion.[155] These GI disorders are often characterized by dysbiosis, including a reduction in *Bifidobacterium* and bacterial richness; however, it is unclear whether the onset of symptoms is due to inherent host factors (eg, genetics), environmental factors (eg, antibiotics, prior infection), or a combination.[155,156] Currently, a gluten-free diet is the only effective means of managing symptoms. In some individuals with celiac disease or gluten sensitivity, FODMAPs may also elicit symptoms, requiring additional targeted restriction. A narrative review of the literature found that a gluten-free diet normalized GI microbiota composition similarly in individuals with celiac disease or nonceliac gluten or wheat sensitivity vs healthy control subjects. Gluten-free diets and gluten-free products are marketed to the general public. Studies in healthy individuals revealed that a gluten-free diet decreases the abundance of commensal taxa, including *Bifidobacterium*, *Lactobacillus*, *Roseburia*, *R bromii*, and *F prausnitzii*, and increases opportunistic pathogens, including Enterobacteriaceae and *Escherichia coli*.[155] No changes in SCFAs or other biomarkers have been observed as a result of a gluten-free diet, though more research is needed using untargeted metabolomics to identify potential changes in microbial metabolite production.[157] In sum, restricting gluten-containing foods may beneficially alter the GI microbiota of people with gluten-related disorders but may negatively affect the GI microbiota of healthy individuals.

Dietary Recommendations for the Gastrointestinal Microbiota and Health

Diet affects the gut microbiota. Furthermore, changes in microbial composition and function have been connected with health outcomes. Yet, the connections between diet, the gut microbiome, and human health outcomes remain an early research area, with few high-quality randomized controlled trials clearly demonstrating causal connections between the microbiota and human health. Fortunately, healthful dietary patterns, such as those detailed in the *2020–2025 Dietary Guidelines for Americans*, support the GI microbiome (see Box 14.5).[158] Following these dietary guidelines can also help individuals consume the recommended amount of daily fiber (14 g per 1,000 kcal). The guidelines recommend eating a variety of plant foods, including vegetables, fruits, grains, nuts, and beans, which provide the gut microbiota with nutrients, including fiber and resistant starch but also phytonutrients and minerals, that are made more bioactive or accessible through actions of the microbiota. Furthermore, certain foods—including bananas, some whole grains, garlic, and onions—provide a source of prebiotic fibers, such as inulin-type fructans (fructo-oligosaccharides and inulin), and yogurts may contain probiotics.

BOX 14.5

Food-Group Recommendations That Support Health and the Gastrointestinal Microbiome[158]

Vegetables: Eating a variety of types of vegetables (dark green; red and orange; beans, peas, and lentils; starchy; and other vegetables) provides a source of dietary fiber, resistant starch, and prebiotics that gut microbes can metabolize. Phytonutrients are converted to bioactive components by the gut microbiota. The microbiota helps facilitate the absorption of micronutrients, such as calcium, that are less bioavailable in plant-based foods.

Fruits: Consuming a variety of whole fruits provides a source of fiber, prebiotics, and phytonutrients for microbial fermentation. The different types of fibers found within fruits provide fermentative substrates for a variety of microorganisms.

Grains: Whole grains provide a source of fiber, resistant starch, and phytonutrients, which gut microbes can metabolize. The microbiota helps facilitate the absorption of micronutrients, such as iron, found in whole grains.

Dairy: Some yogurts and fermented dairy beverages contain probiotics. Eating a fiber-rich diet in combination with calcium-rich dairy foods may also increase calcium absorption and bone mineralization via the promotion of short-chain fatty acid production.

Protein foods: Consumption of beans, peas, and lentils provides the microbiota with a source of fiber and resistant starch. The fiber and fatty acid profiles in nuts and seeds lead to a beneficial metabolite profile. Consumption of phytonutrient-rich plant proteins leads to the production of beneficial metabolites, such as equol from soy isoflavones, via microbiota.

Oils: Vegetable oils, nuts, and seafood provide polyunsaturated fats that help maintain microbial diversity. Individuals should limit their intake of total fat, *trans* fats, and meat-based saturated fat and emphasize the intake of polyunsaturated fats, particularly omega-3 fats.

Considerations for Evaluating the Quality of Diet-Microbiome Studies

The increased interest in the GI microbiome has prompted many new studies on the links between diet, the microbiome, and human health.[159] However, it is often difficult to interpret the significance or relevance of research findings, compare results from different studies, and translate results into actionable practices and recommendations.

Although associations between changes in certain microbes have been linked to diet or health outcomes, this may not necessarily indicate a causal relationship. Combining human clinical studies with animal and in vitro models is a robust way of identifying mechanisms and testing causal relationships between nutrients, microbes, and health outcomes. Studies conducted exclusively in animals or in vitro should be interpreted with caution, as their biological relevance is limited by the differences in murine GI physiology, microbiota composition, genetic background, coprophagy, housing conditions, and feeding, as well as the inability to test systemic effects using in vitro models.[160,161] Regarding intervention trials, adequate and relevant dosage must also be considered. For instance, most prebiotics require a dose of at least 3 g/d to elicit an effect.[74] Conversely, many studies, particularly animal studies, use high doses of compounds that are not relevant to normal levels of human consumption.[83]

Comparison of results between studies is also complicated by the heterogeneity of methods used in study design, sample collection and processing, and bioinformatic and statistical analysis.[159,160,162,163] Study design considerations include the type of dietary intervention (eg, food, nutrient, dietary pattern, dose, and so on), the duration of the intervention, and the study population used. Randomized controlled trials, especially those with a crossover design, are the best for discerning microbiota-health connections.[159] Multiple microbiota samples should also be collected at each time point, at least before and after the intervention, to control for daily intraindividual variability relative to the effects of the intervention.[159,163] Also, although fecal sampling is the most-used method for surveying the GI microbiota, this sample type is an approximation of the intestinal microbiota, containing both live and dead microorganisms. Despite these limitations, fecal sampling remains the preferred method, as it is noninvasive and easy to obtain frequently.[16] Variability introduced by different technological and statistical methods may overwhelm or exceed biological variability, thus masking true effects.[160,163,164] Additionally, differences in study populations based on demographic factors (eg, age, gender, health, or disease status) as well as lifestyle factors (eg, dietary intake, medication use, and exercise) may also introduce variability that makes the comparison of results difficult.[159,163] A lack of robust methods for accurate dietary assessment also remains an obstacle in diet-microbiota research, as self-reported dietary intake is often unreliable. The development of technologies for accurately assessing food intake, including image-assisted methods and biomarkers, and the development of tools such as microbiome-focused food intake questionnaires have the potential to improve our ability to discover meaningful connections between dietary intake and the GI microbiota.[159] In sum, when interpreting or comparing studies, it is important to critically assess the methods used and the study population to determine whether or how they may influence the results.

Emerging Research

Interindividual variability in the way the GI microbiome responds to diet is common. Scientists are increasingly focusing on personalized or precision nutrition as a lens through which to analyze this variability and determine its contribution to differences in health outcomes in response to dietary intake.[160,165] This personalized approach has shown promising results in predicting individuals' metabolic responses to foods based on their GI microbiota composition.[165-167] Most notably, personal and microbiota features enabled accurate prediction of glucose responses to different food items in a large cohort and improved postprandial glucose when used to prescribe personalized dietary recommendations.[166] The GI microbiota may also be used as a biomarker of dietary intake.[115,168]

The prospect of being able to determine what foods a person should eat, should not eat, or has eaten based on their GI microbiota composition is appealing to individuals, clinicians, and public health experts alike. Indeed, companies market kits and products designed to test the microbiota and provide dietary recommendations or to modulate the GI microbiota composition to improve metabolic response. The use of these products is still premature, given the current evidence linking particular features of the GI microbiota to metabolic response and disease risk. Also, lack of regulation or standardization leads to inconsistencies in results and difficulties in interpretation. This can result in unnecessary stress, dietary restriction, or supplementation, which may or may not have any health benefit and could lead to harm.[169] Though not currently a reliable tool for consumers to enact personalized dietary recommendations, GI microbiome testing is useful for increasing consumer awareness of the microbial community. Continued testing will also expand our knowledge base for future research that has the potential to bring personalized nutrition from theory to practice.

Moving forward, research must focus on both the short- and long-term effects of nutrients, foods, and dietary patterns on the GI microbiome, including taxonomic profiles, functional potential, metabolite production, and subsequent effects on human health. This research requires a complex approach involving large sample sizes to account for inter-individual variability and well-controlled interventions that account for different types, amounts, combinations, and preparations of foods and nutrients. Moreover, current databases of the nutrition components of foods focus on essential nutrients, covering only a small fraction of the total number of chemicals present.[170,171] Many of the thousands of other molecules present in foods have documented health effects, which may be mediated via the GI microbiota.[171] Chemical profiling and machine-learning techniques to better understand chemical exposure through the diet could help researchers map the complex effect of diet on the GI microbiota and human health.[170,171] This will allow for the elucidation of microbiome-mediated effects of diet on health and the identification of potential microbiome-targeted therapies and dietary strategies for improving human health.

Summary

The GI microbiome has become recognized as an important factor in human health. The complexity of the GI microbiome has led to the development of a myriad of methods used to measure, analyze, and interpret the composition and function of this community. Intake of specific dietary components or nutrients, specific foods, or dietary patterns has been shown to influence the composition and function of the GI microbiome in ways that may influence human health. Nutrition and other health professionals should be aware of nutrition recommendations to support the GI microbiome. Given the rising popularity of marketing toward the GI microbiome, practitioners should also be aware of the prematurity of specific, targeted recommendations based on GI microbiota composition.

References

1. Fan Y, Pedersen O. Gut microbiota in human metabolic health and disease. *Nat Rev Microbiol*. 2021;19(1):55-71. doi:10.1038/s41579-020-0433-9
2. Sender R, Fuchs S, Milo R. Are we really vastly outnumbered? Revisiting the ratio of bacterial to host cells in humans. *Cell*. 2016;164(3):337-340. doi:10.1016/j.cell.2016.01.013
3. Louis P, Young P, Holtrop G, Flint HJ. Diversity of human colonic butyrate-producing bacteria revealed by analysis of the butyryl-CoA:acetate CoA-transferase gene. *Environ Microbiol*. 2010;12(2):304-314. doi:10.1111/j.1462-2920.2009.02066.x
4. Costea PI, Hildebrand F, Arumugam M, et al. Enterotypes in the landscape of gut microbial community composition. *Nat Microbiol*. 2018;3(1):8-16. doi:10.1038/s41564-017-0072-8
5. Le Chatelier E, Nielsen T, Qin J, et al. Richness of human gut microbiome correlates with metabolic markers. *Nature*. 2013;500(7464):541-546. doi:10.1038/nature12506
6. Villa CR, Ward WE, Comelli EM. Gut microbiota-bone axis. *Crit Rev Food Sci Nutr*. 2017;57(8):1664-1672. doi:10.1080/10408398.2015.1010034
7. Roager HM, Dragsted LO. Diet-derived microbial metabolites in health and disease. *Nutr Bull*. 2019;44(3):216-227. doi:10.1111/nbu.12396
8. Lozupone CA, Stombaugh JI, Gordon JI, Jansson JK, Knight R. Diversity, stability and resilience of the human gut microbiota. *Nature*. 2012;489(7415):220-30. doi:10.1038/nature11550
9. Samarkos M, Mastrogianni E, Kampouropoulou O. The role of gut microbiota in *Clostridium difficile* infection. *Eur J Intern Med*. 2018;50:28-32. doi:10.1016/j.ejim.2018.02.006
10. Hjorth MF, Christensen L, Kjølbæk L, et al. Pretreatment *Prevotella*-to-*Bacteroides* ratio and markers of glucose metabolism as prognostic markers for dietary weight loss maintenance. *Eur J Clin Nutr*. 2020;74(2):338-347. doi:10.1038/s41430-019-0466-1

11. Jeffery I, Claesson M, O'Toole P, et al. Categorization of the gut microbiota: enterotypes or gradients? *Nat Rev Microbiol*. 2012;10(9):591-592. doi:10.1038/nrmicro2859

12. Wang DD, Nguyen LH, Li Y, et al. The gut microbiome modulates the protective association between a Mediterranean diet and cardiometabolic disease risk. *Nat Med*. 2021;27(2):333-343. doi:10.1038/s41591-020-01223-3

13. Ze X, Le Mougen F, Duncan SH, Louis P, Flint HJ. Some are more equal than others: the role of "keystone" species in the degradation of recalcitrant substrates. *Gut Microbes*. 2013;4(3):236-40. doi:10.4161/gmic.23998

14. Shanahan F, Ghosh TS, O'Toole PW. The healthy microbiome—what is the definition of a healthy gut microbiome? *Gastroenterol*. 2021;160(2):483-494. doi:10.1053/j.gastro.2020.09.057

15. Levy M, Kolodziejczyk AA, Thaiss CA, Elinav E. Dysbiosis and the immune system. *Nat Rev Immunol*. 2017;17(4):219-232. doi:10.1038/nri.2017.7

16. Claesson MJ, Clooney AG, O'Toole PW. A clinician's guide to microbiome analysis. *Nat Rev Gastroenterol Hepatol*. 2017;14(10):585-595. doi:10.1038/nrgastro.2017.97

17. Zhang X, Li L, Butcher J, Stintzi A, Figeys D. Advancing functional and translational microbiome research using meta-omics approaches. *Microbiome*. 2019;7(1):154. doi:10.1186/s40168-019-0767-6

18. Dominguez-Bello MG, Godoy-Vitorino F, Knight R, Blaser MJ. Role of the microbiome in human development. *Gut*. 2019;68(6):1108-1114. doi:10.1136/gutjnl-2018-317503

19. Walker RW, Clemente JC, Peter I, Loos RJF. The prenatal gut microbiome: are we colonized with bacteria in utero? *Pediatr Obes*. 2017;12(suppl 1):3-17. doi:10.1111/ijpo.12217

20. Bokulich NA, Chung J, Battaglia T, et al. Antibiotics, birth mode, and diet shape microbiome maturation during early life. *Sci Transl Med*. 2016;8(343):343ra82-343ra82. doi:10.1126/scitranslmed.aad7121

21. O'Toole PW, Claesson MJ. Gut microbiota: changes throughout the lifespan from infancy to elderly. *Int Dairy J*. 2010;20(4):281-291. doi:10.1016/j.idairyj.2009.11.010

22. Yatsunenko T, Rey FE, Manary MJ, et al. Human gut microbiome viewed across age and geography. *Nature*. 2012;486(7402):222-227. doi:10.1038/nature11053

23. Hollister EB, Riehle K, Luna RA, et al. Structure and function of the healthy pre-adolescent pediatric gut microbiome. *Microbiome*. 2015;3(1):36. doi:10.1186/s40168-015-0101-x

24. Johnson AJ, Vangay P, Al-Ghalith GA, et al. Daily sampling reveals personalized diet-microbiome associations in humans. *Cell Host Microbe*. 2019;25(6):789-802. e5. doi:10.1016/j.chom.2019.05.005

25. Costello EK, Lauber CL, Hamady M, Fierer N, Gordon JI, Knight R. Bacterial community variation in human body habitats across space and time. *Science*. 2009;326(5960):1694-1697. doi:10.1126/science.1177486

26. Spor A, Koren O, Ley R. Unravelling the effects of the environment and host genotype on the gut microbiome. *Nat Rev Microbiol*. 2011;9(4):279-290. doi:10.1038/nrmicro2540

27. Claesson MJ, Jeffery IB, Conde S, et al. Gut microbiota composition correlates with diet and health in the elderly. *Nature*. 2012;488(7410):178-184. doi:10.1038/nature11319

28. O'Toole PW, Jeffery IB. Gut microbiota and aging. *Science*. 2015;350(6265):1214-1215. doi:10.1126/science.aac8469

29. Wilmanski, T., Diener, C., Rappaport, N. et al. Gut microbiome pattern reflects healthy ageing and predicts survival in humans. *Nat Metab*. 2021;3(2):274-286. doi:10.1038/s42255-021-00348-0

30. Sonnenburg JL, Backhed F. Diet-microbiota interactions as moderators of human metabolism. *Nature*. 2016;535(7610):56-64. doi:10.1038/nature18846

31. Kelly D, Mulder IE. Microbiome and immunological interactions. *Nutr Rev*. 2012;70(suppl 1):S18-S30. doi:10.1111/j.1753-4887.2012.00498.x

32. Lustgarten MS. The role of the gut microbiome on skeletal muscle mass and physical function: 2019 update. *Front Physiol*. 2019;10:1435. doi:10.3389/fphys.2019.01435

33. Tripathi A, Debelius J, Brenner DA, et al. The gut–liver axis and the intersection with the microbiome. *Nat Rev Gastroenterol Hepatol*. 2018;15(7):397-411. doi:10.1038/s41575-018-0011-z

34. Chen YY, Chen DQ, Chen L, et al. Microbiome-metabolome reveals the contribution of gut–kidney axis on kidney disease. *J Transl Med*. 2019;17(1):1-11. doi:10.1186/s12967-018-1756-4

35. Steinert RE, Lee Y-K, Sybesma W. Vitamins for the gut microbiome. *Trends Mol Med*. 2020;26(2):137-140. doi:10.1016/j.molmed.2019.11.005

36. Sanidad KZ, Zeng MY. Neonatal gut microbiome and immunity. *Curr Opin Microbiol*. 2020;56:30-37. doi:10.1016/j.mib.2020.05.011

37. Kim S, Covington A, Pamer EG. The intestinal microbiota: antibiotics, colonization resistance, and enteric pathogens. *Immunol Rev*. 2017;279(1):90-105. doi:10.1111/imr.12563

38. Cryan JF, O'Riordan KJ, Cowan CSM, et al. The microbiota-gut-brain axis. *Physiol Rev*. 2019;99(4):1877-2013. doi:10.1152/physrev.00018.2018

39. Hawley JA. Microbiota and muscle highway—two way traffic. *Nat Rev Endocrinol*. 2020;16(2):71-72. doi:10.1038/s41574-019-0291-6

40. Hornef M. Pathogens, commensal symbionts, and pathobionts: discovery and functional effects on the host. *ILAR J*. 2015;56(2):159-162. doi:10.1093/ilar/ilv007

41. Dinan TG, Cryan JF. The microbiome-gut-brain axis in health and disease. *Gastroenterol Clin North Am*. 2017;46(1):77-89. doi:10.1016/j.gtc.2016.09.007

42. Dalile B, Van Oudenhove L, Vervliet B, Verbeke K. The role of short-chain fatty acids in microbiota–gut–brain communication. *Nat Rev Gastroenterol Hepatol*. 2019;16(8):461-478. doi:10.1038/s41575-019-0157-3

43. Bostanciklioğlu M. The role of gut microbiota in pathogenesis of Alzheimer's disease. *J Appl Microbiol*. 2019;127(4):954-967. doi:10.1111/jam.14264

44. Holscher HD. Dietary fiber and prebiotics and the gastrointestinal microbiota. *Gut Microbes*. 2017;8(2):172-184. doi:10.1080/19490976.2017.1290756

45. Alexander C, Swanson KS, Fahey GC, Jr, Garleb KA. Perspective: physiologic importance of short-chain fatty acids from nondigestible carbohydrate fermentation. *Adv Nutr*. 2019;10(4):576-589. doi:10.1093/advances/nmz004

46. Frame LA, Costa E, Jackson SA. Current explorations of nutrition and the gut microbiome: a comprehensive evaluation of the review literature. *Nutr Rev*. 2020;78(10):798-812. doi:10.1093/nutrit/nuz106

47. Boets E, Gomand SV, Deroover L, et al. Systemic availability and metabolism of colonic-derived short-chain fatty acids in healthy subjects: a stable isotope study. *J Physiol*. 2017;595(2):541-555. doi:10.1113/JP272613

48. Wu J, Wang K, Wang X, Pang Y, Jiang C. The role of the gut microbiome and its metabolites in metabolic diseases. *Protein Cell*. 2021;12(5):360-373. doi:10.1007/s13238-020-00814-7

49. Yao CK, Muir JG, Gibson PR. Review article: insights into colonic protein fermentation, its modulation and potential health implications. *Aliment Pharmacol Ther*. 2016;43(2):181-196. doi:10.1111/apt.13456

50. Mokkala K, Houttu N, Cansev T, Laitinen K. Interactions of dietary fat with the gut microbiota: evaluation of mechanisms and metabolic consequences. *Clin Nutr*. 2020;39(4):994-1018. doi:10.1016/j.clnu.2019.05.003

51. Laparra JM, Sanz Y. Interactions of gut microbiota with functional food components and nutraceuticals. *Pharmacol Res*. 2010;61(3):219-25. doi:10.1016/j.phrs.2009.11.001

52. Valdes AM, Walter J, Segal E, Spector TD. Role of the gut microbiota in nutrition and health. *BMJ*. 2018;361:k2179. doi:10.1136/bmj.k2179

53. Albenberg L, Esipova TV, Judge CP, et al. Correlation between intraluminal oxygen gradient and radial partitioning of intestinal microbiota. *Gastroenterol*. 2014;147(5):1055-1063.e8. doi:10.1053/j.gastro.2014.07.020

54. Martinez-Guryn K, Leone V, Chang EB. Regional diversity of the gastrointestinal microbiome. *Cell Host Microbe*. 2019;26(3):314-324. doi:10.1016/j.chom.2019.08.011

55. El Aidy S, van den Bogert B, Kleerebezem M. The small intestine microbiota, nutritional modulation and relevance for health. *Curr Opin Biotechnol*. 2015;32:14-20. doi:10.1016/j.copbio.2014.09.005

56. Gropper SS, Smith JL. *Advanced Nutrition and Human Metabolism*. Cengage Learning; 2012.

57. Mandalari G, Parker ML, Grundy MM-L, et al. Understanding the effect of particle size and processing on almond lipid bioaccessibility through microstructural analysis: from mastication to faecal collection. *Nutrients*. 2018;10(2):213. doi:10.3390/nu10020213

58. Scott KP, Gratz SW, Sheridan PO, Flint HJ, Duncan SH. The influence of diet on the gut microbiota. *Pharmacol Res*. 2013;69(1):52-60. doi:10.1016/j.phrs.2012.10.020

59. Yang Q, Liang Q, Balakrishnan B, Belobrajdic DP, Feng Q-J, Zhang W. Role of dietary nutrients in the modulation of gut microbiota: a narrative review. *Nutrients*. 2020;12(2):381. doi:10.3390/nu12020381

60. Korpela K. Diet, microbiota, and metabolic health: trade-off between saccharolytic and proteolytic fermentation. *Ann Rev Food Science Technol*. 2018;9:65-84. doi:10.1146/annurev-food-030117-012830

61. Tomás-Barberán FA, Selma MV, Espín JC. Interactions of gut microbiota with dietary polyphenols and consequences to human health. *Curr Opin Clin Nutr Metab Care*. 2016;19(6):471-476. doi:10.1097/mco.0000000000000314

62. Holscher HD, Guetterman HM, Swanson KS, et al. Walnut consumption alters the gastrointestinal microbiota, microbially derived secondary bile acids, and health markers in healthy adults: a randomized controlled trial. *J Nutr*. 2018;148(6):861-867. doi:10.1093/jn/nxy004

63. Holscher HD, Taylor AM, Swanson KS, Novotny JA, Baer DJ. Almond consumption and processing affects the composition of the gastrointestinal microbiota of healthy adult men and women: a randomized controlled trial. *Nutrients*. 2018;10(2):126. doi:10.3390/nu10020126

64. Kaczmarek JL, Liu X, Charron CS, et al. Broccoli consumption affects the human gastrointestinal microbiota. *J Nutr Biochem*. 2019;63:27-34. doi:10.1016/j.jnutbio.2018.09.015

65. Thompson SV, Bailey MA, Taylor AM, et al. Avocado consumption alters gastrointestinal bacteria abundance and microbial metabolite concentrations among adults with overweight or obesity: a randomized, controlled trial. *J Nutr*. 2021;151(4):753-762. doi:10.1093/jn/nxaa219

66. Wu GD, Chen J, Hoffmann C, et al. Linking long-term dietary patterns with gut microbial enterotypes. *Science*. 2011;334(6052):105-108. doi:10.1126/science.1208344

67. David LA, Maurice CF, Carmody RN, et al. Diet rapidly and reproducibly alters the human gut microbiome. *Nature*. 2014;505(7484):559-63. doi:10.1038/nature12820

68. Merra G, Noce A, Marrone G, et al. Influence of Mediterranean diet on human gut microbiota. *Nutrients*. 2021;13(1):7. doi:10.3390/nu13010007

69. Singh RK, Chang HW, Yan D, et al. Influence of diet on the gut microbiome and implications for human health. *J Transl Med*. 2017;15(1):73. doi:10.1186/s12967-017-1175-y

70. Asnicar F, Berry SE, Valdes AM, et al. Microbiome connections with host metabolism and habitual diet from 1,098 deeply phenotyped individuals. *Nat Med*. 2021;27(2):321-332. doi:10.1038/s41591-020-01183-8

71. Center for Food Safety and Applied Nutrition, US Food and Drug Administration. *Guidance for Industry: Scientific Evaluation of the Evidence on the Beneficial Physiological Effects of Isolated or Synthetic Non-Digestible Carbohydrates Submitted as a Citizen Petition (21 CFR 10.30)*. Docket no. FDA-2016-D-3401. March 2018. Accessed January 21, 2022. www.fda.gov/regulatory-information/search-fda-guidance-documents/guidance-industry-scientific-evaluation-evidence-beneficial-physiological-effects-isolated-or

72. Gill SK, Rossi M, Bajka B, Whelan K. Dietary fibre in gastrointestinal health and disease. *Nat Rev Gastroenterol Hepatol*. 2021;18(2):101-116. doi:10.1038/s41575-020-00375-4

73. Center for Food Safety and Applied Nutrition, US Food and Drug Administration. *Guidance for Industry: The Declaration of Certain Isolated or Synthetic Non-Digestible Carbohydrates as Dietary Fiber on Nutrition and Supplement Facts Labels*. Docket no. FDA-2018-D-1323. June 2018. Accessed January 28, 2021. www.fda.gov/regulatory-information/search-fda-guidance-documents/guidance-industry-declaration-certain-isolated-or-synthetic-non-digestible-carbohydrates-dietary

74. Gibson GR, Hutkins R, Sanders ME, et al. Expert consensus document: the International Scientific Association for Probiotics and Prebiotics (ISAPP) consensus statement on the definition and scope of prebiotics. *Nat Rev Gastroenterol Hepatol*. 2017;14(8):491-502. doi:10.1038/nrgastro.2017.75

75. Hill C, Guarner F, Reid G, et al. The International Scientific Association for Probiotics and Prebiotics consensus statement on the scope and appropriate use of the term probiotic. *Nat Rev Gastroenterol Hepatol*. 2014;11(8):506-514. doi:10.1038/nrgastro.2014.66

76. Swanson KS, Gibson GR, Hutkins R, et al. The International Scientific Association for Probiotics and Prebiotics (ISAPP) consensus statement on the definition and scope of synbiotics. *Nat Rev Gastroenterol Hepatol*. 2020;17(11):687-701. doi:10.1038/s41575-020-0344-2

77. Marco ML, Sanders ME, Gänzle M, et al. The International Scientific Association for Probiotics and Prebiotics (ISAPP) consensus statement on fermented foods. *Nat Rev Gastroenterol Hepatol*. 2021;18(3):196-208. doi:10.1038/s41575-020-00390-5

78. Stiemsma LT, Nakamura RE, Nguyen JG, Michels KB. Does consumption of fermented foods modify the human gut microbiota? *J Nutr*. 2020;150(7):1680-1692. doi:10.1093/jn/nxaa077

79. Taylor BC, Lejzerowicz F, Poirel M, et al. Consumption of fermented foods is associated with systematic differences in the gut microbiome and metabolome. *mSystems*. 2020;5(2):e00901-19. doi:10.1128/mSystems.00901-19

80. Di Rienzi SC, Britton RA. Adaptation of the gut microbiota to modern dietary sugars and sweeteners. *Adv Nutr*. 2019;11(3):616-629. doi:10.1093/advances/nmz118

81. Erickson J, Wang Q, Slavin J. White grape juice elicits a lower breath hydrogen response compared with apple juice in healthy human subjects: a randomized controlled trial. *J Acad Nutr Diet*. 2017;117(6):908-913. doi:10.1016/j.jand.2017.01.020

82. Sen T, Cawthon CR, Ihde BT, et al. Diet-driven microbiota dysbiosis is associated with vagal remodeling and obesity. *Physiol Behav*. 2017;173:305-317. doi:10.1016/j.physbeh.2017.02.027

83. Lobach AR, Roberts A, Rowland IR. Assessing the in vivo data on low/no-calorie sweeteners and the gut microbiota. *Food Chem Toxicol*. 2019;124:385-399. doi:10.1016/j.fct.2018.12.005

84. Ruiz-Ojeda FJ, Plaza-Díaz J, Sáez-Lara MJ, Gil A. Effects of sweeteners on the gut microbiota: a review of experimental studies and clinical trials. *Adv Nutr*. 2019;10(suppl 1):S31-S48. doi:10.1093/advances/nmy037

85. US Food and Drug Administration. Additional information about high-intensity sweeteners permitted for use in food in the United States. February 8, 2018. Accessed January 8, 2021. www.fda.gov/food/food-additives-petitions/additional-information-about-high-intensity-sweeteners-permitted-use-food-united-states

86. Hughes RL, Holscher HD, Davis CD, Lobach AR. An overview of current knowledge of the gut microbiome and low-calorie sweeteners. *Nutr Today*. 2021;56(3):105-113. doi:10.1097/NT.0000000000000481

87. Uebanso T, Ohnishi A, Kitayama R, et al. Effects of low-dose non-caloric sweetener consumption on gut microbiota in mice. *Nutrients*. 2017;9(6):560. doi:10.3390/nu9060560

88. Li S, Chen T, Dong S, Xiong Y, Wei H, Xu F. The effects of rebaudioside A on microbial diversity in mouse intestine. *Food Sci Technol*. 2014;20(2):459-467. doi:10.3136/fstr.20.459

89. Nettleton JE, Klancic T, Schick A, et al. Low-dose stevia (Rebaudioside A) consumption perturbs gut microbiota and the mesolimbic dopamine reward system. *Nutrients*. 2019;11(6):1248. doi:10.3390/nu11061248

90. Rowland I. Optimal nutrition: fibre and phytochemicals. *Proc Nutr Soc*. 1999;58(2):415-419. doi:10.1017/s0029665199000543

91. Kumar Singh A, Cabral C, Kumar R, et al. Beneficial effects of dietary polyphenols on gut microbiota and strategies to improve delivery efficiency. *Nutrients*. 2019;11(9):2216. doi:10.3390/nu11092216

92. Yin R, Kuo H-C, Hudlikar R, et al. Gut microbiota, dietary phytochemicals, and benefits to human health. *Curr Pharmacol Rep*. 2019;5:332-344. doi:10.1007/s40495-019-00196-3

93. Lampe JW, Atkinson C, Hullar MAJ. Assessing exposure to lignans and their metabolites in humans. *J AOAC International*. 2019;89(4):1174-1181. doi:10.1093/jaoac/89.4.1174

94. Romo-Vaquero M, Cortés-Martín A, Loria-Kohen V, et al. Deciphering the human gut microbiome of urolithin metabotypes: association with enterotypes and potential cardiometabolic health implications. *Mol Nutr Food Res*. 2019;63(4):1800958. doi:10.1002/mnfr.201800958

95. Espín JC, González-Sarrías A, Tomás-Barberán FA. The gut microbiota: a key factor in the therapeutic effects of (poly)phenols. *Biochem Pharmacol*. 2017;139:82-93. doi:10.1016/j.bcp.2017.04.033

96. Rusu IG, Suharoschi R, Vodnar DC, et al. Iron supplementation influence on the gut microbiota and probiotic intake effect in iron deficiency—a literature-based review. *Nutrients*. 2020;12(7):1993. doi:10.3390/nu12071993

97. Skrypnik K, Suliburska J. Association between the gut microbiota and mineral metabolism. *J Sci Food Agric*. 2018;98(7):2449-2460. doi:10.1002/jsfa.8724

98. Whisner CM, Martin BR, Nakatsu CH, et al. Soluble maize fibre affects short-term calcium absorption in adolescent boys and girls: a randomised controlled trial using dual stable isotopic tracers. *Br J Nutr*. 2014;112(3):446-456. doi:10.1017/S0007114514000981

99. Whisner CM, Martin BR, Nakatsu CH, et al. Soluble corn fiber increases calcium absorption associated with shifts in the gut microbiome: a randomized dose-response trial in free-living pubertal females. *J Nutr*. 2016;146(7):1298-1306. doi:10.3945/jn.115.227256

100. Whisner CM, Martin BR, Schoterman MHC, et al. Galacto-oligosaccharides increase calcium absorption and gut bifidobacteria in young girls: a double-blind cross-over trial. *Br J Nutr*. 2013;110(7):1292-1303. doi:10.1017/S000711451300055X

101. Asemi Z, Esmaillzadeh A. Effect of daily consumption of probiotic yoghurt on serum levels of calcium, iron and liver enzymes in pregnant women. *Int J Prev Med*. 2013;4(8):949.

102. Asemi Z, Bahmani S, Shakeri H, Jamal A, Faraji AM. Effect of multispecies probiotic supplements on serum minerals, liver enzymes and blood pressure in patients with type 2 diabetes. *Int J Diabetes Dev Ctries*. 2015;35(2):90-95.

103. Abrams SA, Griffin IJ, Hawthorne LM, et al. A combination of prebiotic short- and long-chain inulin-type fructans enhances calcium absorption and bone mineralization in young adolescents. *Am J Clin Nutr*. 2005;82(2):471-476. doi:10.1093/ajcn/82.2.471

104. Wolters M, Ahrens J, Romani-Perez M, et al. Dietary fat, the gut microbiota, and metabolic health—a systematic review conducted within the MyNewGut project. *Clin Nutr*. 2019;38(6):2504-2520. doi:10.1016/j.clnu.2018.12.024

105. Lang JM, Pan C, Cantor RM, et al. Impact of individual traits, saturated fat, and protein source on the gut microbiome. *mBio*. 2018;9(6):e01604-18. doi:10.1128/mBio.01604-18

106. Astrup A, Geiker NRW, Magkos F. Effects of full-fat and fermented dairy products on cardiometabolic disease: food is more than the sum of its parts. *Adv Nutr*. 2019;10(5):924S-930S. doi:10.1093/advances/nmz069

107. Aslam H, Marx W, Rocks T, et al. The effects of dairy and dairy derivatives on the gut microbiota: a systematic literature review. *Gut Microbes*. 2020;12(1):1799533. doi:10.1080/19490976.2020.1799533

108. Hughes RL, Holscher HD. Fueling gut microbes: a review of the interaction between diet, exercise, and the gut microbiome in athletes. *Adv Nutr*. 2021;12(6):2190-2215. doi:10.1093/advances/nmab077

109. Hamaya R, Ivey KL, Lee DH, et al. Association of diet with circulating trimethylamine-*N*-oxide concentration. *Am J Clin Nutr*. 2020;112(6):1448-1455. doi:10.1093/ajcn/nqaa225

110. Cho CE, Caudill MA. Trimethylamine-*N*-oxide: friend, foe, or simply caught in the cross-fire? *Trends Endocrinol Metab*. 2017;28(2):121-130.

111. Cho CE, Taesuwan S, Malysheva OV, et al. Trimethylamine-*N*-oxide (TMAO) response to animal source foods varies among healthy young men and is influenced by their gut microbiota composition: a randomized controlled trial. *Mol Nutr Food Res*. 2017;61(1). doi:10.1002/mnfr.201600324

112. Cho CE, Aardema NDJ, Bunnell ML, et al. Effect of choline forms and gut microbiota composition on trimethylamine-*N*-oxide response in healthy men. *Nutrients*. 2020;12(8):2220.

113. Wilcox J, Skye SM, Graham B, et al. Dietary choline supplements, but not eggs, raise fasting TMAO levels in participants with normal renal function: a randomized clinical trial. *Am J Med*. 2021;134(9):1160-1169.e3. doi:10.1016/j.amjmed.2021.03.016

114. Blachier F, Beaumont M, Portune KJ, et al. High-protein diets for weight management: interactions with the intestinal microbiota and consequences for gut health. A position paper by the My New Gut study group. *Clin Nutr*. 2019;38(3):1012-1022. doi:10.1016/j.clnu.2018.09.016

115. Shinn LM, Li Y, Mansharamani A, et al. Fecal bacteria as biomarkers for predicting food intake in healthy adults. *J Nutr*. 2021;151(2):423-433. doi:10.1093/jn/nxaa285

116. Willis HJ, Slavin JL. The influence of diet interventions using whole, plant food on the gut microbiome: a narrative review. *J Acad Nutr Diet*. 2020;120(4):608-623.

117. Creedon AC, Hung ES, Berry SE, Whelan K. Nuts and their effect on gut microbiota, gut function and symptoms in adults: a systematic review and meta-analysis of randomised controlled trials. *Nutrients*. 2020;12(8):2347.

118. Dhillon J, Li Z, Ortiz RM. Almond snacking for 8 wk increases alpha-diversity of the gastrointestinal microbiome and decreases *Bacteroides fragilis* abundance compared with an isocaloric snack in college freshmen. *Curr Dev Nutr.* 2019;3(8):nzz079. doi:10.1093/cdn/nzz079

119. McDonald D, Hyde E, Debelius JW, et al. American Gut: an open platform for citizen science microbiome research. *mSystems.* 2018;3(3):e00031-18. doi:10.1128/mSystems.00031-18

120. Li F, Hullar MA, Schwarz Y, Lampe JW. Human gut bacterial communities are altered by addition of cruciferous vegetables to a controlled fruit- and vegetable-free diet. *J Nutr.* 2009;139(9):1685-1691.

121. Wu F, Guo X, Zhang J, Zhang M, Ou Z, Peng Y. *Phascolarctobacterium faecium* abundant colonization in human gastrointestinal tract. *Exp Ther Med.* 2017;14(4):3122-3126. doi:10.3892/etm.2017.4878

122. Bess EN, Bisanz JE, Yarza F, et al. Genetic basis for the cooperative bioactivation of plant lignans by *Eggerthella lenta* and other human gut bacteria. *Nat Microbiol.* 2020;5(1):56-66. doi:10.1038/s41564-019-0596-1

123. Mukherjee A, Lordan C, Ross P, Cotter PD. Gut microbes from the phylogenetically diverse genus *Eubacterium* and their various contributions to gut health. *Gut Microbes.* 2020;12(1):1802866. doi:10.1080/19490976.2020.1802866

124. Hiel S, Bindels LB, Pachikian BD, et al. Effects of a diet based on inulin-rich vegetables on gut health and nutritional behavior in healthy humans. *Am J Clin Nutr.* 2019;109(6):1683-1695. doi:10.1093/ajcn/nqz001

125. Shinohara K, Ohashi Y, Kawasumi K, Terada A, Fujisawa T. Effect of apple intake on fecal microbiota and metabolites in humans. *Anaerobe.* 2010;16(5):510-515. doi:10.1016/j.anaerobe.2010.03.005

126. Ravn-Haren G, Dragsted LO, Buch-Andersen T, et al. Intake of whole apples or clear apple juice has contrasting effects on plasma lipids in healthy volunteers. *Eur J Nutr.* 2013;52(8):1875-1889.

127. Jefferson A, Adolphus K. The effects of intact cereal grain fibers, including wheat bran on the gut microbiota composition of healthy adults: a systematic review. *Front Nutr.* 2019;6:33.

128. Van Trijp MPH, Schutte S, Esser D, et al. Minor changes in the composition and function of the gut microbiota during a 12-week whole grain wheat or refined wheat intervention correlate with liver fat in overweight and obese adults. *J Nutr.* 2021;151(3):491-502. doi:10.1093/jn/nxaa312

129. Martínez I, Lattimer JM, Hubach KL, et al. Gut microbiome composition is linked to whole grain-induced immunological improvements. *ISME J.* 2013;7(2):269.

130. Marinangeli CPF, Harding SV, Zafron M, Rideout TC. A systematic review of the effect of dietary pulses on microbial populations inhabiting the human gut. *Beneficial Microbes.* 2020;11(5):457-468.

131. Yao ZD, Cao YN, Peng LX, Yan ZY, Zhao G. Coarse cereals and legume grains exert beneficial effects through their interaction with gut microbiota: a review. *J Agric Food Chem.* 2021;69(3):861-877. doi:10.1021/acs.jafc.0c05691

132. Kratz M, Baars T, Guyenet S. The relationship between high-fat dairy consumption and obesity, cardiovascular, and metabolic disease. *Eur J Nutr.* 2013;52(1):1-24. doi:10.1007/s00394-012-0418-1

133. Guo J, Astrup A, Lovegrove JA, Gijsbers L, Givens DI, Soedamah-Muthu SS. Milk and dairy consumption and risk of cardiovascular diseases and all-cause mortality: dose–response meta-analysis of prospective cohort studies. *Eur J Epidemiol.* 2017;32(4):269-287. doi:10.1007/s10654-017-0243-1

134. Soedamah-Muthu SS, de Goede J. Dairy consumption and cardiometabolic diseases: systematic review and updated meta-analyses of prospective cohort studies. *Curr Nutr Rep.* 2018;7(4):171-182. doi:10.1007/s13668-018-0253-y

135. Sayon-Orea C, Martínez-González MA, Ruiz-Canela M, Bes-Rastrollo M. Associations between yogurt consumption and weight gain and risk of obesity and metabolic syndrome: a systematic review. *Adv Nutr.* 2017;8(1):146S-154S. doi:10.3945/an.115.011536

136. Martinez-Gonzalez MA, Sayon-Orea C, Ruiz-Canela M, de la Fuente C, Gea A, Bes-Rastrollo M. Yogurt consumption, weight change and risk of overweight/obesity: the SUN cohort study. *Nutr Metab Cardiovasc Dis.* 2014;24(11):1189-1196. doi:10.1016/j.numecd.2014.05.015

137. Misselwitz B, Butter M, Verbeke K, Fox MR. Update on lactose malabsorption and intolerance: pathogenesis, diagnosis and clinical management. *Gut.* 2019;68(11):2080-2091. doi:10.1136/gutjnl-2019-318404

138. Li X, Yin J, Zhu Y, et al. Effects of whole milk supplementation on gut microbiota and cardiometabolic biomarkers in subjects with and without lactose malabsorption. *Nutrients.* 2018;10(10):1403. doi:10.3390/nu10101403

139. Heaney RP. Dairy intake, dietary adequacy, and lactose intolerance. *Adv Nutr.* 2013;4(2):151-156. doi:10.3945/an.112.003368

140. Heiman ML, Greenway FL. A healthy gastrointestinal microbiome is dependent on dietary diversity. *Mol Metab.* 2016;5(5):317-320. doi:10.1016/j.molmet.2016.02.005

141. Sze MA, Schloss PD. Looking for a signal in the noise: revisiting obesity and the microbiome. *mBio.* 2016;7(4):e01018-16. doi:10.1128/mBio.01018-16

142. Trichopoulou A, Kouris-Blazos A, Wahlqvist ML, et al. Diet and overall survival in elderly people. *BMJ.* 1995;311(7018):1457-1460.

143. Losasso C, Eckert EM, Mastrorilli E, et al. Assessing the influence of vegan, vegetarian and omnivore oriented westernized dietary styles on human gut microbiota: a cross sectional study. *Front Microbiol.* 2018;9:317. doi:10.3389/fmicb.2018.00317

144. Wu GD, Compher C, Chen EZ, et al. Comparative metabolomics in vegans and omnivores reveal constraints on diet-dependent gut microbiota metabolite production. *Gut*. 2016;65(1):63-72.

145. Glick-Bauer M, Yeh M-C. The health advantage of a vegan diet: exploring the gut microbiota connection. *Nutrients*. 2014;6(11):4822-4838.

146. De Filippis F, Pellegrini N, Vannini L, et al. High-level adherence to a Mediterranean diet beneficially impacts the gut microbiota and associated metabolome. *Gut*. 2016;65(11):1812-1821. doi:10.1136/gutjnl-2015-309957

147. Trimboli P, Castellana M, Bellido D, Casanueva FF. Confusion in the nomenclature of ketogenic diets blurs evidence. *Rev Endoc Metab Disord*. 2020;21(1):1-3. doi:10.1007/s11154-020-09546-9

148. Kossoff EH, Hartman AL. Ketogenic diets: new advances for metabolism-based therapies. *Curr Opin Neurol*. 2012;25(2):173-178. doi:10.1097/WCO.0b013e3283515e4a

149. Ang QY, Alexander M, Newman JC, et al. Ketogenic diets alter the gut microbiome resulting in decreased intestinal Th17 cells. *Cell*. 2020;181(6):1263-1275.e16. doi:10.1016/j.cell.2020.04.027

150. Vandeputte D, Joossens M. Effects of low and high FODMAP diets on human gastrointestinal microbiota composition in adults with intestinal diseases: a systematic review. *Microorganisms*. 2020;8(11):1638.

151. Gibson PR, Halmos EP, Muir JG. Review article: FODMAPS, prebiotics and gut health-the FODMAP hypothesis revisited. *Aliment Pharmacol Ther*. 2020;52(2):233-246. doi:10.1111/apt.15818

152. Staudacher HM, Whelan K. The low FODMAP diet: recent advances in understanding its mechanisms and efficacy in IBS. *Gut*. 2017;66(8):1517-1527.

153. Huaman J-W, Mego M, Manichanh C, et al. Effects of prebiotics vs a diet low in FODMAPs in patients with functional gut disorders. *Gastroenterol*. 2018;155(4):1004-1007. doi:10.1053/j.gastro.2018.06.045

154. Varney J, Barrett J, Scarlata K, Catsos P, Gibson PR, Muir JG. FODMAPs: food composition, defining cutoff values and international application. *J Gastroenterol Hepatol*. 2017;32(S1):53-61. doi:10.1111/jgh.13698

155. Caio G, Lungaro L, Segata N, et al. Effect of gluten-free diet on gut microbiota composition in patients with celiac disease and non-celiac gluten/wheat sensitivity. *Nutrients*. 2020;12(6):1832.

156. Polo A, Arora K, Ameur H, Di Cagno R, De Angelis M, Gobbetti M. Gluten-free diet and gut microbiome. *J Cereal Sci*. 2020;95:103058. doi:10.1016/j.jcs.2020.103058

157. Bonder MJ, Tigchelaar EF, Cai X, et al. The influence of a short-term gluten-free diet on the human gut microbiome. *Genome Med*. 2016;8(1):1-11.

158. US Department of Agriculture, US Department of Health and Human Services. *Dietary Guidelines for Americans, 2020-2025*. 9th ed. US Department of Agriculture and US Department of Health and Human Services; 2020. Accessed February 17, 2022. www.dietaryguidelines.gov/resources/2020-2025-dietary-guidelines-online-materials

159. Johnson AJ, Zheng JJ, Kang JW, Saboe A, Knights D, Zivkovic AM. A guide to diet-microbiome study design. *Front Nutr*. 2020;7:79. doi:10.3389/fnut.2020.00079

160. Hughes RL, Marco ML, Hughes JP, Keim NL, Kable ME. The role of the gut microbiome in predicting response to diet and the development of precision nutrition models—part I: overview of current methods. *Adv Nutr*. 2019;10(6):953-978. doi:10.1093/advances/nmz022

161. Nguyen TL, Vieira-Silva S, Liston A, Raes J. How informative is the mouse for human gut microbiota research? *Dis Model Mech*. 2015;8(1):1-16. doi:10.1242/dmm.017400

162. Knight R, Vrbanac A, Taylor BC, et al. Best practices for analysing microbiomes. *Nat Rev Microbiol*. 2018;16(7):410.

163. Goodrich JK, Di Rienpzi SC, Poole AC, et al. Conducting a microbiome study. *Cell*. 2014;158(2):250-262. doi:10.1016/j.cell.2014.06.037

164. Comin M, Di Camillo B, Pizzi C, Vandin F. Comparison of microbiome samples: methods and computational challenges. *Brief Bioinform*. 2021;22(1):88-95. doi:10.1093/bib/bbaa121

165. Hughes RL, Kable ME, Marco M, Keim NL. The role of the gut microbiome in predicting response to diet and the development of precision nutrition models. Part II: results. *Adv Nutr*. 2019;10(6):979-998. doi:10.1093/advances/nmz049

166. Zeevi D, Korem T, Zmora N, et al. Personalized nutrition by prediction of glycemic responses. *Cell*. 2015;163(5):1079-1094.

167. Mendes-Soares H, Raveh-Sadka T, Azulay S, et al. Assessment of a personalized approach to predicting postprandial glycemic responses to food among individuals without diabetes. *JAMA Netw Open*. 2019;2(2):e188102-e188102.

168. Frankenfeld CL. Fecal bacteria as an addition to the lineup of objective dietary biomarkers. *J Nutr*. 2021;151(2):273-274. doi:10.1093/jn/nxaa359

169. Mills S, Lane JA, Smith GJ, Grimaldi KA, Ross RP, Stanton C. Precision nutrition and the microbiome. Part II: potential opportunities and pathways to commercialisation. *Nutrients*. 2019;11(7):1468.

170. Hooton F, Menichetti G, Barabási A-L. Exploring food contents in scientific literature with FoodMine. *Sci Rep*. 2020;10(1):16191. doi:10.1038/s41598-020-73105-0

171. Barabási A-L, Menichetti G, Loscalzo J. The unmapped chemical complexity of our diet. *Nature Food*. 2020;1(1):33-37. doi:10.1038/s43016-019-0005-1

Prebiotics

Kelly A. Tappenden, PhD, RDN, FASPEN

KEY POINTS

- The consumption of prebiotics is a nutrition strategy that may foster a diverse, robust, and stable intestinal microbiota associated with enhanced health and reduced disease risk or burden. Health-promoting effects of prebiotics often result from the metabolites produced by the microbes that are stimulated.
- Prebiotics and fiber are not synonyms because not all fibers have prebiotic activity, and not all prebiotics are fibers.
- The selection of specific prebiotics and fibers for clinical use should be based on documented clinical outcomes.

Introduction

The intestinal microbiota is critically important to human health, as reviewed in Chapter 14. Much of the current research is focused on strategies to modulate the intestinal microbiota and thereby achieve a microbial community profile associated with health. In contrast, other research efforts seek to mitigate or treat disease.

Diet is a crucial factor affecting the intestinal microbiota; therefore, multiple nutrition strategies have been explored to correct and maintain a beneficial microbiota. Chapter 16 reviews the role of probiotics to support health, in part by influencing the intestinal microbiota. Lesser explored and often misunderstood options to affect the microbiota for health include the consumption of dietary fiber and prebiotics. This chapter reviews the impact of prebiotic consumption on the composition of the intestinal microbiota, its associated metabolic functions, and its effects on human health. Information about dietary fiber is included to provide context for those fibers with prebiotic activity in humans.

Adequate dietary fiber consumption has been a central tenet of human health throughout history. Hippocrates first reported the value of dietary fiber consumption in 300 BC. This key health principle was again advocated centuries later, in the late 1800s, at the world-renowned health resort founded by brothers John and Will Kellogg (the Battle Creek Sanitarium), and it was linked to the prevention of chronic diseases by Denis Burkitt and Hubert Trowell in the 1970s.[1,2] Though it is difficult to separate the protective properties of fiber from the other components of plant foods (eg, micronutrients and phytochemicals), epidemiological studies indicate that dietary fiber intake, especially the intake of whole grains or cereal fiber, protects against the development of obesity, stroke, diabetes, and coronary heart disease.[3] Though not a causal observation, and many other diet and lifestyle changes are likely confounders, dietary fiber intake in the developed world has decreased over the past century, while chronic diseases have increased substantially over the same period.

Prebiotics Defined

The term *prebiotic* was coined in 1995,[4] nearly a century after the term *probiotic* first appeared in publication.[5] Since then, the definition of prebiotic has been reassessed according to shifting views of gastrointestinal (GI) ecology and advances in molecular sequencing methods.[6,7] In 2017, a consensus panel defined a prebiotic as "a substrate that is selectively utilized by host microorganisms conferring a health benefit."[8] This definition expands the concept of prebiotics to

- include noncarbohydrate substances;
- apply to substances that support microbe growth beyond the GI tract;

- include nonfood applications (ie, drugs, topical uses, intravaginal uses); and
- be applicable to animals and not just humans.

Despite the evolution of the concept, one element that remains central to the notion of a prebiotic is that it must confer a health benefit when properly consumed. Unlike *probiotics*, which are live microorganisms, *prebiotics* are the nutrients that support the abundance of the beneficial microbes that ordinarily reside in a particular environment. For dietary applications, prebiotics enrich members of the resident intestinal microbiota (including any resident probiotic strains). Prebiotics, like dietary fibers, are not hydrolyzed by stomach acids or intestinal enzymes; therefore, they generally reach the distal intestine intact and are available for fermentation by the microbes in the distal intestine.

Prebiotics vs Dietary Fiber

Prebiotics and dietary fiber are often considered the same thing, but they are distinct substances, and the terms should not be used interchangeably for two reasons: not all fibers are prebiotics, and not all prebiotics are fiber.

Briefly, many fermentable fibers are preferential fuels used by specific microbes or groups of microbes within the intestinal microbiota. In contrast, other, less fermentable fibers may influence the microbiota overall but do not have prebiotic activity. Similarly, though many prebiotics are indeed considered fibers, other types of nutrients, including specific fatty acids included within plants, may have prebiotic activity (see Figure 15.1).[8]

FIGURE 15.1 What is a prebiotic vs a fiber?

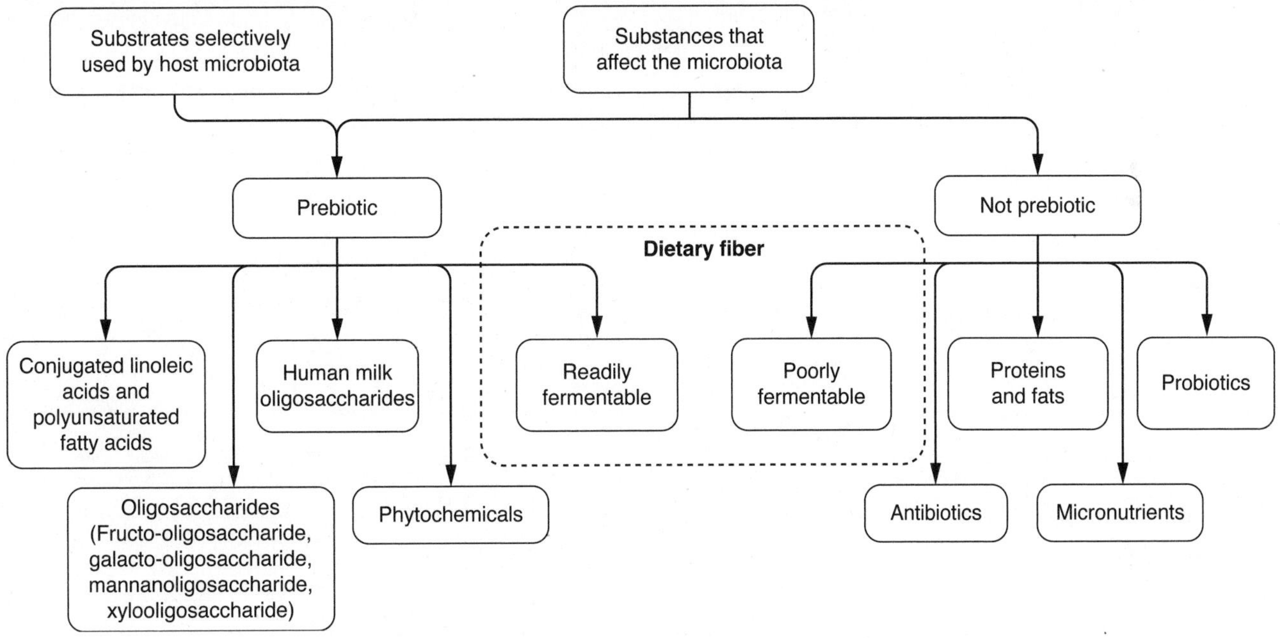

Prebiotics must be selectively utilized by the intestinal microbiota and produce a health benefit. Other substances affect the microbiota (some negatively), but they do not selectively target health-promoting microbes.

Adapted under CC BY 4.0 from Gibson GR, Hutkins R, Sanders ME, et al. Expert consensus document: the International Scientific Association for Probiotics and Prebiotics (ISAPP) consensus statement on the definition and scope of prebiotics. *Nat Rev Gastroenterol Hepatol.* 2017;14(8):491-502.[8]

Fiber Defined

In 2001, after considering the physiological, analytical, regulatory, and projected use in the 21st century, an expert panel of the Institute of Medicine (now the National Academy of Medicine) defined *total fiber* as the sum of two components: *dietary fiber* and *functional fiber* (also known as added fiber). Dietary fiber consists of nondigestible carbohydrates and lignin that are intrinsic and intact in plants, and functional fiber consists of isolated, nondigestible carbohydrates that have beneficial physiological effects in humans.[9]

The definition of total fiber was important because it highlighted the physiological impact of fiber consumption in humans, rather than chemical properties observed in a test tube (ie, soluble vs insoluble) as stratified in the gold standard analytical definition of fiber from the Association of Official Analytical Chemists (now AOAC International). Central to the National Academy of Medicine concept is that the physiological effect of fiber varies among food sources, fiber fraction, and chemical structures. For the purposes of this chapter, strict distinctions will not be made between dietary fiber and functional fiber, but the discussion will relate primarily to the physiological and health effects associated with all fiber consumed by humans, regardless of the categories defined by the National Academy of Medicine. The impact of fiber that is consumed with other nutrients and in the context of food matrixes vs the impact of fiber that is isolated and supplemented for functional purposes is acknowledged and important, but is beyond the scope of this discussion. Similarly, this chapter does not discuss other recent descriptions and terms that involve dietary fiber, such as microbiota-accessible carbohydrate.[10]

The Institute of Medicine expert panel recommended reliance on more meaningful physiochemical properties of dietary fiber that affect human health, specifically viscosity and fermentability. The classification of dietary fibers based on solubility was developed in accordance with fiber's longstanding chemical definition by the AOAC. Though relevant for product formulation, the attribute of solubility is less important in the human body. In addition, the oversimplification of physiological functions historically aligned with solubility is not factual. For example, generations of registered dietitian nutritionists were taught that soluble fiber was fermentable and that insoluble fiber was not fermentable. Though a tidy concept, solubility and fermentability are not strictly aligned, and soluble fibers vary in fermentability. For example, pectin is a soluble fiber that is readily fermented.[11] In contrast, methylcellulose is a soluble fiber that is not easily fermented by the human intestinal microbiota.[12] In fact, fermentability does not depend on solubility and occurs along a spectrum that is influenced by the intestinal microbiota present and intestinal transit time. As such, the fermentability of fiber in the body differs from species to species (eg, humans vs cows) based on attributes of the GI anatomy, transit time, enzyme expression, and the intestinal microbiota.

Prebiotics in the Human Diet

Prebiotics can be consumed via certain plants that are part of our diet, or they can be isolated for their functional value and consumed alone or supplemented in products.[13] Ample reports of human health benefits associated with galacto-oligosaccharides and fructo-oligosaccharides exist in the peer-reviewed literature, and other prebiotic substrates are under study.[14] The selection of a prebiotic for therapeutic use should be specific and based on peer-reviewed, published evidence because prebiotic effects cannot be generalized across various compounds. For example, fructans, which are incorporated into many consumer and medical-nutrition foods, are prebiotics that occur in differing degrees of polymerization (ie, in different chain lengths). The therapeutic use of prebiotics must be based on well-controlled, peer-reviewed evidence for the target population.

Some fermentable fibers, without prebiotic action, may affect the intestinal microbiota by inducing changes in transit time and interactions with other nutrients within the chyme.

This contrasts with prebiotics that provide targeted support to selective health-promoting microbes within the microbiota (see Figure 15.1). As such, prebiotics are not metabolized broadly by microbial community members but rather stimulate the abundance, or activity, of specific health-promoting microbial groups, such as *Bifidobacterium*, *Lactobacillus*, and other microbial groups associated with a defined health benefit.[8]

Health-Promoting Benefits of Prebiotics

The health-promoting effects of prebiotics often result from the metabolites produced by the microbes that are stimulated. For example, fermentation is the primary pathway by which most intestinal microbes make use of the prebiotic substrates. The major fermentation end products include the short-chain fatty acids (acetate, propionate, and butyrate), which have beneficial health effects relating to colonocyte function, metabolism, immune function, blood lipids, renal physiology, and appetite regulation.[15-18] In addition, metabolites produced from prebiotic metabolism, as well as partially digested prebiotics, may serve as substrates for other microbes, a concept called cross-feeding. Thus, rather than affecting only a single microbe or small groups of microbes, the intestinal microbiota exists as a complex, competitive ecosystem involving a community of microbes that ultimately influences the overall function of the intestinal microbiota.[19] Furthermore, metabolites produced by the microbial community likely play an important role in the observed health benefits, supporting the value of metabonomic assessment (ie, global dynamic metabolic responses of the microbial community) rather than the simple identification of species present in the intestinal microbiota.[20]

The details of well-designed clinical trials demonstrating the health benefits and reduced disease risk or burden associated with prebiotics are reported elsewhere.[8] Box 15.1 provides a summary of the health impacts of orally administered prebiotics reported in human clinical trials.[21-51] The remainder of this section discusses systematic reviews and meta-analyses of the benefit of prebiotic consumption for various populations or conditions, with a focus on how it effectively reduces disease risk or burden. A great deal of variation exists among prebiotic type, dose, duration, and mode of consumption in the current literature, and analysis of these issues is beyond the scope of this chapter. Readers should refer to the references cited for details regarding specific prebiotic treatment protocols for the conditions discussed.

BOX 15.1

Health Impacts Reported in Human Trials of Orally Administered Prebiotics[21-51]

Health end point	Prebiotics used
Reduced incidence of necrotizing enterocolitis in preterm infants[23]	Galacto-oligosaccharides (GOS), fructo-oligosaccharides (FOS)
Long-term improvement of colonization in intestinal microbiota of formula-fed infants[24-26]	GOS, FOS
Bowel habit and general gastrointestinal health in infants[27,28]	GOS, FOS

Box continues

BOX 15.1 (CONTINUED)

Health end point	Prebiotics used
Reduced incidence of infection and fever during first 6 months through 2 years of life in formula-fed infants[29,30]	GOS, FOS
Less manifestation of allergic symptoms (eczema, hives, wheezing, atopic dermatitis) during first 2 years of life in formula-fed infants[30,31]	GOS, FOS
Improved absorption of various minerals, including calcium, enhancing bone health[32-35]	GOS
Improved skin health and hydration, reduced erythema[36]	GOS
Enhanced satiety, decreased appetite[37-40]	FOS
Improved metabolic health[21,22,38,41-43] • reduced overweight and obesity • control of type 2 diabetes mellitus • diminished metabolic syndrome and dyslipidemia • decreased inflammation	FOS, oligofructose, inulin, GOS
Reduced severity of symptoms in irritable bowel syndrome[44]	GOS
Relief of constipation[45,46]	Inulin
Relief and prevention of traveler's diarrhea[47]	GOS
Improved urogenital health[48]	GOS
Reduced recurrence of *Clostridioides difficile*–associated diarrhea[49]	Oligofructose
Enhanced immune function in elderly individuals[50,51]	GOS

Infant Health Benefits

The value of prebiotic consumption has been demonstrated for vulnerable populations early in life. One meta-analysis reported that preterm infants who were given prebiotics showed significant decreases in the incidence of sepsis, mortality, length of hospital stay, and time to full enteral feeding, compared to infants in control groups.[52] Furthermore, when these investigators evaluated the impact of *Lactobacillus* and *Bifidobacterium* probiotics on these outcomes in preterm infants, necrotizing enterocolitis morbidity and mortality were significantly reduced when prebiotics were coadministered.[53] Though the mechanism has not yet been elucidated, prebiotic consumption in preterm infants increases the relative abundance of bifidobacteria,[54] which is beneficial and predominant in healthy infants consuming human milk.[55] Reduced mortality in children hospitalized with severe, acute malnutrition is associated with prebiotic treatment (vs control measures).[56]

A prominent ailment in healthy infants is the atopic march—the pattern in which atopic dermatitis develops early in life and is later followed by food allergies, allergic rhinitis, and allergic asthma. The potential for prebiotic therapy to mitigate the dysbiotic intestinal microbiota associated with these infants has been of interest in reducing disease susceptibility and severity. Prebiotic consumption in healthy term infants, without a family history of atopy, has been found to reduce the incidence of eczema and asthma.[57] Similarly, incidences of eczema and systemic sensitization during the first 2 years of life in healthy children are reduced with prebiotic consumption, according to a meta-analysis.[58] Although research into the value of probiotics on the development of childhood asthma revealed no difference between children receiving probiotics and children receiving placebo, prebiotic consumption was observed to lower the incidence of asthma development.[59]

Improved Immune Function

Strong and appropriate immune responses are a physiological function necessary for human health. Given that dysbiosis is often associated with impaired immune function (see Chapter 14), prebiotic therapy has been investigated for its impact on the incidence of infections, vaccine efficacy, and systemic inflammation. A systematic review and meta-analysis reported that prebiotic consumption in children aged 0 to 24 months prevented acute infectious disease, as evidenced by fewer overall infections and infectious episodes requiring antibiotic therapy.[60]

Vaccine efficacy is reported to be enhanced with prebiotic consumption. Healthy adult study subjects who consumed prebiotics had enhanced seroconversion (B strain influenza) and seroprotection (H1N1 and H3N2 influenza strains) after being inoculated with influenza vaccines, compared to those who were given a placebo.[61] Similarly, study subjects who took prebiotic supplements had higher influenza hemagglutination inhibition antibody titers (A/H1N1, A/H3N2, B strains) after vaccination than control subjects.[62] Prebiotic interventions also affect infectious susceptibility, as evidenced by decreased viral load, less-severe symptoms, fewer infections, and reduced mortality rate associated with respiratory viral infections.[63] The prebiotic effects in these studies were associated with beneficial changes in key mediators of host defense, including interferon-α, interferon-γ, interleukin-12, interleukin-1γ, tumor necrosis factor α (TNF-α), and interleukin-6.

Decreased Inflammation

Though a vital aspect of the human defense mechanism and healing process, inflammation can be associated with poor outcomes when presenting acutely (ie, bronchitis, appendicitis, trauma) and chronically (ie, autoimmune disorders, metabolic syndrome). Biomarkers of systemic inflammation in humans, such as C-reactive protein (CRP) and TNF-α, are reduced with prebiotic treatment compared to placebo.[64] In studies of adult subjects with overweight and obesity, prebiotic consumption decreased systemic inflammatory markers (CRP, TNF-α, interleukin-1β, and lipopolysaccharide) compared to control subjects.[64]

Metabolic Disorder Benefits

Because of the link between metabolic syndrome and the intestinal microbiota, the potential impact of prebiotics in individuals with metabolic disorders has been of potential therapeutic interest. Prebiotic supplementation reduced the plasma concentration of total cholesterol and low-density lipoprotein cholesterol (LDL-C) in individuals with obesity and diabetes, according to one systematic review and meta-analysis.[65] Furthermore, when adults with diabetes were analyzed alone, reduced serum triglyceride levels and increased high-density lipoprotein cholesterol (HDL-C) concentrations also occurred.[65] Individuals with metabolic syndrome are at increased risk for nonalcoholic fatty liver disease (NAFLD), a condition in which excess fat is stored in the liver. Prebiotic supplementation in adults with NAFLD reduced BMI, hepatic enzyme levels (alanine aminotransferase, aspartate aminotransferase, and γ-glutamyltransferase), and serum lipid levels (total cholesterol, LDL-C, and triglycerides), according to a 2018 meta-analysis.[66] A more recent report in adults with NAFLD confirmed that prebiotic supplements result in favorable changes in anthropometric, metabolic, and liver-related biomarkers (BMI; serum insulin concentration and insulin resistance; and alanine aminotransferase and aspartate aminotransferase, respectively).[67] The benefit of prebiotic consumption is also reported in healthy adult subjects by improving satiety and reducing postprandial glucose and insulin concentrations.

Gastrointestinal Disorder Benefits

Functional bowel disorders, such as irritable bowel syndrome, functional dyspepsia, and chronic idiopathic constipation, are the most common GI disorders in the general population, estimated to be present in one in four Americans.[68] Given that dysbiosis of the intestinal microbiota is commonly associated with pathophysiology, the use of microbial-directed therapies, such as prebiotic consumption, is of considerable interest.[69] Limited clinical trials investigating the therapeutic efficacy of prebiotic use in irritable bowel syndrome currently preclude systematic reviews and meta-analyses.[70-72] Whereas prebiotic consumption is reported to mitigate symptom severity associated with functional dyspepsia, a troubling problem arises, wherein recurring signs and symptoms of indigestion occur.[73] Prebiotic use also benefits chronic idiopathic constipation, as evidenced by increasing stool frequency, improving stool consistency, and normalizing intestinal transit time.[74]

Chronic Kidney Disease Benefits

Chronic kidney disease is a leading public health problem worldwide. It is characterized by a gradual loss of kidney function over time and is associated with diabetes, hypertension, heart disease, and a family history of kidney failure. Among patients with chronic kidney disease, prebiotic therapy improved markers of inflammation (CRP), oxidative stress (malondialdehyde, glutathione, and total antioxidant capacity), and lipid profiles (total cholesterol, LDL-C, HDL-C).[75-77] Further, prebiotic use also reduces the formation of the uremic toxin, *para*-cresol, blood urea, and serum phosphate concentrations; effects are hypothesized to occur by virtue of increasing intestinal *Bifidobacterium* and *Lactobacillus* abundance.[77]

Recommended Intake of Prebiotics

Most prebiotics studied to date require an oral consumption of 3 to 20 g/d to elicit a benefit; however, effectiveness depends on dietary fiber intake and the abundance of specific species within the intestinal microbiota.[78,79] Further, dosage recommendations should be made based on evidence relating to the specific prebiotic and clinical population, as supported by clinical evidence. Products containing quantities below this level should not be called prebiotics unless such a low dose is proven to stimulate selective effects in the microbiota and concomitant health aspects.[8] Similarly, prebiotic consumption of more than 20 g/d can have negative consequences, such as excess flatus.[80]

Summary

Recent and ongoing developments demonstrating the importance of the microbiota to human health are driving research aimed at microbiota-targeted interventions that foster, and in other instances correct, this active and influential community of microbes within the human intestine. Prebiotic and fiber consumption may be effective strategies for specific health and disease outcomes. Nutrition and other health professionals should ensure they are well-armed with knowledge of the different prebiotics and the associated effects on health and the intestinal microbiota.

References

1. Korczak R, Slavin JL. Definitions, regulations, and new frontiers for dietary fiber and whole grains. *Nutr Rev.* 2020;78(suppl 1):6-12. doi:10.1093/nutrit/nuz061

2. Burkitt DP, Trowell HC. Dietary fibre and western diseases. *Ir Med J.* 1977;70(9):272-277.

3. Reynolds A, Mann J, Cummings J, Winter N, Mete E, Te Morenga L. Carbohydrate quality and human health: a series of systematic reviews and meta-analyses. *Lancet.* 2019;393(10170):434-445. doi:10.1016/s0140-6736(18)31809-9

4. Gibson GR, Roberfroid MB. Dietary modulation of the human colonic microbiota: introducing the concept of prebiotics. *J Nutr.* 1995;125(6):1401-1412. doi:10.1093/jn/125.6.1401

5. Mackowiak PA. Recycling Metchnikoff: probiotics, the intestinal microbiome and the quest for long life. *Front Public Health.* 2013;1:52. doi:10.3389/fpubh.2013.00052

6. Bindels LB, Delzenne NM, Cani PD, Walter J. Towards a more comprehensive concept for prebiotics. *Nat Rev Gastroenterol Hepatol.* 2015;12(5):303-310. doi:10.1038/nrgastro.2015.47

7. Cunningham M, Azcarate-Peril MA, Barnard A, et al. Shaping the future of probiotics and prebiotics. *Trends Microbiol.* 2021;29(8):667-685. doi:10.1016/j.tim.2021.01.003

8. Gibson GR, Hutkins R, Sanders ME, et al. Expert consensus document: the International Scientific Association for Probiotics and Prebiotics (ISAPP) consensus statement on the definition and scope of prebiotics. *Nat Rev Gastroenterol Hepatol.* 2017;14(8):491-502. doi:10.1038/nrgastro.2017.75

9. Institute of Medicine (US) Panel on the Definition of Dietary Fiber; Standing Committee on the Scientific Evaluation of Dietary Reference Intakes. *Dietary Reference Intakes Proposed Definition of Dietary Fiber.* National Academies Press; 2001.

10. Sonnenburg ED, Sonnenburg JL. Starving our microbial self: the deleterious consequences of a diet deficient in microbiota-accessible carbohydrates. *Cell Metab.* 2014;20(5):779-786. doi:10.1016/j.cmet.2014.07.003

11. Cui J, Lian Y, Zhao C, et al. Dietary fibers from fruits and vegetables and their health benefits via modulation of gut microbiota. *Compr Rev Food Sci Food Saf.* 2019;18(5):1514-1532. doi:10.1111/1541-4337.12489

12. Bliss DZ, Weimer PJ, Jung HJ, Savik K. In vitro degradation and fermentation of three dietary fiber sources by human colonic bacteria. *J Agric Food Chem.* 2013;61(19):4614-4621. doi:10.1021/jf3054017

13. Brownawell AM, Caers W, Gibson GR, et al. Prebiotics and the health benefits of fiber: current regulatory status, future research, and goals. *J Nutr.* 2012;142(5):962-974. doi:10.3945/jn.112.158147

14. Rastall RA, Gibson GR. Recent developments in prebiotics to selectively impact beneficial microbes and promote intestinal health. *Curr Opin Biotechnol.* 2015;32:42-46. doi:10.1016/j.copbio.2014.11.002

15. Blaak EE, Canfora EE, Theis S, et al. Short chain fatty acids in human gut and metabolic health. *Benef Microbes.* 2020;11(5):411-455. doi:10.3920/bm2020.0057

16. O'Keefe SJ. Diet, microorganisms and their metabolites, and colon cancer. *Nat Rev Gastroenterol Hepatol.* 2016;13(12):691-706. doi:10.1038/nrgastro.2016.165

17. Roberfroid M, Gibson GR, Hoyles L, et al. Prebiotic effects: metabolic and health benefits. *Br J Nutr.* 2010;104(suppl 2):S1-S63. doi:10.1017/s0007114510003363

18. Pluznick JL. Gut microbiota in renal physiology: focus on short-chain fatty acids and their receptors. *Kidney Int.* 2016;90(6):1191-1198. doi:10.1016/j.kint.2016.06.033

19. Litvak Y, Byndloss MX, Bäumler AJ. Colonocyte metabolism shapes the gut microbiota. *Science.* 2018;362(6418):eaat9076. doi:10.1126/science.aat9076

20. Nicholson JK, Lindon JC. Systems biology: metabonomics. *Nature.* 2008;455(7216):1054-1056. doi:10.1038/4551054a

21. Beserra BT, Fernandes R, do Rosario VA, Mocellin MC, Kuntz MG, Trindade EB. A systematic review and meta-analysis of the prebiotics and synbiotics effects on glycaemia, insulin concentrations and lipid parameters in adult patients with overweight or obesity. *Clin Nutr.* 2015;34(5):845-858. doi:10.1016/j.clnu.2014.10.004

22. Kellow NJ, Coughlan MT, Reid CM. Metabolic benefits of dietary prebiotics in human subjects: a systematic review of randomised controlled trials. *Br J Nutr*. 2014;111(7):1147-1161. doi:10.1017/s0007114513003607

23. Armanian AM, Sadeghnia A, Hoseinzadeh M, et al. The effect of neutral oligosaccharides on reducing the incidence of necrotizing enterocolitis in preterm infants: a randomized clinical trial. *Int J Prev Med*. 2014;5(11):1387-1395.

24. Moro G, Minoli I, Mosca M, et al. Dosage-related bifidogenic effects of galacto- and fructooligosaccharides in formula-fed term infants. *J Pediatr Gastroenterol Nutr*. 2002;34(3):291-295. doi:10.1097/00005176-200203000-00014

25. Nakamura N, Gaskins HR, Collier CT, et al. Molecular ecological analysis of fecal bacterial populations from term infants fed formula supplemented with selected blends of prebiotics. *Appl Environ Microbiol*. 2009;75(4):1121-1128. doi:10.1128/aem.02359-07

26. Wopereis H, Sim K, Shaw A, Warner JO, Knol J, Kroll JS. Intestinal microbiota in infants at high risk for allergy: effects of prebiotics and role in eczema development. *J Allergy Clin Immunol*. 2018;141(4):1334-1342.e5. doi:10.1016/j.jaci.2017.05.054

27. Giovannini M, Verduci E, Gregori D, et al. Prebiotic effect of an infant formula supplemented with galacto-oligosaccharides: randomized multicenter trial. *J Am Coll Nutr*. 2014;33(5):385-393. doi:10.1080/07315724.2013.878232

28. Radke M, Picaud JC, Loui A, et al. Starter formula enriched in prebiotics and probiotics ensures normal growth of infants and promotes gut health: a randomized clinical trial. *Pediatr Res*. 2017;81(4):622-631. doi:10.1038/pr.2016.270

29. Arslanoglu S, Moro GE, Boehm G. Early supplementation of prebiotic oligosaccharides protects formula-fed infants against infections during the first 6 months of life. *J Nutr*. 2007;137(11):2420-2424. doi:10.1093/jn/137.11.2420

30. Arslanoglu S, Moro GE, Schmitt J, Tandoi L, Rizzardi S, Boehm G. Early dietary intervention with a mixture of prebiotic oligosaccharides reduces the incidence of allergic manifestations and infections during the first two years of life. *J Nutr*. 2008;138(6):1091-1095. doi:10.1093/jn/138.6.1091

31. Arslanoglu S, Moro GE, Boehm G, Wienz F, Stahl B, Bertino E. Early neutral prebiotic oligosaccharide supplementation reduces the incidence of some allergic manifestations in the first 5 years of life. *J Biol Regul Homeost Agents*. 2012;26(3 suppl):49-59.

32. Abrams SA, Griffin IJ, Hawthorne KM, et al. A combination of prebiotic short- and long-chain inulin-type fructans enhances calcium absorption and bone mineralization in young adolescents. *Am J Clin Nutr*. 2005;82(2):471-476. doi:10.1093/ajcn.82.2.471

33. Firmansyah A, Chongviriyaphan N, Dillon DH, et al. Fructans in the first 1000 days of life and beyond, and for pregnancy. *Asia Pac J Clin Nutr*. 2016;25(4):652-675. doi:10.6133/apjcn.092016.02

34. Holloway L, Moynihan S, Abrams SA, Kent K, Hsu AR, Friedlander AL. Effects of oligofructose-enriched inulin on intestinal absorption of calcium and magnesium and bone turnover markers in postmenopausal women. *Br J Nutr*. 2007;97(2):365-372. doi:10.1017/s000711450733674x

35. McCabe L, Britton RA, Parameswaran N. Prebiotic and probiotic regulation of bone health: role of the intestine and its microbiome. *Curr Osteoporos Rep*. 2015;13(6):363-371. doi:10.1007/s11914-015-0292-x

36. Kano M, Masuoka N, Kaga C, et al. Consecutive intake of fermented milk containing *Bifidobacterium breve* strain Yakult and galacto-oligosaccharides benefits skin condition in healthy adult women. *Biosci Microbiota Food Health*. 2013;32(1):33-39. doi:10.12938/bmfh.32.33

37. Cani PD, Knauf C, Iglesias MA, Drucker DJ, Delzenne NM, Burcelin R. Improvement of glucose tolerance and hepatic insulin sensitivity by oligofructose requires a functional glucagon-like peptide 1 receptor. *Diabetes*. 2006;55(5):1484-1490. doi:10.2337/db05-1360

38. Cani PD, Lecourt E, Dewulf EM, et al. Gut microbiota fermentation of prebiotics increases satietogenic and incretin gut peptide production with consequences for appetite sensation and glucose response after a meal. *Am J Clin Nutr*. 2009;90(5):1236-1243. doi:10.3945/ajcn.2009.28095

39. Parnell JA, Reimer RA. Weight loss during oligofructose supplementation is associated with decreased ghrelin and increased peptide YY in overweight and obese adults. *Am J Clin Nutr*. 2009;89(6):1751-1759. doi:10.3945/ajcn.2009.27465

40. Verhoef SP, Meyer D, Westerterp KR. Effects of oligofructose on appetite profile, glucagon-like peptide 1 and peptide YY3-36 concentrations and energy intake. *Br J Nutr*. 2011;106(11):1757-1762. doi:10.1017/s0007114511002194

41. Barengolts E. Gut microbiota, prebiotics, probiotics, and synbiotics in management of obesity and prediabetes: review of randomized controlled trials. *Endocr Pract*. 2016;22(10):1224-1234. doi:10.4158/ep151157.Ra

42. Dewulf EM, Cani PD, Claus SP, et al. Insight into the prebiotic concept: lessons from an exploratory, double blind intervention study with inulin-type fructans in obese women. *Gut*. 2013;62(8):1112-1121. doi:10.1136/gutjnl-2012-303304

43. Fernandes R, do Rosario VA, Mocellin MC, Kuntz MGF, Trindade E. Effects of inulin-type fructans, galacto-oligosaccharides and related synbiotics on inflammatory markers in adult patients with overweight or obesity: a systematic review. *Clin Nutr*. 2017;36(5):1197-1206. doi:10.1016/j.clnu.2016.10.003

44. Silk DB, Davis A, Vulevic J, Tzortzis G, Gibson GR. Clinical trial: the effects of a trans-galactooligosaccharide prebiotic on faecal microbiota and symptoms in irritable bowel syndrome. *Aliment Pharmacol Ther*. 2009;29(5):508-518. doi:10.1111/j.1365-2036.2008.03911.x

45. Christodoulides S, Dimidi E, Fragkos KC, Farmer AD, Whelan K, Scott SM. Systematic review with meta-analysis: effect of fibre supplementation on chronic idiopathic constipation in adults. *Aliment Pharmacol Ther*. 2016;44(2):103-116. doi:10.1111/apt.13662

46. Closa-Monasterolo R, Ferré N, Castillejo-DeVillasante G, et al. The use of inulin-type fructans improves stool consistency in constipated children. A randomised clinical trial: pilot study. *Int J Food Sci Nutr*. 2017;68(5):587-594. doi:10.1080/09637486.2016.1263605

47. Drakoularakou A, Tzortzis G, Rastall RA, Gibson GR. A double-blind, placebo-controlled, randomized human study assessing the capacity of a novel galacto-oligosaccharide mixture in reducing travellers' diarrhoea. *Eur J Clin Nutr*. 2010;64(2):146-152. doi:10.1038/ejcn.2009.120

48. Coste I, Judlin P, Lepargneur JP, Bou-Antoun S. Safety and efficacy of an intravaginal prebiotic gel in the prevention of recurrent bacterial vaginosis: a randomized double-blind study. *Obstet Gynecol Int*. 2012;2012:147867. doi:10.1155/2012/147867

49. Lewis S, Burmeister S, Brazier J. Effect of the prebiotic oligofructose on relapse of *Clostridium difficile*–associated diarrhea: a randomized, controlled study. *Clin Gastroenterol Hepatol*. 2005;3(5):442-448. doi:10.1016/s1542-3565(04)00677-9

50. Vulevic J, Drakoularakou A, Yaqoob P, Tzortzis G, Gibson GR. Modulation of the fecal microflora profile and immune function by a novel trans-galactooligosaccharide mixture (B-GOS) in healthy elderly volunteers. *Am J Clin Nutr*. 2008;88(5):1438-1446. doi:10.3945/ajcn.2008.26242

51. Vulevic J, Juric A, Walton GE, et al. Influence of galacto-oligosaccharide mixture (B-GOS) on gut microbiota, immune parameters and metabonomics in elderly persons. *Br J Nutr*. 28 2015;114(4):586-595. doi:10.1017/s0007114515001889

52. Chi C, Buys N, Li C, Sun J, Yin C. Effects of prebiotics on sepsis, necrotizing enterocolitis, mortality, feeding intolerance, time to full enteral feeding, length of hospital stay, and stool frequency in preterm infants: a meta-analysis. *Eur J Clin Nutr*. 2019;73(5):657-670. doi:10.1038/s41430-018-0377-6

53. Chi C, Li C, Buys N, Wang W, Yin C, Sun J. Effects of probiotics in preterm infants: a network meta-analysis. *Pediatrics*. 2021;147(1):e20200706. doi:10.1542/peds.2020-0706

54. Srinivasjois R, Rao S, Patole S. Prebiotic supplementation of formula in preterm neonates: a systematic review and meta-analysis of randomised controlled trials. *Clin Nutr*. 2009;28(3):237-242. doi:10.1016/j.clnu.2009.03.008

55. Moro G, Arslanoglu S, Stahl B, Jelinek J, Wahn U, Boehm G. A mixture of prebiotic oligosaccharides reduces the incidence of atopic dermatitis during the first six months of age. *Arch Dis Child*. 2006;91(10):814-819. doi:10.1136/adc.2006.098251

56. Noble CCA, Sturgeon JP, Bwakura-Dangarembizi M, Kelly P, Amadi B, Prendergast AJ. Postdischarge interventions for children hospitalized with severe acute malnutrition: a systematic review and meta-analysis. *Am J Clin Nutr*. 2021;113(3):574-585. doi:10.1093/ajcn/nqaa359

57. Osborn DA, Sinn JK. Prebiotics in infants for prevention of allergy. *Cochrane Database Syst Rev*. 2013;(3):CD006474. doi:10.1002/14651858.CD006474.pub3

58. Dang D, Zhou W, Lun ZJ, Mu X, Wang DX, Wu H. Meta-analysis of probiotics and/or prebiotics for the prevention of eczema. *J Int Med Res*. 2013;41(5):1426-1436. doi:10.1177/0300060513493692

59. Wawryk-Gawda E, Markut-Miotła E, Emeryk A. Postnatal probiotics administration does not prevent asthma in children, but using prebiotics or synbiotics may be the effective potential strategies to decrease the frequency of asthma in high-risk children—a meta-analysis of clinical trials. *Allergol Immunopathol (Madr)*. 2021;49(4):4-14. doi:10.15586/aei.v49i4.69

60. Lohner S, Küllenberg D, Antes G, Decsi T, Meerpohl JJ. Prebiotics in healthy infants and children for prevention of acute infectious diseases: a systematic review and meta-analysis. *Nutr Rev*. 2014;72(8):523-531. doi:10.1111/nure.12117

61. Lei WT, Shih PC, Liu SJ, Lin CY, Yeh TL. Effect of probiotics and prebiotics on immune response to influenza vaccination in adults: a systematic review and meta-analysis of randomized controlled trials. *Nutrients*. 2017;9(11):1175. doi:10.3390/nu9111175

62. Yeh TL, Shih PC, Liu SJ, et al. The influence of prebiotic or probiotic supplementation on antibody titers after influenza vaccination: a systematic review and meta-analysis of randomized controlled trials. *Drug Des Devel Ther*. 2018;12:217-230. doi:10.2147/dddt.S155110

63. Wang F, Pan B, Xu S, et al. A meta-analysis reveals the effectiveness of probiotics and prebiotics against respiratory viral infection. *Biosci Rep*. 2021;41(3):BSR20203638. doi:10.1042/bsr20203638

64. McLoughlin RF, Berthon BS, Jensen ME, Baines KJ, Wood LG. Short-chain fatty acids, prebiotics, synbiotics, and systemic inflammation: a systematic review and meta-analysis. *Am J Clin Nutr*. 2017;106(3):930-945. doi:10.3945/ajcn.117.156265

65. Qu H, Song L, Zhang Y, Gao ZY, Shi DZ. The effect of prebiotic products on decreasing adiposity parameters in overweight and obese individuals: a systematic review and meta-analysis. *Curr Med Chem*. 2021;28(2):419-431. doi:10.2174/0929867327666191230110128

66. Loman BR, Hernández-Saavedra D, An R, Rector RS. Prebiotic and probiotic treatment of nonalcoholic fatty liver disease: a systematic review and meta-analysis. *Nutr Rev*. 2018;76(11):822-839. doi:10.1093/nutrit/nuy031

67. Stachowska E, Portincasa P, Jamioł-Milc D, Maciejewska-Markiewicz D, Skonieczna-Żydecka K. The relationship between prebiotic supplementation and anthropometric and biochemical parameters in patients with NAFLD—a systematic review and meta-analysis of randomized controlled trials. *Nutrients*. 2020;12(11):3460. doi:10.3390/nu12113460

68. Talley NJ. Functional gastrointestinal disorders as a public health problem. *Neurogastroenterol Motil*. 2008;20(suppl 1):121-129. doi:10.1111/j.1365-2982.2008.01097.x

69. Kurokawa S, Kishimoto T, Mizuno S, et al. The effect of fecal microbiota transplantation on psychiatric symptoms among patients with irritable bowel syndrome, functional diarrhea and functional constipation: an open-label observational study. *J Affect Disord*. 2018;235:506-512. doi:10.1016/j.jad.2018.04.038

70. Asha MZ, Khalil SFH. Efficacy and safety of probiotics, prebiotics and synbiotics in the treatment of irritable bowel syndrome: a systematic review and meta-analysis. *Sultan Qaboos Univ Med J*. 2020;20(1):e13-e24. doi:10.18295/squmj.2020.20.01.003

71. Ford AC, Harris LA, Lacy BE, Quigley EMM, Moayyedi P. Systematic review with meta-analysis: the efficacy of prebiotics, probiotics, synbiotics and antibiotics in irritable bowel syndrome. *Aliment Pharmacol Ther*. 2018;48(10):1044-1060. doi:10.1111/apt.15001

72. Ford AC, Quigley EM, Lacy BE, et al. Efficacy of prebiotics, probiotics, and synbiotics in irritable bowel syndrome and chronic idiopathic constipation: systematic review and meta-analysis. *Am J Gastroenterol*. 2014;109(10):1547-1561; quiz 1546, 1562. doi:10.1038/ajg.2014.202

73. Zhang J, Wu HM, Wang X, et al. Efficacy of prebiotics and probiotics for functional dyspepsia: a systematic review and meta-analysis. *Medicine (Baltimore)*. 2020;99(7):e19107. doi:10.1097/md.0000000000019107

74. Collado Yurrita L, San Mauro Martín I, Ciudad-Cabañas MJ, Calle-Purón ME, Hernández Cabria M. Effectiveness of inulin intake on indicators of chronic constipation; a meta-analysis of controlled randomized clinical trials. *Nutr Hosp*. 2014;30(2):244-252. doi:10.3305/nh.2014.30.2.7565

75. Zheng HJ, Guo J, Wang Q, et al. Probiotics, prebiotics, and synbiotics for the improvement of metabolic profiles in patients with chronic kidney disease: a systematic review and meta-analysis of randomized controlled trials. *Crit Rev Food Sci Nutr*. 2021;61(4):577-598. doi:10.1080/10408398.2020.1740645

76. Bakhtiary M, Morvaridzadeh M, Agah S, et al. Effect of probiotic, prebiotic, and synbiotic supplementation on cardiometabolic and oxidative stress parameters in patients with chronic kidney disease: a systematic review and meta-analysis. *Clin Ther*. 2021;43(3):e71-e96. doi:10.1016/j.clinthera.2020.12.021

77. Lopes RCSO, Balbino KP, Jorge MP, Ribeiro AQ, Martino HSD, Alfenas RCG. Modulation of intestinal microbiota, control of nitrogen products and inflammation by pre/probiotics in chronic kidney disease: a systematic review. *Nutr Hosp*. 2018;35(3):722-730. doi:10.20960/nh.1642

78. Holscher HD, Bauer LL, Gourineni V, Pelkman CL, Fahey GC Jr, Swanson KS. Agave inulin supplementation affects the fecal microbiota of healthy adults participating in a randomized, double-blind, placebo-controlled, crossover trial. *J Nutr*. 2015;145(9):2025-2032. doi:10.3945/jn.115.217331

79. Tandon D, Haque MM, Gote M, et al. A prospective randomized, double-blind, placebo-controlled, dose-response relationship study to investigate efficacy of fructo-oligosaccharides (FOS) on human gut microflora. *Sci Rep*. 2019;9(1):5473. doi:10.1038/s41598-019-41837-3

80. Bouhnik Y, Vahedi K, Achour L, et al. Short-chain fructo-oligosaccharide administration dose-dependently increases fecal bifidobacteria in healthy humans. *J Nutr*. 1999;129(1):113-116. doi:10.1093/jn/129.1.113

Probiotics

Malissa Warren, RDN, LDN, CNSC
Robert Martindale, MD, PhD

KEY POINTS

- The human microbiota is described as a virtual organ composed of commensal microorganisms (eubacteria, archaea, filamentous fungi, yeasts, protozoa, viruses) that coexist in symbiosis with the body and that have a major impact on digestion, immune system development, cognitive functions, and longevity, as well as maintaining good health.
- Recommendations for probiotics should be based on national practice guidelines or, when not available, rigorous clinical trials that have tested specific probiotics or probiotic combinations using well-defined dosing, mode of administration, and patient population.
- Careful probiotic selection in the form of food or supplement can be a helpful adjunct to a diet that contains a wide variety of minimally processed foods, fiber, and prebiotics in maintaining a healthy microbiome and preventing dysbiosis.

Introduction

Since antiquity, live microbes in the form of fermented foods have been used for health purposes, yet the concept of a probiotic was not formally introduced until the early 1900s, when Élie Metchnikoff, a Russian Nobel Prize–winning scientist, proposed that consuming live microbes may benefit human health and prolong life. The word *probiotic* was first used in the 1950s by a German bacteriologist to describe various organic and inorganic supplements that were thought to restore the health of malnourished patients. Various definitions of the term have been proposed since then.[1] The currently accepted definition of probiotics by the International Scientific Association for Probiotics and Prebiotics is "live microorganisms that, when administered in adequate amounts, confer a health benefit on the host."[2] The minimum criteria that qualify a microorganism as a "probiotic" for use in food and dietary supplements are as follows[1,3]:

- The microorganism must be sufficiently characterized by strain identification and naming.
- It must be safe for the intended use.
- Its effectiveness must be supported by at least one positive human clinical trial conducted according to generally accepted scientific standards.
- The microorganism must be alive in the product at an efficacious dose throughout the shelf life.

Probiotic consumption continues to grow in the general public and the hospital setting. Experts in probiotics urge the use of the stated criteria to ensure that the term *probiotic* is used accurately and responsibly in scientific publications, dietary supplement product labels, clinical practice, and communication to the general public.[3] Experts estimate that the value of the global probiotics market will exceed $64 billion by 2022.[4]

The commercial market for fermented foods is growing substantially. Although fermented foods contribute an array of microbes to the diet that may be associated with health benefits, the International Scientific Association for Probiotics and Prebiotics clarified in a recent consensus statement (published in 2021) that fermented foods are not equivalent to probiotics. The bacterial composition of fermented foods is rarely defined, and established evidence for their health benefits is often lacking, with the exception of some yogurts and cultured dairy products for which there is a long history of research.[5] Box 16.1 provides a list of common fermented foods that provide live and active cultures; however, unless they meet minimum criteria, they may not be considered probiotics.[3]

BOX 16.1

Fermented Foods With Live and Active Cultures[a,3]

[a] Strains must be identified and labeled to be considered a probiotic.

Fermented dairy foods

Yogurt

Kefir

Aged cheeses (Swiss, provolone, Gouda, cheddar, Edam, Gruyère, and cottage cheese)

Fermented soy foods

Miso

Natto

Tempeh

Other fermented foods

Most kombuchas

Nonheated fermented vegetables (sauerkraut, pickles, kimchi)

Cultured nondairy yogurts

In the United States, oversight of probiotic dietary supplements is provided by the US Food and Drug Administration (FDA) under the Dietary Supplement Health and Education Act of 1994. Evidence of safety and current good manufacturing practice is required under the act. The FDA dictates that no product can be marketed to cure, mitigate, treat, or prevent disease. For this reason, manufacturers of probiotic supplements maintain general claims on product labels such as "supports digestive and immune health." It is the manufacturer's responsibility to demonstrate product safety and purity; premarket approval of safety and efficacy is not required by the FDA. Though medical foods must comply with food regulations, they are not required to obtain FDA approval before going to market.[6] Given the current process, the burden is placed on the consumer and clinician to distinguish between marketed probiotic products that are supported by high-quality evidence and those with poor-quality evidence. A US regulatory framework requiring FDA premarket approval of safety and efficacy would provide additional scrutiny. On the other hand, when probiotics are used for research purposes, they are frequently viewed as drugs by the FDA, in which case safety and efficacy studies within the FDA's Investigational New Drug framework are required.[7] The field of probiotics would benefit from more rigorous clinical trials that meet established quality standards (such as the Consolidated Standards of Reporting Trials, or CONSORT) to provide evidence in support of the efficacy and safety of well-characterized probiotic products with a clear rationale.[4]

Probiotics and Gastrointestinal Microbiota

Understanding probiotics requires knowledge of the gastrointestinal (GI) microbiota, the subject of Chapter 14. The focus of this chapter is on probiotics and their effect on the GI microbiota, which undoubtedly has repercussions on overall health and disease. According to a 2021 review article, the human microbiota is aptly described as a "virtual organ composed of commensal micro-organisms (eubacteria, archaea, filamentous fungi, yeasts, protozoa, viruses) that coexist in symbiosis with our body and have a major impact on digestion, immune system development, cognitive functions, even longevity, as well as maintaining good health."[8] Some probiotic bacteria that have been incorporated into foods or supplements are members of species found in the GI tract, but others have been isolated from food or animal sources and are not members of the typical human microbiota.

Whole-genome shotgun metagenomics has identified the dominant microbiota phyla in the GI tract as Firmicutes and Bacteroidetes, though Actinobacteria, Proteobacteria, Fusobacteria, and Verrucomicrobia are also present. In clinical studies, the microorganisms that make up the human GI microbiota are usually identified by their phylum, genus, and species. Box 16.2 provides the taxonomy for several examples of dominant bacteria in the GI microbiota, as well as their function.[9]

BOX 16.2

Taxonomy and Function of Several Dominant Bacteria in the Human Gastrointestinal Microbiota[9]

Phylum	Genus	Species	Function
Bacteroidetes (Gram-negative bacteria)	*Bacteroides*	*Bacteroides fragilis* *Bacteroides uniformis*	Polysaccharide fermentation and short-chain fatty acid production
	Prevotella	*Prevotella* spp	
Firmicutes (Gram-positive bacteria)	*Limosilactobacillus*	*Limosilactobacillus reuteri*	Energy resorption from colonic fermentation and short-chain fatty acid production
	Clostridium	*Clostridum* spp	
	Enterococcus	*Enterococcus faecium*	
	Ruminococcus	*Ruminococcus faecis*	

Lactic acid bacteria and bifidobacteria are commonly used microbes in dietary supplements. Other commonly used probiotics are from the *Bacillus* and *Saccharomyces* genuses.[10] Probiotics are identified by genus and species, as are all microbes. Probiotics are also identified by an alphanumeric strain designation. The strain designation ties a specific probiotic to evidence that supports any claimed benefits.[11] Box 16.3 on page 268 provides examples of common probiotic nomenclature.

The efficacy of a probiotic depends on several factors, including the specific strain or blend of strains used, the dose of those strains, the mode of administration, and the clinical endpoint, which may be prevention of a disease, treatment of a disease, or maintenance of health. The mechanisms that drive clinical efficacy are often unknown, but many are proposed. Not all mechanisms involve direct interaction with the resident microbiota. When considering evidence for probiotic efficacy, it is important to recognize that results are specific to the intervention, the study population, and the clinical endpoint. For example, certain probiotics are helpful in maintaining remission of ulcerative colitis but not in Crohn's disease. In making evidence-based recommendations, it is important to remember that not all strains of a species have the same clinical efficacy.[12] Lastly, recommendations should be tied to the specific dose or doses of a strain that was shown to be effective in clinical studies. Many commercial probiotic products contain 1 billion to 10 billion colony-forming units

(CFU) per dose or more, but some probiotics may be more effective at lower or higher doses for their intended use. Dosing recommendations should be dictated by the evidence.[12]

Beneficial Effects of Probiotics

The beneficial effects of probiotics can be attributed to three mechanisms of action: competitive exclusion, intestinal barrier function, and immune modulation.[13] These mechanisms of probiotic action do not function independently of one another, but rather they overlap to contribute to the efficacy of probiotics.

In some instances of competitive exclusion, probiotic bacteria produce antimicrobial substances, short-chain fatty acids, and biosurfactants and also modify the luminal pH, creating an unfavorable environment for pathogenic bacteria.[13-15] In other instances, certain probiotic strains coaggregate and form a protective barrier, keeping pathogenic bacteria from colonizing the gut epitheliums. Still others produce vitamins, scavenge superoxide radicals, and modify toxins produced by pathogens. In addition, probiotic bacteria may compete with other microbes for nutrients that favor the survival of the beneficial bacteria in the GI tract. Competitive exclusion by probiotics increases the adhesion of probiotics, enabling them to colonize the GI tract and promote further benefits to the host.[11,13-15]

The second mechanism by which probiotics benefit GI function is via promotion of gut barrier defense. Probiotics stimulate and increase the number of goblet cells and mucin expression, reinforcing the mucus layer of the epithelium that protects against pathogenic bacteria and antigens.[16] Some strains of Lactobacillus, Bifidobacterium, and Streptococcus stimulate and protect tight junction proteins from disruption by toxins and pathogens.[13] Epithelial cells produce antimicrobial peptides, and the integrity of tight junctions between the epithelial cells are strengthened, contributing to gut barrier strength and function.[11,15] Studies have shown that lactobacilli reduce proinflammatory cytokine production by pathogenic bacteria and repair intestinal barrier damage.[13]

The third and likely most complex mechanism of probiotic action is modulation of the host's immune system. Probiotics interact and communicate with immune cells that initiate signaling and production of immune mediators. Toll-like receptors, retinoic acid–inducible gene-I–like receptors, nucleotide oligomerization domain–like receptors, and C-type lectin receptors are pattern recognition receptors expressed by epithelial cells.[13] Immune activation occurs when the epithelial cells express pattern recognition receptors that interact with the pathogen-associated molecular patterns distributed on the bacteria in the GI tract (commensal and pathogenic bacteria). This interaction results in a cascade of molecular signaling and cellular response against microbes. Dendritic cells, in addition to epithelial cells, are activated by probiotics and can mediate an inflammatory response by T-cell differentiation, downregulation of toll-like receptor expression, and inhibition of nuclear factor κB signaling in the enterocytes. Probiotics also modulate the immune response by mediating release of cytokines, including interferons, interleukins, transforming growth factor, and tumor necrosis factors. Certain probiotic strains are known to decrease inflammatory cytokine release and increase anti-inflammatory cytokine production.[13] The immune-modulating effects of probiotics are complex and only briefly described here. Considering the plethora of information regarding the benefits of probiotics, it is not surprising that attention has turned to their potential as therapeutic alternatives or adjuncts in the management of many chronic GI diseases and disorders. However, it is crucial to remember that specific probiotic species and strains have individual effects, and each GI disease and disorder may be influenced differently by probiotics. No single probiotic is a magic bullet for all GI diseases and disorders. Figure 16.1 summarizes the beneficial effects of probiotics.

FIGURE 16.1 Probiotic mechanisms

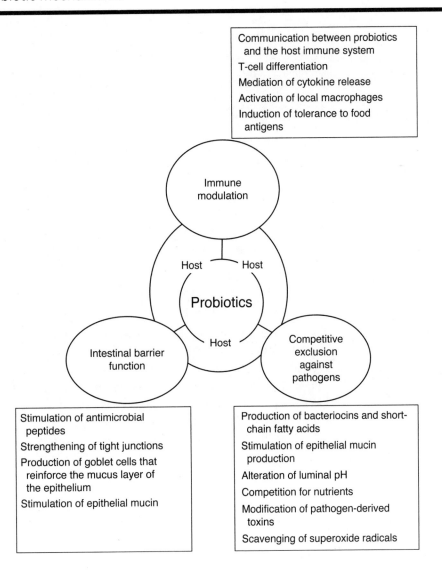

Probiotics in Gastrointestinal Disease

Diarrhea

Antibiotic-Associated Diarrhea

Adults Antibiotic-associated diarrhea (AAD) is a well-known side effect of antibiotic treatment that occurs in 3.2% to 29% of patients taking antibiotics.[17] Risk factors for AAD include advanced age, use of more than one antibiotic, use of proton pump inhibitors, prolonged hospital stays, previous hospital stays, and prior GI surgery.[18] Data indicate that 10% to 20% of cases are associated with *Clostridioides difficile* infection (discussed in detail shortly). Evidence indicates that probiotics may be able to alter microbial dysbiosis caused by antibiotics and reduce the risk of AAD.

In a 2017 systematic review and meta-analysis, probiotics were found to have a protective effect as adjunct therapy for the prevention of AAD in outpatients of all ages.[19] In 17 studies (a total of more than 3,600 patients), the risk of AAD was reduced by 51% (relative risk, 0.49; 95% confidence interval [CI], 0.36–0.66; I^2 = 58%) with probiotic use. The number needed to treat to prevent one case of AAD was 11 (95% CI, 6–13). According to the Grading of Recommendations Assessment, Development and Evaluation working group criteria, the quality of evidence to support the use of probiotics to prevent AAD is moderate due to heterogeneity and high risk of bias in certain trials.[19] *Lacticaseibacillus rhamnosus* GG (LGG) was found to be the most effective probiotic strain for the prevention of AAD in combined study results.

In another systematic review and meta-analysis, which included hospitalized patients and outpatients in the Netherlands, pooled results of 32 studies revealed that the treatment containing the probiotic strain LGG (single or multistrain probiotic) was most effective when compared to placebo for prevention of AAD.[20] The largest trial conducted in elderly hospitalized patients on the effectiveness of high-dose, multistrain probiotic formulation in the prevention of AAD and *C difficile*, the PLACIDE trial, did not show any benefit to probiotic treatment over placebo.[18] This study has been critiqued for its timing of probiotic treatment in relation to antibiotic therapy. Patients were reported to be on antibiotics for up to 7 days before starting probiotic treatment.

Determining the optimal protocol to prevent AAD remains difficult because of the heterogeneity of studies using varying probiotic strains, doses, timing, and types of study participants. In 2018, researchers evaluated the evidence in 59 randomized controlled trials on the prevention of AAD and reported strong evidence for three probiotic types—two single strains (*Saccharomyces boulardii* CNCM I-745 and *Lactobacillus rhamnosus* CLR2) and one mixture of three probiotic strains (*Lactobacillus acidophilus* CL1285, *Lactobacillus casei* LBC80R, and *Lactobacillus rhamnosus* CLR2).[12] Effectiveness is affected by dose and timing of probiotic consumption, starting within 1 to 2 days of antibiotic initiation and doses greater than 10 billion CFU per day continued for 1 to 4 weeks after antibiotic treatment appears optimal.[12] The most recently published meta-analysis (July 2021), including 36 studies and more than 9,300 adult participants, concluded that probiotics reduce the incidence of AAD by 38%. Adverse effects of probiotics were reported in less than half of the studies; however, adverse effects (mainly GI dysfunction) were not substantially increased in the probiotic group vs the placebo group. Not enough data are available to determine the exact dose and duration of probiotic treatment, though it is thought that probiotic treatment should continue for the duration of antibiotic therapy.[21]

In summary, for adults, *Lactobacillus*-containing probiotic therapy may help reduce the risk of AAD when administered within 2 days of antibiotic initiation. More specific recommendations for probiotic strain, dose, duration, and selection of adult patient population cannot be made at this time but are likely to be forthcoming as more clinical trials are performed.

Children The incidence of AAD in children is estimated at 5% to 30%.[22] As in adults, studies in children suggest that probiotics can play an important role in preventing AAD. In a 2019 Cochrane review that included 33 studies and a total of more than 6,300 children, the incidence of AAD in children receiving probiotics was 8% compared to 19% in the placebo group (number needed to benefit, 9 [95% CI 7–13]).[22] High-dose probiotics (more than 5 billion CFU per day) were more effective than lower doses.[22] Guidelines published in 2016 by the Working Group for Probiotics and Prebiotics of the European Society for Paediatric Gastroenterology, Hepatology, and Nutrition (ESPGHAN) recommend LGG and *S boulardii* for AAD prevention based on a review of 21 randomized controlled trials conducted in the pediatric population.[23] The suggested doses are 10 to 20 billion CFU per day for LGG and 5 to 10 billion CFU per day for *S boulardii*.[23]

The World Gastroenterology Organisation global guidelines for probiotics and prebiotics, published in 2017, mirror the recommendations of ESPGHAN.[11] That probiotics are safe to use for the prevention of AAD in healthy children is clear; however, a systematic review of case reports, randomized studies, and nonrandomized studies noted serious (though reversible) adverse events in severely debilitated or immunocompromised children.[24] In sum, LGG given at doses of 10 to 20 billion CFU daily, or *S boulardii* given at doses of 5 to 10 billion CFU daily, is recommended for the prevention of AAD in children who are not severely ill or immunocompromised.[24]

Clostridioides difficile Infection

C difficile was responsible for more than 450,000 cases of infection and approximately 29,000 deaths in the United States in 2011.[25] *C difficile* infection (CDI) is one of the most common health care–associated infections in US hospitals and currently accounts for 15% to 25% of AAD in hospital cases. In addition to the hospital infections, the prevalence and severity of community-associated CDI have been increasing. *C difficile* colonization can result in a wide range of clinical symptoms and outcomes, from asymptomatic carriers reporting mild diarrhea to symptomatic carriers with severe diarrhea, pseudomembranous colitis, toxic megacolon, and even death. The pathogenic potential of *C difficile* is most commonly associated with an alteration in the host's microbiome by antibiotics.[26] Risk factors, aside from recent antibiotic use, include being older than 65 years, recent hospitalization, being a resident of a nursing home, having a compromised immune system, and previous CDI.

Probiotics have been proposed as a preventive measure and as a treatment for CDI.[27] Multiple randomized controlled trials, and now several large meta-analyses, have reported that probiotics can reduce the incidence of CDI. The most recent meta-analysis, including nearly 7,000 study participants, reported that probiotic prophylaxis decreased the incidence of CDI by almost 60% and that using multispecies probiotics was more beneficial than using single species.[27] Adverse events were minimal. The importance of probiotic efficacy, specifically strain specificity, was demonstrated in the PLACIDE trial. Patients were randomly assigned to receive one yogurt per day containing 60 billion CFU *Lactobacillus acidophilus* and *Bifidobacterium bifidum* or placebo for 21 days to prevent AAD and CDI. Based on their findings, the authors concluded that the trial produced no evidence that the multistrain preparation was effective in prevention of AAD or CDD. Rather than conclude that probiotics are not beneficial in AAD and CDI, it is more likely that these strains in this combination are not effective for the prevention of AAD and CDI.[18]

Recurrent CDIs are associated with increased morbidity and mortality and with a severalfold increase in the cost of management, and they occur in one in six patients who initially suffer from CDI. Multiple studies have attempted to evaluate the effectiveness of probiotics in the prevention of recurrent CDI with variable success. It appears probiotics are clearly beneficial in *preventing* recurrent CDI, but once again, the benefit is likely disease-specific, as the benefit in *treating* recurrent CDI remains in question.[28] The 2020 American

Gastroenterological Association (AGA) practice guidelines on the role of probiotics in the management of GI disorders do not make a recommendation for probiotics in the treatment of CDI; however, they do suggest certain probiotic strains and strain combinations for the prevention of CDI in adults and children taking antibiotic therapy.[29] The AGA Institute's Clinical Guidelines Committee concluded, with a low level of evidence, that four preparations—the single-strain *S boulardii*; the two-species combination of *L acidophilus* CL1285 and *Lactobacillus casei* LBC80R; the three-strain combination of *L acidophilus*, *Lactobacillus delbrueckii* subsp *bulgaricus*, and *B bifidum*; and the four-strain combination of *L acidophilus*, *L delbrueckii* subsp *bulgaricus*, *B bifidum*, and *Streptococcus salivarius* subsp *thermophilus*—may have a beneficial effect in preventing CDI in patients (adults and children) with very high baseline risk compared to placebo.[29]

In summary, certain probiotics may be beneficial as an adjunct treatment in combination with antibiotics for preventing CDI in patients with the highest risk factors (advanced age, recent hospitalization, resident of a long-term-care facility, immunosuppression, and previous CDI). Large placebo-controlled, randomized clinical trials with standardized study designs are necessary to further define the role of probiotics in the treatment and prevention of CDI.[29] Recommendations should be based on clinical trials.

Radiation-Induced Diarrhea

A common consequence of cancer therapy toxicity is radiation-induced diarrhea, or GI mucositis. Radiation-induced diarrhea can result in nutritional compromise and the cessation or delay of cancer treatment. Probiotic treatment has been studied mainly in patients with cancer who were undergoing pelvic or abdominal radiation. The studies are critiqued for having small numbers of participants and for their variable use of probiotic species, strain, and dosages.

In a multicenter, randomized, placebo-controlled trial, 56 participants with endometrial adenocarcinoma or cervical squamous cell carcinoma consumed a probiotic drink containing 10 billion CFU *L casei* DN-114 001 three times daily. The researchers determined that the probiotic delayed the onset of diarrhea compared to placebo but provided only modest improvement in stool consistency.[30] In a dosing study, using a commercial product in capsule form containing *Lactobacillus acidophilus* 361 and *Bifidobacterium longum*, investigators randomly assigned participants to a standard dose (0.3–1.3 billion CFU administered twice per day), high dose (10 billion CFU administered three times per day), and placebo. Severe diarrhea was reduced in the participants who received the standard dose of probiotics compared to those who received the placebo.[31] A larger randomized trial found a significant reduction ($P=.001$) in the incidence and severity of diarrhea in the treatment group using the probiotic preparation VSL#3 (450 billion CFU/g; a combination of *Streptococcus thermophilus*, four lactobacilli strains, and three bifidobacterial strains) administered three times daily, for a total of more than 1 trillion CFU per day.[32] In a meta-analysis including 917 study participants with abdominal or pelvic cancer, probiotic treatment was associated with a reduced incidence of radiation-induced diarrhea (RR, 0.55; 95% CI, 0.34–0.88; $P=.01$).[33]

Though some studies have provided positive results, limitations mainly related to study heterogeneity make it difficult to provide recommendations for the treatment or prevention of radiation-induced diarrhea with probiotics.[33] Probiotics containing *Lactobacillus* and *Bifidobacterium* can be effective in minimizing the side effects of antitumor treatment; however, there are not enough data to specify dose. Limited safety data indicate that infections related to these strains in patients are extremely rare and are most often the result of underlying disease. Patients with cancer are considered to have impaired immune function, though recent evidence suggests that probiotics may promote intestinal homeostasis in patients undergoing hematopoietic stem cell transplantation or with attenuating consequences of graft-versus-host disease.[34] The benefit of probiotics for reducing antitumor side effects is promising, but experts remain concerned for a higher incidence of infection in patients with severely impaired immune function, so the use of probiotics should be carefully evaluated. Large-scale trials are still needed to define specific recommendations for the use of probiotics in patients with cancer.

Helicobacter pylori Infection

Helicobacter pylori infection is one of the most common bacterial infections globally and is a substantial risk factor for gastric cancer. Eradication of the pathogen *H pylori* may require multimodal treatment, including antibiotics and a proton pump inhibitor regimen. The proposed mechanisms for probiotics in the treatment of *H pylori* infection include adhesion inhibition, mucus barrier enhancement, antibacterial secretion, and immune modulation that alters and inhibits *H pylori* colonization of the gastric mucosa.[35] Studies to date have applied different probiotic preparations (single-strain and multistrain), mainly including *Lactobacillus*, *Bifidobacterium*, and *Saccharomyces*, in the treatment of *H pylori*. A large meta-analysis concluded that only four select individual strains (*L acidophilus*, *L casei* DN-114 001, *Lactobacillus gasseri*, and *Bifidobacterium infantis* 20036) were more effective in eradicating *H pylori* in patients when the antibiotic therapies were considered ineffective (an eradication rate of less than 80%).[36]

The major side effects of multimodal treatment for *H pylori* infection include antibiotic-associated diarrhea, vomiting, and abdominal pain, and they often lead to nonadherence to eradication treatment regimens.[37] The positive evidence for probiotic therapy in *H pylori* infection may be related to its effectiveness in reducing these adverse GI effects associated with *H pylori* treatment.[37] Evidenced-based guidance describes two probiotic strains with strong efficacy for preventing adverse side effects of *H pylori* treatment—*S boulardii* I-745 (a yeast) and a blend of *Lactobacillus helveticus* R52 and *Lacticaseibacillus rhamnosus* R11.[12] Despite positive results to date in clinical trials, the 2021 AGA clinical practice update on the management of refractory *H pylori* infection concludes that probiotic use as a nonantibiotic adjunct should be considered experimental because there are limited data to guide the timing, formulation, dose, and appropriate patient selection.[38]

Inflammatory Bowel Disease

Inflammatory bowel disease (IBD) is characterized by inflammation in the GI tract that contributes to periods of intensified symptoms (diarrhea, obstruction, abdominal cramps and pain, weight loss, fever, weakness, fatigue, and malnutrition) with phases of remission.[39] In comparison to the microbiota of a healthy individual, the microbiota of patients with IBD is characterized by an abundance of pathogenic bacteria (*Escherichia coli*, *Clostridium*) and a reduced number of beneficial bacteria (*Bifidobacterium* and *Lactobacillus*), resulting in altered microbial activity, specifically decreased synthesis of short-chain fatty acids and increased toxins in the GI tract.[40] Probiotic studies in IBD are focused on modulating the GI microbiota and downregulating intestinal inflammation, as it relates to inducing and maintaining remission of disease. Unfortunately, the majority of clinical trials on the use of probiotics in IBD have been based on animal models. The few human clinical trials have not yet demonstrated induction and maintenance of remission of IBD, particularly in the case of Crohn's disease.[40]

Crohn's Disease

To date, there are limited studies on probiotics in Crohn's disease. Research suggests an immunomodulating benefit, specifically for *Bifidobacterium* genus and the yeast *S boulardii*, by reducing relapse rate, improving the disease activity index scores, and reducing intestinal permeability.[40] In a randomized, double-blind, placebo-controlled trial to evaluate the combination of 1,000 mg *S boulardii* with 3 g mesalamine per day compared with 3 g mesalamine per day alone in 32 adult patients with Crohn's disease in remission for a 6-month period, researchers determined that the *S boulardii*–mesalamine group had a 6% relapse rate (1 in 16 patients) compared with a rate of 38% in the mesalamine-only group (6 in 16 patients).[41]

In a much larger prospective study of 165 patients who experienced remission after treatment with steroids or salicylates, patients were randomly assigned to *S boulardii* (1 g/d) or placebo for 52 weeks. There were no significant differences between the two groups in mean Crohn's disease activity index scores, erythrocyte sedimentation rates, or median levels of C-reactive protein.[42] A single-center, double-blind, randomized, placebo-controlled trial in adult patients with asymptomatic IBD, published in 2019, assessed the efficacy of a multistrain probiotic in quality-of-life issues and intestinal inflammation after 4 weeks of use. No significant changes were seen for patients with Crohn's disease in quality-of-life results, disease activity scores, and laboratory measures.[43]

Several studies have assessed the potential for probiotic therapy to prevent recurrence of Crohn's disease following surgical resection, using mixed *Lactobacillus* probiotic species and prebiotics as well as a single *Lactobacillus* strain (*L johnsonii* LA1), but no therapeutic effect of probiotic supplementation has been shown.[40] In a 2020 Cochrane review, only two studies met the inclusion criteria to assess effectiveness of probiotics compared to placebo for remission of Crohn's disease in adults. Due to a lack of evidence and the very small size of the studies (a total of 46 participants), no recommendations could be made.[44] The 2020 AGA clinical practice guidelines on the role of probiotics in the management of GI disorders identified 11 clinical trials for the use of probiotics for induction of remission in Crohn's disease.[29] Only one of the 11 studies included children. The guidelines committee concluded that probiotic use in adults and children could only be recommended in the context of a clinical trial.[29] In other words, no specific recommendation was provided because of the small number of studies and low level of evidence for probiotics and the lack of effect for induction or maintenance of remission in Crohn's disease.[29] Additional well-designed human trials are needed. In sum, due to a lack of data and controversial existing data, the use of probiotics in Crohn's disease is not recommended at this time.[29]

Ulcerative Colitis and Pouchitis

Studies for probiotic use in ulcerative colitis have shown more promising results than in Crohn's disease. The probiotic preparation VSL#3, which has 450 billion live bacteria in each dose, is the most extensively studied probiotic for this purpose. VSL#3 is a multistrain preparation including *Bifidobacterium breve*, *B longum*, *B infantis*, *L acidophilus*, *L plantarum*, *L paracasei*, *L bulgaricus*, and *S thermophilus*. A number of well-designed clinical trials have shown that VSL#3 can facilitate both the induction and maintenance of remission in patients with ulcerative colitis better than when medication is used alone.[45-48] In a 2010 meta-analysis of the effects of administering probiotics in the treatment of ulcerative colitis, disease maintenance was generally improved with the probiotic compared with placebo, though the same was not true for induction of remission.[49] A randomized, double-blind, placebo-controlled trial showed that a multistrain probiotic (*Lactobacillus rhamnosus* NCIMB 30174, *Lactobacillus plantarum* NCIMB 30173, *L acidophilus* NCIMB 30175, and *Enterococcus faecium* NCIMB 30176) was associated with significantly decreased intestinal inflammation (P<.015), as measured by fecal calprotectin, in patients with ulcerative colitis when compared to placebo.[43] A 2021 systematic review and meta-analysis explored the clinical effects and GI microbiota changes in IBD. As with some previous reviews, the results corroborated that probiotics, particularly *Lactobacillus* and *Bifidobacterium* species or multistrain preparations, may be effective for maintenance of remission and reduction of the ulcerative colitis disease activity index.[50] Finally, the 2020 AGA clinical practice guidelines reviewed 11 studies meeting rigorous criteria for the use of probiotics for induction or maintenance of remission in adults and children with ulcerative colitis, but the guidelines committee was unable to make a specific recommendation due to the low quality of the evidence. Though there may be multiple studies that show potential for probiotic benefit—for example, VSL#3 studies—they are small and limited by heterogeneity in design.[29]

When patients have undergone surgery for ulcerative colitis to remove their colon and rectum, a pouch made from a loop of small intestine takes the place of the rectum. Unfortunately, patients can develop pouchitis—inflammation of the pouch that leads to diarrhea, fecal urgency, and abdominal cramping. A 2019 Cochrane review evaluated 15 studies to determine effective therapies for the treatment and prevention of pouchitis.[51] Half of the studies evaluated the use of probiotics in treatment (one study), remission (two studies), and prevention of pouchitis (four studies). It was concluded that a benefit of probiotics was not clear due to the small number of participants in each study, with the largest study including only 40 patients.[51] The 2020 AGA clinical practice guidelines identified seven studies.[29] Like the Cochrane review, the AGA guidelines also note the overall low quality of evidence due to small sample sizes, risk of bias, and heterogeneity in patient selection and modes of therapy.[29] However, they recognize that the majority of studies were performed using the eight-strain probiotic VSL#3. On the basis of very low-quality evidence, the AGA suggests the use of VSL#3 in adults and children with pouchitis over no probiotic or any other probiotic preparation.[29]

Irritable Bowel Syndrome

Irritable bowel syndrome (IBS) is a chronic GI disorder characterized by abdominal pain and altered bowel habits that negatively affects quality of life in approximately 5% to 20% of the general population.[50] Probiotics are commonly used by people suffering from IBS in an effort to improve symptoms. IBS is a heterogenous disorder with four diagnostic subtypes classified by symptoms: IBS with constipation, IBS with diarrhea, IBS of mixed type, and unclassified IBS.[52] The two most common probiotic genuses used in the studies of IBS include *Lactobacillus* and *Bifidobacterium*; however, doses, strains, and single-vs-multistrain preparations vary considerably. In 2016, the British Dietetic Association published a systematic review of systematic reviews (nine reviews) and evidenced-based practice guidelines for the use of probiotics in adults with IBS.[52]

The systematic review included more than 3,400 adults from 35 randomized control trials performed around the world in various health care settings.[52] Twenty-nine different probiotics were used to compare probiotics to placebo for global and individual symptom improvement and quality-of-life outcomes. Eight trials analyzed *Lactobacillus* and three analyzed *Bifidobacterium*. Evidence statements for the clinical efficacy of certain probiotics and their dosing shown in single studies, as well as a statement identifying 12 probiotics that were not effective, were published.[52] Despite some clinic evidence of improved outcomes for certain strains and doses in single studies, the conclusion was that there is no consistency of efficacy between different probiotics; therefore, specific recommendations for the use of probiotics in clinical practice for patients with IBS could not be made.[52]

A 2020 systematic review of 35 randomized controlled trials involving a total of 3,452 adult patients with IBS demonstrated that probiotics, especially combination probiotics, have greater potential to improve IBS symptoms than placebo.[53] Global symptom, abdominal pain, bloating, and flatulence scores were improved for subjects taking probiotics when compared to placebo. The reviewers also concluded, however, that exact species, strain, dose, and duration of probiotic therapy are still unclear.[53] Another meta-analysis showed similar results, in that combination probiotic treatment was found to improve overall IBS symptoms and scores.[54] The 2020 AGA clinical practice guidelines reviewed 55 trials that tested 44 different probiotic formulations (species, strains, and combinations).[29] As with previous systematic reviews, many of the probiotics were found to be beneficial in single trials for certain IBS outcomes in adults. However, the certainty of evidence across all outcomes for the use of probiotics in IBS (adults and children) was low or very low.[29] See Box 16.4 for a summary of probiotic efficacy in single trials for IBS.[29]

BOX 16.4

Efficacy of Probiotics in Irritable Bowel Syndrome: Single Trials[29]

Population: adults

Outcome: improved global symptoms

Single strains

Lactobacillus plantarum 299v

Saccharomyces cerevisiae CNCM I-3856160

Eschirichia coli DSM 17252130

Three-strain combination

L plantarum CECT7484

L plantarum CECT7485

Pediococcus acidilactici CECT7483

Four-strain combination

Streptococcus salivarius subsp thermophilus

Lactobacillus delbrueckii subsp bulgaricus

Lactobacillus acidophilus

Bifidobacterium longum subsp longum

Four-strain combination

Bifidobacterium animalis subsp *lactis* Bb12

L acidophilus LA-5

L delbrueckii subsp *bulgaricus* LBY-27

Streptococcus salivarius subsp *thermophilus*

Seven-strain combination

L acidophilus KCTC 11906BP

L plantarum KCTC 11876BP

Lactobacillus rhamnosus KCTC 11868BP

Bifidobacterium breve KCTC 11858BP

B animalis subsp lactis KCTC 11903BP

B longum subsp *longum* KCTC 11860BP

S salivarius subsp *thermophilus* KCTC 11870BP

14-strain combination

Bacillus subtilis PXN 21

Bifidobacterium bifidum PXN 23

B breve PXN 25

B longum subsp *infantis* PXN 27

Box continues

BOX 16.4 (CONTINUED)

B longum subsp *longum* PXN 30

L acidophilus PXN 35

L delbrueckii subsp *bulgaricus* PXN 39

Lactobacillus casei PXN 37

Lactobacillus plantarum PXN 47

Lactobacillus rhamnosus PXN 54

Lactobacillus helveticus PXN 45

Lactobacillus salivarius PXN 57

Lactococcus lactis PXN 63

S salivarius subsp *thermophilus* PXN 66166

Outcome: improved global symptoms

Single strains

L plantarum 299v

L rhamnosus ATCC 53103119

Bacillus coagulans MTCC 5856168

Two-strain combination

L acidophilus SDC 2012 and SDC 2013128

E coli DSM 17252130

Two-strain combination

B longum subsp *longum*

L acidophilus

Three-strain combination

B longum subsp *infantis* M-63

B breve M-16V

B longum Reuter ATCC BAA-999162

Four-strain combination

S salivarius subsp *thermophilus*

L delbrueckii subsp *bulgaricus*

L acidophilus

B longum subsp *longum*

Four-strain combination

L rhamnosus NCIMB 30174

L plantarum NCIMB 30173

L acidophilus NCIMB 30175

Enterococcus faecium NCIMB 30176153

Box continues

BOX 16.4 (CONTINUED)

Population: children

Outcome: improved global symptoms

Single strains

L rhamnosus ATCC 53103

B coagulans Unique IS2

Eight-strain combination

L paracasei subsp *paracasei*

L plantarum

L acidophilus

L delbrueckii subsp *bulgaricus*

B longum subsp *longum*

B breve

B longum subsp *infantis*

S salivarius subsp *thermophilus*

Though the clinical research for probiotic use in IBS is vast, the studies suffer from substantial disease heterogeneity as well as heterogeneity in their probiotic preparations, strains, doses, and outcomes used in the studies.[29,52] In summary, the 2020 AGA clinical practice guidelines conclude that there is not sufficient evidence to make specific recommendations for the use of probiotics in IBS.[29,52] See Chapter 5 for additional discussion of the use of probiotics in IBS.

Safety Considerations

Most probiotics are intended for use in healthy individuals and have been derived from fermented food or nonpathogenic species that colonize the healthy human GI tract. Adverse effects of probiotics, though rare, have been noted in severely ill or vulnerable patients, such as neonates or immunocompromised adults. Studies of probiotics have been criticized for lack of safety assessments, lack of adverse effects reporting, and lack of quality control of commercial probiotics being studied.[55] The safety of probiotics depends on their intended use, the health status of the target patient (for which they have been studied), the dose, and mode of administration. A 2018 systematic review examined harms-related data reporting in 384 trials conducted in either healthy volunteers or patients with medical conditions who were using probiotics, prebiotics, or synbiotics; the studies of probiotics accounted for 69% of the total trials. Harms reporting was nonexistent in 28% of all trials included in the systematic review, and there was no mention of adverse events in 81% of studies. In over 90% of included studies, adverse and severe adverse events were not defined, nor were methods for collecting harm-related information described. This systematic review identified serious shortcomings related to safety data reporting in probiotic studies.[56]

Safety assessments in studies must consider the risk of bacterial translocation from the GI tract, virulence factors of the probiotic used, and transfer of antibiotic-resistant genes.[55] More recent studies do a much better job of reporting adverse events in clinical trials, an essential development for the probiotic field. It is imperative for clinicians to know the safety data for the practice recommendations that are made. The use of probiotic foods or dietary supplements—products designed for healthy consumers—in vulnerable populations must be done with caution.[57] Products must be composed of strains that are safe for the target population and must be manufactured using quality standards rigorous enough for the target population. In current times, with advanced technology, responsible manufacturing processes that include annotated genome sequencing should guarantee avoidance of contamination and the absence of transferable antibiotic resistance genes from the probiotic strains.[55]

Summary

Drawing conclusions about the benefit of probiotics in the treatment of GI disease is complex for several reasons. Studies use differing probiotic strains with variable doses, variable timing of administration, and diverse probiotic combinations, making it difficult to compare clinical trials. Many trials to date have small sample sizes and methodological problems, such as questionable randomization and blinding. In addition, many trials lack adequate safety data and adverse event reporting. For these reasons, most conclusions in the literature on the effectiveness of probiotics are based on meta-analyses, and finding specific recommendations is difficult.[57] Recommendations for probiotics should be based on national practice guidelines and, when those are not available, on rigorous clinical trials that have tested specific probiotics or probiotic combinations and use well-defined dosing, mode of administration, and patient population. It is also important to avoid oversimplification and extrapolation of recommendations based on single-study results. To identify effective probiotic strains and doses for specific GI conditions, all positive and null probiotic studies must be examined. "One probiotic does not work for all indications or sub-populations."[1] What most professional societies and experts can agree on is that more well-controlled human efficacy trials are needed, and the careful selection of a probiotic in the form of a food or supplement can be a helpful adjunct to a diet that contains a wide variety of unprocessed foods—with fiber, prebiotics, and minimal additives—in maintaining a healthy microbiome and preventing dysbiosis.[1]

References

1. International Scientific Association for Probiotics and Prebiotics. The ISAPP quick guide to probiotics for health professionals: history, efficacy, and safety. December 2019. Accessed February 2021. https://isappscience.org/for-clinicians/resources/probiotics

2. Hill C, Guarner F, Reid G, et al. The International Scientific Association for Probiotics and Prebiotics consensus statement on the scope and appropriate use of the term probiotics. *Nat Rev Gastroenterol Hepatol.* 2014;11(8):506-514. doi:10.1038/nrgastro.2014.66

3. Binda S, Hill C, Johansen E, et al. Criteria to qualify microorganisms as "probiotic" in foods and dietary supplements. *Front Microbiol.* 2020;11:1-9. doi:10.3389/fmicb.2020.01662

4. Quigley, EMM. Prebiotics and probiotics in digestive health. *Clin Gastroenterol Hepatol.* 2019;17(2):333-344. doi:10.1016/j.cgh.2018.09.028

5. Marco ML, Sanders ME, Gänzle M, et al. The International Scientific Association for Probiotics and Prebiotics (ISAPP) consensus statement on fermented foods. *Nat Rev Gastroenterol Hepatol.* 2021;18:196-208. doi:10.1038/s41575.020.00390.5

6. US Food and Drug Administration. Dietary supplements. August 16, 2019. Accessed July 2020. www.fda.gov/food/dietary-supplements

7. de Simone C. The unregulated probiotic market. *Clin Gastroenterol Hepatol.* 2019;17:809-817. doi:10.1016/j.cgh.2018.01.018

8. Ailioaie LM, Litscher G. Probiotics, photobiomodulation, and disease management: controversies and challenges. *Int J Mol Sci.* 2021;22(9):4942. doi:10.3390/ijms22094942

9. Thursby E, Juge N. Introduction to the human gut microbiota. *Biochem J.* 2017;474:1823-1836. doi:10.1042/BCJ20160510

10. Fenster K, Freeburg B, Hollard C, Wong C, Rønhave Laursen R, Ouwehand AC. The production and delivery of probiotics: a review of a practical approach. *Microorganisms.* 2019;7(3):83. doi:10.3390/microorganisms7030083

11. World Gastroenterology Organisation. World Gastroenterology Organisation global guidelines: probiotics and prebiotics. February 2017. Accessed March 2021. www.worldgastroenterology.org/guidelines/probiotics-and-prebiotics/probiotics-and-prebiotics-english

12. Sniffen JC, McFarland LV, Evean CT, Goldstein EJC. Choosing an appropriate probiotic product for your patient: an evidenced-based practical guide. *PLoS ONE.* 2018;13(12):e0209205. doi:10.10371/journal.pone.0209205

13. Raheem A, Liang L, Zhang G, Cui S. Modulatory effects of probiotics during pathogenic infections with emphasis on immune regulation. *Front Immunol.* 2021;13:616713. doi:10.3389/fimmu.2021.616713

14. Markowiak P, Slizewska K. Effects of probiotics, prebiotics and synbiotics on human health. *Nutrients.* 2017;9:1021. doi:10.3390.nu9091021

15. Simon E, Calinoiu LF, Mitrea L, Vodnar DC. Probiotics, prebiotics, and synbiotics: implications and beneficial effects against irritable bowel syndrome. *Nutrients.* 2021;13(6):2112. doi:10.3390/nu13062112

16. Galdeano CM, Cazorla SI, Dumit JML, et al. Beneficial effects of probiotic consumption on the immune system. *Ann Nutr Metab.* 2019;74:115-124. doi:10.1159/000496426

17. Elseviers MM, Van Camp Y, Nayaert S, et al. Prevalence and management of antibiotic-associated diarrhea in general hospitals. *BMC Infect Dis.* 2015;15:129-138. doi:10.1186/s12879-015-0869-0

18. Allen SJ, Wareham K, Wang D, et al. Lactobacilli and bifidobacterial in the prevention of antibiotic-associated diarrhoea and *Clostridium difficile* diarrhoea in older inpatients (PLACIDE): randomised, double-blind, placebo-controlled, multicenter trial. *Lancet.* 2013;382(9900):1249-1257. doi:10.1016/S0140-6736(13)61218-0

19. Blaabjerg S, Artzi DM, Aabenhus R. Probiotics for the prevention of antibiotic-associated diarrhea in outpatients—a systematic review and meta-analysis. *Antibiotics.* 2017;6(4):21-38. doi:10.3390/antibiotics6040021

20. Agamennone V, Crul CAM, Rijkers G, Kort R. A practical guide for probiotics applied to the case of antibiotic associated diarrhea in the Netherlands. *BMC Gastroenterol.* 2018;18(1):103-115. doi:10.1186/s12876-018-0831-x

21. Liao W, Chen C, Wen T, Zhao Q. Probiotics for the prevention of antibiotic-associated diarrhea in adults: a meta-analysis of randomized placebo-controlled trials. *J Clin Gastroenterol.* 2021;55(6):469-480. doi:10.1097MCG.0000000000001464

22. Guo Q, Goldenberg JZ, Humphrey C, et al. Probiotics for the prevention of pediatric antibiotic-associated diarrhea. *Cochrane Database Syst Rev.* 2019;(4):CD004827.

23. Szajewska H, Canani RB, Guarino A, et al; ESPGHAN Working Group for Probiotics and Prebiotics. Probiotics for the prevention of antibiotic-associated diarrhea in children. *J Pediatr Gastroenterol Nutr.* 2016;62(3):495-506. doi:10.1097/MPG0000000000001081

24. Whelan K, Myers CE. Safety of probiotics in patients receiving nutrition support: a systematic review of case reports, randomized controlled trials, and nonrandomized trials. *Am J Clin Nutr.* 2010;91(3)687-703. doi:10.3945/ajcn.2009.28759

25. Lessa FC, Mu Y, Bamberg WM, et al. Burden of *Clostridium difficile* infection in the United States. *N Engl J Med.* 2015;372(9):825-834. doi:10.1056/NEJMoa1408913

26. Robinson JI, Weir WH, Crowley JR, et al. Metabolomic networks connect host-microbiome processes to human *Clostridioides difficile* infections. *J Clin Invest.* 2019;129(9):3792-3806. doi:10.1172/JCI126905

27. Johnston BC, Lo CK, Allen SJ, et al. Microbial preparations (probiotics) for the prevention of *Clostridium difficile* infection in adults and children: an individual patient data meta-analysis of 6,851 participants. *Infect Control Hosp Epidemiol.* 2018;39(7):771-781. doi:10.1017/ice.2018.84

28. Madoff SE, Urquiaga M, Alonso CD, Kelly CP. Prevention of recurrent *Clostridium difficile* infection: a systematic review of randomized controlled trials. *Anaerobe.* 2020;61:102098. doi:10.1016/j.anaerobe.2019.102098

29. Su GL, Ko CW, Bercik P, et al. AGA clinical practice guidelines on the role of probiotics in the management of gastrointestinal disorders. *Gastroenterol.* 2020;159:697-705. doi:10.1053/j.gastro.2020.05.059

30. Giralt J, Regadera JP, Verges R, et al. Effects of probiotic *Lactobacillus casei* DN-114 001 in prevention of radiation induced diarrhea: results from a multicenter, randomized, placebo-controlled nutritional trial. *Int J Radiat Oncol Biol Phys.* 2008;71(4):1213-1219. doi:10.1016/j.ijrobp.2007.11.009

31. Demers M, Dagnault A, Desjardins J. A randomized double-blind controlled trial: impact of probiotics on diarrhea in patients treated with pelvic radiation. *Clin Nutr.* 2014;33:761-767. doi:10.1016/j.clnu.2013.10.015

32. Delia P, Sansotta G, Donato V, et al. Use of probiotics for prevention of radiation induced diarrhea. *World J Gastroenterol.* 2007;6:912-915. doi:10.3748/wjg.v13.i6.912

33. Liu M, Li S, Shu Y, Zhan H. Probiotics for prevention of radiation-induced diarrhea: a meta-analysis of randomized controlled trials. *PLoS ONE*. 2017;12:1-15. doi:10.1371/journal.pone.0178870

34. Lu K, Dong S, Wu X, Jin R, Chen H. Probiotics in cancer. *Front Oncol*. 2021;11:638148. doi:10.3389/fonc.2021.638148

35. Ji Y, Yang H. Using probiotics as supplementation for *Helicobacter pylori* antibiotic therapy. *Int J Mol Sci*. 2020;21(3):1136. doi:10.3390/ijms21031136

36. Dang Y, Reinhardt JD, Zhou X, Zhang G. The effect of probiotics supplementation on *Helicobacter pylori* eradication rates and side effects during eradication therapy: a meta-analysis. *PLoS ONE*. 2014;9(11):e111030. doi:10.1371/journal.pone.0111030

37. McFarland LV, Huang Y, Wang L, Malferheiner P. Systematic review and meta-analysis: multi-strain probiotics as adjunct therapy for *Helicobacter pylori* eradication and prevention of adverse events. *United Euro J Gastroenterol*. 2016;4(4):546-561. doi:10.1177/2050640615617358

38. Shah SC, Iyer PG, Moss SF. AGA clinical practice update on the management of refractory *Helicobacter pylori* infection: expert review. *Gastroenterol*. 2021;160:1831-1841. doi:10.1053/j.gastro.2020.11.059

39. Jakubczyk D, Leszczynska K, Gorska S. The effectiveness of probiotics in the treatment of inflammatory bowel disease (IBD)—a critical review. *Nutrients*. 2020;12:1973. doi:10.3390/nu12071973

40. Coqueiro AY, Raizel R, Bonvini A, et al. Probiotics for inflammatory bowel diseases: a promising adjuvant treatment. *Int J Food Sci Nutr*. 2019;70(1)20-29. doi:10.1080/09637486.2018.1477123

41. Guslandi M, Mezzi G, Sorghi M, Testoni PA. *Saccharomyces boulardii* in maintenance treatment of Crohn's disease. *Dig Dis Sci*. 2000;45:1462-1464. doi:101023/a:1005588911207

42. Bourreille A, Cadiot G, Le Dreau G, et al. *Saccharomyces boulardii* does not prevent relapse of Crohn's disease. *Clin Gastroenterol Hepatol*. 2013;11:982-987. doi:10.1016/j.cgh.2013.02.021

43. Bjarnason I, Sission G, Hayee B. A randomized, double-blind, placebo-controlled trial of a multi-strain probiotic in patients with asymptomatic ulcerative colitis and Crohn's disease. *Inflammopharmacology*. 2019;27(3):465-473. doi:10.1007/s10787-019-00595-4

44. Limketkai BN, Akobeng AK, Gordon M, Adepoju AA. Probiotics for induction of remission in Crohn's disease (review). *Cochrane Database Syst Rev*. 2020;(7):CD006634. doi:10.1002/14651858.CD004826.pub2

45. Bibiloni R, Fedorak RN, Tannock GW, et al. VSL#3 probiotic-mixture induces remission in patients with active ulcerative colitis. *Am J Gastroenterol*. 2005;100(7):1539-1546. doi:10.1111/j.1572-0241.2005.41794.x

46. Miele E, Pascarella F, Giannetti E, et al. Effect of a probiotic preparation (VSL#3) on induction and maintenance of remission in children with ulcerative colitis. *Am J Gastroenterol*. 2009;104(2):437-443. doi:10.1038/ajg.2008.118

47. Sood A, Midha V, Makharia GK, et al. The probiotic preparation, VSL#3 induces remission in patients with mild-to-moderately active ulcerative colitis. *Clin Gastroenterol Hepatol*. 2009;7(11):1202-1209. doi:10.1016/j.cgh.2009.07.016

48. Tursi A. Balsalazide plus high-potency probiotic preparation (VSL#3) in the treatment of acute mild-to-moderate ulcerative colitis and uncomplicated diverticulitis of the colon. *J Clin Gastroenterol*. 2008;42(suppl 3 pt 1):S119-S122. doi:10.1097/MCG.0b013e31815f5ac7

49. Sang LX, Chang B, Zhang WL, et al. Remission induction and maintenance effect of probiotics on ulcerative colitis: a meta-analysis. *World J Gastroenterol*. 2010;16(15):1908-1915. doi:10.3748/wjg.v16.i15.1908

50. Zhang XF, Guan XX, Tang YJ, et al. Clinical effects and gut microbiota changes of using probiotics, prebiotics or synbiotics in inflammatory bowel disease: a systematic review and meta-analysis. *Eur J Nutr*. 2021;60(5):2855-2875. doi:10.1007/s00394-021-02503-5

51. Nguyen N, Zhang B, Holubar SD, Pardi DS, Singh S. Treatment and prevention of pouchitis after ileal pouch-anal anastomosis for chronic ulcerative colitis. *Cochrane Database Syst Rev*. 2019;(11):CD001176. doi:10.1002/14651858.CD001176.pub5

52. McKenzie YA, Thompson J, Gulia P, Lomer MCE; IBS Dietetic Guideline Review Group on behalf of Gastroenterology Specialist Group of the British Dietetic Association. British Dietetic Association systematic review of systematic reviews and evidenced-based practice guidelines for the use of probiotics in the management of irritable bowel syndrome in adults (2016 update). *J Hum Nutr Diet*. 2016;29(5):576-592. doi:10.1111/jhn.12386

53. Niu HL, Xiao JY. The efficacy and safety of probiotics in patients with irritable bowel syndrome: evidenced based on 35 randomized clinical trials. *Int J Surgery*. 2020;75:116-127. doi:10.1016/j.ijsu.2020.01.142

54. Sun JR, Kong CF, Qu XK, Deng C, Lou YN, Jia LQ. Efficacy and safety of probiotics in irritable bowel syndrome: a systematic review and meta-analysis. *Saudi J Gastroenterol*. 2020;26(2):66-77. doi:10.4103/sjg.SJF_384_19

55. Sanders ME, Akkermans LMA, Haller D, et al. Safety assessment of probiotics for human use. *Gut Microbes*. 2010;1(3):164-185. doi:10.4161/gmic.1.3.12127

56. Bafeta A, Koh M, Riveros C, Ravaud P. Harms reporting in randomized controlled trials of interventions aimed at modifying microbiota. *Ann Intern Med*. 2018;169:240-247. doi:10.7326/M18-0343

57. Sanders ME, Merenstein DJ, Ouwehand AC, et al. Probiotic use in at-risk populations. *J Am Pharm Assoc (2003)*. 2016;56(6):680-686. doi:10.1016/j.japh.2016.07.001

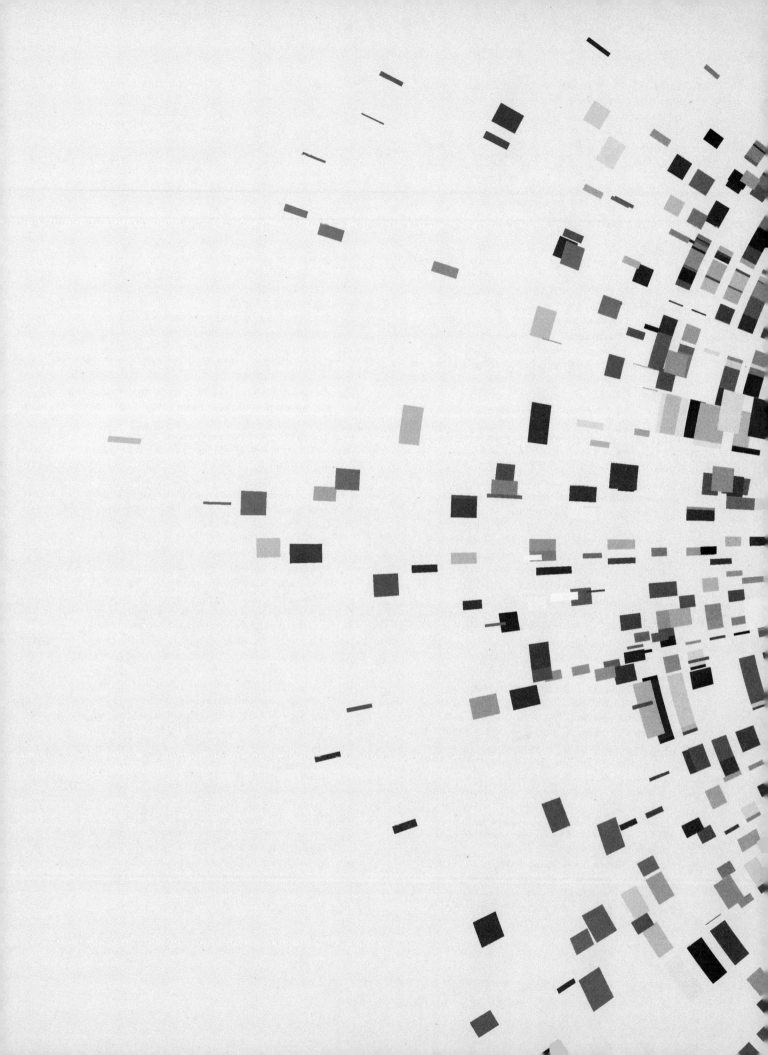

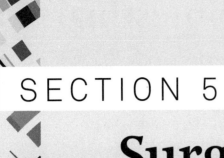

Surgical and Therapeutic Interventions for Gastrointestinal Disorders

Gastrointestinal Tract Surgery

Gail A. Cresci, PhD, RD, LD
Ezra Steiger, MD, FACS, FASPEN, AGAF

KEY POINTS

- The nutrition needs of surgical patients vary according to patient-specific factors, such as disease process, type of surgery being performed, existing comorbidities, and baseline nutritional status.
- Each type of gastrointestinal tract surgery affects nutrition intake and absorption differently, and surgery may be associated with a variety of adverse nutritional consequences. Preoperative nutrition care of the malnourished patient can help improve postoperative outcomes.
- Postoperative nutrition care focuses on the delivery of appropriate amounts of energy, fluids, macronutrients, and micronutrients. Some patients may need long-term nutrition interventions, ranging from avoidance of certain foods to nutrient supplementation to enteral or parenteral nutrition in the home care setting

Introduction

The nutrition needs of patients undergoing surgical procedures vary according to patient-specific factors, such as disease process, type of surgery being performed, existing comorbidities, and baseline nutritional status. This chapter reviews recommendations for the perioperative nutrition care of undernourished patients, both before gastrointestinal (GI) tract surgery—particularly surgery involving the esophagus, stomach, and small intestine—and after surgery.

Preoperative Nutrition

Patients undergoing surgery of the GI tract often have suboptimal preoperative nutritional status as a result of the disease process that precedes the surgery (eg, cancer, obstruction). The patient's disease process may also cause a hypermetabolic state, placing the patient at nutritional risk. Preoperative malnutrition is associated with altered immune function, poor wound healing, and increased morbidity and mortality.[1,2]

Ideally, for optimal postoperative outcomes, a mildly malnourished patient should be nutritionally repleted for 7 to 10 days before surgery; severely malnourished patients often require a longer period of conditioning.[2,3] Unless the GI tract is nonfunctional, nutrition should be provided enterally rather than parenterally.[3] In cases of elective surgery, the provision of an immune-modulated enteral formula for 5 to 7 days preoperatively (a component of the Enhanced Recovery After Surgery protocol, also referred to as ERAS), as a means of minimizing catabolism and supporting anabolism, has been associated with improved postoperative outcomes.[2] A key nutritional aspect of the ERAS protocol is the use of perioperative nutrition strategies to minimize long periods of fasting. In addition to preoperative oral supplementation, the protocol recommends reestablishment of an oral postoperative diet within hours of surgery and rapid advancement to a GI soft diet, with early initiation of nutrition therapy as soon as a nutritional risk becomes apparent—as, for example, in malnourished patients who are unable to consume on their own at least 50% of the recommended intake for more than 7 days.[2]

Energy

Patients should receive adequate energy, with carbohydrates constituting the majority of the energy intake (50%–60%), to supply sufficient glucose for optimal glycogen storage and to prevent lean muscle and adipose tissue catabolism (see Table 17.1).[4]

TABLE 17.1 Energy and Protein Requirements of Surgical Patients[4]

Patient status	Energy, kcal/kg/d	Protein, g/kg/d
Adequately nourished, preoperative	25	0.8-1.0
Adequately nourished, postoperative	25	1.0-1.1
Adequately nourished, stressed, postoperative	25-30	1.2-2.0
Nutritionally depleted, nonstressed, preoperative	25	1.0-1.2
Nutritionally depleted, nonstressed, postoperative	25	1.2-1.5
Nutritionally depleted, stressed	25-30	1.5-2.0

Protein

Most surgical patients do not require extra protein before surgery, but their needs should be assessed individually. Patients who are nutritionally depleted have slightly elevated protein requirements and should be given adequate protein along with adequate total energy (see Table 17.1).[4]

Micronutrients and Fluids

Any deficiency state, such as anemia, should be corrected. Electrolytes and fluids should be normalized and in balance; if the patient is dehydrated or has acidosis or alkalosis, these conditions should be resolved before surgery.[4] A patient who has been unable to consume or retain adequate nutrients because of their disease process (eg, GI obstruction) or GI symptoms (eg, nausea, vomiting, diarrhea) for a prolonged period may be at risk for refeeding syndrome. Laboratory test results should be assessed for the intracellular electrolytes potassium, phosphorus, and magnesium.[5] Low electrolyte levels should be corrected before initiating nutrition intervention, including intravenous glucose, and levels should be continually monitored and electrolytes replenished as nutrition therapy is provided.[5]

The appropriate approach to providing postoperative nutrition depends on the following factors:

- the surgical procedure performed and the anticipated time before the patient can resume oral intake
- any surgical complications and the patient's postoperative clinical status
- the patient's preoperative nutritional status

The well-nourished patient who has undergone elective surgery typically resumes oral feeding with liquids as soon as 12 hours after surgery, and with solids by postoperative days 2 to 5. In this situation, nutrition therapy in the form of enteral nutrition (EN) or parenteral nutrition (PN) is not indicated.

Postoperative Nutrition

Malnourished patients undergoing elective or emergent procedures who are not expected to meet their nutritional needs orally for 7 to 10 days should receive specialized nutrition support.[3] If feasible, this nutrition therapy should be provided enterally rather than parenterally, to minimize the incidence of complications. Therapy should begin 24 to 48 hours after surgery, and the patient should be advanced to the goal energy intake over the subsequent 48 to 72 hours.[3] The duration of the nutrition therapy depends on the patient's clinical status and transition to adequate oral diet consumption and tolerance. See specific sections in this chapter on intestinal surgery, and see Chapters 19 and 20, respectively, for more information on EN and PN.

In the immediate postoperative period, especially in patients who are critically ill, the goal of nutrition therapy is to attenuate the patient's metabolic response to stress, prevent oxidative cellular injury, and favorably modulate the immune response.[3] Nutrition care includes providing appropriate macronutrients and micronutrients.

Energy

The energy requirements of surgical patients are generally higher postoperatively than preoperatively (see Table 17.1)[4] and may be affected by complications including infection, fever, sepsis, and wounds. These conditions alter the patient's metabolism and catabolism and thus elevate energy and protein requirements. If indirect calorimetry is not available to determine the patient's resting energy expenditure, predictive equations can be used to estimate energy requirements, though only a few equations have been validated (see Chapter 1). When it is not feasible to provide a patient's full energy requirements, efforts should be made to provide at least 60% to 80% of the goal energy requirements in order to achieve the clinical benefits of nutrition therapy within the first week after surgery.[3]

Protein

Postoperative patients have elevated protein requirements, particularly if they are critically ill.[2] Reasons for elevated requirements include increased catabolism and protein turnover and the need for tissue synthesis and wound healing. In patients who are critically ill, metabolic stress results in a loss of lean body mass, which leads to elevated protein requirements for all age groups (see Chapter 1). Protein tolerance, as opposed to protein requirements, often determines the amount of protein provided. Patients with impaired renal or hepatic function may not be able to tolerate the standard recommended levels of protein.

Fluids

A variety of methods can be used to estimate normal body fluid requirements. The Food and Nutrition Board of the National Academies of Sciences, Engineering, and Medicine recommends 1 mL fluid per kcal of energy expenditure for adults with average energy expenditures who live in average environmental conditions.[6] Fluid requirements increase with fever, high altitude, low humidity, profuse sweating, watery diarrhea, vomiting, hemorrhage, diuresis, surgical drains, and loss of skin integrity (eg, open wounds, burns).[7] Therefore, fluid status is of vital concern postoperatively. It is common for large volumes of fluids to be provided intraoperatively. Patients will typically diurese these volumes postoperatively; however, some patients may require diuretics.

To ensure fluid balance, surgical patients are typically provided with intravenous fluids until they can resume and tolerate oral intake. A patient's daily weight can be monitored to assess fluid balance; a fluctuation of 1 kg in body weight roughly reflects 1 L of fluid gain or loss.

Micronutrients

Adequate micronutrient nourishment is important for optimal postoperative recovery. Vitamins and minerals support many metabolic processes in the body, many of which are altered as a result of surgery (see Box 17.1). Surgical patients who experience excessive GI losses through nasogastric tube suctioning or surgical drains, diarrhea, and high ostomy or fistula outputs may be at risk for many vitamin and mineral deficiencies.[8] If a patient's fluid losses exceed 800 mL/d, micronutrient supplementation should be considered.[4,9]

BOX 17.1

Selected Vitamins and Minerals of Concern in Surgical Patients

Folate

Functions as a coenzyme in the transfer of single-carbon fragments from one compound to another for amino acid metabolism and nucleic acid synthesis

Recommended daily intake: 400 mcg

Thiamin

Facilitates energy transformation; synthesis of pentoses and nicotinamide adenine dinucleotide phosphate (NADPH); and membrane and nerve conduction

As thiamin pyrophosphate: serves as a magnesium-coordinated coenzyme for the oxidative decarboxylation of α-keto acids involved in carbohydrate metabolism

Involved in the activity of transketolase in the pentose phosphate pathway

Recommended daily intake: 1.0 to 1.2 mg

Vitamin A

Forms of vitamin A are important for reproduction (retinol), vision (retinaldehyde), and normal structure and function of epithelial cells (retinoic acid)

Recommended daily intake: 700 to 900 RE

Vitamin B12

Involved in the metabolism of every cell of the body; especially affects DNA synthesis and regulation and fatty acid synthesis and energy production

Recommended daily intake: 2.4 mcg

Vitamin C

Antioxidant; reacts with superoxide, hydroxyl radicals, and singlet oxygen

Provides reducing equivalents for a variety of reactions

Acts as a cofactor for reactions requiring a reduced metal

Required for synthesis of collagen, carnitine, and neurotransmitters

Enhances intestinal absorption of nonheme iron, cholesterol hydroxylation into bile acids, reduction of toxic transition metals, reductive protection of folate and vitamin E, and immune-mediated and antibacterial functions of white blood cells

Recommended daily intake: 65 to 90 mg

Box continues

BOX 17.1 (CONTINUED)

Vitamin D

Maintains serum calcium and phosphorus levels to support neuromuscular function, bone calcification, and other cellular processes; anti-inflammatory agent

Recommended daily intake: 5 to 15 mcg

Vitamin E

Maintains membrane integrity in body cells via its role as an antioxidant

Recommended daily intake: 15 mg α-tocopherol

Vitamin K

Functions in the posttranslational gamma-carboxylation of clotting factors (II, VII, IX, X) and anticoagulant proteins (C and S)

May benefit bone health

Recommended daily intake: 75 to 120 mcg

Copper

Copper enzymes (superoxide dismutase, ceruloplasmin, copper thioneins): function in oxidation-reduction and electron transfer reactions involving oxygen

Ceruloplasmin: also responsible for manganese oxidation and oxidation of ferrous iron to ferric iron

Other copper-dependent enzymes:

- lysyl oxidase—forms cross linkages found in collagen and elastin
- dopamine β-monooxygenase—needed to convert dopamine to norepinephrine
- peptidylglycine α-amidating monooxygenase—needed to activate and deactivate various peptide hormones
- others—used to form myelin

Necessary for cholesterol and glucose metabolism and the formation of melatonin pigment

Recommended daily intake: 700 to 900 mcg

Iron

Is an essential component of hemoglobin (facilitates oxygen transport), myoglobin (facilitates muscle iron storage), and cytochromes (facilitates oxidative production of cellular energy as adenosine triphosphate [ATP])

Recommended daily intake: 8 to 18 mg

Selenium

Has antioxidant activity

Essential for thyroid hormone synthesis and metabolism

Recommended daily intake: 55 mcg

Box continues

Specific Types of Surgery and Their Related Nutritional Concerns

The digestive tract is a metabolically active organ involved in digestion, absorption, and metabolism of many nutrients. For this reason, various surgical interventions involving the GI tract can result in malabsorption and maldigestion and lead to nutritional deficiencies. To appreciate the magnitude of the nutrient alterations that can occur as a result of surgery, one must be familiar with both the anatomy of the GI tract and sites of nutrient absorption (see Figure 17.1 on page 290). Practitioners should monitor patients for potential deficiencies of specific nutrients according to the type of surgical resection performed or the location of the nonfunctioning GI tract that remains.

Head and Neck Surgery

Preoperative patients with head and neck cancer are usually malnourished as a result of their disease state. Often, the tumor inhibits the patient's ability to chew and swallow normally, which typically is what makes the patient seek medical attention. Also, preoperative treatment may involve radiation, chemotherapy, or a combination of both to reduce tumor bulk, and these therapies may diminish the patient's ability to swallow. Even if the patient can consume some liquids and soft foods, oral intake is often not enough to support nutritional needs. Furthermore, many patients with head and neck cancer have a long history of alcohol and tobacco use, which may also negatively affect their nutrient intake (see Chapter 10 for more information on head and neck cancer).

Preoperative improvements in nutritional status are important for optimal postoperative recovery. Oral supplementation may be indicated, and in some cases liquid supplements with altered consistency may be necessary because of dysphagia. Preoperative PN may be appropriate if the esophagus is obstructed. Patients with head and neck cancer typically require postoperative nutrition support, particularly if they receive chemotherapy, radiation therapy, or both, which can further delay their return to adequate oral nutrient consumption. Before surgery, a plan should be developed for how nutrition therapy will be provided postoperatively to avoid the use of PN, if feasible (see Chapter 20). If the tumor size permits, a percutaneous endoscopic gastrostomy (PEG) tube can be placed preoperatively to allow for perioperative EN. A feeding tube (PEG, open gastrostomy or jejunostomy, or nasoenteric) may also be placed intraoperatively to provide postoperative EN. If enteral access is not obtained intraoperatively, then PN is indicated because patients may not resume oral intake for 7 to 10 days.[3]

FIGURE 17.1 Nutrient absorption in the gastrointestinal tract

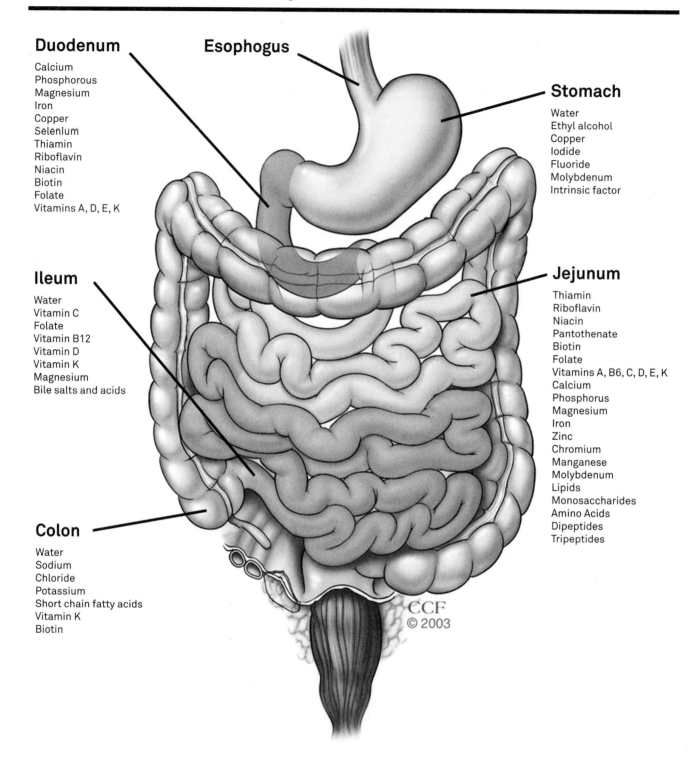

Duodenum

Calcium
Phosphorous
Magnesium
Iron
Copper
Selenium
Thiamin
Riboflavin
Niacin
Biotin
Folate
Vitamins A, D, E, K

Esophogus

Stomach

Water
Ethyl alcohol
Copper
Iodide
Fluoride
Molybdenum
Intrinsic factor

Ileum

Water
Vitamin C
Folate
Vitamin B12
Vitamin D
Vitamin K
Magnesium
Bile salts and acids

Jejunum

Thiamin
Riboflavin
Niacin
Pantothenate
Biotin
Folate
Vitamins A, B6, C, D, E, K
Calcium
Phosphorus
Magnesium
Iron
Zinc
Chromium
Manganese
Molybdenum
Lipids
Monosaccharides
Amino Acids
Dipeptides
Tripeptides

Colon

Water
Sodium
Chloride
Potassium
Short chain fatty acids
Vitamin K
Biotin

CCF
© 2003

Esophageal Surgery

Several medical conditions, such as corrosive injuries and perforation, achalasia, gastro-esophageal reflux disease, and partial or full obstruction caused by cancer, strictures, or congenital abnormalities, affect the esophagus and inhibit the ability to swallow. When surgical intervention is required to correct the abnormality, it involves removal of a segment of or the entire esophagus. The esophageal tract is then replaced with either the stomach (gastric pull-up) or the intestine (colonic or jejunal interposition). A gastric pull-up procedure (see Figure 17.2A) results in displacement of the stomach in the thoracic cavity. Patients having this procedure will have a reduced stomach capacity, with the potential for delayed gastric emptying and dumping syndrome (see Box 17.2 on page 292 for more on dumping syndrome). Another option for reestablishing esophageal continuity is to interpose a segment of colon (see Figure 17.2B) or jejunum between the distal esophageal remnant and the stomach or the duodenum after subtotal gastrectomy. Complications following this procedure include dysphagia, strictures, and leakage at the anastomotic site. Patients with dysphagia or strictures may be limited to a soft or liquid diet postoperatively. If the patient is unable to consume adequate nutrients orally, then a nasoenteric feeding tube may be placed, if feasible. A gastrostomy tube is not indicated if a gastric pull-up procedure is planned because the stomach is used to make the esophageal conduit, and a hole resulting from a gastrostomy tube would be contraindicated.

A Nissen fundoplication procedure is the most common antireflux operation for patients with chronic gastroesophageal reflux disease that is refractory to medical management. This procedure involves wrapping the stomach around the base of the esophagus (near the lower

FIGURE 17.2 Options for surgical reconstruction after esophagectomy

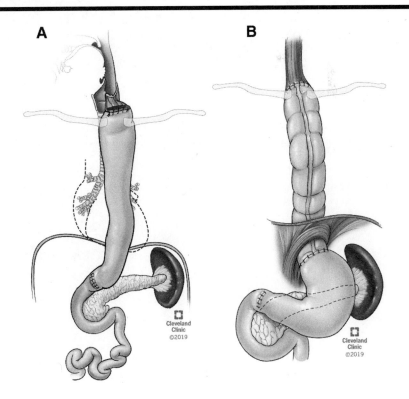

A   B

Reproduced with permission from Cleveland Clinic Center for Medical Art & Photography ©2020. All Rights Reserved.

Dumping syndrome is a constellation of postprandial symptoms that result from rapid emptying of hyperosmolar gastric contents into the small intestine. The hypertonic load in the small intestine promotes reflux of vascular fluid into the bowel lumen. A rapid decrease in circulating blood volume results. Early symptoms begin 10 to 30 minutes after eating or drinking. Late symptoms occur 1 to 4 hours after eating or drinking.

Symptoms include:

- abdominal cramping
- nausea
- vomiting
- palpitations
- sweating
- weakness
- hypotension
- tremors
- osmotic diarrhea

Dumping syndrome can result from insulin hypersecretion in response to carbohydrate loads being dumped into the small intestine. Following carbohydrate absorption, the hyperinsulinemia causes hypoglycemia, which results in vasomotor symptoms, such as diaphoresis, weakness, flushing, and palpitations.

esophageal sphincter) to place pressure in this region and narrow the lower esophageal opening in order to prevent reflux (see Figure 17.3). Because esophageal swelling occurs postoperatively and produces a feeling of tightness and dysphagia, patients are typically placed on a pureed diet for 2 to 4 weeks after this procedure until the swelling is reduced. Patients who undergo a Nissen fundoplication should subsequently avoid foods that can become lodged in the lower esophagus (eg, nuts, rice, and seeds). See Box 17.3 for other dietary guidelines.

FIGURE 17.3 Nissen fundoplication

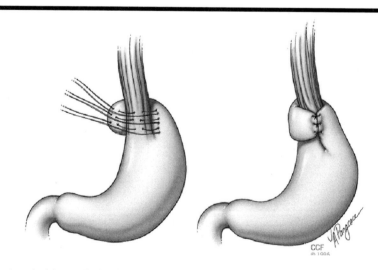

Eat pureed and moist foods for 2 to 4 weeks.

Avoid nuts, seeds, fresh bread, rice, tough meats, and foods with sharp edges (eg, chips, hard raw vegetables and fruits, pretzels, crackers).

Consume small, frequent meals.

Do not gulp fluids or food; chew and eat slowly.

Avoid use of straws.

Avoid gas-causing foods.

Avoid carbonated beverages, onions, cabbage, and beans.

Gastric Surgery

There are several indications for gastric surgery (see Box 17.4). A vagotomy is a surgical procedure in which one or more of the branches of the vagus nerve are cut, often done to eliminate gastric acid secretion. Vagotomy at certain levels can alter the normal physiologic function of the stomach, small intestine, pancreas, and biliary system (see Box 17.5 on page 295).[8,9] Vagotomy procedures are commonly accompanied by a drainage procedure (antrectomy or pyloroplasty) that aids with gastric emptying. Dumping syndrome, steatorrhea, and small intestinal bacterial overgrowth may be associated with these procedures.

A total gastrectomy involves removal of the entire stomach, whereas only a portion of the stomach is removed in a subtotal gastrectomy. A gastrectomy is accompanied by a reconstructive procedure. A Billroth I procedure (gastroduodenostomy) involves removal of the pylorus or antrum (or both) and an anastomosis of the proximal end of the duodenum to the distal end of the remnant stomach (see Figure 17.4 on page 294). A Billroth II procedure (gastrojejunostomy) involves removal of the stomach antrum and an anastomosis of the remnant stomach to the side of the jejunum, which creates a blind loop (see Figure 17.5 on page 294).

Patients who undergo any gastric surgical procedure are at risk for postoperative malnutrition (see Box 17.5 on page 295). Dietary modifications are a key component of the medical therapy after these surgical procedures (see Box 17.6 on page 296).[4] Many patients only require an antidumping diet for several weeks after surgery, but some patients may need to restrict their diet indefinitely.

Gastric tumor resection

Ulcer disease

Gastric perforation

Gastric hemorrhage

Zollinger-Ellison syndrome

Gastric polyposis

Ménétrier disease

Pylorotomy for gastroparesis

FIGURE 17.4 Gastroduodenostomy (Billroth I procedure)

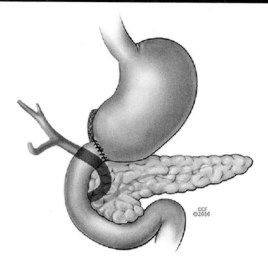

FIGURE 17.5 Gastrojejunostomy (Billroth II procedure)

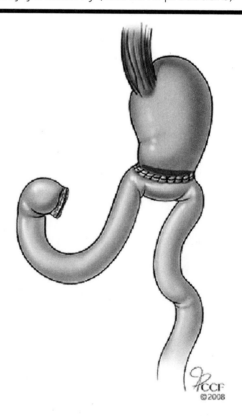

BOX 17.5

Gastric Surgical Procedures and Their Potential Complications[8,9]

[a] A bezoar is a retained concretion of indigestible foreign material that can accumulate in the stomach and cause a partial or complete blockage. A phytobezoar is a bezoar consisting of nondigestible food material. A pharmacobezoar is a bezoar consisting of medications. Precautions to prevent bezoar formation are to avoid nondigestible food ingredients and to crush medications or use liquid medications.

Procedure	Potential complications
Vagotomy: total gastric and truncal vagotomy	Impaired proximal and distal motor function of the stomach
	Delayed digestion and emptying of solids
	Accelerated emptying of liquids
Total gastrectomy	Early satiety, nausea, vomiting
	Weight loss
	Inadequate bile acid and pancreatic enzyme availability due to anastomotic changes
	Malabsorption
	Protein-energy malnutrition
	Anemia
	Dumping syndrome
	Bezoar[a] formation
	Vitamin B12 deficiency
	Metabolic bone disease
Subtotal gastrectomy with vagotomy	Early satiety
	Delayed gastric emptying
	Rapid emptying of hypertonic fluids

When a patient is malnourished preoperatively, a small bowel feeding tube may be placed intraoperatively so that low-rate enteral feedings can be initiated in the early postoperative phase. Enteral feedings can then be adjusted according to the patient's clinical progress and tolerance of an oral diet. It is not unusual to discharge patients to home care with tube feedings until their oral diet is optimal (see Chapter 22 for more information on EN in the home setting). Oral supplements may be provided to increase nutrient intake; however, to avoid dumping, the supplements need to be isotonic and should not contain simple sugars.[9] Unfortunately, many oral supplements contain simple sugars and are hyperosmolar, which means they are not tolerated well postoperatively. PN is indicated only if enteral access is not available, the patient is malnourished, and unable to tolerate adequate nutrients orally.

Anemia is a common long-term consequence of gastric surgery. It may be a result of a deficiency or malabsorption of one or more nutrients, including iron, folate, and vitamin B12 (see Box 17.7 on page 297).[8] Patients who have had a total gastrectomy, and some who have had a subtotal gastrectomy, require periodic intramuscular vitamin B12 injections.

Metabolic bone disease (eg, osteoporosis)—an abnormality of bones that is commonly caused by deficiencies in minerals such as calcium, phosphorus, magnesium, and vitamin D, and which increases the risk of bone failure—can also be a late complication of gastric surgery. For that reason, in addition to consuming dietary calcium, patients require calcium and vitamin D supplementation (see Box 17.7).[9]

Principles of the diet

Postoperatively, some discomfort (gas, bloating, cramping) and diarrhea may occur. To reduce the likelihood of these symptoms, patients should follow a healthy, nutritionally complete diet. Each patient may react to foods differently. Foods should be reintroduced into the diet slowly.

Diet guidelines for patients

Eat small, frequent meals.

Limit fluids to 4 oz (½ c) at a meal—just enough to "wash down" food.

Drink remaining fluids at least 30 to 40 minutes before and after meals.

Eat slowly and chew foods thoroughly.

Avoid extreme temperatures of foods (very hot or very cold).

Use seasonings and spices as tolerated (but consider avoiding pepper and hot sauce).

Remain upright while eating and for at least 30 minutes after eating.

Avoid simple sugars in foods and drinks. Examples of foods and ingredients to avoid: fruit juice, sport drinks, fruit-flavored drinks, sweet tea, sucrose, honey, jelly, corn syrup, cookies, pie, and doughnuts.

Eat complex carbohydrates, such as bread, pasta, rice, potatoes, and vegetables, as desired; these foods do not need to be limited.

Include a protein-containing food at each meal.

Limit fats to less than 30% of total energy intake. Avoid fried foods, gravies, fat-containing sauces, mayonnaise, fatty meats (sausage, hot dogs, ribs), chips, biscuits, and pancakes.

Because lactose in milk and dairy products may not be tolerated, introduce dairy foods slowly into the diet if they were tolerated preoperatively. Lactose-free milk or soy milk is suggested.

Avoid sugar alcohols (eg, sorbitol in beverages, candies, and medications).

Intestinal Surgery

If an excessive length of a patient's intestine is removed, nutritional consequences can arise depending on the location resected (see Box 17.8 on page 298). Short bowel syndrome may occur if more than 50% of the small intestine is removed. This syndrome is characterized by severe diarrhea or steatorrhea, malabsorption, and malnutrition (see Chapter 4). Patients with short bowel syndrome often require long-term PN to maintain nutritional status and fluid and electrolyte balance.

Pancreaticoduodenectomy (Whipple Procedure)

In cases of ampullary, duodenal, and pancreatic malignancy, a pancreaticoduodenectomy (Whipple procedure) may be performed. This procedure is one of the most technically difficult and challenging of GI surgical procedures and involves resecting the distal stomach, the distal common bile duct, the pancreatic head, and the duodenum. Three anastomoses must be done: (1) pancreaticojejunostomy, (2) choledochojejunostomy, or hepaticojejunostomy

BOX 17.7

Nutrient Deficiency–Related Complications of Gastric Surgery[8,9]

Microcytic anemia (iron deficiency or malabsorption)

Surgery-related causes or mechanisms

With a total and subtotal gastrectomy the following may occur:

- Achlorhydria leads to insufficient cleavage of iron from food sources.
- Reduction and solubilization of ferric iron to the ferrous form.
- *Note:* Anemia is more common with the Billroth II procedure than with the Billroth I because Billroth II bypasses the primary sites of iron absorption.

Food intolerance and reduced gastric capacity lead to reduced intake of iron-rich foods.

Management

Supplementation with 325 mg ferrous sulfate twice daily and coadministration of vitamin C

Macrocytic anemia (folate or vitamin B12 deficiency or malabsorption)

Surgery-related causes or mechanisms

Achlorhydria leads to insufficient liberation of vitamin B12 from protein food sources.

Decreased intrinsic factor leads to decreased binding of vitamin B12.

Reduced intake of protein-rich foods that supply vitamin B12 and/or their intolerance and reduced gastric capacity.

Management

Monthly intramuscular vitamin B12 injections (1,500 mcg)

Metabolic bone disease (calcium deficiency or malabsorption)

Surgery-related causes or mechanisms

Rapid gastric emptying can reduce calcium absorption.

Fat malabsorption can lead to insoluble calcium soap formation.

Vitamin D malabsorption may accompany fat malabsorption, which can impair calcium and phosphorus metabolism.

Note: Metabolic bone disease is more common with the Billroth II procedure than with Billroth I because Billroth II bypasses the duodenum and proximal jejunum.

Management

Daily supplementation with 1,500 mg calcium and 800 IU vitamin D

BOX 17.8

Nutritional Consequences of Intestinal Surgery

Surgical location	Potential consequences
Stomach (gastric bypass)	Protein-energy malnutrition from malabsorption due to dumping or unavailability of bile acids and pancreatic enzymes related to anastomotic changes
	Bezoar formation
Proximal small intestine	Malabsorption of calcium, magnesium, iron, vitamin A, and vitamin D
Distal small intestine	Malabsorption of water-soluble vitamins (folate, vitamins B12, thiamin, riboflavin, vitamin B6, and vitamin C)
	Protein-energy malnutrition due to dumping
	Fat malabsorption
	Bacterial overgrowth if ileocecal valve is resected
Colon	Fluid malabsorption
	Electrolyte (potassium, sodium, chloride) malabsorption

if a cholecystectomy was performed before or as part of the Whipple procedure, and (3) gastrojejunostomy (Billroth II). In some cases, the pylorus-sparing pancreatoduodenectomy has become the preferred variation because it has fewer postoperative nutritional consequences (Figure 17.6).

Common complications after these procedures include delayed gastric emptying, dumping syndrome, weight loss, diabetes, and malabsorption due to pancreatic exocrine insufficiency or asynchrony. Nutrient guidelines for the period following these procedures are similar to those following a gastrectomy and proximal small bowel resection.

Ileostomy and Colostomy

An ileostomy or colostomy may be required in patients with intestinal lesions, obstruction, necrosis, or inflammatory bowel disease of the distal small intestine or colon, or when diversion of fecal matter is necessary. These procedures involve the creation of an artificial anus on the abdominal wall by cutting into the colon or ileum and bringing it out to the surface, forming a stoma. A pouch is placed externally over the stoma to collect the fecal matter.

In general, patients should consume a modified diet consisting of mostly bland, low-fiber foods for the first few weeks after an ostomy in order to avoid stoma blockage; then, after this initial period, patients with ostomies should eat regular diets. Patients may wish to avoid foods that are gas-forming or difficult to digest in order to reduce adverse effects (see Box 17.9). In the case of high-output ostomies (>800 mL/d), patients may need to avoid hypertonic, simple sugar–containing liquids and foods, fatty foods, and foods high in insoluble fiber.

FIGURE 17.6 Pancreaticoduodenectomy (Whipple procedure)

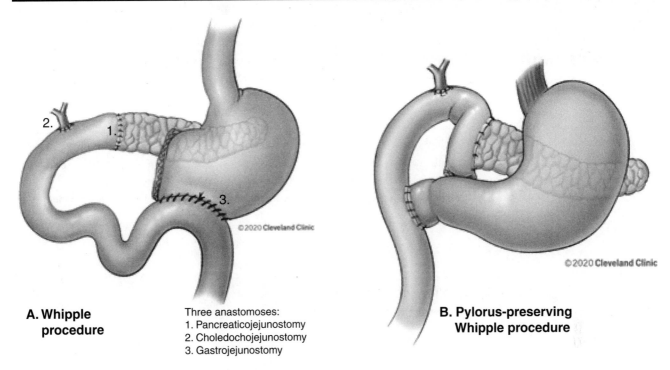

A. Whipple procedure

Three anastomoses:
1. Pancreaticojejunostomy
2. Choledochojejunostomy
3. Gastrojejunostomy

B. Pylorus-preserving Whipple procedure

©2020 Cleveland Clinic

©2020 Cleveland Clinic

Reproduced with permission from Cleveland Clinic Center for Medical Art & Photography ©2020. All Rights Reserved.

BOX 17.9

Foods and Their Effects for Patients With an Ostomy

Food effect	Foods
Produces odor[a]	Asparagus, beans, brussels sprouts, cabbage, coffee, cucumber, eggs, fish, garlic, green peppers, milk, onions, prunes, radishes, turnips
Decreases odor	Buttermilk, cranberry juice, parsley, spinach, yogurt
Produces gas[b]	Apples (raw), asparagus, beans, broccoli, cabbage, carbonated beverages, cauliflower, corn, cucumber, dairy foods, eggs, melons, mushrooms, onions, peas, spicy foods, spinach
Thickens stools[c]	Applesauce, bananas (the greener the better), breads, cheeses, marshmallows, milk, peanut butter (creamy), starches (rice, pasta, potatoes, tapioca), yogurt
Thins stools	Apple juice, chocolate, fresh fruits, fried foods, grape juice, green beans, highly seasoned foods, prune juice

[a] *Vitamin supplements may also contribute to odor production.*
[b] *Chewing gum and the use of straws (swallowing air) may also cause gas.*
[c] *Soluble fiber supplements may also help thicken stools.*

Surgical Procedures for Short Bowel Syndrome and Intestinal Failure

Strictureplasty

Some patients, especially those with Crohn's disease, can develop strictures or have an area of narrowing in chronically inflamed areas of their small intestine. This can lead to abdominal pain with eating and result in a small bowel obstruction. In previous eras, this would lead to resection and, if recurrent, the eventual development of short bowel syndrome and intestinal failure. Current techniques help to preserve intestinal length. One technique, the Heineke-Mikulicz strictureplasty, involves incising horizontally through the area of stricture and closing the incision vertically in order to enlarge the constricted area and simultaneously relieve the intestinal obstruction (see Figure 17.7). Another technique, the Jaboulay strictureplasty, involves creating a side-to-side anastomosis that bypasses the obstructing segment and preserves intestinal length (see Figure 17.8). These procedures have reduced the need for intestinal resections in patients with intestinal strictures and can potentially prevent the iatrogenic development of short bowel syndrome in patients with recurrent or multiple strictures.[10,11]

FIGURE 17.7 Heineke-Mikulicz strictureplasty

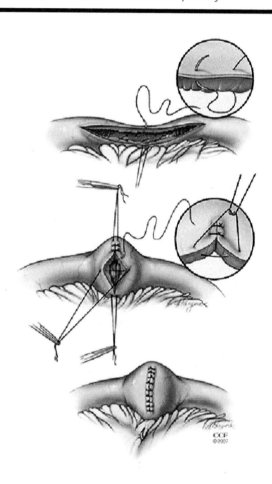

FIGURE 17.8 Jaboulay strictureplasty

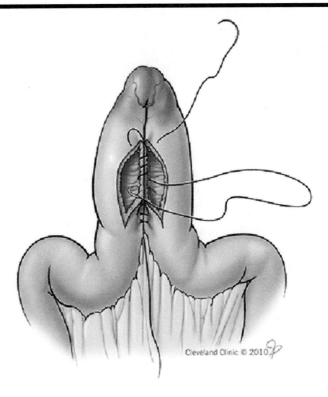

Intestinal Lengthening

Patients with short bowel syndrome and intestinal failure may have their intestinal absorption improved by intestinal lengthening procedures. These procedures are done on dilated segments of remnant small intestine. It is not clear if the benefit comes from the actual lengthening of the intestine or from the reduction in stasis in the dilated segment. The Bianchi procedure, which creates two smaller cylindrical tubes from a dilated segment, is technically demanding and has been replaced in many medical centers by serial transverse enteroplasty, or STEP (see Figure 17.9 on page 302).[10,11] In STEP, a serrated edge on opposite sides of the intestine is created by serial applications of a stapling and cutting device to form an accordion-like bowel segment that increases the length of the small bowel. A repeat STEP procedure on the same segment of intestine can be done if additional lengthening is needed. Patients who undergo these procedures may have less need for PN.[10,11]

Visceral Transplantation

Transplantation of GI organs has become a lifesaving surgical option for the management of selected patients with intestinal failure (see Box 17.10 on page 302).[10,11] After a visceral transplant, patients must take immunosuppressive medications to prevent organ rejection. Patients are gradually weaned off PN as enteral feedings and diet are advanced and tolerated. An oral diet should be initiated within 2 weeks of the transplant, starting with small, frequent meals of a regular diet. The end goal is for the patient to have full nutrition autonomy, making healthy food choices and being mindful of food safety and potential drug–nutrient interactions.

FIGURE 17.9 Intestinal lengthening procedure: STEP

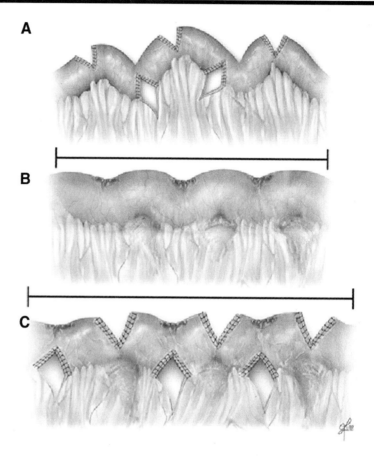

BOX 17.10

Indications for Intestinal Transplant in Patients Who Can No Longer Be Safely Maintained on Parenteral Nutrition[10,11]

- Impending or overt liver failure
- Inability to secure, or difficulty in securing, central venous access
- Frequent central-line infections requiring intensive care or hospital admissions
- Frequent episodes of severe dehydration

The type of transplant procedure performed depends on the organs to be transplanted and the type of intestinal failure. The four major types of visceral transplant procedures are as follows[10,11]:

1. isolated intestinal transplant for patients with intestinal failure and whose liver demonstrates adequate function and architecture (Figure 17.10a)
2. combined intestinal and liver transplant for patients with intestinal failure in whom the prime indication for transplant is impending or actual severe liver disease (Figure 17.10b)
3. full multivisceral transplant for patients with intestinal failure, severe liver disease, and diffuse GI disorders, including trauma and polyposis (Figure 17.10c)
4. modified multivisceral transplant for patients with diffuse GI disorders and good liver function (Figure 17.10d)

FIGURE 17.10 Four types of visceral transplantation

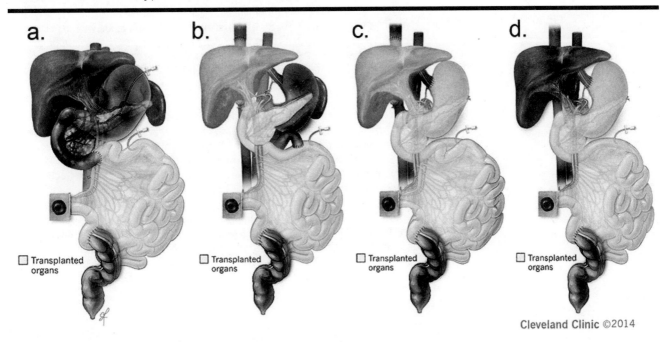

a. b. c. d.

☐ Transplanted organs   ☐ Transplanted organs   ☐ Transplanted organs   ☐ Transplanted organs

Cleveland Clinic ©2014

Summary

Preoperative nutrition care of the malnourished patient undergoing GI surgery can help improve postoperative outcomes. Postoperative nutrition care must focus on the delivery of appropriate amounts of energy, fluids, macronutrients, and micronutrients. The nutrition needs of patients will depend in part on the type of GI tract surgery performed—the various types affect intake and absorption differently and may be associated with a variety of adverse nutritional consequences. Some patients will need long-term nutrition interventions, ranging from avoidance of certain foods to nutrient supplementation to EN or PN in the home care setting.

References

1. White JV, Guenter P, Jensen G, Malone A, Schofield M; A.S.P.E.N. Malnutrition Task Force; A.S.P.E.N. Board of Directors. Consensus statement: Academy of Nutrition and Dietetics and American Society for Parenteral and Enteral Nutrition: characteristics recommended for the identification and documentation of adult malnutrition (undernutrition). *JPEN J Parenter Enteral Nutr*. 2012;36(3):275-283. doi:10-1177/0148607112440285

2. Weimann A, Braga M, Carli F, et al. ESPEN guideline: clinical nutrition in surgery. *Clin Nutr*. 2017;36(3):623-650. doi:10-1016/j-clnu-2017-02-013

3. McClave SA, Taylor BE, Martindale RG, et al; Society of Critical Care Medicine; American Society for Parenteral and Enteral Nutrition. Guidelines for the provision and assessment of nutrition support therapy in the adult critically ill patient: Society of Critical Care Medicine (SCCM) and American Society for Parenteral and Enteral Nutrition (A.S.P.E.N.). *JPEN J Parenter Enteral Nutr*. 2016;40:159-211.

4. Cresci GAM, MacGregor JM, Harbison SP. Surgical nutrition. In: Lawrence PF, ed. *Essentials of General Surgery and Surgical Specialties*. 6th ed. Wolters Kluwer; 2019:23-38.

5. Da Silva JSV, Seres DS, Sabino K, et al. ASPEN consensus recommendations for refeeding syndrome. *Nutr Clin Pract*. 2020;35:178-195.

6. Langley G, Tajchman S, Canada T. Fluids, electrolytes, and acid-base disorders. In: Mueller CM, ed. *The A.S.P.E.N. Adult Nutrition Support Core Curriculum*. 3rd ed. American Society for Parenteral and Enteral Nutrition; 2017:99-120.

7. Food and Nutrition Board, Institute of Medicine. *Dietary Reference Intakes for Water, Potassium, Sodium, Chloride, and Sulfate*. National Academies Press; 2004.

8. McKeever L. Vitamins and trace elements. In: Mueller CM, ed. *The A.S.P.E.N. Adult Nutrition Support Core Curriculum*. 3rd ed. American Society for Parenteral and Enteral Nutrition; 2017:121-148.

9. Palmer LB, Janas R, Sprang M. Gastrointestinal disease. In: Mueller CM, ed. *The A.S.P.E.N. Adult Nutrition Support Core Curriculum*. 3rd ed. American Society for Parenteral and Enteral Nutrition; 2017:426-453.

10. Fujiki M, Parekh N, Abu-Elmagd KM. Intestinal transplantation. In: Corrigan M, Roberts K, Steiger E, eds. *Adult Short Bowel Syndrome*. Elsevier, 2019:chap 16.

11. Abu-Elmagd KM, Armanyous SR, Fujiki M, et al. Management of five hundred patients with gut failure at a single center. *Ann Surg*. 2019;270:656.

CHAPTER 18

Bariatric Surgery

Jacqueline P. Dziuba, MS, RDN, LDN
Eric J. DeMaria, MD, FACS, FASMBS
Maria S. Altieri, MD, MS
Walter J. Pories, MD, FACS

KEY POINTS

- The prevalence of obesity among adults is increasing, with the causes rooted in genetics, health behaviors, psychological factors, environmental factors, disease prevalence, and medication use.
- Obesity and its associated comorbidities contribute to increased morbidity and mortality, increased health care costs, and decreased quality of life.
- Bariatric surgery is the most effective treatment for morbid obesity, as it provides the benefits of long-term weight loss, the improvement or remission of obesity-related comorbidities, and increased quality of life.

Introduction

Obesity is a chronic disease that is defined as a BMI of 30 or higher. The rates of obesity continue to rise in the United States, as evidenced by an increase of 11.9% in the prevalence of obesity from 1999–2000 through 2017–2018.[1] The causes of obesity are rooted in genetics, health behaviors (increased consumption of nonnutritive energy-dense foods, decreased physical activity), psychological factors (depression, disordered eating), environmental factors (lack of access to healthy food resources, food insecurity), disease prevalence (polycystic ovary syndrome, Cushing syndrome, hypothyroidism), and medication use (steroids, antidepressants).[1,2] The impact of obesity and its associated comorbidities contribute to increased morbidity and mortality, increased health care costs, and decreased quality of life (see Box 18.1).[1-3]

BMI has its limitations as an indicator of obesity, necessitating good clinical judgment. BMI is calculated using a simple formula—a person's weight in kilograms divided by the

---

BOX 18.1

Obesity-Related Comorbidities[2]

Cancer: breast, colon, endometrial, prostate, renal cell

Cardiovascular: coronary artery disease, congestive heart failure, hypertension, peripheral vascular disease

Endocrine: dyslipidemia, type 2 diabetes mellitus, gestational diabetes mellitus, metabolic syndrome, polycystic ovary syndrome

Gastrointestinal: cholelithiasis, nonalcoholic steatohepatitis, gastroesophageal reflux disease, hiatal hernia

Genitourinary: female infertility, urinary incontinence

Musculoskeletal: degenerative joint disease, gout, osteoarthritis

Neurologic: pseudotumor cerebri

Psychological: depression, eating disorders

Pulmonary: obstructive sleep apnea, asthma, hypoventilation syndrome

square of the person's height in meters (kg/m²)—and, as such, it excludes critical details of lean body mass vs adiposity, sex, age-related muscle loss, and ethnic and racial population differences.[4] Lean muscle mass weighs up to 18% more than nonlean mass or adipose tissue. A physical assessment of a patient's body composition should be performed to determine the presence of nonlean mass and adiposity. The distribution of adipose tissue should be categorized as android (visceral) or gynoid (subcutaneous). Sex differences should be considered, as males tend to have more android adiposity and females tend to have more gynoid adiposity. Android adiposity poses a greater risk for insulin resistance than gynoid adiposity does. As we age, lean muscle loss increases, and lean muscle is often replaced with nonlean mass. BMI does not consider ethnic and racial differences outside of European descent, meaning it does not consider Asian, African, or Aboriginal descent. BMI can be a useful screening tool, but a person-centered approach is best for ultimately determining whether a patient is at risk for obesity and its related comorbidities and whether that patient is a potential candidate for metabolic and bariatric surgery.[4]

Metabolic and bariatric surgery is the most effective treatment for obesity, as it provides the benefits of long-term weight loss, the improvement or remission of obesity-related comorbidities, and increased quality of life.[1] Patients with obesity may lose substantial percentages of their body weight in response to metabolic and bariatric surgical procedures, as follows[2,5]:

- adjustable gastric banding (AGB): 40% to 50%
- vertical sleeve gastrectomy (SG): more than 50%
- Roux-en-Y gastric bypass (RYGB): a mean of 60% to 80%
- biliopancreatic diversion with duodenal switch (BPD/DS): up to 70%

See Box 18.2 for equations to calculate excess body weight and estimate weight loss in adults undergoing metabolic and bariatric procedures.

The National Institutes of Health consensus statement for gastrointestinal (GI) surgery for severe obesity identifies potential candidates of metabolic and bariatric surgery as having a BMI of 40 or higher without comorbidity or a BMI of 35 or higher with at least one comorbidity.[6] See Table 18.1 for rates of resolved or improved comorbidities after bariatric surgery. Because this patient population has complex needs, a multidisciplinary team approach is recommended to ensure comprehensive preoperative screening and patient education, as well as postoperative care with continuation of long-term follow-up.

BOX 18.2

Calculating Excess Body Weight and Estimating Weight Loss in Adults Undergoing Bariatric Surgery

Excess body weight

Excess weight = Preoperative weight − Desirable weight

where: Desirable weight = Weight at BMI of 25

Weight loss

Excess weight loss (%) = (Weight loss ÷ Excess weight) × 100

Total weight loss (%) = (Weight loss ÷ Preoperative weight) × 100

To estimate weight loss expected with each procedure:

Estimated weight loss = Excess weight × Mean % of excess weight loss expected per procedure

Estimated weight loss expected with each procedure = Preoperative weight − Estimated weight loss

TABLE 18.1 Resolution or Improvement of Obesity-Related Comorbidities After Bariatric Surgery[2,5]

Comorbidity	Resolved or improved	Resolved
Hyperlipidemia	78.5%	61.7%
Hypertension	78.5%	61.7%
Obstructive sleep apnea	85.7%	83.6%
Type 2 diabetes mellitus	86%	76.8%

Patient Screening and Selection for Bariatric Surgery

The evaluation process consists of medical (including cardiac and pulmonary), psychological, nutritional, and surgical evaluations for metabolic and bariatric surgery. The process can take from several months to more than a year to complete, and the time needed often depends on the requirements of the candidate's insurance company. Potential candidates for metabolic and bariatric surgery must be well informed about the types of surgeries, the risks involved, the responsibilities of the patient, and weight-loss expectations according to the mean weight loss associated with each procedure. Candidates must demonstrate sufficient motivation to make lifelong diet and behavior changes to sustain weight loss, and they must have previously attempted nonsurgical approaches to weight loss without success. Additional criteria for patient screening and selection are listed in Box 18.3.

BOX 18.3

Screening and Selection Criteria for Metabolic and Bariatric Surgery[5]

Characteristic or issue	Criteria
Age	No universally accepted guidelines for age
	No minimum or maximum age identified
Clinically severe obesity	BMI of 40 or greater, or BMI of 35 or greater with obesity-related comorbidities
Previous weight loss	History of multiple weight-loss attempts without successful weight maintenance
Medical and surgical clearance	Absence of diseases associated with increased risk for complications or mortality
Psychological evaluation	Absence of eating disorders, major depression, or psychosis
	No drug or alcohol abuse
	Ability to comprehend behavioral and lifestyle changes
Other considerations	Cessation of smoking for at least 2 months prior to surgery
	Pregnancy not planned for at least 2 years after surgery
	Mobility and potential for physical activity
	Commitment to lifelong nutritional supplementation and medical monitoring after surgery

Nutrition Management Before Bariatric Surgery

The registered dietitian nutritionist (RDN) plays an integral role in the care of patients undergoing metabolic and bariatric surgery, helping to ensure positive health outcomes and sustained weight loss.[6] The RDN provides medical nutrition therapy according to the four steps of the Academy of Nutrition and Dietetics Nutrition Care Process—nutrition assessment, diagnosis, intervention, and monitoring and evaluation[7]—as guided by current practice recommendations in the Academy of Nutrition and Dietetics position paper on weight management.[8]

Most candidates are required to complete a preoperative medically supervised weight management program involving diet education and behavior modification to achieve optimal postoperative success. Preoperative weight-loss goals are provided at the discretion of the bariatric multidisciplinary team but are not a standardized requirement.

A preoperative diet is often recommended to improve the patient's glycemic control, produce rapid weight loss, reduce liver size, shorten surgical time, and reduce postoperative complications, such as bleeding, anastomotic leak, abscess, and wound infections. Use of the very low-calorie diet (400–800 kcal/d) or low-calorie diet (less than 1,000 kcal/d) for 2 weeks before surgery may aid in reducing weight, BMI, visceral adiposity, and liver size.[9] The American Society for Metabolic and Bariatric Surgery (ASMBS) does not provide a consensus on the length of a preoperative diet but recommends limiting restrictions to less than 3 months for greater adherence.[10]

The preoperative diet, as recommended by the treating health care providers, must be differentiated from the preoperative supervised weight management program mandated by many health insurers for authorization to proceed with metabolic and bariatric surgery. The 2016 updated ASMBS position statement on insurance-mandated preoperative weight-loss requirements has concluded that there is no evidence-based need for these requirements or benefit to patient outcome, and they are generally viewed as a barrier to patient care imposed by insurance carriers and the cause of needless delays in treatment.[10]

Types of Metabolic and Bariatric Surgical Procedures

Minimally invasive surgical techniques are most commonly used in metabolic and bariatric surgery. Laparoscopic procedures, using multiple small incisions, speed the patient's recovery and return to normal activities and decrease operative morbidity and mortality.

When a laparoscopic approach is not an option, surgical access is obtained through an upper midline incision, which is referred to as an open approach. Patients undergoing an open procedure may have a longer hospital stay and higher incidence of some complications, such as infections, hernias, and wound dehiscence.[11]

Metabolic and bariatric surgical procedures (see Figure 18.1 on page 310) are classified as follows[2]:

- restrictive (AGB)
- restrictive with some metabolic aspects (SG)
- restrictive with some malabsorption (RYGB)
- primarily malabsorptive with some restriction and metabolic aspects (BPD/DS)

SG and RYGB are the most common weight-loss surgeries in the United States. The AGB procedure has generally faded from popularity for several reasons, including a high repeat operation rate and relatively poor weight loss overall. It has also faded because of the emergence of the SG procedure, which has gained tremendous popularity as a primary procedure in recent years and is now the most commonly performed metabolic and bariatric surgical procedure in the United States. SG provides rapid weight loss similar to RYGB, does not require a foreign object (as in AGB) or a bypass of the GI tract (as in RYGB), and requires a shorter hospital stay.[5]

RYGB has greater long-term weight-loss results and less risk of reflux, but it has a higher rate of complications than SG. BPD/DS has better weight-loss outcomes and is more effective in treating type 2 diabetes mellitus than either AGB, SG, or RYGB, but it comes with a higher mortality rate, more complications, and more macronutrient and micronutrient deficiencies.[5] Selecting the most appropriate procedure for a patient requires a surgical consultation and the consideration of several variables, including the patient's BMI, operative risk, and comorbidities.

Adjustable Gastric Banding

AGB is a gastric restrictive procedure that is used to create an early sense of satiety in the patient, limit food intake, and cause weight loss. The band is placed just below the gastroesophageal junction, creating a small pouch with a narrow opening to the larger lower stomach (see Figure 18.1). The gastric pouch is less than 30 mL in volume. An access port, placed deep under the patient's skin, is connected to the band by tubing. Saline solution is used to add fluid to the interior lumen of the band, restricting the flow of food from the pouch to the lower stomach. Adjustments are made to increase or decrease the diameter of the stoma to affect satiety and oral intake.[12]

Sleeve Gastrectomy

SG is a considered a restrictive and metabolic procedure that, in part, restricts how much food the stomach can hold (see Figure 18.1). During the surgery, a long, sleeve-shaped tube is created along the lesser curvature of the stomach using a 36-French to 42-French bougie to "size" the gastric diameter, and 75% to 80% of the remaining stomach, including the greater curvature, is removed. The macronutrients and micronutrients in food are absorbed normally; however, food intake is limited due to gastric restriction or neurohumoral changes (the reduction of ghrelin by removal of the gastric fundus) caused by the procedure. SG has evolved over time to a stand-alone procedure from its original role as a component of the BPD/DS (see Figure 18.1), a malabsorptive bariatric surgery for the superobese. It is now considered a primary operation for managing weight and has been widely adopted. However, a second procedure (either RYGB or BPD/DS) is occasionally needed if more weight loss is desired or for complications such as gastroesophageal reflux.[5]

Roux-en-Y Gastric Bypass

The RYGB procedure restricts food intake by creating a small gastric pouch, causes malabsorption of micronutrients by bypassing a portion of the intestines, and affects GI neuronal and hormonal signals (see Figure 18.1 on page 310).[13] The major feature of the RYGB is the proximal gastric pouch (<50 mL in volume) made from the lesser curvature of the stomach. This part of the stomach is less distensible and provides the restriction necessary for optimal long-term weight management. A gastrojejunostomy is made to connect the gastric pouch to the jejunum. This anastomosis, only 12 to 15 mm in diameter, limits the rate at which food flows through the pouch. The portion of the jejunum brought up to the pouch creates the alimentary (or Roux) limb. The length of the Roux limb can vary from 75 to 150 cm. A longer Roux limb may enhance the malabsorptive effects of the operation, which can produce greater weight loss. A longer Roux limb length may be indicated for patients with a BMI of more than 50. With the creation of the pouch and gastrojejunostomy, the larger distal stomach (or gastric remnant), the duodenum, and a small portion of the jejunum, referred to as the biliopancreatic limb, are bypassed. To permit gastric juices, as well as bile and pancreatic secretions, to mix with food, another anastomosis, a jejunojejunostomy, is created to connect the biliopancreatic limb to the Roux limb.

FIGURE 18.1 Bariatric surgical procedures

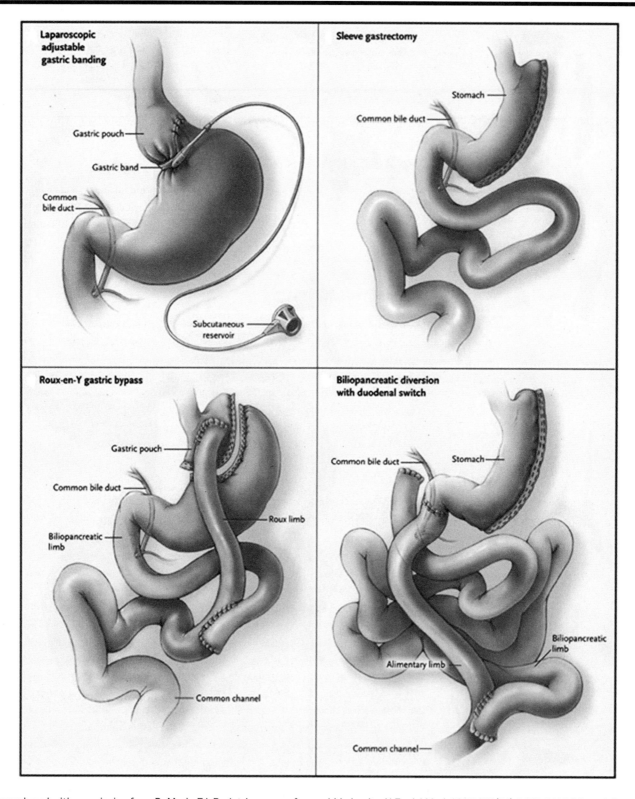

Biliopancreatic Diversion With Duodenal Switch

The BPD/DS is a restrictive, metabolic, and malabsorptive procedure that restricts how much food the stomach can hold, much like the SG procedure. Just as in the SG, a sleeve-shaped tube is created along the lesser curvature of the stomach and the duodenal stump is closed. The bypassed intestine (segment between the ligament of Treitz and the ileocecal valve) is connected from the stomach to the distal bowel, creating an alimentary limb. The biliopancreatic limb is connected to the alimentary limb above the ileocecal valve, forming a common channel that allows bile and pancreatic enzymes to mix with food.[14]

The metabolic and malabsorptive aspects are achieved via bypassing a portion of the intestines, thus affecting GI neuronal and hormonal signals (see Figure 18.1). Macronutrient malabsorption includes malabsorption of energy, largely via protein and fat, due to reduced bile and pancreatic enzymes. Micronutrient malabsorption includes malabsorption of fat-soluble vitamins, iron, zinc and copper.[14] One study concluded that BPD with DS does not improve weight loss or reduce macro- or micronutrient deficiency over BPD alone.[14]

Stages of the Postoperative Diet

Currently, there is no evidence-based recommendation for postoperative diet protocol following metabolic and bariatric surgery. The stages of the postoperative diet and diet progression can vary among medically supervised weight management programs. It is important for patients to strictly follow the directions given to them by their surgical team because the team takes a patient-centered approach, and general recommendations or other resources may not meet their individual nutrient and food-texture needs. Box 18.4 on page 312 summarizes the possible stages of the postoperative diet.[15-17]

Management of Adjustable Gastric Banding

Early Postoperative Management

Standard intravenous fluids are administered while the patient's status is nothing by mouth (npo). Consultation with an RDN is recommended to provide nutrition assessment, education, and recommendations for the patient's plan of care. As noted in Box 18.4 on page 312, patients usually advance to a bariatric clear liquid diet on postoperative day 1. Patients should be monitored for symptoms of postoperative stoma obstruction and gastric edema. After demonstrating tolerance to liquids, most patients are discharged within 24 hours of their AGB procedure, depending on their medical status, pain control, and presence or absence of nausea. The diet progresses to a bariatric full-liquid diet once the patient is at home and then advances as outlined in Box 18.4 on pages 312 and 313.

Patients should be cautioned to strictly adhere to dietary guidelines to prevent vomiting in the early postoperative period. If persistent vomiting occurs before the stomach has healed, the lower stomach may prolapse above the band. Patients may experience hunger for approximately 1 week postoperatively. They should be encouraged to consume protein-containing foods to increase satiety.

Diet-Related Concerns and Symptoms

Dysphagia to Solid Food

Dysphagia, also called "sticking" or "plugging," occurs in up to 12% of patients and can be caused by eating too quickly, taking too big a mouthful, not chewing the food enough, eating food that is not easily masticated, or eating doughy foods.[18] Some patients report dysphagia early in the day, with improvement over the course of the day. Food tends to be regurgitated from the esophagus rather than coughed up, as seen in patients with aspiration.

BOX 18.4

Postoperative Diet Stages Following Metabolic and Bariatric Surgery[15-17]

Stage 1: Bariatric clear-liquid diet

Indications	The clear-liquid diet is used to initiate oral intake after surgery and can usually be started within 24 hours of any bariatric procedure.
Duration	1 to 2 days. If clear liquids are required for a longer period of time, low-insoluble-fiber, high-protein nutritional supplements should be added and appropriate micronutrient supplements started, if not contraindicated.
Foods and fluids	Noncarbonated, caffeine-free, sugar-free beverages, as well as foods that are liquid at body temperature, are allowed. These include sugar-free gelatin, broth, sugar-free popsicles, decaffeinated or herbal teas, and artificially sweetened beverages.

Stage 2: Bariatric full-liquid diet

Indications	A full-liquid diet is indicated for the bariatric patient who has demonstrated tolerance to clear liquids for two meals or for patients being discharged from the hospital. The full-liquid diet permits further healing and is an intermediate step in the progression from clear liquids to a pureed diet. This stage approximates the energy and protein equivalent of a very low-calorie diet (less than 800 kcal/d). Patients, however, are not encouraged to "count calories" during this time but should instead focus on tolerance of oral intake.
Duration	10 to 14 days (postoperative weeks 1 and 2).
Foods and fluids	Low-fat milk products and milk alternatives, strained milk-based soups, vegetable juice, and low-energy liquid protein supplements are allowed. Some medically supervised weight management programs permit thin, refined hot cereals and low-fat or light Greek yogurt and custards on the full-liquid diet, whereas other programs introduce these foods on the pureed diet.
Vitamin and mineral supplementation	Patients should begin chewable or liquid supplements in accordance with protocol.

Stage 3: Bariatric pureed diet

Indications	A pureed diet is often indicated for the bariatric patient as an intermediate step in the progression from full liquids to a soft diet. Pureed foods gradually increase gastric residue and decrease the risk of obstruction due to improperly masticated foods.
Duration	Approximately 10 to 14 days, as tolerated.
Foods and fluids	Allowed foods and fluids include blended or liquefied foods that are low in sugar and fat; scrambled eggs and egg substitutes; pureed meat and beans; flaked, water-packed tuna or salmon, and meat alternatives; light or Greek yogurt; sugar-free pudding supplemented with protein powder; cottage cheese; soft cheeses; and hot and cold cereal. Pureed fruit or vegetables can be introduced, but protein-containing foods and beverages should be consumed first in the meal. Patients should continue taking liquid low-calorie protein supplements.
Vitamin and mineral supplementation	Patients should continue taking supplements according to protocol.

Box continues

BOX 18.4 (CONTINUED)

Stage 4: Bariatric soft diet

Indications	A soft diet is indicated for the bariatric patient as an intermediate step in the progression from pureed foods to a regular diet. The diet focuses on foods with a "soft" or "fork tender" texture that decrease the risk of obstruction due to improperly masticated foods.
Duration	Adjustable gastric banding: 14 days or more (starting in postoperative weeks 5 and 6). Roux-en-Y gastric bypass: 14 days (starting in postoperative weeks 5 and 6). Patients often remain on a soft diet for a longer period of time. Vertical sleeve gastrectomy: Progress as tolerated.
Foods and fluids	Allowed foods and fluids include ground or chopped tender cuts of meat and poultry; fish; cooked beans and lentils; meat alternatives; low-fat dairy products; well-cooked vegetables and canned fruits; soft, fresh fruit without peels or skins; and toasted whole grain bread and crackers as tolerated.
Vitamin and mineral supplementation	Patients should continue taking supplements according to protocol.

Stage 5: Bariatric regular diet (maintenance diet)

Indications	A regular diet is appropriate starting at 2 to 3 months (or more) postprocedure in patients who are able to tolerate foods of regular consistency.
Duration	Initiated approximately 2 months after surgery or when tolerated, maintained for life.
Foods and fluids	Allowed foods and fluids include solid and whole foods instead of processed; lean proteins; low-fat dairy products; fresh fruits and vegetables; whole grain bread and cereals. Patients should follow the MyPlate guide for variety among food groups and the Dietary Reference Intakes for vitamins and minerals.

A liquid meal replacement or protein-containing beverage may help these patients maintain appropriate nutrition and decrease their feelings of anxiety associated with dysphagia.

Obstruction of the Outlet of the Pouch

The prevalence of stoma obstruction is unknown. Severe pain and increased salivation can occur if the outlet of the pouch is obstructed. Vomiting or regurgitation may relieve the obstruction. If symptoms persist and liquid, including saliva, is not tolerated, all fluid in the band should be removed to permit the food bolus obstruction in the stoma to pass. If deflating the band does not work, endoscopy may be required to remove the obstruction.

Reflux

Up to 7% of patients experience reflux if the band is too tight or has slipped or if the stomach prolapses above the band.[18] Treatment may include removing the fluid from the band or undergoing another surgical procedure to reposition the band. The following behaviors may help reduce the risk of reflux:

- consuming lean sources of protein and limiting intake of fat to minimize delayed gastric emptying
- following appropriate diet advancement and consuming appropriate portion sizes to prevent overeating
- sitting upright at about a 90-degree angle after eating to reduce pressure on the esophageal sphincter

Band Adjustments

The process of incrementally adding fluid to the band is called an adjustment or fill. Several bands are approved for use in the United States. The type of band used will determine the total amount of fluid that can be added. Fill adjustments may be made per provider discretion.

If needed, the band can be adjusted at 6 weeks postoperatively. Multiple adjustments every 4 to 6 weeks may be needed in the first postoperative year for the patient to achieve optimal restriction and produce early satiety.

Patients should frequently be asked about their appetites, portion sizes, eating behaviors, and weight loss. An adjustment may be needed if the patient reports any the following:

- hunger between meals,
- increased appetite,
- ability to eat larger portions,
- increased snacking, or
- weight gain or weight plateau.

Fluid may need to be removed from the band if the patient reports any of the following:

- dysphagia,
- reflux or heartburn symptoms,
- night cough,
- regurgitation of food and liquids, or
- maladaptive eating behaviors, such as consuming soft foods and high-calorie liquids that digest easier through the tight band than do solid foods.

Adjustments can be made in the physician's office with or without the use of fluoroscopy. Accessing the port under fluoroscopy permits visualization of the esophagus, stomach, band, and the outlet of the pouch, and helps to diagnose complications.

After an adjustment of the band, a modified diet progression (see Box 18.5 on page 318) is followed to give the patient the opportunity to slowly experience drinking and eating with more fluid in the band. Weight loss should be slow and steady (1 to 2 lb [0.45 to 0.9 kg] per week in the first 24 to 36 months after surgery).[5]

The patient's commitment to frequent follow-up can positively influence weight loss.[19] Ongoing dietary and behavioral counseling, in addition to evaluating the need for an adjustment, are essential components of AGB outpatient monitoring.

Management of Sleeve Gastrectomy

Early Postoperative Management

Postoperative dietary management includes npo status for the first few hours. Standard intravenous fluids are administered until the patient demonstrates tolerance to liquids. Patients should consult with an RDN.

Patients usually advance to a bariatric clear-liquid diet within a day (see Box 18.4) and are typically hospitalized for 1 to 2 days. After demonstrating tolerance to liquids, most patients are discharged, depending on their medical status, pain control, and presence or absence of nausea.

The diet progresses to a bariatric full-liquid diet at home and advances as outlined in Box 18.4. Patients should be cautioned to strictly adhere to dietary guidelines to prevent dehydration and vomiting in the early postoperative period. Patients may not be hungry for weeks or months after surgery and need to be counseled on the importance of following diet instructions to develop positive eating behaviors and good dietary habits.

Diet-Related Concerns and Symptoms

Gastroesophageal Reflux

Up to 47% of patients experience symptoms of gastroesophageal reflux.[20] Over time, the incidence of reflux substantially decreases or completely resolves.[5] Dietary behaviors to manage reflux are the same as mentioned for AGB.

Nausea and Vomiting

Nausea and vomiting have been reported in 30% to 60% of patients postoperatively.[5] This may be related to specific food intolerances or caused by eating or drinking too quickly, too much, or not chewing food well enough.

Constipation

Constipation occurs postoperatively in 7% to 39% of patients.[5] It may be caused by decreased food and fluid intake. Patients should be advised to use appropriate fiber supplements and make dietary modifications to increase their fluid and fiber consumption. Patients may use stool softeners and laxatives when indicated. Frequent, light physical activity, such as walking each hour, can help stimulate GI motility and aid in bowel movement.

Early Dumping Syndrome

Early dumping syndrome occurs in up to 30% of patients after SG.[5] Refer to Management of Roux-en-Y Gastric Bypass.

Management of Roux-en-Y Gastric Bypass

Early Postoperative Management

Dietary management following RYGB includes npo status for the first few hours. Standard intravenous fluids are administered until the patient demonstrates tolerance to liquids. Consultation with an RDN is recommended.

Patients usually advance to a bariatric clear-liquid diet on postoperative day 1. Patients are typically hospitalized for 1 to 3 days. After demonstrating tolerance to liquids, most patients are discharged, depending on their medical status, pain control, and presence or absence of nausea.

The diet progresses to a bariatric full-liquid diet at home and advances as outlined in Box 18.4. Patients must follow the postoperative diet stages and advance as directed by their surgical team to meet hydration and protein needs and reduce the risk of complications. Patients may not feel hungry for weeks after their procedure, so the importance of following diet instructions, including a consistent, structured meal and fluid intake plan, must be stressed. Consistent and structured meal and fluid intake will help patients develop proper eating behaviors and maintain long-term success.

Diet-Related Concerns and Symptoms

Nausea and Vomiting

Refer to Management of Sleeve Gastrectomy.

Constipation

Refer to Management of Sleeve Gastrectomy.

Diarrhea and Flatulence

Diarrhea and flatulence following RYGB have been reported in up to 40% of patients.[5] Symptoms vary from two to three bowel movements a day to as many as 20 bowel movements a day.[6] Flatulence tends to be more common in patients who have had malabsorptive procedures. The general recommendations for managing diarrhea include increasing fluid intake and limiting the intake of lactose, insoluble fiber, and fat. Recommendations for managing flatulence include slowing the pace of eating, limiting sugar alcohols and gas-producing foods (cruciferous vegetables and legumes), and considering the use of probiotics, pancreatic enzymes, and bile chelators.

Early Dumping Syndrome

Early dumping syndrome occurs in 40% to 76% of patients following RYGB.[5] Early dumping usually occurs within 30 minutes of eating or drinking and can last for up to 60 minutes after eating a food or drinking a beverage that contains simple sugars or refined carbohydrates. The tolerable amount of sugar has not been identified. After ingestion, the hyperosmolar sugar particles rapidly empty into the jejunum, causing an influx of fluid into the intestine and triggering a gut neuroendocrine response that produces symptoms such as nausea, vomiting, abdominal cramping, diarrhea, dizziness, diaphoresis, and tachycardia. Often, patients need to lie down until symptoms resolve. Ingesting foods that are high in fat may cause GI symptoms similar to those observed with dumping syndrome due to delayed gastric emptying. The patient's fat intake should mostly consist of unsaturated fats, but overall fat intake should be limited due to its higher energy density.

Late Dumping Syndrome (Hyperinsulinemic Hypoglycemia)

Late dumping (postprandial hyperinsulinemic hypoglycemia) occurs 1 to 3 hours after eating. Symptoms usually include flushing, dizziness, palpitation, and light-headedness. In severe cases, loss of consciousness or other neurologic symptoms, including seizures, may occur.

Late dumping syndrome does not usually present until 1 to 2 years after RYGB. It is hypothesized to be the result of altered or increased beta cell function, exaggerated release in insulin, and decreased release of glucagon secondary to direct passage of oral intake (particularly high carbohydrate intake) into the small intestine.[21] Another theory suggests increased insulin sensitivity secondary to substantial weight loss following metabolic and bariatric surgery.[22]

General recommendations for managing late dumping syndrome include a meal structure consisting of four to six meals per day, spaced 3 to 4 hours apart, and refraining from fluid intake for 30 minutes postprandially. Since there is no standard for the tolerable amount of sugar intake, recommendations focus on limiting the intake of simple sugars and refined carbohydrates overall.[19] Carbohydrate intake should consist mainly of foods with a low glycemic index that are rich in fiber, such as fruits, vegetables, and whole grains.[5,23,24]

One study suggests that carbohydrate intake should be limited to 30 g per meal and 15 g per snack, as in a reduced-carbohydrate diet.[25] A clinical trial found that patients eating a high-protein, reduced-carbohydrate diet had greater hypoglycemic control than patients on a reduced-carbohydrate diet alone.[26]

Lactose Intolerance

Lactose is a sugar found in dairy products (milk, ice cream, cheese, and yogurt) and in protein supplements containing whey protein concentrates. Lactose digestion is initiated by the lactase enzyme, which hydrolyzes lactose (a disaccharide) into the monosaccharides galactose and glucose. Lactose intolerance is caused by reduced expression or activity of lactase in the small intestine. Reduced lactase activity allows lactose to pass into the large intestine, where gut flora cleave lactose into short-chain fatty acids and hydrogen, carbon dioxide, or methane gas, causing GI symptoms such as flatulence, bloating, and cramps. Some undigested lactose may persist and cause diarrhea.[27]

Lactose intolerance is most likely to occur in patients who have undergone malabsorptive RYGB because the site of the highest lactase activity in the small intestine is surgically bypassed. This allows more lactose to pass directly into the latter portions of small and large intestines, where less lactose activity is present.[27]

Patients with suspected lactose intolerance should consume lactose-free milk products, soy-based protein drinks, or protein supplements that contain whey protein isolates (lactose has been extracted from the product). Some milk alternatives, such as almond, cashew, and rice milks, do not contain as much protein as dairy or soy products, and patients opting for these lactose-free alternatives may need protein supplementation.

Micronutrient Deficiencies

Refer to the section on micronutrient (vitamin and mineral) requirements beginning on page 321.

Stricture of the Gastrojejunostomy

A gastrojejunal stricture is the most common stricture and occurs in 3% to 7% of patients within 1 to 3 months of RYGB.[28] Patients may experience vomiting and an inability to advance their diet or notice that they are only able to tolerate fluids. Treatment for a stricture is endoscopic balloon dilatation of the anastomosis. Several dilatations may be required before the stricture resolves and the patient can tolerate diet advancement. During this time, patients should receive dietary guidance to ensure that their nutrition goals are met. Patients may also develop a fear of eating and require psychological or emotional support.

Marginal Ulcers

The incidence of ulcers is higher in patients who resume smoking or who use nonsteroidal analgesics or aspirin after RYGB. Symptoms include vomiting, epigastric pain, and GI bleeding. Endoscopy is indicated for evaluation and treatment. Ulcers may compromise the patient's ability to meet nutrition goals. They are managed with acid-suppression medications and sucralfate before meals. Patients with severe ulcers may require bowel rest and parenteral nutrition.

Internal Hernia or Bowel Obstruction

Bowel obstruction can occur in up to 5% of patients in the immediate postoperative period or many years after RYGB.[28] An internal hernia occurs when the bowel herniates across a patent defect in the small bowel mesentery as a result of the surgical rerouting of intestine. Patients may experience intermittent or severe abdominal pain. Vomiting may not occur until late in the progression of obstruction. Emergency evaluation is indicated, including computed tomography of the abdomen. Reoperation is often necessary for hernia repair and to relieve the obstruction.

Leak of the Staple Line

Leaks of the staple line can be a life-threatening complication of RYGB if not diagnosed early. Reoperation is often necessary, and patients may require nutrition support in the postoperative period.

Management of Biliopancreatic Diversion With Duodenal Switch

Early Postoperative Management

Postoperative dietary management in BPD/DS includes npo status for the first few hours. Standard intravenous fluids are administered until the patient demonstrates tolerance to liquids. An RDN consult is recommended to provide nutrition assessment, education, and recommendations for the patient's plan of care.

Patients usually advance to a bariatric clear-liquid diet on postoperative day 1. See the section on postoperative dietary principles and modifications later in this chapter for more details.

Patients are typically hospitalized for 1 to 3 days. After demonstrating tolerance to liquids, most patients are discharged, depending on their medical status, pain control, and presence or absence of nausea.

The diet progresses to a bariatric full-liquid diet at home and advances as outlined in Box 18.5. Patients must follow the postoperative diet stages and advance as directed by their surgical team to meet their hydration and protein needs and reduce the risk of complications. Patients may not feel hungry for weeks after their procedure, so the importance of following diet instructions, including a consistent, structured meal and fluid intake plan, must be stressed. Consistent and structured meal and fluid intake will help patients develop proper eating behaviors and maintain long-term success.

Diet-Related Concerns and Symptoms

Following BPD/DS, 7% of patients experience nausea and vomiting, up to 19% experience diarrhea, and up to 5% experience anastomotic leak.[14] Other postoperative diet-related concerns include internal hernia or bowel obstruction, and a leak of the staple line. See the relevant topics under Management of Roux-en-Y Gastric Bypass for details.

Micronutrient Deficiencies

Refer to the section on micronutrient (vitamin and mineral) requirements beginning on page 321.

BOX 18.5	**Indications:** The postadjustment diet is used to gradually introduce solid foods after the band is filled.
Adjustable Gastric Banding: Postadjustment Diet Progression[15-17]	**Progression:** Full liquids for 1 to 2 days; pureed and soft foods for 3 days; regular foods as tolerated by day 5. **Foods and fluids:** As described in stages 2 through 5 in Box 18.4. **Other restrictions and considerations:** Patients should be reminded to chew foods well to facilitate digestion through a tighter stoma and to decrease the likelihood of an obstruction.

Dietary Principles and Modifications Following Bariatric Surgery

During the preoperative evaluation phase, patients must be educated about the postoperative diet stages they will go through and need for protein and micronutrient supplementation. Specific counseling on both *how* to eat and *what* to eat is essential for safe and successful weight loss.

The goals of the postoperative bariatric diet are as follows:

- Ensure adequate hydration.
- Consume high-quality protein in order to decrease loss of lean body mass, promote wound healing, maintain visceral protein stores, and support metabolic processes.
- Facilitate and promote weight loss by focusing on low-energy foods and beverages.
- Use the recommended vitamin and mineral supplements to ensure that micronutrient needs are met.
- Maximize food digestibility and tolerance with a gradual diet progression.

Initiating Postoperative Fluid Intake

Patients will need to learn to sip liquids slowly, beginning with 1 to 2 oz over 15 minutes. They should be instructed to increase their rate of fluid intake as tolerated, progressing from 4 oz per hour to 6 oz per hour to 8 oz per hour, eventually establishing a new "normal" pace of drinking. Drinking too quickly may cause patients to experience fluid stacking in their esophagus, foaming of saliva in the back of the throat, nausea, and vomiting. Recommended sources of fluid intake include:

- sugar-free or low-energy beverages,
- decaffeinated beverages (because caffeine is a GI irritant and diuretic that can increase the risk of dehydration),
- noncarbonated beverages (because carbonated beverages may cause cramping, bloating, nausea, and vomiting), and
- protein-containing liquids, including low-fat and nonfat milk, lactose-free milk, soy milk, and liquid protein supplements meeting the dietary criteria.

Fluid requirements are 48 to 64 oz of total fluid per day. Protocols vary based on provider and program.

Initiating Postoperative Food Intake

Approaches to initiate postoperative eating may vary by program or individual patient. Recommendations may include separating fluid intake and meals, limiting the volume of intake, pacing oral intake, and learning hunger and satiety cues.

Eating and drinking at the same time after metabolic and bariatric surgery may cause rapid gastric emptying, rapid gut transit, and rapid digestion of food, leading to increased consumption. It may also cause dumping symptoms in patients who have undergone RYGB. For these reasons, an important diet principle for all patients is to separate eating from drinking. Patients should be instructed to refrain from drinking during a meal and to wait at least 30 minutes after eating to drink.

Patients must also be taught to limit their food volume appropriately. Food volume is initially limited to ¼ cup (2 oz) per meal. Meal sizes gradually increase with tolerance, as the patient progresses through the postoperative diet stages, to a maximum of 1 cup (8 oz) per meal.

Because of volume limitations, patients are encouraged to eat three to six small meals daily, based on their estimated nutrition needs. The pace of eating is very important. Food should be consumed slowly over a 20- to 30-minute period. A bite, forkful, or spoonful of food should be quite small. Using an infant spoon and small-pronged fork can help remind patients to take small mouthfuls. Food must be chewed until it is of a semiliquid or pureed consistency. Examples of behavioral techniques to achieve this may include reciting phrases such as "chew for 42" or "the more you chew, the better you will do." Resting the eating utensil on the table in between bites may help slow the pace of eating. Patients should be advised to limit distractions, such as the television, computer, music, or other environmental stimuli, during meals so they can focus on appropriate eating behavior.

It is essential for patients to learn to recognize the signs of fullness (satiety), such as pressure, pain, or nausea, and to stop eating as soon as signs of fullness occur. Patients may feel like food is getting "stuck" if they eat too quickly. If the bolus of food cannot be digested, the body may expel the obstruction through vomiting or regurgitation. In a patient with an adjustable gastric band, slippage or prolapse of the stomach through the gastric band may occur if overeating causes frequent vomiting. If the obstruction persists, patients should be instructed to contact their physician.

Macronutrient Recommendations

Protein

The recommended daily goal for protein intake may be 60 to 80 g/d or 1.1 to 1.5 g per kg of ideal body weight, and up to 1.5 to 2 g per kg of ideal body weight in patients following BPD/DS.[5,15] It may be difficult for patients to meet their protein goals initially, but that will improve with tolerance of oral intake during the postoperative diet progression.

Commercially produced liquid or powder protein supplements of high biological value (whey, casein, soy protein, and egg albumin) are recommended until patients are able to meet their protein needs with food alone. Collagen-based products with added casein or another complete protein may not provide sufficient amounts of several indispensable amino acids; therefore, collagen-based products should not be used as the sole protein source after weight-loss surgery. Whey protein isolates are lactose-free; whey concentrates contain lactose in varying amounts. Patient adherence may be influenced by supplement taste, texture, convenience, ease of mixing, and price, as well as the patient's diet preference (eg, veganism). Before surgery, it is imperative that patients find a protein supplement they find palatable.

Patients should select foods that contain protein of high biological value, such as eggs, lean meats, poultry, fish, low-fat dairy products, and plant-based foods including green peas, nuts, beans, lentils, soy products, and other meat alternatives. The development of food intolerance to meat, poultry, or dairy foods may compromise protein intake. Patients should start each meal with protein-containing foods before consuming vegetables, grains, and fruit.

Fat

Experts recommend that patients select low-fat foods to minimize their energy intake. Patients who have undergone an RYGB procedure should also understand that eating high-fat foods may cause dumping-like symptoms. Patients should be encouraged to choose healthy sources of essential fatty acids and limit their intake of saturated fats.

Carbohydrates

The recommended daily carbohydrate intake is 130 g, which provides sufficient glucose to the central nervous system.[29] Consuming nutrient-dense, low-glycemic-index, fiber-rich carbohydrates, such as fruit, vegetables, and whole grains, is best, as is limiting the intake of carbohydrates with a high glycemic index. Patients should also avoid concentrated sweets because of their simple-sugar and nonnutritive energy content.[25]

Sugar alcohols may have a laxative effect in certain individuals who are sensitive; therefore, foods containing high concentrations of sugar alcohols should be avoided.

The fiber content prescribed in the early stages of the postoperative diet is suboptimal. Powder fiber supplements may be added to liquids or pureed foods (eg, applesauce) if the current diet stage restricts high-fiber foods, such as raw fruits and vegetables and whole grains.

Alcohol

There is no standardized recommendation on alcohol intake postoperatively, but most medically supervised weight management programs recommend limitation or avoidance in the initial postoperative diet stages or for longer. Recommendations vary based on program and provider. The 2016 ASMBS position statement on alcohol use before and after bariatric surgery states that some individuals are at risk for developing new onset or relapse of alcohol use disorder, particularly after RYGB.[30]

Following RYGB, patients are at higher risk for alcohol use disorder because of accelerated alcohol absorption, higher maximum concentration (blood alcohol content), and increased time needed to eliminate alcohol from the body. Data are inconclusive regarding altered alcohol metabolism in patients with SG and showed no effect on alcohol metabolism in those with AGB.

Although a history of alcohol use disorder is not a contraindication to metabolic and bariatric surgery, recommendations are to counsel patients about the risk and possibility of postoperative alcohol use disorder. Preoperative screening, assessment, and preparation, including treatment and abstinence, may be required as well.

Micronutrient Recommendations

Micronutrient supplementation may start as early as postoperative day 1, if tolerated, in chewable or liquid form. Transition from chewable or liquid form to tablet or capsule may depend on the discretion of the surgical team based on concerns of adequate absorption, size, and individual tolerance. Education about supplementation should begin in the preoperative stages. The RDN should review products with the patient to ensure that they meet ASMBS guidelines because over-the-counter supplements do not follow standardized formulas.

Barriers to adherence to micronutrient supplementation may include the high cost of products, intolerance to products, unpleasant taste, and forgetting to take the supplements. If cost or access to specialty products is limited, doubling the daily serving of a standard daily multivitamin is a more acceptable alternative than not taking any supplement. Vitamins may cause nausea or discomfort, and recommendations to improve tolerance include taking the supplements in smaller doses throughout the day and crushing or mixing tablets or the contents of capsules in unsweetened applesauce or a liquid. Liquid supplements may be better tolerated by patients who do not like chewable products or capsules. Taking supplements at the same time every day can help patients remember to take them, as can setting a reminder or alarm on a telephone, watch, or other device with a clock.

Patients may be advised to search for products that received a certification of quality from the United States Pharmacopeial Convention (USP). The USP performs manufacturing facility audits, evaluates product quality-control processes, and tests products to ensure the quality, potency, and purity of products.[31]

The risk of micronutrient deficiency is high following metabolic and bariatric surgery because of the restrictive, malabsorptive, or combined nature of the procedures. The lengthy postoperative diet advancement and patient intolerances to foods or food groups may also contribute to the risk of deficiency. Screening and repletion of an existing micronutrient deficiency should be done before surgery. Adherence to postoperative micronutrient supplementation according to the ASMBS guidelines is imperative to prevent deficiency and negative consequences on overall health. See Tables 18.2 to 18.5 (pages 322–323) for the ASMBS guidelines for postoperative micronutrient supplementation following AGB, SG, RYGB, and BPD/DS.[5,32]

TABLE 18.2 American Society for Metabolic and Bariatric Surgery Guidelines for Postoperative Micronutrient Supplementation After Adjustable Gastric Banding[5,32]

Nutrient	Supplementation to prevent deficiency
Calcium	1,200-1,500 mg/d
Copper	1 mg/d
Folate	400-800 mcg/d 800-1,000 mcg/d[a]
Iron	18 mg/d[b] 45-60 mg/d[c]
Thiamin	≥12 mg/d 500 mg/d titrated down to 100 mg/d[d]
Vitamin A	5,000 IU/d
Vitamin B12	350-500 mcg/d or 1,000 mcg/mo intramuscular
Vitamin D	≥ 3,000 IU/d
Vitamin E	15 mg/d
Vitamin K	90-120 mcg/d
Zinc	8-11 mg/d

[a] Potential birth parent
[b] Low-risk patients: people without history of anemia
[c] High-risk patients: menstruating people or those with history of anemia before surgery
[d] At-risk patients: vomiting, excessive alcohol intake, neuropathy, encephalopathy, heart failure, parenteral nutrition

TABLE 18.3 American Society for Metabolic and Bariatric Surgery Guidelines for Postoperative Micronutrient Supplementation After Sleeve Gastrectomy[5,32]

Nutrient	Supplementation to prevent deficiency
Calcium	1,200-1,500 mg/d
Copper	1 mg/d
Folate	400-800 mcg/d 800-1,000 mcg/d[a]
Iron	18 mg/d[b] 45-60 mg/d[c]
Thiamin	≥12 mg/d 500 mg/d titrated down to 100 mg/d[d]
Vitamin A	5,000-10,000 IU/d
Vitamin B12	350-500 mcg/d or 1,000 mcg/mo intramuscular
Vitamin D	≥3,000 IU/d
Vitamin E	15 mg/d
Vitamin K	90-120 mcg/d
Zinc	8-11 mg/d

[a] Potential birth parent
[b] Low-risk patients: people without history of anemia
[c] High-risk patients: menstruating people or those with history of anemia before surgery
[d] At-risk patients: vomiting, excessive alcohol intake, neuropathy, encephalopathy, heart failure, parenteral nutrition

TABLE 18.4 American Society for Metabolic and Bariatric Surgery Guidelines for Postoperative Micronutrient Supplementation After Roux-en-Y Gastric Bypass[5,32]

Nutrient	Supplementation to prevent deficiency
Calcium	1,200-1,500 mg/d
Copper	2 mg/d
Folate	400-800 mcg/d 800-1,000 mcg/d[a]
Iron	18 mg/d[b] 45-60 mg/d[c]
Thiamin	≥12 mg/d 500 mg/d titrated down to 100 mg/d[d]
Vitamin A	5,000-10,000 IU/d
Vitamin B12	350-500 mcg/d or 1,000 mcg/mo intramuscluar
Vitamin D	≥3,000 IU/d
Vitamin E	15 mg/d
Vitamin K	90-120 mcg/d
Zinc	8-22 mg/d

[a] Potential birth parent
[b] Low-risk patients: people without history of anemia
[c] High-risk patients: menstruating people or those with history of anemia before surgery
[d] At-risk patients: vomiting, excessive alcohol intake, neuropathy, encephalopathy, heart failure, parenteral nutrition

TABLE 18.5 American Society for Metabolic and Bariatric Surgery Guidelines for Postoperative Micronutrient Supplementation After Biliopancreatic Diversion/Duodenal Switch[5,32]

Nutrient	Supplementation to prevent deficiency
Calcium	1,800-2,400 mg/d
Copper	2 mg/d
Folate	400-800 mcg/d 800-1,000 mcg/d[a]
Iron	18 mg/d[b] 45-60 mg/d[c]
Thiamin	≥12 mg/d 500 mg/d titrated down to 100 mg/d[d]
Vitamin A	10,000 IU/d
Vitamin B12	350-500 mcg/d or 1,000 mcg/mo intramuscluar
Vitamin D	≥3,000 IU/d
Vitamin E	15 mg/d
Vitamin K	300 mcg/d
Zinc	16-22 mg/d

[a] Potential birth parent
[b] Low-risk patients: people without history of anemia
[c] High-risk patients: menstruating people or those with history of anemia before surgery
[d] At-risk patients: vomiting, excessive alcohol intake, neuropathy, encephalopathy, heart failure, parenteral nutrition

Special Considerations Regarding Bioavailability of Micronutrients

Calcium citrate is recommended over calcium carbonate because it is more readily absorbed. Intake should be limited to 500 to 600 mg per individual dose and paired with vitamin D for optimal absorption. Separate patient intake of calcium supplements from their intake of iron supplements by at least 2 hours because calcium and iron compete for absorption, and taking them too close together may make them less effective. Pairing 250 mg of vitamin C with iron aids in the absorption of iron supplementation.

Iron supplements may cause GI side effects, including constipation, dark stool, nausea, vomiting, metallic taste in the mouth, stomach pain, and headache. Ferrous iron is the most absorbable form, but patients may need to try different supplements to find the most tolerable form. Some of the iron supplements available include ferrous gluconate, ferrous fumarate, sulfate extended-release with mucoproteose, ferrous sulfate without mucoproteose, ferrous glycine sulfate, and iron protein succinylate. Other options for increasing tolerance of iron supplements may include taking smaller doses throughout the day or trying extended-release supplements or liquid formulas.[33]

Micronutrient Deficiency

Micronutrient deficiency can be identified by the patient's reporting of symptoms, observed by nutrition focused physical examination, and confirmed by abnormal laboratory values. Table 18.6 summarizes the signs, symptoms, and laboratory indexes of the various micronutrient deficiencies.[32, 34]

Evaluating Laboratory Markers of Nutritional Status

Box 18.6 on page 327 presents nutrition-related laboratory data that should be periodically assessed in patients who have undergone metabolic and bariatric surgery.[5] Monitoring of these markers should occur at 3 months, 6 months, 9 months, and then annually or as needed.[5] Treat deficiencies in accordance with established protocols.

Outpatient Monitoring After Bariatric Surgery

To achieve optimal results after bariatric surgery, patients should seek regular follow-up with an RDN, adhere to dietary recommendations, and commit to an active lifestyle. Nutrition visits are suggested at 1 to 2 weeks, 1 month, 3 months, 6 months, 9 months, and 12 months to monitor diet tolerance and progression. Appointments can be more frequent, if needed for an adjustment or other medical or nutritional indication.[5]

Evaluating Weight Changes

In the first 3 months after malabsorptive procedures, substantial weight loss (40 to 90 lb [18.2 to 40.9 kg]) may be observed. This translates into a loss of 0.5 to 1 lb (0.45 to 0.9 kg) per day. Weight loss is more gradual at 6 to 9 months postprocedure, with the goal being 1 to 2 lb (0.45 to 0.9 kg) per week.[35]

Maximum weight loss after RYGB is achieved within 12 to 18 months and averages 60% to 80% of body weight.[5] A more gradual weight loss is observed with AGB—goal weight may be achieved after 2 to 3 years and averages 48% of body weight.[5] Weight loss after SG can be achieved in 1 to 2 years and is similar to the weight loss observed with the RYGB (approximately 60%).[5] After BPD/DS, weight loss is achieved within 2 years and averages 70% of body weight.[14]

TABLE 18.6 Signs, Symptoms, and Laboratory Indexes of Possible Micronutrient Deficiencies After Bariatric Surgery[32,34]

Micronutrient deficiency	Prevalence	Early signs and symptoms	Advanced signs and symptoms	Laboratory indexes
Calcium	≤100%	Osteoporosis Osteomalacia Muscle weakness Cramping Excitability		Serum calcium, 9.0-10.5 mg/dL Diagnostic testing: DXA scan—current gold standard Assays for bone turnover markers, including bone formation markers (C-terminal P1CP N-terminal P1NP, alkaline phosphatase, osteocalcin) Assays for bone resorption markers assays (measurements of urinary excretion of N- and C- terminal cross-linked telopeptides and serum C-terminal telopeptides)
Copper	RYGB, 10%-20% SG, one case report BPD/DS ≤90%	Hypochromic anemia Neutropenia Pancytopenia Hypopigmentation of skin, nails, and hair Hypercholesterolemia	Gait ataxia	Plasma copper, 11.8-22.8 nmol/L Ceruplasmin, 75-145 mcg/dL
Folate	≤65%	Fatigue Physical changes in pigmentation Skin and oral ulcers		Serum folate, 34-1,020 ng/mL RBC folate count, <305 nmol/L
Iron	At 3 mo to 10 yr after surgery: AGB, 14% SG, <18% RYGB, 20%-55% BPD/DS, 13%-62%	Fatigue Microcytic anemia Glossitis Cardiac palpitations Decreased immunity Spoon-shaped nails Vertical nail ridges		Serum iron, 60-170 mcg/dL Serum transferrin, 200-230 mcg/dL Transferrin saturation, 20%-50% Serum ferritin[a]: male, 12-300 ng/mL; female, 12-150 ng/mL
Thiamin (B1)[b]	1%-49%	Anorexia Delayed gastric emptying Gait ataxia Upper and lower extremity weakness With dry beriberi: peripheral neuropathy With wet beriberi: pitting edema in lower extremities, heart failure, tachycardia, bradycardia, dyspnea	Wernicke encephalopathy Psychosis Hallucinations Nystagmus	Plasma thiamin, 4-15 nmol/L Whole blood thiamin, 70-180 nmol/L

Table continues

AGB = adjustable gastric banding | BPD/DS = biliopancreatic diversion with duodenal switch | DXA = dual-energy x-ray absorptiometry | P1CP = C-terminal propeptide of type 1 procollagen | P1NP = N-terminal propeptide of type 1 procollagen | PT = prothrombin time | RBC = red blood cell | RYGB = Roux-en-Y gastric bypass | SG = sleeve gastrectomy

[a] Ferritin varies based on inflammation, infection, and age

[b] Thiamin deficiency is also called beriberi

TABLE 18.6 Signs, Symptoms, and Laboratory Indexes of Possible Micronutrient Deficiencies After Bariatric Surgery[32,34] (continued)

Micronutrient deficiency	Prevalence	Early signs and symptoms	Advanced signs and symptoms	Laboratory indexes
Vitamin A	Within 4 yr of surgery: ≤70%	Night blindness Poor wound healing Bitot spots Loss of taste	Blindness Corneal damage Xerosis Keratomalacia	Plasma retinol, 20-80 mcg/dL
Vitamin B12 (cobalamin)	At 2-5 yr after surgery: RYGB, <20% SG, 4%-20%	Pernicious anemia Megaloblastic anemia Muscle stiffness and weakness Neuropathy Tinnitus Cardiac palpitations Red "beefy" tongue (magenta tongue)	Angina Irritability Psychosis	Serum cobalamin, 200-1,000 pg/mL
Vitamin D	≤100%	Muscle cramping Hypocalcemia Tingling in extremities Cognitive impairment		Plasma 25-hydroxyvitamin D, >30 ng/mL
Vitamin E	Uncommon	Muscle weakness Hyporeflexia Gait ataxia Hemolytic anemia Nystagmus		Plasma α-tocopherol, >5 mcg/mL
Vitamin K	Uncommon	Hemorrhage Bleeding gum Nose bleeding Delayed clotting		PT, 10-13 s
Zinc	AGB, ≤34% RYGB, ≤40% SG, ≤19% BPD/DS, ≤70%	Rash Acne Loss of taste Infertility Decreased growth	Hypogonadism Alopecia Skin lesions Anorexia Delayed wound healing Night blindness	Plasma zinc, 60-130 mcg/dL

AGB = adjustable gastric banding | BPD/DS = biliopancreatic diversion with duodenal switch | DXA = dual-energy x-ray absorptiometry | P1CP = C-terminal propeptide of type 1 procollagen | P1NP = N-terminal propeptide of type 1 procollagen | PT = prothrombin time | RBC = red blood cell | RYGB = Roux-en-Y gastric bypass | SG = sleeve gastrectomy

Complete blood count with platelets

Hemoglobin and hematocrit

Electrolytes

Glucose

Hemoglobin A1c

Iron

Ferritin

Lipid profile

Liver function

25-hydroxyvitamin D

Vitamin B12

Optional studies:

- Red blood cell folate concentration
- Intact parathyroid hormone
- Thiamin (measuring via whole blood reflects body stores; measuring via plasma reflects recent intake)

Weight loss alone should not be the only parameter used to define success after bariatric surgery. Resolution or improvement in comorbid conditions (Table 18.1) and an improved sense of well-being and quality of life are also important factors to consider when evaluating surgical outcomes.

Multiple tools are available to assess quality of life. These tools have evolved from being generic to allowing for more specific measures in people who are overweight with a comorbidity vs people with obesity. A few examples of such tools include the Medical Outcomes Study 36-Item Short-Form Health Survey and the RAND-36 are two similar tools that assess eight health concepts in order to measure quality of life: physical functioning, role limitations caused by physical health problems, role limitations caused by emotional problems, social functioning, emotional well-being, energy and fatigue, pain, and general health perceptions.[36]

The Obesity and Weight Loss Quality of Life questionnaire and the Weight-Related Symptom Measure were developed to incorporate culturally sensitive measures of quality of life, including culturally influenced aspects of living, interactions with others, and health-related behaviors.[36]

Reviewing Diet and Ability to Meet Nutrition Goals

Patients should be instructed to keep daily diet diaries for self-monitoring and for review by the RDN. In this review, the RDN should do the following:

- Assess fluid and protein intake, portion size, food texture and tolerance, frequency of eating, and overall dietary quality.
- Evaluate adherence to diet principles and progression and readiness to advance the diet.
- Evaluate the frequency of protein supplementation and daily use of vitamin and mineral supplements.

- Assess hunger and satiety.
- Review for symptoms of stricture, obstruction (reflux, vomiting, or pain) or other complications.
- Ensure that nutrition needs are being met, in accordance with the MyPlate guide[37] and Dietary Reference Intakes,[29] in order to promote health and prevent chronic disease across the patient's life span.

Assessing and Treating Nutrition-Related Complications

Box 18.7 provides a list of conditions and behaviors that may cause nutrition-related complications. Protein malnutrition, or protein-energy malnutrition, after metabolic and bariatric surgery is not common but may occur if the patient's dietary intake is suboptimal because of confounding circumstances or medical conditions or because weight loss is prolonged for more than 2 years postoperatively.[5]

BOX 18.7

Conditions and Behaviors That Can Negatively Affect Nutritional Status After Bariatric Surgery

Alcohol or drug abuse

Anorexia

Depression

Diarrhea

Fear of regaining weight

Food intolerance

Limited resources for food or supplements

Nonadherence

Prolonged vomiting

Prolonged weight loss

Protein-energy malnutrition

Nutrition Support

The implementation of enteral or parenteral nutrition should be considered following bariatric surgery when patients who are high risk and critically ill cannot tolerate oral nutrition for more than 5 to 7 days, and when patients who are not critically ill cannot tolerate oral nutrition for more than 7 to 10 days.[2] Standard nutrition-support protocols should be followed.

Pregnancy After Weight-Loss Surgery

Patients should be advised to avoid pregnancy for 18 months after surgery or until their weight loss has plateaued and nutritional intake is stable. Fertility increases with weight loss, and patients should be counseled regarding appropriate contraception methods.

Patients who are planning to become pregnant should be cared for by a multidisciplinary team that includes the patient's dietitian and surgeon. Baseline nutritional status should be assessed before pregnancy for micronutrient deficiencies and treated as needed to support the mother and fetal development. The recommendations for weight gain during pregnancy are based on the patient's ideal body weight and BMI, and are as follows: 28 to 40 lb (12.7 to 18.2 kg) if BMI indicates the patient is underweight; 25 to 35 lb (11.4 to 15.9 kg) if BMI indicates the patient is of normal weight; 15 to 25 lb (6.8 to 11.4 kg) if BMI indicates the patient is overweight; and 11 to 20 lb (5 to 9.09 kg) if BMI indicates the patient is obese.[38]

Nonsurgical Therapies for Overweight and Obesity

Endoscopic Therapy

The US Food and Drug Administration (FDA) has approved nonsurgical, endoscopic therapies to treat overweight and obesity by reducing gastric volume.

A volume-occupying device, or intragastric balloon, functions to increase satiety by occupying volume in the stomach and may also affect gut neuroendocrine signals. Some limitations include abdominal pain, nausea, vomiting, and food intolerance.[39]

An endoscopic suturing procedure called endoscopic sleeve gastroplasty is a more effective procedure than an intragastric balloon, but it is less effective than SG. Some limitations of endoscopic sleeve gastroplasty are that it is an experimental procedure, it is less effective for long-term weight loss, postoperative weight gain is more likely, and it is expensive.[40]

Aspiration therapy involves aspirating roughly 30% of energy from food contents in a meal. Food contents are aspirated from the stomach via a percutaneous gastrostomy tube. Some limitations are abdominal pain and discomfort, and peristomal irritation.[41]

These nonsurgical therapies produce short-term weight loss and require much additional research to investigate their safety and effects on long-term obesity management.

Pharmacotherapy

Weight-loss medications have been approved by the FDA for overweight (BMI ≥27 with comorbidity) and obese (BMI ≥30) individuals. Combination phentermine and topiramate is an appetite suppressant that stimulates the release of norepinephrine. A low dose is sustained for 14 days and can be increased to a moderate dose and high dose to pursue therapeutic effect. If a 5% weight loss is not achieved within 12 weeks of use, the medication is discontinued. Liraglutide is a glucagon-like peptide-1 (GLP-1) receptor agonist that slows gastric emptying and increases satiety.[42] Combination naltrexone and bupropion increases satiety, reduces food intake, and enhances energy expenditure via manipulation of the hypothalamus and mesolimbic system. Naltrexone is an opioid receptor antagonist, and bupropion is a dopamine and norepinephrine reuptake inhibitor. The exact synergistic mechanisms are not fully understood but the agents have been proven to be more effective for weight loss when taken together than when taken separately.[43] These medications can be used before or after metabolic and bariatric surgery in patients who have been unable to lose weight or who have regained substantial weight postprocedure. See Chapter 11 for additional information on medical and pharmacotherapy management of obesity.

Summary

Metabolic and bariatric surgery can help people who are morbidly obese lose substantial amounts of weight and improve or resolve comorbidities of obesity. After a bariatric procedure, patients must commit to lifelong changes to their eating practices, food choices, and physical activity and be prepared to address nutrient deficiencies and adverse effects of surgery, which can vary depending on the type of surgical procedure. Regular follow-up with an RDN and other members of the health care team is essential for the patient's long-term success.

Additional areas of research should include preventing and treating micronutrient deficiency before and after metabolic and bariatric surgery; the bioavailability and absorption of macronutrients and micronutrients in patients (to prevent nutrition gaps); reported changes in taste sensation and food and protein supplement tolerance following surgery; and finally, barriers to maintaining a commitment to lifestyle changes that will ensure weight loss and health care success.

References

1. Adult obesity facts. Centers for Disease Control and Prevention. Accessed August 3, 2020. www.cdc.gov/obesity/data/adult.html

2. DeMaria EJ. Bariatric surgery for morbid obesity. *N Engl J Med.* 2007;356(21):2176-2183. doi:10.1056/NEJMct067019

3. Ramasamy A, Laliberte F, Aktavoukian SA, et al. Direct and indirect cost of obesity among the privately insured in the United States: a focus on the impact on type of industry. *J Occup Environ Med.* 2019;61(11)877-886.

4. Moore EC, Pories WJ. The BMI: is it time to scratch for a more accurate assessment of metabolic dysfunction? *Curr Obes Rep.* 2014;3(2):286-90.

5. Mechanick JI, Apovian CA, Brethauer S, et al. Clinical practice guidelines for the perioperative nutrition, metabolic, and nonsurgical support of patients undergoing bariatric procedures—2019 update: cosponsored by American Association of Clinical Endocrinologists/American College of Endocrinology, The Obesity Society, American Society for Metabolic and Bariatric Surgery, Obesity Medicine Association, and American Society of Anesthesiologists. *Surg for Obesity and Rel Dis.* 2020;16:175-247.

6. Gastrointestinal surgery for severe obesity. *Consens Statement.* 1991;9(1)1-20.

7. Academy of Nutrition and Dietetics. Nutrition Care Process. Accessed September 10, 2021. www.eatrightpro.org/practice/quality-management/nutrition-care -process

8. Raynor HA, Champagne CM. Position of the Academy of Nutrition and Dietetics: interventions for the treatment of overweight and obesity in adults. *J Acad Nutr Diet.* 2016;116(1):129-147.

9. Colles SL, Dixon JB, Marks P, Strauss BJ, O'Brien PE. Preoperative weight loss with a very-low-energy diet: quantitation of changes in liver and abdominal fat by serial imaging. *Am J Clin Nutr.* 2006;84:304-311.

10. Kim JJ, Rodgers AM, Bellem N, Schirmer B. ASMBS updated position statement on insurance mandated preoperative weight loss requirements. *Surg Obes Relat Dis.* 2016:12;955-959.

11. Guidelines for laparoscopic and open surgical treatment of morbid obesity. American Society for Bariatric Surgery. Society of American Gastrointestinal Endoscopic Surgeons. *Obes Surg.* 2000;10(4):378-379.

12. Dixon AF, Dixon JS, O'Brien PE. Laparoscopic adjustable gastric banding induces prolonged satiety: a randomized blind crossover study. *J Clin Endocrinol Metab.* 2005;(90)813-819.

13. Beckman L, Beckman T, Earthman C. Changes in gastrointestinal hormones and leptin after Roux-en-Y gastric bypass procedure: a review. *J Am Diet Assoc.* 2010;110:571-584.

14. Dolan K, Hatzifotis M, Newbury L, Lowe N, Fielding N. A clinical and nutritional comparison of biliopancreatic diversion with and without duodenal switch. *Ann Surg.* 2004;240(1):51-56.

15. Kushner R, Cummings S, Herron DM. Bariatric surgery: postoperative nutritional management. UpToDate. 2019. Accessed January 18, 2021. www.uptodate.com /contents/bariatric-surgery-postoperative-nutritional-management

16. Isom KA, Majumdar MM, eds. *Academy of Nutrition and Dietetics Pocket Guide to Bariatric Surgery.* 3rd ed. Academy of Nutrition and Dietetics; 2022.

17. Allied Health Sciences Section Ad Hoc Nutrition Committee, Aillis L, Blankenship L, Buffinton C, Furtado M, Parrott J. ASMBS Allied Health nutrition guidelines for the surgical weight loss patient. *Surg Obes Relat Dis.* 2008;(5):73-108.

18. Kodner C, Hartman D. Complications of adjustable gastric banding surgery for obesity. *Am Fam Physician.* 2014; 89(10):813-818.

19. Shen R, Dugay G, Rajaram K, Cabrera I, Siegel N, Ren CJ. Impact of patient follow-up on weight loss after bariatric surgery. *Obes Surg.* 2004;14:514–519.

20. Althuwaini S, Bamehriz F, Aldohayan A, et al. Prevalence and predictors of gastroesophageal reflux disease after laparoscopic sleeve gastrectomy. *Obes Sur.* 2018;(28)916-922.

21. Goldfine AB, Mun EC, Devine E, et al. Patients with neuroglycopenia after gastric bypass surgery have exaggerated incretin and insulin secretory responses to a mixed meal. *J Clin Endocrinol Metab.* 2007; 92(12):4678-4685.

22. Jørgensen NB, Jacobsen SH, Dirksen C, et al. Acute and long-term effects of Roux-en-Y gastric bypass on glucose metabolism in subjects with type 2 diabetes and normal glucose tolerance. *Am J Physiol Endocrinol Metab.* 2012;303(1):E122-E131.

23. Dagan SD, Goldenshluger A, Globus I, et al. Nutrition recommendations for adult bariatric surgery patients: clinical practice. *Adv Nutr.* 2017;8:382-394.

24. Garvey WT, Mechanick JI, Brett EM, et al. American Association of Clinic Endocrinologists and American College of Endocrinology comprehensive clinical practice guidelines for medical care of patients with obesity. *Endocr Pract.* 2016;22 (Suppl 3):1-203. doi:10.4158/EP161365.GL

25. Suhl E, Anderson-Haynes SE, Mulla C, Patti M. Medical nutrition therapy for post-bariatric hypoglycemia: practical insights. *Surg Obes Relat Dis.* 2017;13:888-898.

26. Kandel D, Bojsen-Møller KN, Svane MS, et al. Mechanisms of action of a carbohydrate-reduced, high protein diet in reducing the risk of postprandial hypoglycemia after Roux-en-Y gastric bypass. *Am J Clin Nutr.* 2019; 110(2):296-304.

27. Misselwitz B, Pohl D, Fruhauf H, Fried M, Vavricka S, Fox M. Lactose malabsorption and intolerance: pathogenesis, diagnosis and treatment. *United European Gastroenterol J.* 2013;1(3):151-159.

28. Seeras K, Acho R, Lopez P. Roux-en-Y gastric bypass chronic complications. In: *StatPearls* (online). StatPearls Publishing; 2021. NCBI Bookshelf. Accessed February 14, 2021. www.ncbi.nlm.nih.gov/books/NBK519489

29. Nutrient recommendations: Dietary Reference Intakes (DRI). Office of Dietary Supplements, National Institutes of Health. Accessed January 2021. https://ods.od.nih.gov/HealthInformation/Dietary_Reference_Intakes.aspx

30. Parikh M, Johnson J, Ballem N. ASMBS position statement on alcohol use before and after bariatric surgery. *Surg Obes Relat Dis.* 2016;12(2):225-230.

31. United States Pharmacopeial Convention. Search and buy Reference Standards. Accessed January 2021. www.usp.org/reference-standards/reference-standards-catalog

32. Parrott J, Frank L, Rabena R, Craggs-Dino L, Isom KA, Greiman L. American Society for Metabolic and Bariatric Surgery integrated health nutritional guidelines for the surgical weight loss patient 2016 update: micronutrients. *Surg Obes Relat Dis.* 2017; 13(5):727-741. doi:10.1016/j.soard.2016.12.018

33. Cancelo-Hidalgo MJ, Castelo-Branco C, Palacios S, et al. Tolerability of different oral iron supplements: a systematic review. *Curr Med Res Opin.* 2013;29(4):291-303.

34. Shetty S, Kapoor N, Bondu J, Thomas N, Paul T. Bone turnover markers: emerging tool in the management of osteoporosis. *Indian J Endo Metab.* 2016; 20(6):846-852.

35. Gerber P, Anderin C, Gustafsson UO, Thorell A. Weight loss before gastric bypass and postoperative weight change: data from the Scandinavian Obesity Registry. *Surg Obes Relat Dis.* 2016;12(3):556-562.

36. Niero M, Martin M, Finger T, et al. A new approach to multicultural item generation in the development of two obesity-specific measures: the Obesity and Weight Loss Quality of Life (OWLQOL) questionnaire and the Weight-Related Symptom Measure (WRSM). *Clin Ther.* 2002;24(4):690-700.

37. United States Department of Agriculture. MyPlate. Accessed January 2021. www.myplate.gov

38. Ellis E. Healthy weight during pregnancy. Academy of Nutrition and Dietetics. July 9, 2019. Accessed September 12, 2020. www.eatright.org/health/pregnancy/prenatal-wellness/healthy-weight-during-pregnancy

39. Kim S, Chun H, Choi, H, Kim E, Keum B, Jeen Y. Current status of intragastric balloon for obesity treatment. *World J Gastroenterol.* 2016; 22(24):5495-5504.

40. Wang W, Chen C. Current status of endoscopic sleeve gastroplasty: an opinion review. *World J Gastroenterol.* 2020; 26(11):1107-1112.

41. Thompson CC, Abu Dayyeh BK, Kushner R, et al. Percutaneous gastrostomy device for the treatment of class II and class III obesity: results of a randomized controlled trial. *Am J Gastroenterol.* 2017; 12(3):447-457.

42. Mehta A, Marso SP, Neeland. IJ. Liraglutide for weight management: a critical review of the evidence. *Obes Sci Pract.* 2017;3(1):3-14.

43. Sherman MM, Ungureanu S, Rey JA. Naltrexone/bupropion ER (Contrave): newly approved treatment option for chronic weight management in obese adults. *P T.* 2016;41(3):164-172.

Enteral Nutrition

Angela A. MacDonald, DCN, RD
Jennifer R. Bridenbaugh, MS, RD, CNSC

KEY POINTS

- Enteral nutrition is a safe and beneficial method of supporting the nutritional status of patients who are unable to take food orally.
- Enteral nutrition is associated with improved clinical outcomes and reduced infectious complications and, therefore, is the preferred method of nutrition support if the gastrointestinal tract is functional and of sufficient length, unless its use is otherwise contraindicated.
- Complications associated with enteral nutrition can be prevented or managed with thoughtful initiation, delivery, and monitoring.

Introduction

Nutrition support has progressed from adjunctive care provided solely to prevent malnutrition to a proactive therapy designed to prevent oxidative cellular injury and to favorably modulate the immune response.[1] Enteral nutrition (EN), also known as tube feeding, delivers nutrition directly to the stomach or small intestine. EN should usually be attempted before parenteral nutrition (PN) because EN is generally considered safer and more efficacious. See Chapter 20 for additional information on PN. Chapter 21 considers issues related to the use of nutrition support in pediatric patients, and Chapter 22 addresses the use of EN and PN in home care.

Indications for the Use of Enteral Nutrition

The use of EN is preferred because of its many physiological and practical advantages. The proposed benefits of EN include the prevention of adverse structural and functional alterations of the gut barrier, increased epithelial proliferation, maintenance of mucosal integrity, decreased gut permeability, improved mesenteric blood flow, and improved local and systemic immune responsiveness.[2-4] When compared to PN, EN has been shown to reduce cost, septic morbidity, and the rate of infectious complications.[5,6] However, current guidelines state that during the first week of critical illness, no significant difference in outcomes are found when EN or PN is provided; therefore, both are acceptable.[7] Clinical judgment is still recommended when the decision of initiating nutrition support is necessary. EN is appropriate for patients who cannot consume food by mouth or are unable to support their energy and protein requirements with adequate oral intake. Before starting EN, the patient must have access to a functional gastrointestinal (GI) tract and be hemodynamically stable. Hemodynamic stability is defined as having a mean arterial pressure of more than 60 mm Hg and a stable or weaning dose of catecholamine agents (pressors). Fluid resuscitation is a priority for patients who are hemodynamically unstable. When stable, trophic feeding (10–20 mL/h) is an ideal approach for initiation of EN.[1,8]

Contraindications to Enteral Nutrition

EN is absolutely contradicted in individuals without a functional GI tract—for example, in patients with a mechanical obstruction that cannot be bypassed. Relative contraindications include the following[1-3,7]:

- intractable vomiting or diarrhea that is refractory to medical management
- short bowel syndrome (≤100 cm of the small bowel remaining)

- paralytic ileus without postpyloric access
- high-output fistula (>500 mL)[9,10]
- peritonitis
- major GI bleeding
- inability to access the GI tract
- hemodynamic instability

EN may also be contraindicated for ethical reasons, as in the case of a patient with imminently terminal disease who does not desire aggressive intervention such as artificial nutrition. See Chapter 25 for more information on ethical issues.

Potential Complications of Enteral Nutrition

If EN is not managed appropriately, it can be associated with serious and potentially fatal complications, including the following[11-13]:

- enteral tube misconnection
- device misplacements or displacements
- bronchopulmonary aspiration
- GI intolerance
- drug-nutrient interactions
- electrolyte abnormalities
- GI ischemia
- stoma and tube-site infection

Complications of EN can be minimized when attention is paid to proper selection of the appropriate site for delivery as well as confirmation of the device placement. In addition, proper timing for initiation and delivery of EN can also decrease complications. Careful selection and ordering of the appropriate EN product, as well as safe preparation and delivery of EN, decreases complications. Finally, safe and accurate monitoring, including care for the access site and feeding tube, is essential to reducing the incidence of complications.

Selecting the Appropriate Tube Type and Site for Enteral Nutrition Delivery

The success of EN depends on the careful selection of an appropriate enteral access device and placement technique, along with proper maintenance and care. Considerations for an enteral access device include its intended use, individual patient outcomes, and the length of time EN will be required. In addition, comorbidities and any prior GI surgery must be considered, as these may affect the condition of the GI anatomy (eg, the condition of the abdominal wall), the degree of motility, and the patency of the upper GI tract.[11,13] Finally, if the patient has any risk factors for anesthesia or may be unable to correct coagulopathies, this will influence the choice of EN access.

EN administered into the stomach is acceptable for most patients; however, postpyloric placement may benefit patients with two or more of the following risk factors[14,15]:

- prior aspiration
- decreased level of consciousness
- neuromuscular disease and structural abnormalities of the aerodigestive tract
- endotracheal intubation
- vomiting
- risk of persistently high gastric residual volumes
- need for supine, flat positioning

Short-Term Feeding Tubes

Short-term feeding tubes are for patients who are expected to receive EN for less than 4 weeks or in whom a long-term feeding tube cannot be placed. Decisions about the placement of the tube should be based on the desired tip location and the ability to place the tube nasally or orally (see Box 19.1 and Box 19.2 for more information). For most patients, gastric feeding is acceptable even during critical illness.[14-17]

BOX 19.1

Comparison of Short-Term Feeding Tubes

	Gastric	Postpyloric
Types of tubes	Nasogastric	Nasoenteric
	Orogastric	Oroenteric
Advantages	Easier to place	Safe for patients with gastric dysmotility
	Less expensive	May allow enteral nutrition (EN) feeding in patients who are high risk
	Tube feeding initiated more quickly	Small bowel feedings result in increased total intake and decreased time to reach feeding goal
Disadvantages	May increase risk of aspiration[a]	Requires special training to place
	Cannot use in patients with obstruction or the need for gastric decompression	May delay start of EN
		Unable to provide bolus feeding

[a] *One meta-analysis showed increased risk of ventilator-associated pneumonia with gastric feedings, whereas others showed no associations.*[17,18]

Once the tube has been placed, several methods can be used to determine whether the tip is in the desired location (see Box 19.3 on page 336).[2,13,18-22] There are also several indicators that the tube tip may have migrated after placement (see Box 19.4 on page 336).[13,18,19,23] In patients who are at high risk for pulling out their nasogastric feeding tube—for example, patients with altered mental status, facial burns, or the need for frequent positional changes—a nasal bridle may be used.[24] The nasal bridle technique secures the feeding tube to the nasal septum; this way, if the patient pulls on the tube, the resulting discomfort prevents them from dislodging the tube.[3] A meta-analysis of studies evaluating the use of nasal bridles in adult patients concluded that securing a feeding tube with a nasal bridle is more effective than the traditional method of using adhesive tape alone.[24] Skin complications may occur with the nasal bridle, but there appears to be no difference in the incidence of sinusitis.[24] A nasal bridle should not be used for more than 4 weeks.[13]

BOX 19.2

Methods for Placing Short-Term Feeding Tubes

	Advantages	Disadvantages
Overall blind placement	Less expensive Can be placed at bedside Lower skill level required to place Nurses and dietitians can be trained to place	Increased risk for bronchopulmonary placement Requires x-ray for confirmation Typically is difficult to place postpyloric tubes No direct or indirect visualization used with insertion
Magnetically guided (blind placement)	May not require x-ray for confirmation Can be placed at bedside Allows for postpyloric placement	Requires specialized equipment Requires trained personnel Requires more expensive tubes
Fluoroscopic	Does not require x-ray for confirmation Allows for postpyloric placement Direct visualization technique	Typically requires transport to fluoroscopy Requires trained personnel More expensive than blind placement
Endoscopic	Allows for postpyloric placement Direct visualization technique	Typically requires transport to endoscopy Requires trained personnel Requires x-ray, as endoscope can displace tube when removed More expensive than blind placement
Surgical	Can be placed at time of surgery Does not require x-ray for confirmation Allows for gastric or postpyloric placement Direct visualization technique	Requires anesthesia and poses risks associated with surgery Requires trained personnel More expensive, if tube placement is the sole reason for surgery

BOX 19.3

Methods for Checking Placement of Blindly Placed Feeding Tubes[2,13,17-22]

Radiography[18,20]

Radiography is the gold standard for checking blindly placed feeding tubes.

A disadvantage is that repeated exposure to radiation can be dangerous.

Aspirate pH

Aspirates from different locations in the gastrointestinal tract have different appearances and pH.

Aspirate pH is less reliable than radiography for distinguishing between gastric and bronchopulmonary placement.[13]

- Pleural space aspirate: pale yellow, serous appearance; $pH \geq 7$
- Gastric fluid: clear, colorless, or grassy green appearance (in fasting patients); $pH \leq 5$ (without gastric acid suppression therapy)
- Small bowel aspirate, bile stained: $pH \geq 6$

For patients taking gastric acid inhibitors, aspirate pH may not distinguish tube location but can be used to assess bronchopulmonary vs gastric placement.[18,20]

Auscultation

Auscultation relies on sound differences between the stomach and lung.

It is often not accurate.

Testing for enzymes in fluid aspirated from tube

Carbon dioxide detectors (capnography)[2]:

- Can detect carbon dioxide when the tube has been placed inadvertently into the lung
- Cannot distinguish between placement in the esophagus vs the stomach

Electromagnetic placement device

The US Food and Drug Administration recommends that electromagnetic placement devices (EMPDs) be used by properly trained and credentialed clinical personnel.[21]

The use of an EMPD is a safe alternative for confirming the placement of small-bore feeding tubes in adults and can reduce the need for routine radiographs.[17-19]

The evidence to support EMPD use with nasogastric tube placement in the pediatric population is limited but promising, especially with postpyloric feeding tube placement.[18,22]

BOX 19.4

Indicators That the Short-Term Feeding Tube Tip Has Been Displaced[13,18,19,23]

If external length of tubing is increased, tube may have withdrawn from stomach into esophagus

If external length of tubing is decreased, tube may have migrated into small bowel

If unable to withdraw fluids from tube, tube may have migrated into small bowel

Unexpected change in residual volumes

Long-Term Feeding Tubes

Long-term feeding tubes are for patients requiring either full or supplemental EN for more than 4 weeks. These tubes are generally placed by a physician. Box 19.5 provides more information on the various types of long-term feeding tubes and their advantages and disadvantages.[3]

BOX 19.5

Comparison of Long-Term Feeding Tubes[3]

	Types of tubes	Advantages	Disadvantages
Gastric	Percutaneous endoscopic gastrostomy	Easier to place	Cannot be used in patients with obstruction or the need for gastric decompression
	Gastrostomy	Less expensive	
	Radiologically inserted gastrostomy	Easier to maintain	
Postpyloric	Percutaneous endoscopic jejunostomy	Safe for patients with gastric dysmotility	May clog more easily because they are typically smaller in diameter
	Jejunostomy	May allow enteral feeding in high-risk patients	
	Jejunal extension of percutaneous endoscopic gastrostomy		

Complications Associated With Feeding Tubes

A number of complications can develop both during and after the placement of short-term and long-term feeding tubes (see Box 19.6).[3,12] Among these complications are aspiration, which can be potentially fatal, and the common problem of tube occlusion. Box 19.7 on page 338 and Box 19.8 on page 339 provide more information on aspiration and tube occlusion, respectively.[2,9,11-13,25-29]

BOX 19.6

Potential Complications Associated With Enteral Feeding Tubes[3,12]

[a] The use of a nasal bridle decreases dislodgement rates but may increase the risk of nasal septal and nasal tissue trauma.

Short-term

Placement complications	Postprocedure complications
Epistaxis	Inadvertent bronchopulmonary placement
Aspiration	Inadvertent tube dislodgement[a]
Esophageal or gastric perforation	Tube malfunction: breaking, cracking, or kinking
Circulatory and respiratory compromise (eg, pneumothorax, inadvertent lung placement)	Tube occlusion
	Aspiration
	Intestinal ischemia

Box continues

BOX 19.6

(CONTINUED)

Long-term

Placement complications	Postprocedure complications
Aspiration	Peristomal infection[b]
Hemorrhage	Inappropriate equipment usage, such as enteral misconnections
Perforation of the gastrointestinal lumen	Premature or inadvertent tube removal, with increased risk of peritonitis within the first few weeks of insertion
Peritonitis or necrotizing fasciitis	Accidental catheter tip malposition, leading to leakage of intestinal secretions, gastric or intestinal obstruction, or aspiration
Prolonged ileus	Excessive traction of feeding device, leading to "buried bumper syndrome," pain, tube obstruction, peritonitis, or stomal site drainage

[b] *Reduced risk and successful treatment of infection may be achieved with prophylactic antibiotics, early recognition of wound infections, treatment with antibiotics, local wound care, and debridement when indicated.*

BOX 19.7

Aspiration: Risk Factors and Prevention[9,11-13,26,27]

Risk factors

Previous aspiration events

Decreased level of consciousness

Significant neuromuscular disease

Contaminated oropharyngeal environment

Structural abnormalities of the aerodigestive tract

Supine, flat positioning

Advanced age

Need for sedation

Neurological impairment

Presence and size of nasogastric tube

Malposition of feeding tube

Mechanical ventilation

Bolus feeding delivery

Presence of high-risk disease or injury (eg, neurological disorders, dysphagia, traumatic brain injury, vomiting, gastroesophageal reflux disease)

Nursing-related factors such as understaffing, lack of training, and enteral feeding protocols not being in place

Prevention

Infusion of enteral feeding into the small bowel instead of the stomach

Elevation of the head of the bed to more than 30-45 degrees[9]

Minimized use of sedatives[11]

Oral mouth care, including use of chlorhexidine mouthwashes

Use of prokinetic agents to increase gastrointestinal motility

BOX 19.8

Tube Occlusion: Risk Factors, Prevention, and Treatment[2,12,13,25,28,29]

Risk Factors

Feeding tube diameter: greater risk with small bore vs large bore

Inadequate routine water flushing before and after interruptions and following all medication administration

Improper administration of medications:
- Medications should not be mixed with tube-feeding formulas.
- Diluted liquid medications should be used when available and tolerated.
- Feeding tube should be flushed with 30 mL water before and after administration of medications.

Concentration of the enteral formula: greater risk with concentrated formula vs standard formula

Use of ENFit connector with blenderized tube feeding (BTF)[28]

Rate of infusion: greater risk with slow infusion vs fast infusion

Addition of fiber supplements to nonfiber formulas (increases risk)

Feeding tube material: greater risk with silicone vs polyurethane

Tip location: greater risk with gastric location vs small bowel location (low pH of stomach may cause formula to coagulate)

Tube length: greater risk with long tubes vs short tubes

Prevention

Flushing of tube with at least 30 mL water every 4 hours during continuous feeding, or before and after infusion during intermittent feedings

Possible additional free-water flushes in patients with BTF if allowed within the nutrition prescription[28]

Flushing of tube with at least 30 mL water if checking gastric residual volumes

Flushing of tube with at least 30 mL water before and after each medication

Avoidance of carbonated beverages and cranberry juice[25]

Treatment

Flushing of tube with warm water using a small-bore syringe (5–10 mL)

Use of a solution of one uncoated pancreatic enzyme (pancrealipase) and 375 mg sodium bicarbonate to dissolve clog[29]

Use of a cytology brush

Use of an endoscopic retrograde cholangiopancreatography catheter

Use of a commercial corkscrew device

Timing of Enteral Nutrition

Timing in Critical Illness

In the critically ill, EN should be started within 24 to 48 hours of admission to the intensive care unit. Do not wait for bowel sounds, passing of flatus, or stool to initiate feeds.[1] Early EN is associated with many benefits, including reduced infectious complications, maintaining gut integrity, potential reduction in disease severity, potential reduction in total length of hospital stay, and improved patient outcomes.[1,16,30] If the gastrointestinal tract is not functioning and EN cannot be initiated, PN should be initiated. Current guidelines recommend that both EN and PN are acceptable in adults during the first week of critical illness.[7]

Timing After Percutaneous Endoscopic Gastrostomy Tube Placement

The placement of a percutaneous endoscopic gastrostomy (PEG) tube is the preferred method of EN delivery for individuals requiring support for more than 3 to 4 weeks. Despite some manufacturer instructions, which recommend delaying the initiation of EN for 24 hours after PEG tube placement, the American Society for Gastrointestinal Endoscopy clinical guidelines support the initiation of EN within 4 hours of placement.[31-33] Studies of patients whose EN is started within 3 to 4 hours of PEG tube placement show no difference in short-term mortality or complications and suggest that this timing could lead to improved outcomes, such as cost savings and less intravenous medication and intravenous nutrition (ie, PN) use.[33]

Timing After Surgery

Traditionally, clinicians require the return of bowel function before initiating EN postoperatively, and this often leads to a prolonged delay. The use of aggressive but careful perioperative nutrition interventions, as described in the Enhanced Recovery After Surgery (ERAS) protocols, has been shown to benefit the patient.[34] Positive outcomes—such as earlier progression to oral feeding, improved metabolic control (eg, blood glucose), reduction of stress response, fewer infectious complications, and reduced length of stay—are some of the benefits seen with early EN and ERAS protocols in some surgical patients.[30,34] However, individuals with extensive GI surgery, especially in the small bowel, may not tolerate early EN; therefore, consultation with the surgical team is suggested. Tolerance must be monitored closely to avoid serious complications, such as bowel necrosis. The presence of abdominal distension, sepsis, or a worsening condition should prompt immediate evaluation.[13]

Enteral Formula Selection

Many categories of enteral formulas, targeted for specific patient populations, are available on the market (see Box 19.9).[1,3,35-50] Almost all formulas are nutritionally complete when administered in sufficient quantities. Box 19.10 on page 344 provides more detail on the ingredients in specialty formulas.[1,3,5,11,47,51-67]

Nutrient Composition of Formulas

Carbohydrate

Carbohydrate is the primary macronutrient and energy source in EN formulas, constituting 40% to 90% of the energy content. Corn syrup solids are the main form of carbohydrate in polymeric EN formulas. In hydrolyzed EN formulas, carbohydrate in the form of hydrolyzed corn starch or maltodextrin is used. Carbohydrate contributes to osmolality, digestibility, and sweetness. Most formulas are lactose-free and gluten-free.[3,41]

BOX 19.9

Enteral Formula Categories[1,3,35-50]

	Composition	Specialty ingredients	Uses, contraindications, and other notes
Standard	1.0 to 1.2 kcal/mL Protein: 14% to 19% Carbohydrate: 51% to 57% Fat: 29% to 33% Free water: 82% to 85% Fiber: 0 g/L	Contains intact nutrients without the addition of fiber	Standard formulas without fiber are used for patients who do not tolerate a formula with fiber or for those at risk for bowel ischemia or severe dysmotility.[1]
Standard with fiber	1.0 to 1.2 kcal/mL Protein: 16% to 19% Carbohydrate: 51% to 53% Fat: 29% to 33% Free water: 81% to 84% Fiber: 10 to 18 g/L	Contains intact nutrients with the addition of insoluble or soluble fiber	Standard formulas with fiber are used for patients who do not require a specialty formula or one without fiber.[1,35] Using a mixed fiber formula is not recommended for the prevention of diarrhea.[1] However the use of guar gum may reduce diarrhea.[1,35]
Concentrated	1.5 to 2.0 kcal/mL Protein: 16% to 18% Carbohydrate: 39% to 54% Fat: 29% to 45% Free water: 70% to 78% Fiber: 0 to 22 g/L	Based on a typical healthy diet without additional free water	Concentrated formulas are used for patients who need a reduced volume due to enteral nutrition (EN) intolerance, cycled feeds, fluid overload, congestive heart failure, renal failure, ascites, or syndrome of inappropriate antidiuretic hormone.
Real-food	1 to 1.5 kcal/mL Protein: 18% to 20% Carbohydrate: 36% to 48% Fat: 34% to 45% Free water: 59% to 83% Fiber: 8 to 12 g/L	Contains blenderized whole foods Some with peptides and medium-chain triglycerides (MCTs)	Real-food formulas are a convenient alternative to homemade blenderized formulas. They provide the nutritional compounds found in whole foods.
Low carbohydrate (for glucose intolerance)	1.0 to 1.2 kcal/mL Protein: 17% to 20% Carbohydrate: 31% to 40% Fat: 42% to 49% Free water: 81% to 85% Fiber: 14 to 21 g/L	Lower in carbohydrate and higher in fat Some with added arginine or α-linolenic acid	If the initial use of standard formulas plus insulin does not adequately manage a patient's glucose levels, use of a low-carbohydrate formula may be warranted.[41] The use of low-carbohdrate formulas for individuals who are critically ill with type 2 diabetes mellitus may improve the patient's total insulin requirement and glucose profile.[42-45]

Box continues

BOX 19.9 (CONTINUED)

	Composition	Specialty ingredients	Uses, contraindications, and other notes
Pulmonary	1.5 kcal/mL Protein: 17% to 18% Carbohydrate: 27% to 28% Fat: 55% Free water: 78% to 79% Fiber: 0 g/L	Lower in carbohydrate and higher in fat to minimize carbon dioxide production	Research does not support the use of formulas designed to reduce carbon dioxide production. Emphasis should be placed on the prevention of overfeeding.[1]
Renal	1.8 to 2.0 kcal/mL Protein: 7% to 18% Carbohydrate: 34% to 58% Fat: 35% to 48% Free water: 70% to 73% Fiber: 0 to 16 g/L	Lower in protein Concentrated to reduce volume Lower in potassium, phosphorus, and magnesium Some with added arginine	Renal formulas may benefit patients who cannot tolerate standard formulas due to electrolyte abnormalities.[1,37] Very low-protein formulas should only be used when the goal of care is to avoid renal replacement therapy.[3,37,46] Often, the protein content of these products is too low to meet the higher protein needs of the patient on renal replacement therapy. Higher-protein formulas will address the increased protein needs of patients with chronic kidney disease.[37,47]
Liver	1.5 kcal/mL Protein: 11% Carbohydrate: 77% Fat: 12% Free water: 76% Fiber: 0 g/L	Higher in branched-chain amino acids (BCAAs) and lower in aromatic amino acids	American Society for Parenteral and Enteral Nutrition (ASPEN), Society of Critical Care Medicine, and American College of Gastroenterology do not support the use of BCAA-containing formulas in patients with liver disease who have hepatic encephalopathy. Hepatic encephalopathy should be addressed with medical treatment. The lower total protein content of these products may not benefit patients with liver disease who are malnourished.[1,3,37,48]

Box continues

BOX 19.9 (CONTINUED)

	Composition	Specialty ingredients	Uses, contraindications, and other notes
Immune-enhancing	1.0 to 1.5 kcal/mL Protein: 17% to 25% Carbohydrate: 28% to 53% Fat: 25% to 55% Free water: 85% to 87% Fiber: 0 to 10 g/L	May contain arginine, glutamine, eicosapentaenoic acid (EPA), docosahexaenoic acid (DHA), γ-linolenic acid, nucleotides, antioxidants	Immune-enhancing products may be beneficial and used in hospitalized patients with trauma or traumatic brain injury, and in postoperative patients requiring EN in the surgical intensive care unit (ICU).[1,3] Their use may be associated with increased mortality in patients with severe sepsis or medical ICU patients.[1,3] Currently, formulas enriched with EPA, DHA, γ-linolenic acid, and antioxidants are not recommended for patients who are critically ill on mechanical ventilation with acute respiratory distress syndrome or acute lung injury. Such patients should not be given these formulas until further evidence is available.[1]
Elemental	1 kcal/mL Protein: 8% to 20% Carbohydrate: 70% to 90% Fat: 1% to 10% Free water: 85% to 86% Fiber: 0 g/L	Completely hydrolyzed nutrients May contain increased amounts of MCTs May contain arginine, glutamine	Elemental products may be beneficial for patients with malabsorptive syndromes, food allergies, or pancreatic insufficiency who are unable to tolerate a standard formula.[3,37,49]

Box continues

BOX 19.9 (CONTINUED)

	Composition	Specialty ingredients	Uses, contraindications, and other notes
Semielemental	1.0 to 1.5 kcal/mL Protein: 16% to 25% Carbohydrate: 36% to 74% Fat: 9% to 39% Free water: 77% to 85% Fiber: 0 to 10 g/L	Contains small peptides May contain increased amounts of MCTs Some with fiber and fish oil	No substantial difference has been found in outcome parameters in patients who are critically ill receiving semi-elemental vs polymeric formulas.3,37,49 In patients with acute pancreatitis, a semi-elemental formula has not shown to be preferred over a standard polymeric formula.[36,39,40,50]

BOX 19.10

Specialized Nutrients in Enteral Formulas[1,3,5,41,47,51-67]

Glutamine

Glutamine is a conditionally essential amino acid during times of metabolic stress.[51]

It has a trophic effect on the intestinal epithelium by stimulating the proliferation of epithelial cells, which maintains gut integrity.[51]

It stimulates the release of heat-shock proteins, which reduces heat shock–associated cell death (stabilizes organ function at distant sites).[51]

Enteral glutamine may decrease mortality and infectious complications in patients with burn injuries; however, it is *not* recommended as a supplement in patients who are critically ill at this time. More outcome studies are needed.[1,52-54]

Supplemental parenteral glutamine at higher doses (>0.5 g/kg of body weight per day) is not recommended for patients who are critically ill.[1,55]

Arginine

Arginine is a conditionally essential amino acid.

It is important for cell growth and proliferation; wound healing; collagen synthesis; immunity through the proliferation of T cells; and as a precursor to nitric oxide.[56]

Increased production of nitric oxide can lead to vasodilation; therefore, arginine is not recommended for patients who are hemodynamically unstable or have sepsis.[1,56]

Arginine-containing enteral nutrition (EN) formulas are not recommended for patients in the medical intensive care unit (ICU).[1]

Arginine-containing EN formulas with eicosapentaenoic acid (EPA) or docosahexaenoic acid (DHA) may be beneficial in patients with traumatic brain injury who are postoperative in the surgical ICU, or in patients with trauma.[1]

Box continues

BOX 19.10 (CONTINUED)

Fish oils

Fish oils promote anti-inflammatory cascade under stress conditions by competing with arachidonic acid for the conversion to lipid mediators.[56]

EN formulas containing fish oils are not recommended for patients in the medical ICU or patients with acute respiratory distress syndrome or severe acute lung injury.[1]

Fish oil–containing EN formulas including arginine may be beneficial in patients with traumatic brain injury who are postoperative in the surgical ICU, or in patients with trauma.[1,56]

Nucleotides

Nucleotides are essential in DNA and RNA production during high turnover induced by illness.[56]

Selenium

Decreased selenium plasma concentrations have been observed in patients who are critically ill, especially those with septic shock.[57]

Currently, there is no evidence to support the use of high-dose selenium to improve mortality, and supplementing with selenium is not recommended in patients with sepsis.[1,57-59]

Probiotics

It has been postulated that immunomodulation results from the interaction of gastrointestinal microbiota, the gut mucosa, and underlying mucosal lymphoid elements. Dysbiosis occurs in critical illness, which can lead to poor outcomes.[60-62]

Outcomes with probiotic supplements vary with species and strain. Supplements may reduce infection for patients who are critically ill.[5] *Lactobacillus rhamnosus* GG is associated with a reduction in ventilator-associated pneumonia and ICU length of stay.[1,63,64]

Probiotic species may have different effects with variable impact on patient outcomes. Lack of homogeneity in type of probiotic and populations studied makes broad recommendations difficult.[1,64]

Fiber

Fiber increases short-chain fatty acids (SCFAs) and fecal microbiota.[65] SCFAs are a fuel for the colonocytes and help increase intestinal mucosal growth and promote water and sodium absorption.[41,65]

A mixed-fiber formula may be beneficial in preventing or treating persistent diarrhea in fully resuscitated, hemodynamically stable patients who are critically ill receiving EN.[1,3]

Patients who are critically ill at risk for bowel ischemia or significant dysmotility should not receive EN with soluble or insoluble fiber.[1]

Insoluble fiber has not been shown to decrease diarrhea but may help decrease transit time by increasing fecal weight.[3]

Fructo-oligosaccharides are poorly absorbed carbohydrates that may help maintain large bowel integrity and promote growth of beneficial bacteria. However, they may not be tolerated by some patients and can cause bloating and gas.[3,66]

Fiber-containing formulas have been associated with lower glucose levels.[67]

Fiber-containing formulas may be associated with bowel obstructions in high-risk populations.[1]

Adequate fluid must be delivered to promote bowel regularity and prevent constipation.[47]

Fat

Fats are a concentrated energy source. Types of fats found in enteral formulas include the following[3,41]:

- long-chain triglycerides (LCTs)
- medium-chain triglycerides (MCTs)
- structured lipids
- omega-3 fatty acids and omega-6 fatty acids

LCTs are a source of the essential fatty acids linoleic acid and linolenic acid; corn and soybean oil are the most common sources of LCTs used in EN formulas. MCTs are absorbed in portal circulation (they do not need bile salts and lipase) and provide no essential fatty acids; palm kernel and coconut oil are most common sources of MCTs used. Structured lipids are a mixture of LCTs and MCTs on the same glycerol molecule; MCTs combined with a higher ratio of omega-3 LCTs may reduce infection and produce fewer inflammatory eicosanoids compared to LCTs alone. Omega-3 fatty acids have greater anti-inflammatory properties compared to omega-6 fatty acids.

Protein

Protein is a source of nitrogen. The types of protein in enteral formulas are[41]:

- intact proteins,
- hydrolyzed proteins (dipeptides and tripeptides), and
- free amino acids.

Intact proteins require normal levels of pancreatic enzymes for digestion and absorption; casein and soy protein isolates are the most common types. Hydrolyzed proteins may improve nitrogen absorption better than free amino acids.

Vitamins and Minerals

Enteral products provide adequate amounts of vitamins and minerals in 1,000 to 1,500 mL of formula to meet Dietary Reference Intakes. Disease-specific formulations may contain more or less of specific nutrients depending on the disease state.[41]

Water

Enteral products are 70% to 85% water. The amount of water in EN formulas typically does not provide enough fluid to completely meet hydration needs.[41]

Osmolality of Enteral Formulas

An enteral formula has an established osmolality, which is the concentration of molecules, free particles, or ions in a solution.[3] Enteral formulas range from 280 to 875 mOsm/kg.[3] The normal range of osmolality for body fluids is 285 to 290 mOsm/kg. Any formula with an osmolality of 320 mOsm/kg or higher is considered hypertonic.[3,7] The osmolality of EN formulas is generally not related to formula tolerance; in fact, selected clear-liquid food items and medications have substantially greater osmolalities than EN formulas.[3,41]

Modular Products

Modular products are available to provide additional energy, protein, or fiber. Typically, modulars are added to meet nutritional needs in patients who have disproportionate requirements for nutrients such as protein.[3,41]

Considerations for Formula Selection

Product-Related Considerations

When selecting a formula for a patient, relevant product-related considerations include the digestibility or availability of nutrients, nutritional adequacy, viscosity, osmolality, ease of use, and cost.[3,37]

Patient-Related Considerations

Aspects of the patient's medical status must be taken into account when choosing the appropriate enteral formula and infusion prescription.[2,3,37] Patient- and medical-related considerations include the patient's organ system function (eg, kidney and digestive or absorptive capacity), the need for a disease-specific formula, nutritional status of the patient and estimated nutrient requirements, the need for volume restriction, the route of administration, and the timing and dosage of medications. [2,3,37]

Placing the Formula Order

The EN formula order should contain the following elements[13]:

- patient demographics, including name, location, date of birth, and medical record number,
- formula (either specific name or generic type) and any modulars or additives,
- route and site of delivery (tube type and location),
- administration method, infusion rate and volume, and time for infusion, and
- any additional orders for advancement, transitions, water flushes, head elevations, and monitoring parameters.

The American Society for Parenteral and Enteral Nutrition (ASPEN) Safe Practices for Enteral Nutrition Therapy Task Force recommends the use of standardized order sets to help prescribers meet a patient's individual nutritional needs and to improve order clarity.[13]

Delivery of Enteral Nutrition

EN can be delivered by various methods, depending on the medical condition, tolerance to feedings, and needs of the patient (see Box 19.11 on page 349).[1,2,7,48,68-70] Most products are available as "ready-to-hang," with no reconstitution necessary. Formulas should not be diluted, as the risk for microbial contamination is high due to the low osmolality and high pH of the formulas.[13] A few products come in powder form and need to be mixed with water before administration. These powders are not sterile and have a high risk for contamination.

Closed EN systems are available for most formulations. These products are prepackaged in 1-L or 1.5-L containers that can be hung at room temperature for 24 to 48 hours after the container is spiked.[13] These systems are associated with less bacterial contamination and decreased incidence of diarrhea in patients who are critically ill.[4,13] If the containers are opened, the formula can be infused for a maximum of 8 hours or unused formula from the opened container must be refrigerated, with any remaining formula discarded after 24 hours.

Open systems require a feeding container to be filled with formula (either ready-to-hang or reconstituted) and can be hung at room temperature for a maximum of 4 to 8 hours in the hospital setting or 12 hours at home.[11] The recommended maximum hang time for formulas that are reconstituted from powder or contain powder modular additives is 4 hours.[13]

Contamination can occur at several points in the preparation process. To decrease the risk of contamination, follow the steps outlined in Box 19.12 and Box 19.13 (see pages 350 and 351).[11,13,71] Safe delivery of EN requires that clinicians use aseptic techniques when hanging the containers of EN and avoid touch contamination throughout the infusion process.

BOX 19.11

Types of Enteral Nutrition Delivery[1,2,7,48,68-70]

Continuous

Infused for 24 hours with minimal interruptions

Initiation and advancement	Initiate at 25 to 50 mL/h, or less.
	Increase by 25 to 50 mL/h every 4 to 8 hours.
	Do not exceed 150 mL/h (maximum rate).
	Divide goal volume over the desired number of hours for infusion (ie, 12 hours, 20 hours, 24 hours).
Advantages	May reduce diarrhea occurrence and abdominal distension in patients who are critically ill
	Requires less time for nursing care in hospitalized patients
Disadvantages	Requires a pump and tubing for accurate infusion

Volume-based[68,69]

A continuous method, infused over time based on goal volume

Initiation and advancement	Initiate as for continuous infusion.
	Determine the goal volume and adjust the infusion rate throughout the day to compensate for scheduled and unscheduled interruptions.
	Adjust the rate based on volume goal, remaining volume, and number of hours left in the day to meet goal.
Advantages	Improves efficiency of enteral nutrition (EN) delivery in meeting energy and protein goals
	Is best achieved when driven by a validated protocol
Disadvantages	Requires additional time for the nurse to calculate the adjustment of EN infusion rate
	Poses risk for gastrointestinal intolerance at higher infusion rates

Cycled

Infused at higher rates during a period of 10 to 12 hours (usually at night)

Initiation and advancement	Start with continuous infusion over 24 hours, and slowly increase the rate and decrease the number of hours infused.
Advantages	Allows the patient to have time away from the EN pump
	Allows for transition to oral intake during the day
Disadvantages	Higher rates may not be well tolerated

Box continues

BOX 19.11 (CONTINUED)

Intermittent

Larger volumes (240–480 mL) administered three to six times per day, infused over periods of 30 to 60 minutes

Initiation and advancement	Initiate at 120 to 240 mL per feeding.
	Increase by 120 mL per feeding per day to goal volume.
Advantages	Mimics meal schedule
	Allows time off from feedings
	May result in more adequate volumes being administered
	Gravity feeding system is less expensive than pump
Disadvantages	Higher rates may not be well tolerated
	May require pump for larger volume and slower infusions
	Requires more time for nurse care in hospitalized patients

Bolus

Larger volumes (240– 480 mL) administered three to six times per day over short periods of time (10–15 min)

Initiation and advancement	Initiate at 120 to 240 mL per feeding.
	Increase by 120 mL per feeding per day to goal volume.
Advantages	Mimics meal schedule
	Allows time off from feedings
	Is the quickest administration method
	Requires fewest supplies
	Is the least expensive
Disadvantages	Larger volume may not be well tolerated
	Gastrointestinal symptoms may occur with faster infusion
	Requires more time for nurse care in hospitalized patients

Conversion of gravity drip to an hourly rate

Total goal volume delivered via drop method without a pump but with the use of a feeding bag, clamp, and tubing[70]

Initiation and advancement	Goal rate	Drops per minute
	60 mL/h	14
	80 mL/h	19
	100 mL/h	23
	120 mL/h	28
	140 mL/h	33
Advantages	Removes the need for a pump	
Disadvantages	Requires manual adjustment for drops per minute	
	Is less accurate in delivery of EN rate	

BOX 19.12

Steps for Reducing Contamination Risk When Preparing Enteral Formulas[11,13]

Open systems

1. Practice proper hand hygiene before touching the cans or bottles of enteral formula.
2. Clean the tops of all cans or bottles with isopropyl alcohol, and allow them to dry before opening.
3. Use a sterile enteral nutrition (EN) container.
4. Pour enough formula into the container to last for a maximum of 4 to 8 hours.
5. Label the product (see labeling guidelines at end of this box).
6. Refrigerate any remaining formula immediately for a maximum of 24 hours or for use within this time frame.
7. Infuse the product for 4 hours (reconstituted formulas and modulars) to 8 hours (sterile formulas). Home EN can hang for 12 hours. Discard any remaining formula after this time frame.
8. *Never* add more formula to the container to allow for a longer infusion.
9. Change the delivery device (the container and administration set) according to the manufacturer's recommendations.
10. Discard the container after 24 hours.

Blenderized tube feeding

1. Use safe food-handling techniques when preparing blenderized tube feeding (BTF).
2. Store the BTF in the refrigerator after preparation and discard any unused formula after 24 hours.
3. Limit the hang time of BTF to 2 hours or less.
4. If the BTF is to be delivered via gastrostomy tube, use a tube that is at least 14 French in size.
5. Do not use BTF in patients with intolerance to bolus feeding, who are medically unstable, and who do not have a mature gastrostomy site that is free of infection.
6. Involve a registered dietitian nutritionist or certified nutrition support practitioner to ensure adequate nutrient composition and delivery of the BTF.
7. Sanitize all mechanical devices (mixers, blenders) used to prepare the BTF after each use in accordance with an established protocol.

Labeling

Properly label both open and closed systems. Labels should include the following information:

- patient identifiers (name, medical record number)
- name and strength of the formula
- date and time the formula was prepared
- date and time the formula was hung
- site of the enteral access device
- administration route
- administration rate, expressed as "____ mL/h over 24 hours" if continuous; "rate not to exceed ____"; or "formula not to exceed ____"
- administration duration, rate, and time, if cycled or using an intermittent schedule
- water flush type, volume, and frequency
- initials of the individuals responsible for preparation and hanging
- appropriate hang time (expiration date and time)
- dosing weight, if necessary
- the words "Not for IV Use"

BOX 19.13

Steps for Reducing the Contamination Risk in Closed System Enteral Delivery Systems[13,71]

1. Practice proper hygiene and thoroughly wash hands with soap and water before handling the container or feeding set.
2. Obtain the proper feeding set for the ready-to-hang container.
3. Label the product as described in Box 19.12.
4. Mix well and turn the container upside down and shake vigorously, using a twisting motion, for at least 10 seconds.
5. Without removing the safety screw cap, remove the dust cover from the enteral formula container.
6. Remove the dust cover from the safety screw connector set, and make sure nothing touches the tip of the connector that will come in contact with the formula.
7. Insert the safety screw connector set into the port on the ready-to-hang safety screw cap. Push down on the safety screw connector until the inner foil is punctured.
8. Turn and tighten the safety screw connector clockwise until securely fastened.
9. To assure proper flow of formula, close the clamp on the set, invert the container and suspend it, using the hanging feature on the bottom of the container.
10. Follow the pump priming and operation directions provided with the feeding set.
11. Discard any open, unused formula within 24 to 48 hours. A 48-hour hang time is safe if only one new feeding set is used.
12. To avoid contamination, change all ancillary feeding supplies (flushing syringes, adapter covers, and so on) at least every 24 hours.

Reminders:

If the feeding set is disconnected from the feeding tube, cover the adapter at the distal end of the set with the provided adapter cover to reduce the risk of touch contamination.

If the pump has a holder for the adapter cover, store the cover in the holder during feeding. Discard the cover when the feeding set is discarded.

Store unopened containers between 32° and 95° F (0° and 35° C) in the box in a dry area or in closed cabinets.

If there is potential for contact with bodily fluids (eg, gastric contents) while connecting the feeding set to the feeding tube, use universal precautions.

Never add any substances to the container. They may interact with the formula, introduce contaminants, and compromise the integrity of the container, all of which drastically reduces safe hang time.

Enteral misconnections—connections between an enteral and a nonenteral system, such as an intravenous access—should also be avoided to prevent potentially fatal errors.[13,72] One approach to preventing enteral misconnections is to use equipment with connectors that comply with the International Organization for Standardization standard 80369-3 (ie, ENFit connectors).[13,72] ENFit connectors are available for enteral equipment including feeding tubes, syringes, and administration sets. The design includes a screw type connector but may require some adjustments to medication administration, maintenance, and delivery of blenderized tube feedings.[28]

Box 19.14 on page 352 summarizes the ASPEN "Be A.L.E.R.T." campaign for educating practitioners on EN safety.[73]

Monitoring of Enteral Nutrition

Adequate monitoring is required to ensure feeding tube patency and location, prevent bronchopulmonary aspiration, make sure the patient is tolerating EN and manage any adverse effects of intolerance, and to provide the patient with adequate nutritional intake.

Monitoring for Tube Patency and Location

For proper monitoring of feeding tube patency and location, see the discussion of tube types and site selection for EN delivery earlier in this chapter (see Boxes 19.1 and 19.2).

Monitoring for Bronchopulmonary Aspiration

To prevent bronchopulmonary aspiration in patients receiving EN:

- Elevate the head of the bed at least 30 to 45 degrees.[1,13]
- Use prokinetic medications to promote gastric motility when feasible.[1,13]
- Use chlorhexidine mouthwash twice daily to potentially reduce the risk of ventilator-associated pneumonia.[1]
- Place the feeding tube in the distal jejunum if the patient is at high risk for aspiration.[1]
- Consider continuous method of delivery.[1,13]
- Do not check gastric residual volumes (GRVs) as part of routine care for monitoring patients receiving EN.[1] If GRVs are checked, EN should not be held for any GRV below 500 mL in the absence of signs of intolerance (ie, abdominal distension, diarrhea, vomiting).[1,13]
- Evaluate the abdominal status of patients in the prone position every 4 hours to assess GI motility. Consider using prokinetic agents if indicated, and consider transpyloric feeding access for patients at higher risk for aspiration.[13]
- Recognize that checking tracheal secretions with glucose oxidase strips is *not* specific or sensitive.[20] Do not use blue dye. The presence of blue dye in tracheal aspirations is not a sensitive indicator of aspiration, and the harm from blue dye outweighs its potential benefits.[3,74]

Monitoring for Tolerance and Managing Intolerance

Patients should be carefully monitored to make sure they are tolerating EN and to manage any adverse effects of intolerance, such as:

- diarrhea (osmotic, secretory, infectious, and noninfectious types, including medication-induced)[3,75,76]
- constipation,[77]
- GI dysmotility,[78]
- abdominal distension or pain,
- nausea and vomiting,[12] or
- metabolic complications.[1,3,12,13,79-82]

For detailed management techniques for improving tolerance to EN, see Box 19.15.[1,3,12,41,75,78] Constipation is more common than diarrhea in patients receiving EN[77]; for a list of medications that slow GI motility and lead to constipation, see Box 19.16 on page 355.[75,76] Nausea and vomiting occur in 12% to 20% of patients on EN and may increase the risk of pulmonary aspiration, pneumonia, and sepsis.[12] Most metabolic complications from EN are related to malnutrition or an underlying disease process and are not caused by the EN infusion itself; however, infusion of EN can result in metabolic complications due to preexisting deficiencies or increased demands to metabolize nutrients. Box 19.17 on page 356 describes common metabolic complications associated with EN.[1,3,12,13,79-82]

BOX 19.15

Management Techniques for Improving Tolerance to Enteral Nutrition[1,3,12,41,75,78]

Diarrhea[12,75]

>500 mL every 24 h or more than three stools per day for at least 2 consecutive days

Potential causes	Potential solutions
Osmotic: medications (liquid medications containing sorbitol, lactulose, potassium, magnesium, or phosphates); hyperosmolar enteral nutrition (EN)	Avoid medications containing sorbitol.
	Check for infectious causes.
Secretory: enterotoxins, inflammatory bowel disease (IBD), celiac disease, Zollinger-Ellison syndrome, collagen vascular diseases, intestinal resection, bile acid malabsorption, fatty acid malabsorption, gastric hypersecretion, intestinal motility disorders, laxative abuse	Start antidiarrheal medication if no infectious cause is found.
	Add or remove fiber.
	Use continuous feeds.
	Use probiotics.
	Consider alternate enteral formulas (isotonic, semielemental, or elemental).
Infectious: *Clostridioides difficile*[a]; contaminated enteral formula	Ensure proper procedure is followed for preparation and administration of EN.
Noninfectious: medications (antibiotics, H$_2$ blockers, antineoplastics, quinidine, prokinetic agents), bolus feeding, hyperosmolar EN, malnutrition, hypoalbuminemia, partial small bowel obstruction	

[a] *Previously known as* Clostridium difficile.

Box continues

BOX 19.15 (CONTINUED)

Constipation[3,75]

Excessive waste in the colon causing difficulty with fecal elimination

Potential causes	Potential solutions
Dehydration	Provide adequate fluid.
Decreased gastrointestinal motility	Provide adequate fiber.
Inadequate fiber	Medication-related: Add stool softeners, bowel stimulants, laxatives, enemas. Avoid drugs that decrease motility.
Excessive fiber	
Inactivity	
Medications (see Box 19.16)	Treat by disimpaction.
Advanced age	Recommend increased physical activity.

Abdominal pain, abdominal distension

Potential causes	Potential solutions
Constipation or impaction	Manage constipation and diarrhea.
Obstruction	Change fiber content of formula.
Ileus	Start a prokinetic agent.
Obstipation	Decrease or hold EN.
Ascites	
Diarrhea	
Use of fiber-containing formulas	
Rapid feeding or feeding with very cold formula	

Nausea and vomiting

Potential causes	Potential solutions
Constipation or impaction	Manage constipation.
Partial obstruction	Reduce, change, or discontinue all narcotic medications.
Diabetic gastropathy	
Some autoimmune diseases	Start a prokinetic agent.
Pancreaticoduodenectomy	Switch to a low-fat, isotonic or low-fiber formula.
Hypotension	
Sepsis	Infuse feeding at room temperature.
Anesthesia and surgery	Reduce rate of infusion.
Opiate analgesic medications	Use a postpyloric feeding tube.
Anticholinergics	Consider an antiemetic agent.
Excessive rapid infusion of formula	
Infusion of a very cold solution or one containing a large amount of fat	

Box continues

BOX 19.15 (CONTINUED)

Maldigestion, malabsorption

Potential causes

Lactose intolerance

Steatorrhea

Short bowel syndrome

Crohn's disease

Diverticular disease

Radition enteritis

HIV

Pancreatic insufficiency

Celiac disease

Enteric fistulas

Small intestinal bacterial overgrowth

Potential solutions

Use a peptide-based formula with a greater percentage of fat from medium-chain triglycerides.

Consider formulas with specialty ingredients such as omega-3 fatty acids and prebiotics.[43]

Consider parenteral nutrition (PN) or a combination of EN and PN, if severe.

BOX 19.16

Medications That May Slow Gastrointestinal Motility[75,76]

Sedatives

Opioid analgesics (morphine, fentanyl, hydromorphone, methadone)

Catecholamine vasopressors (dopamine, epinephrine, norepinephrine, phenylephrine)

α2-Adrenergic receptor agonists (clonidine, dexmedetomidine)

Anticholinergics (antihistamines, tricyclic antidepressants, antiparkinsonian agents, phenothiazines)

Calcium channel blockers

Oral or enteral calcium supplements

Oral or enteral iron supplements

Calcium- or aluminum-containing antacids

Diuretics

BOX 19.17

Common Metabolic Complications of Enteral Nutrition[1,3,12,13,79-82]

Hyperglycemia

Causes	Diabetes mellitus
	Insulin resistance
	Excess carbohydrate intake
	Stress
	Infection
	Trauma
	Glucocorticoids
Goal	Maintain blood glucose control (140–180 mg/dL) in patients who are critically ill. Tight control (levels of 80–110 mg/dL) is *not* associated with reductions in length of hospital stay, days on mechanical ventilation, infectious complications, mortality, or cost of medical care, and it increases the risk of hypoglycemia.[80]
	Tight control using a monitoring system can reduce morbidity in some perioperative, cardiac surgery, posttrauma, and neurologically injured patients.[81]
	Hyperglycemia (blood glucose level >180 mg/dL) should be avoided in patients who are critically ill, as it is associated with increased mortality.[81]
Prevention or correction	Treat the underlying disease.
	Use insulin to maintain optimal blood glucose levels between 140 and 180 mg/dL.[1]
	Provide oral hypoglycemic agents as needed.
	Monitor serum glucose every 6 hours.
	Provide 30% of total energy as fat.
	Consider use of a fiber-containing formula.

Hypoglycemia

Causes	Holding enteral nutrition (EN) in patients receiving insulin or oral hypoglycemic agents
Goal	Do not allow blood glucose level to fall below 70 mg/dL.
Prevention or correction	Taper EN gradually vs abruptly stopping formula.
	Add dextrose to intravenous (IV) fluids.
	Continue basal insulin, but hold bolus or carbohydrate coverage insulin if EN is held.

Hypernatremia

Causes	Inadequate fluid intake
	Increased fluid loss
	Increased sodium intake (rare)
Goal	Maintain serum sodium level within normal range for institution.
Prevention or correction	Increase free water administration.
	Decrease exogenous sodium administration from IV solutions.
	Monitor fluid intake and output.
	Monitor changes in daily weight.

Box continues

BOX 19.17 (CONTINUED)

Refeeding syndrome[79]

Causes	Chronic malnutrition
	Inadequate nutritional intake before starting EN
Goal	Maintain serum phosphorus, magnesium, potassium levels within normal range for institution.
Prevention or correction	Assess laboratory values; correct abnormal electrolyte levels before starting EN.
	Initiate and advance feedings slowly. Start high-risk patients at 100 to 150 g dextrose or 10 to 20 kcal/kg of body weight for the first 24 hours, then advance by 33% every 1 to 2 days.
	Supplement thiamin, 100 mg, before feeding or before infusion of IV dextrose.
	Supplement thiamin, 100 mg/d, for 5 to 7 days in patients with severe starvation, chronic alcoholism, or high risk for deficiency.
	Supplement with multivitamin for 10 days.
	Monitor phosphorus, magnesium, and potassium every 12 hours for the first 3 days for high-risk patients.
	Monitor cardiopulmonary function for congestive heart failure, pulmonary edema.
	Check weight daily, with close monitoring of intake and output.

Hyperphosphatemia

Causes	Renal insufficiency
Goal	Maintain serum phosphorus level within normal range for institution.
Prevention or correction	Use a low-phosphorus formula.
	Start a phosphate binder.

Essential fatty acid deficiency[3]

Causes	Inadequate linoleic acid intake
	Inadequate absorption due to gastronintestinal disease
	Conditions requiring severe fat restriction (eg, chylothorax, familial hypertriglyceridemia)
Goal	Supply adequate fat to meet requirements for essential fatty acids.
Prevention or correction	Provide at least 4% of energy needs as linoleic acid.
	Provide soybean oil via enteral access (1.1–1.6 g/d based on age and sex).[82]

Monitoring for Adequate Nutritional Intake

To ensure adequate nutritional intake in patients receiving EN:

- Initiate EN within 24 to 48 hours in patients who are critically ill, and advance toward the estimated goal within the first week in the critical care unit.[1] Patients who are in stable condition will tolerate advancing to their established goal within 24 to 48 hours.[2]
- Use institution-specific strategies and nurse-driven EN feeding protocols to initiate, advance, and deliver nutrition support.[1]
- Use full-strength enteral formulas. Do not dilute formulas, as diluting is not a requirement and may increase the incidence of bacterial contamination.[13]
- Monitor actual infused volumes vs prescribed or desired volumes.
- Monitor holding times and rationales for appropriateness. Do not use GRVs for routine care monitoring, as this leads to unnecessary interruption of EN.[1] If GRVs are used, EN should not be held for any value below 500 mL in the absence of signs of GI intolerance.[1]
- Improve the efficiency of enteral delivery through the use of volume-based feeding protocols. Volume-based protocols focus on target volume instead of the target rate. Daily volume goals are met through adjustments of the infusion rates by nursing staff. This protocol improves the total amount of EN formula delivered.[1,68,69]

Additional strategies for improving nutritional intakes may include initiating the EN of a stable patient at the target rate, using prokinetics to improve GI motility, and initiating the EN using a postpyloric access.[1,78]

Enteral Feeding Protocols

Enteral feeding protocols assist in the appropriate ordering, delivery, and monitoring of EN. Protocols that are nurse-driven result in an earlier start of EN and overall nutritional adequacy and may be associated with a reduction in hospital mortality and length of stay.[1,2,48,83] Effective nurse-driven EN protocols should include the initial EN infusion rate, instructions for management of the GRV, a prescription for proper flushing, and orders for when the EN should be held.[1,48] Volume-based feeding protocols, in which a daily target volume is prescribed instead of a target rate, have also proven to be an efficient way to improve overall EN delivery.[68,69,84,85] Often, multifaceted practice-change strategies must be implemented to achieve compliance with evidence-based nutrition support guidelines. Volume-based protocols may incorporate multiple strategies for improving success with initiation and progression, including the use of prokinetics at initiation or the placement of a postpyloric feeding tube.[1,48,68] This strategy may increase GI transit, improve feeding tolerance and EN delivery, and potentially reduce the risk of aspiration.[68] Improvements in compliance with protocols can be achieved using simple algorithms and personalized protocols based on staffing, patient population, and resources.

Summary

Enteral nutrition is clearly regarded as the safest and most beneficial method of supporting the nutritional status of patients who are unable to eat orally. It is associated with improved clinical outcomes and reduced infectious complications and, therefore, is the preferred method of nutrition support when the patient's GI tract is functional and of sufficient length, unless its use is otherwise contraindicated. Complications associated with EN can be prevented or managed with thoughtful initiation, delivery, and monitoring of EN. Skilled clinicians play an integral role in ensuring that early and adequate EN is achieved in patients who are critically ill in order to minimize complications and improve outcomes.

References

1. McClave SA, Taylor BE, Martindale RG, et al; Society of Critical Care Medicine; American Society for Parenteral and Enteral Nutrition. Guidelines for the provision and assessment of nutrition support therapy in the adult critically ill patient: Society of Critical Care Medicine (SCCM) and American Society for Parenteral and Enteral Nutrition (A.S.P.E.N.). *JPEN J Parenter Enteral Nutr.* 2016;40(2):159-211. doi:10.1177/0148607115621863

2. Doley J, Phillips W. Overview of enteral nutrition. In: Mueller C, ed. *The A.S.P.E.N. Nutrition Support Core Curriculum: A Case Based Approach—The Adult Patient.* American Society for Parenteral and Enteral Nutrition; 2017:213-225.

3. Malone A, Carney LN, Carrera AL, Mays A. *ASPEN Enteral Nutrition Handbook.* 2nd ed. American Society for Parenteral and Enteral Nutrition; 2019.

4. Ukleja A, Gilbert K, Mogensen KM, et al. Standards for nutrition support: adult hospitalized patients. *Nutr Clin Pract.* 2018;33(6):906-920.

5. Academy of Nutrition and Dietetics. Enteral nutrition vs. parenteral nutrition (2012). Evidence Analysis Library. Accessed February 10, 2021. www.andeal.org/topic.cfm?menu=4063&cat=4884

6. Toulson Davisson Correia MI, Castro M, de Oliveira Toledo D, et al. Nutrition therapy cost-effectiveness model indicating how nutrition may contribute to the efficiency and financial sustainability of the health systems. *JPEN J Parenter Enteral Nutr.* 2021;45(7):1542-1550. doi:10.1002/jpen.2052

7. Compher C, Bingham AL, McCall M, et al. Guidelines for the provision of nutrition support therapy in the adult critically ill patient: The American Society for Parenteral and Enteral Nutrition. *JPEN J Parenter Enteral Nutr.* 2022;46(1):12-41.

8. Yang S, Wu X, Yu W, Li J. Early enteral nutrition in critically ill patients with hemodynamic instability: an evidence-based review and practical advice. *Nutr Clin Pract.* 2014;29(1):90-96.

9. Couper C, Doriot A, Siddiqui MTR, Steiger E. Nutrition management of the high-output fistulae. *Nutr Clin Pract.* 2021;36(2):282-296. doi:10.1002/ncp.10608

10. Arebi N, Forbes A. High-output fistula. *Clin Colon Rectal Surg.* 2004;17(2):89-98.

11. Fang J, Kinikini M. Enteral access devices. In: Mueller CM, ed. *The A.S.P.E.N. Nutrition Support Core Curriculum: A Case Based Approach—The Adult Patient.* American Society for Parenteral and Enteral Nutrition; 2017:251-264.

12. Malone A, Seres D, Lord L. Complications of enteral nutrition In: Mueller CM, ed. *The A.S.P.E.N. Nutrition Support Core Curriculum: A Case Based Approach—The Adult Patient.* American Society for Parenteral and Enteral Nutrition; 2017:265-283.

13. Boullata JI, Carrera AL, Harvey L, et al. ASPEN safe practices for enteral nutrition therapy [formula: see text]. *JPEN J Parenter Enteral Nutr.* 2017;41(1):15-103.

14. McClave SA, DeMeo MT, DeLegge MH, et al. North American Summit on Aspiration in the Critically Ill Patient: consensus statement. *JPEN J Parenter Enteral Nutr.* 2002;26(6 suppl):S80-S85.

15. Alkhawaja S, Martin C, Butler RJ, Gwadry-Sridhar F. Post-pyloric versus gastric tube feeding for preventing pneumonia and improving nutritional outcomes in critically ill adults. *Cochrane Database Syst Rev.* 2015;(8):CD008875.

16. Academy of Nutrition and Dietetics. Optimizing enteral nutrition delivery 2012. Evidence Analysis Library. Accessed February 17, 2021. www.andeal.org/template.cfm?template=guide_summary&key=3256&highlight=Enteral&home=1

17. Powers J, Luebbehusen M, Aguirre L, et al. Improved safety and efficacy of small-bore feeding tube confirmation using an electromagnetic placement device. *Nutr Clin Pract.* 2018;33(2):268-273.

18. Irving SY, Rempel G, Lyman B, Sevilla WMA, Northington L, Guenter P. Pediatric nasogastric tube placement and verification: best practice recommendations from the NOVEL Project. *Nutr Clin Pract.* 2018;33(6):921-927.

19. McCutcheon KP, Whittet WL, Kirsten JL, Fuchs JL. Feeding tube insertion and placement confirmation using electromagnetic guidance: a team review. *JPEN J Parenter Enteral Nutr.* 2018;42(1):247-254.

20. Metheny NA, Dahms TE, Stewart BJ, Stone KS, Frank PA, Clouse RE. Verification of inefficacy of the glucose method in detecting aspiration associated with tube feedings. *Medsurg Nurs.* 2005;14(2):112-119, 121; discussion 120.

21. Feeding tube placement systems—letter to health care providers. US Food and Drug Administration. Published 2018. Accessed June 15, 2021. www.fda.gov/medical-devices/letters-health-care-providers/feeding-tube-placement-systems-letter

22. Goggans M, Pickard S, West AN, Shah S, Kimura D. Transpyloric feeding tube placement using electromagnetic placement device in children. *Nutr Clin Pract.* 2017;32(2):233-237.

23. Metheny NA, Krieger MM, Healey F, Meert KL. A review of guidelines to distinguish between gastric and pulmonary placement of nasogastric tubes. *Heart Lung.* 2019;48(3):226-235.

24. Bechtold ML, Nguyen DL, Palmer LB, Kiraly LN, Martindale RG, McClave SA. Nasal bridles for securing nasoenteric tubes: a meta-analysis. *Nutr Clin Pract.* 2014;29(5):667-671.

25. Dandeles LM, Lodolce AE. Efficacy of agents to prevent and treat enteral feeding tube clogs. *Ann Pharmacother.* 2011;45(5):676-680.

26. Darawad MW, Alfasfos N, Zaki I, Alnajar M, Hammad S, Samarkandi OA. ICU nurses' perceived barriers to effective enteral nutrition practices: a multicenter survey study. *Open Nurs J.* 2018;12:67-75.

27. Huang J, Yang L, Zhuang Y, Qi H, Chen X, Lv K. Current status and influencing factors of barriers to enteral feeding of critically ill patients: a multicenter study. *J Clin Nurs.* 2019;28(3-4):677-685.

28. Guenter P, Lyman B. ENFit enteral nutrition connectors: benefits and challenges. *Nutr Clin Pract.* 2016;31(6):769-772.

29. Klang MG, Gandhi UD, Mironova O. Dissolving a nutrition clog with a new pancreatic enzyme formulation. *Nutr Clin Pract.* 2013;28(3):410-412.

30. Lewis SJ, Andersen HK, Thomas S. Early enteral nutrition within 24 h of intestinal surgery versus later commencement of feeding: a systematic review and meta-analysis. *J Gastrointest Surg.* 2009;13(3):569-575.

31. Dubagunta S, Still CD, Kumar A, et al. Early initiation of enteral feeding after percutaneous endoscopic gastrostomy tube placement. *Nutr Clin Pract.* 2002;17(2):123-125.

32. Jain R, Maple JT, Anderson MA, et al. The role of endoscopy in enteral feeding. *Gastrointest Endosc.* 2011;74(1):7-12.

33. Shellnutt C. The evidence on feeding initiation after percutaneous endoscopic gastrostomy tube placement. *Gastroenterol Nurs.* 2019;42(5):420-427.

34. Weimann A, Braga M, Carli F, et al. ESPEN guideline: clinical nutrition in surgery. *Clin Nutr.* 2017;36(3):623-650.

35. Academy of Nutrition and Dietetics. Critical illness. Evidence Analysis Library. Updated December 15, 2020. Accessed March 19, 2021. www.andeal.org/topic.cfm?menu=5302

36. Endo A, Shiraishi A, Fushimi K, Murata K, Otomo Y. Comparative effectiveness of elemental formula in the early enteral nutrition management of acute pancreatitis: a retrospective cohort study. *Ann Intensive Care.* 2018;8(1):69.

37. Escuro AA, Hummell AC. enteral formulas in nutrition support practice: is there a better choice for your patient? *Nutr Clin Pract.* 2016;31(6):709-722.

38. García de Acilu M, Leal S, Caralt B, Roca O, Sabater J, Masclans JR. The role of omega-3 polyunsaturated fatty acids in the treatment of patients with acute respiratory distress syndrome: a clinical review. *Biomed Res Int.* 2015;2015:653750.

39. Lakananurak N, Gramlich L. Nutrition management in acute pancreatitis: clinical practice consideration. *World J Clin Cases.* 2020;8(9):1561-1573.

40. Tiengou LE, Gloro R, Pouzoulet J, et al. Semi-elemental formula or polymeric formula: is there a better choice for enteral nutrition in acute pancreatitis? Randomized comparative study. *JPEN J Parenter Enteral Nutr.* 2006;30(1):1-5.

41. Roberts S, Kirsch R. Enteral formulations. In: Mueller CM, ed. *The A.S.P.E.N. Nutrition Support Core Curriculum: A Case Based Approach—The Adult Patient.* American Society for Parenteral and Enteral Nutrition; 2017:217-249.

42. Singer P, Blaser AR, Berger MM, et al. ESPEN guideline on clinical nutrition in the intensive care unit. *Clin Nutr.* 2019;38(1):48-79.

43. Mesejo A, Montejo-González JC, Vaquerizo-Alonso C, et al. Diabetes-specific enteral nutrition formula in hyperglycemic, mechanically ventilated, critically ill patients: a prospective, open-label, blind-randomized, multicenter study. *Crit Care.* 2015;19:390.

44. Han Y-Y, Lai S-R, Partridge JS, et al. The clinical and economic impact of the use of diabetes-specific enteral formula on ICU patients with type 2 diabetes. *Clinical Nutrition.* 2017;36(6):1567-1572.

45. Doola R, Deane AM, Tolcher DM, et al. The effect of a low carbohydrate formula on glycaemia in critically ill enterally-fed adult patients with hyperglycaemia: a blinded randomised feasibility trial. *Clin Nutr ESPEN.* 2019;31:80-87.

46. American Society for Parenteral and Enteral Nutrition. Enteral nutrition formula guide. Accessed October 25, 2020. www.nutritioncare.org/Guidelines_and_Clinical_Resources/EN_Formula_Guide/Enteral_Nutrition_Formula_Guide

47. Malone A, Hamilton C. The Academy of Nutrition and Dietetics/the American Society for Parenteral and Enteral Nutrition consensus malnutrition characteristics: application in practice. *Nutr Clin Pract.* 2013;28(6):639-650.

48. McClave SA, DiBaise JK, Mullin GE, Martindale RG. ACG clinical guideline: nutrition therapy in the adult hospitalized patient. *Am J Gastroenterol.* 2016;111(3):315-334; quiz 335.

49. Brown B, Roehl K, Betz M. Enteral nutrition formula selection: current evidence and implications for practice. *Nutr Clin Pract.* 2015;30(1):72-85.

50. Lodewijkx PJ, Besselink MG, Witteman BJ, et al. Nutrition in acute pancreatitis: a critical review. *Expert Review of Gastroenterology and Hepatology.* 2016;10(5):571-580.

51. Cruzat V, Macedo Rogero M, Noel Keane K, Curi R, Newsholme P. Glutamine: metabolism and immune function, supplementation and clinical translation. *Nutrients.* 2018;10(11):1564.

52. Moreira E, Burghi G, Manzanares W. Update on metabolism and nutrition therapy in critically ill burn patients. *Med Intensiva.* 2018;42(5):306-316.

53. van Zanten AR, Dhaliwal R, Garrel D, Heyland DK. Enteral glutamine supplementation in critically ill patients: a systematic review and meta-analysis. *Crit Care.* 2015;19(1):294.

54. Heyland D, Muscedere J, Wischmeyer PE, et al. A randomized trial of glutamine and antioxidants in critically ill patients. *N Engl J Med*. 2013;368(16):1489-1497.

55. Wischmeyer PE. The glutamine debate in surgery and critical care. *Curr Opin Crit Care*. 2019;25(4):322-328.

56. McCarthy MS, Martindale RG. Immunonutrition in critical illness: what is the role? *Nutr Clin Pract*. 2018;33(3):348-358.

57. Forceville X, Vitoux D, Gauzit R, Combes A, Lahilaire P, Chappuis P. Selenium, systemic immune response syndrome, sepsis, and outcome in critically ill patients. *Crit Care Med*. 1998;26(9):1536-1544.

58. De Waele E, Malbrain M, Spapen H. Nutrition in sepsis: a bench-to-bedside review. *Nutrients*. 2020;12(2):395.

59. Bloos F, Trips E, Nierhaus A, et al. Effect of sodium selenite administration and procalcitonin-guided therapy on mortality in patients with severe sepsis or septic shock: a randomized clinical trial. *JAMA Intern Med*. 2016;176(9):1266-1276.

60. Cresci GA, Bawden E. Gut microbiome: what we do and don't know. *Nutr Clin Pract*. 2015;30(6):734-746.

61. Wang C, Li Q, Ren J. Microbiota-immune interaction in the pathogenesis of gut-derived infection. *Front Immunol*. 2019;10:1873.

62. Wischmeyer PE, McDonald D, Knight R. Role of the microbiome, probiotics, and "dysbiosis therapy" in critical illness. *Curr Opin Crit Care*. 2016;22(4):347-353.

63. Su M, Jia Y, Li Y, Zhou D, Jia J. Probiotics for the prevention of ventilator-associated pneumonia: a meta-analysis of randomized controlled trials. *Respir Care*. 2020;65(5):673-685.

64. Kothari D, Patel S, Kim SK. Probiotic supplements might not be universally-effective and safe: a review. *Biomed Pharmacother*. 2019;111:537-547.

65. Fu Y, Moscoso DI, Porter J, et al. Relationship between dietary fiber intake and short-chain fatty acid-producing bacteria during critical illness: a prospective cohort study. *JPEN J Parenter Enteral Nutr*. 2020;44(3):463-471.

66. Kamarul Zaman M, Chin KF, Rai V, Majid HA. Fiber and prebiotic supplementation in enteral nutrition: a systematic review and meta-analysis. *World J Gastroenterol*. 2015;21(17):5372-5381.

67. Silva FM, Kramer CK, de Almeida JC, Steemburgo T, Gross JL, Azevedo MJ. Fiber intake and glycemic control in patients with type 2 diabetes mellitus: a systematic review with meta-analysis of randomized controlled trials. *Nutr Rev*. 2013;71(12):790-801.

68. Heyland DK, Murch L, Cahill N, et al. Enhanced protein-energy provision via the enteral route feeding protocol in critically ill patients: results of a cluster randomized trial. *Crit Care Med*. 2013;41(12):2743-2753.

69. Taylor B, Brody R, Denmark R, Southard R, Byham-Gray L. Improving enteral delivery through the adoption of the "Feed Early Enteral Diet adequately for Maximum Effect (FEED ME)" protocol in a surgical trauma ICU: a quality improvement review. *Nutr Clin Pract*. 2014;29(5):639-648.

70. Abbott Laboratories. Gravity tube feeding overview. American Society for Parenteral and Enteral Nutrition website. March 2020. Accessed December 3, 2020. www.nutritioncare.org/uploadedFiles/Documents /Guidelines_and_Clinical_Resources/COVID19/Gravity %20Tube%20Feeding%20Overview_Abbott.pdf

71. Abbott Laboratories. Ready-to-Hang suggested setup procedure. Abbott Nutrition website. January 2015. Accessed June 15, 2021. https://static.abbottnutrition .com/cms-prod/abbottnutrition-2016.com/img/RTH %20setup%20procedure_tcm1411-57850.pdf

72. Guenter P, Lyman B. ENFit enteral nutrition connectors: benefits and challenges. *Nutr Clin Pract*. 2016;31(6):769-772.

73. Guidelines and resources: related publications and tools: BE ALERT campaign. American Society for Parenteral and Enteral Nutrition website. Accessed April 10, 2021. www.nutritioncare.org/Guidelines _and_Clinical_Resources/Toolkits/Enteral_Nutrition _Toolkit/Related_Publications_and_Tools

74. Metheny NA, Dahms TE, Stewart BJ, et al. Efficacy of dye-stained enteral formula in detecting pulmonary aspiration. *Chest*. 2002;122(1):276-281.

75. Tatsumi H. Enteral tolerance in critically ill patients. *J Intensive Care*. 2019;7:30.

76. Bharucha AE, Lacy BE. Mechanisms, evaluation, and management of chronic constipation. *Gastroenterology*. 2020;158(5):1232-1249.e1233.

77. Bittencourt AF, Martins JR, Logullo L, et al. Constipation is more frequent than diarrhea in patients fed exclusively by enteral nutrition: results of an observational study. *Nutr Clin Pract*. 2012;27(4):533-539.

78. Deane AM, Chapman MJ, Reintam Blaser A, McClave SA, Emmanuel A. Pathophysiology and treatment of gastrointestinal motility disorders in the acutely ill. *Nutr Clin Pract*. 2019;34(1):23-36.

79. da Silva JSV, Seres DS, Sabino K, et al. ASPEN consensus recommendations for refeeding syndrome. *Nutr Clin Pract*. 2020;35(2):178-195.

80. Academy of Nutrition and Dietetics. Recommendations summary—CI: blood glucose control 2012. Evidence Analysis Library. Accessed April 14, 2021. www.andeal.org /template.cfm?template=guide_summary&key=3204

81. Jacobi J, Bircher N, Krinsley J, et al. Guidelines for the use of an insulin infusion for the management of hyperglycemia in critically ill patients. *Crit Care Med*. 2012;40(12):3251-3276.

82. Hise M, Brown JC. Lipids. In: Mueller CM, ed. *The ASPEN Adult Nutrition Support Core Curriculum*. 3rd ed. American Society for Parenteral and Enteral Nutrition; 2017.

83. Martin CM, Doig GS, Heyland DK, Morrison T, Sibbald WJ. Multicentre, cluster-randomized clinical trial of algorithms for critical-care enteral and parenteral therapy (ACCEPT). *CMAJ*. 2004;170(2):197-204.

84. Heyland DK, Patel J, Bear D, et al. The effect of higher protein dosing in critically ill patients: a multicenter registry-based randomized trial: the EFFORT trial. *JPEN J Parenter Enteral Nutr*. 2019;43(3):326-334.

85. Sachdev G, Backes K, Thomas BW, Sing RF, Huynh T. Volume-based protocol improves delivery of enteral nutrition in critically ill trauma patients. *JPEN J Parenter Enteral Nutr*. 2020;44(5):874-879.

Parenteral Nutrition

Jennifer Lefton, MS, RD-AP, CNSC, FAND

KEY POINTS

- Parenteral nutrition is indicated for patients who require nutrition support but whose needs cannot be met through oral or enteral nutrition.
- Nutrition assessment, nutrition monitoring, and evaluation of the patient receiving parenteral nutrition are essential to ensuring the safe and efficacious use of this nutrition therapy.
- Parenteral nutrition is a complex therapy that requires knowledge of the patient's disease process, the type and location of the catheter, and the appropriate macronutrients, micronutrients, fluid and electrolytes, and medications. Practitioners must ensure the stability of the parenteral solution, write orders for intravenous replacements of electrolytes and minerals, prevent and monitor for complications, and know how and when to wean.

Introduction

This chapter briefly reviews the topic of parenteral nutrition (PN), which is "the infusion of intravenous nutrients via peripheral or central veins."[1] A more detailed discussion of patient selection and the initiation, advancement, and monitoring of PN is beyond the scope of this publication. For information about the use of PN in pediatric patients, see Chapter 21. Chapter 22 covers home PN, and Chapter 25 discusses the legal and ethical considerations related to nutrition support.

Indications for the Use of Parenteral Nutrition

Traditionally, indications for the use of PN included medical conditions such as malabsorption, bowel obstruction, and gastrointestinal (GI) fistulas. Recent guidelines on the appropriate use of PN, however, suggest that a full evaluation of the patient's nutritional status and ability to be fed enterally is necessary before initiating PN. The guidelines also suggest that PN is not indicated solely on the basis of a diagnosis or condition.[2] This is because some patients with conditions that were traditionally thought to be managed with PN may actually be able to tolerate enteral feedings. For example, some patients with a proximal fistula can be fed distally to the fistula site. Additionally, patients who exhibit intolerance to gastric feedings may be able to tolerate small bowel feedings well. PN is generally reserved for patients who cannot be fed enterally.[3,4] However, current guidelines state that during the first week of critical illness, no significant difference in outcomes are found when EN or PN is provided; therefore, both are acceptable.[5] Clinical judgment is still recommended when the decision of initiating nutrition support is necessary. (See Chapter 19 for more information on enteral nutrition.)

PN is appropriate for patients who are[1]:

- malnourished,
- at risk of becoming malnourished,
- not candidates for enteral feedings,
- unable to meet their nutritional needs with enteral feedings alone, or
- without adequate bowel length or function to maintain or improve their nutritional status.

Timing of Initiation

Some guidelines suggest that if patients who are critically ill cannot be fed enterally, then no nutrition support should be provided for the first 7 days following admission to the intensive care unit.[6] However, if patients have preexisting malnutrition or if their Nutrition Risk in the Critically Ill (NUTRIC) or Nutrition Risk Screening 2002 (NRS-2002) scores indicate they are at high risk for malnutrition, it is appropriate to initiate PN as soon as possible once the patient has been adequately resuscitated. PN can be started in 3 to 5 days for patients who are at nutritional risk or who are unlikely to receive adequate intake via the enteral route.[6] For metabolically unstable patients, PN should be delayed until the patient is more stable. Table 20.1 summarizes laboratory values that warrant caution when considering the start of PN.[2] Additionally, PN should be initiated in patients postoperatively only if the patient is expected to need nutrition support for at least 7 days.[4]

TABLE 20.1 Laboratory Values Warranting Cautious Initiation of Parenteral Nutrition[a,2]

Laboratory test	Value that may warrant delaying initiation
Sodium	<130 mEq/L or >150 mEq/L
Potassium	<3 mEq/L
Blood urea nitrogen	>100 mg/dL
Glucose	>180 mg/dL
Magnesium	<1.3 mEq/L
Phosphorus	<2 mg/dL
Calcium (ionized)	<4.5 mg/dL
Triglycerides	>200 mg/dL

[a] For adults

Supplemental Parenteral Nutrition

For patients who are critically ill who are at nutritional risk and have been unable to meet at least 60% of their nutrient needs with enteral feedings for 7 to 10 days, supplemental PN can be initiated. Initiating before the 7 to 10 days is not recommended, as it can lead to worse outcomes.[4,6]

Venous Access for Parenteral Nutrition

PN may be infused via a peripheral or central line. Peripheral PN often delivers less than adequate nutrients in large amounts of fluid because of constraints in the osmolarity of the solution. Patients must have good peripheral venous access and be able to tolerate large volumes of fluid to receive peripheral PN. For these reasons, patients with renal, cardiac, or hepatic failure or who are elderly are not good candidates for peripheral PN.

Most patients have PN administered through a central line. It is ideal to have a dedicated line for delivery of PN. The tip of the catheter should be confirmed to be in the superior vena cava before administering a central PN formulation.

Box 20.1 on page 364 summarizes selected factors to consider when deciding on a venous access route for PN infusion.[1]

BOX 20.1

Factors to Consider in Selecting an Access Route for Parenteral Nutrition

Available access route and length of therapy

Peripheral venous access

Peripheral catheters access the peripheral vessels and are among the simplest catheters to place for short-term access (≤10–14 days). To minimize the risk of phlebitis, peripheral catheters are rotated every 72 hours. Peripheral access should only be used for parenteral nutrition (PN) solutions with low osmolarity (<900 mOsm/L). The inclusion of intravenous lipid emulsions in the PN formula may also minimize the risk of phlebitis.

Central venous access

Central venous catheters (CVCs) access large veins, and their distal tip lies in the distal vena cava or right atrium. CVCs are most commonly placed in the jugular, subclavian, femoral, cephalic, and basilic veins. They may be single-lumen or multilumen. The three categories of CVC are as follows:

- **Nontunneled:** Percutaneous nontunneled CVCs are used in the acute setting for short-duration therapies. They are most often placed in the subclavian, jugular, and femoral veins. Higher infection risk is present with these catheters, so they are not recommended for home care. Peripherally inserted central catheter (PICC) lines are a form of nontunneled CVC used in acute and home care settings. They are inserted into the basilic, cephalic, or brachial vein and threaded up so that the tip lies in the superior vena cava. Although peripherally inserted, PICCs are considered central lines.
- **Tunneled:** Tunneled CVCs are surgically tunneled through the skin so that the exit point of the catheter is remote from the actual vein entry point. They are used when long-term vascular access is required. Broviac, Hickman, and Groshong are commonly used types of tunneled catheters. Tunneled CVCs have a cuff with antimicrobial qualities that also acts to prevent migration of the catheter. Access to tunneled catheters is external.
- **Implanted:** Implanted ports are entirely internal and are accessed by piercing the skin with a specially designed needle. They are best for long intermittent therapies, such as chemotherapy, but can be used for PN.

Osmolarity and concentration of solution

PN solutions with a final dextrose concentration of more than 10% are extremely hypertonic and must be infused into a large vein to avoid damage to the vein.

Solutions with osmolarity of 900 mOsm/L or more should be infused via CVC.

Anatomical considerations

Consider ease of access to desired site.

Practitioner expertise

PICCs may be placed by specially trained nurses.

Implanted ports and tunneled catheters are placed by surgical staff or interventional radiology staff.

Box continues

Considerations for home PN^a

For patients receiving PN at home, consider the following patient characteristics when determining the insertion site and the catheter type:

- activity level
- lifestyle
- quality of life
- need for additional intravenous therapies

Parenteral Nutrition Formulation

A PN formulation is a very complex mixture containing as many as 40 different components. Recommendations for safe practices for ordering, compounding, and administering PN have been published by the American Society for Parenteral and Enteral Nutrition (ASPEN).[7,8]

PN formulations may vary. Some hospitals may use premixed formulations, whereas others compound custom formulations on-site or at a compounding pharmacy. Premixed solutions provide set amounts of macronutrients and come with or without electrolytes added. These formulations may offer some cost and efficiency advantages. Disadvantages of premixed formulations are that they often cannot meet the energy, protein, or electrolyte needs of patients who are critically ill. Custom formulations can be designed to meet patients' nutrient needs.[7]

The practitioner must also consider whether to use a 2-in-1 or a 3-in-1 formulation. A 3-in-1 formulation, also known as a total nutrient admixture, has an intravenous lipid emulsion (ILE) added to the dextrose and amino acids, whereas a 2-in-1 formulation keeps the ILE separate. Advantages and disadvantages of a 3-in-1 formulation are shown in Box 20.2.[8,9]

ASPEN has published guidelines stating that there is no evidence to suggest a clinical difference in infectious complications between the two systems.[8] For 3-in-1 formulations, macronutrient dosing limits have been recommended to provide the most stable solution (see Box 20.3 on page 366).[8]

BOX 20.2

Advantages and Disadvantages of 3-in-1 Parenteral Nutrition Formulations[8,9]

Advantages	Disadvantages
Less nursing time required	May be less stable over time
Less supply and equipment expense	More sensitive to destabilization
Slower bacterial growth	More prone to lipid separation
Less contamination risk	Requires a larger pore-size filter
More convenient storage	More likely to cause catheter occlusion
Less system manipulation required	
More efficient preparation	
More cost-effective overall	

BOX 20.3

Recommended Macronutrient Dosing Limits for 3-in-1 Parenteral Nutrition Formulations[8]

Amino acids ≥4% final concentration

Dextrose ≥10% final concentration

Lipid ≥2% final concentration

Amino Acids

Crystalline amino acids provide 4 kcal/g and are available in concentrations of 3% to 15%. Specialized amino acid formulations targeted toward patients with hepatic and renal failure patients are available but are rarely used because of a lack of research demonstrating their efficacy. See Table 20.2 for additional information on amino acid PN products. There is no need to start with lesser amounts of amino acids and incrementally increase toward a goal. Amino acids can be prescribed in goal amounts with the initial PN order.

TABLE 20.2 Amino Acid Products for Parenteral Nutrition

Product[a]	Indication	Amino acid concentration
Aminosyn[b]	Standard	3.5%, 8.5%, 10%
Aminosyn II[b]	Standard	8.5%, 10%, 15%
FreAmine	Standard	10%
Travasol[b]	Standard	10%
Synthamin	Standard	10%
Aminosyn—HBC	Metabolic stress	7%
FreAmine HBC	Metabolic stress	6.9%
Clinisol[b]	Fluid restriction	15%
ProSol	Fluid restriction	20%
Plenamine	Fluid restriction	15%
HepatAmine	Hepatic failure	8%
Aminosyn—RF	Renal failure	5.2%
NephrAmine	Renal failure	5.4%
Aminosyn—PF	Pediatric	7%, 10%
Premasol	Pediatric	6%, 10%
TrophAmine	Pediatric	6%,10%

HBC = high branched-chain | PF = pediatric formula | RF = renal formula

[a] Refer to manufacturer for most up-to-date product information. Baxter International: Clinisol, Premasol, Prosol, Synthamin, Travasol; B. Braun Medical, Inc: FreAmine, FreAmine HBC, HepatAmine, NephrAmine, Plenamine, TrophAmine; Pfizer: Aminosyn products

[b] Preferred for use in adults; available for use in pediatric patients.

Dextrose

Anhydrous dextrose monohydrate provides 3.4 kcal/g. Dextrose is typically initiated at half of the goal requirement in order to monitor the patient's glucose tolerance and avoid the electrolyte disturbances that may occur when initiating nutrition support with excessive amounts of dextrose. Once the patient's glucose levels are in a normal range and stable, dextrose amounts in the PN can be adjusted toward goal requirements.

See Box 20.4 for an example of dextrose calculations. Glucose infusion rates (GIR) of more than 4 to 5 mg/kg of body weight per minute should be avoided in the critically ill population.[10]

BOX 20.4

Sample Dextrose Calculations

Calculating the maximum dextrose tolerance

Patient weight (kg) × desired GIR[a] (mg/kg/min) × 1,440 min/d ÷ 1,000 g/kg = grams of dextrose per day

For example: 65 kg × 4 mg/kg/min × 1,440 min/d ÷ 1,000 g/kg = 374 g dextrose per day

Calculating the glucose infusion rate

Dextrose (g) ÷ patient weight (kg) ÷ 1,440 min/d × 1,000 g/kg = infusion rate (mg/kg/min)

For example: 400 g dextrose ÷ 65 kg ÷ 1,440 (min/d) × 1,000 g/kg = 4.3 mg/kg/min

a GIR = glucose infusion rate.

Lipid

An ILE is the fat source added to a PN formulation to provide energy and essential fatty acids. ILEs provide 10 kcal/g. From 1% to 4% of total energy should be provided as linoleic acid and 0.25% to 0.5% as α-linolenic acid in order to prevent essential fatty acid deficiency. Fat intake should be limited to 20% to 35% of total energy, or less than 1 g/kg of body weight per day.

There are circumstances under which an ILE should not be added to the PN formulation. It is contraindicated in patients with egg allergy. Patients receiving propofol for sedation may not require additional ILE because propofol is delivered in a 10% lipid emulsion that provides 1.1 kcal of lipids per milliliter. Additionally, ILE should be avoided in patients with hypertriglyceridemia-induced pancreatitis or a triglyceride level in excess of 400 mg/dL.[11] See Table 20.3 on page 368 for information on ILE products.

In recent years, several new ILE products have received US Food and Drug Administration approval for use in the United States. Clinicians should be familiar with all of the available products and their indications for use. For example, SMOFlipid and Clinolipid are approved for use in adults, whereas Omegaven is approved for use in pediatric patients with cholestasis.

Electrolytes

Sodium, potassium, chloride, acetate, phosphorus, calcium, and magnesium can all be added to PN solutions in various amounts, as determined by the individual patient's requirements. Standard electrolyte requirements are shown in Table 20.4 on page 368.

TABLE 20.3 Intravenous Lipid Emulsion Products for Use in Parenteral Nutrition

Product[a]	Oil source	Concentration
Clinolipid[b]	80% olive oil 20% soybean oil	20%
Intralipid[c]	100% soybean oil	20%, 30%
Liposyn III[c]	100% soybean oil	10%, 20%, 30%
Nutrilipid[c]	100% soybean oil	20%
Omegaven[d]	100% fish oil	10%
SMOFlipid[b]	30% soybean oil 30% medium-chain triglyceride oil 25% olive oil 15% fish oil	20%

[a] Refer to manufacturer for most up-to-date product information. Baxter International: Clinolipid, Intralipid; Hospira: Liposyn III; B. Braun Medical, Inc: Nutrilipid; Fresenius Kabi: Omegaven, SMOFlipid
[b] Approved for adults only.
[c] Approved for use in both adult and pediatric patients.
[d] Approved for use in pediatric patients.

TABLE 20.4 Standard Electrolyte Requirements for Parenteral Nutrition Formulas[7]

Sodium	1-2 mEq/kg/d
Potassium	1-2 mEq/kg/d
Calcium	10-15 mEq/d
Magnesium	8-20 mEq/d
Phosphorus	20-40 mmol/d

Sodium and potassium may be added as chloride, acetate, or phosphate salts. The amount of chloride and acetate added to PN is adjusted to maintain acid-base balance. Bicarbonate is never added to PN solutions because it poses stability concerns. Acetate is provided for base needs, and it is converted into bicarbonate once in the body. The amounts of phosphorus and calcium that can be added to PN solutions also are of concern for PN stability, and institution-specific guidelines should be followed.

Vitamins and Minerals

Vitamins and minerals should be added to PN solutions daily. Table 20.5 and Table 20.6 show parenteral content for select vitamin and trace element products, respectively. In some instances, changes to the formulation may be necessary. For example, patients with excessive small bowel losses from fistula or ostomies should receive an additional 12 mg zinc per liter of loss,[12] and patients with hepatobiliary disease may need to have the copper and manganese removed from the PN solution because of impaired excretion.[7] Iron is not routinely added to PN formulations. If iron supplementation is needed, oral supplements are suggested; but if an intravenous source is needed, it can be added to lipid-free PN.

TABLE 20.5 Vitamin Content of Commercially Available Parenteral Nutrition Products[14,15]

Vitamin	Infuvite	MVI-12
Thiamin	6 mg	6 mg
Riboflavin 5-phosphate	3.6 mg	3.6 mg
Vitamin B3 (niacinamide)	40 mg	40 mg
Folic acid	600 mcg	600 mcg
Pantothenic acid (D-pantothenyl alcohol)	15 mg	15 mg
Vitamin B6 (pyridoxine HCl)	6 mg	6 mg
Vitamin B12 (cyanocobalamin)	5 mcg	5 mcg
Biotin	60 mcg	60 mcg
Ascorbic acid	200 mg	200 mg
Vitamin A	3,300 IU (palmitate)	1 mg (retinol)[a]
Vitamin D	200 IU (cholecalciferol)	5 mcg (ergocalciferol)[b]
Vitamin E (DL-α-tocopherol acetate)	10 IU	10 mg[c]
Vitamin K (phylloquinone)	150 mcg	0-150 mcg[d]

[a] 1 mg vitamin A = 3,300 United States Pharmacopeia (USP) units
[b] 5 mcg ergocalciferol = 200 USP units
[c] 10 mg vitamin E = 10 USP units.
[d] MVI-12 is available with or without vitamin K

TABLE 20.6 Trace Element Content of Commercially Available Parenteral Nutrition Products[16,17]

Trace element[a]	Multitrace-4 concentrate	Tralement
Chromium	10 mcg	0
Copper	1 mg	0.3 mg
Manganese	0.5 mg	55 mcg
Selenium	0	60 mcg
Zinc	5 mg	3 mg

[a] Amount contained in 1 mL

Formulation Calculations

PN may be ordered as stock solutions, final concentrations, or actual amounts of the macronutrients in grams. This can be confusing for patients who transfer between facilities or to home with PN. For this reason, ASPEN recommends prescribing PN in grams per day for macronutrients and milliequivalents or millimoles per day for electrolytes.[8,13]

Box 20.5 shows how to calculate the nutrition provided in a formulation that is essentially the same but has been ordered differently.[18] Refer to Box 20.6 for an example of how to calculate the PN prescription for a critically ill female patient.

BOX 20.5

Calculating Nutrition Provided From Parenteral Nutrition Prescriptions[18]

PN order	Calculations	Amount in grams	Converting to kcal	Amount in kcal
As a 2-in-1 stock solution:				
1,000 mL 30% dextrose	1,000 × 0.30	300	300 g × 3.4 kcal/g	1,020
800 mL 10% amino acid	800 × 0.10	80	80 g × 4 kcal/g	320
250 mL 20% ILE			250 mL × 2 kcal/mL[a]	500
				1,840 total
As a 2-in-1 in percentage final concentration:				
1,800 mL total fluid				
16.5% dextrose	1,800 mL × 0.165	297	297 g × 3.4 kcal/g	1,009
4.5% amino acid	1,800 mL × 0.045	81	81 g × 4 kcal/g	324
250 mL 20% ILE			250 mL × 2 kcal/mL[a]	500
				1,833 total
As a 3-in-1 in total amounts per day[b]:				
1,800 mL total fluid				
80 g amino acid		80	80 g × 4 kcal/g	320
300 g dextrose		300	300 g × 3.4 kcal/g	1,020
50 g ILE		50	50 g × 10 kcal/g	500
				1,840 total

Abbreviations: ILE, intravenous lipid emulsion; PN, parenteral nutrition.
[a] 20% ILE = 2 kcal/mL. This calculation is used with 2-in-1 solutions.
[b] Recommended way to order PN formulation.
Reproduced with permission from Lefton J, Figueiroa S, Betzold A. The basics of macronutrients in parenteral nutrition. Support Line. 2018;40(1):2-9.

BOX 20.6

Sample Parenteral Nutrition Calculation for a 3-in-1 Formulation

A critically ill female patient requires parenteral nutrition (PN). She weighs 64 kg and is 170 cm tall. Her energy needs are estimated to be 25 kcal/kg of body weight per day (1,600 kcal/d) and her protein requirements are 1.5 g/kg/d (roughly 100 g/d).[a]

To calculate the daily PN prescription, the following steps are suggested:

1. Determine grams of protein (as amino acids) and calculate energy provided as protein:

$$100 \text{ g protein} \times 4 \text{ kcal/g} = 400 \text{ kcal as protein}$$

2. Determine energy left to be provided as dextrose and intravenous lipid emulsion:

$$1,600 \text{ kcal desired} - 400 \text{ protein kcal} = 1,200 \text{ kcal}$$

3. Determine amount of energy to be provided as fat (usually about 30% or less of nonprotein energy):

$$1,200 \text{ kcal} \times 0.30 = 360 \text{ kcal as fat}$$

$$360 \text{ kcal} \div 10 \text{ kcal/g} = 36 \text{ or } {\sim}35 \text{ g lipids}$$

4. Determine energy left to be provided as dextrose:

$$1,600 \text{ kcal desired} - (400 \text{ protein kcal} + 360 \text{ fat kcal}) = 840 \text{ kcal as dextrose}$$

$$840 \text{ kcal} \div 3.4 \text{ kcal/g} = 247 \text{ or } {\sim}250 \text{ g dextrose}$$

The final PN prescription would include:

- 100 g amino acids
- 35 g lipids
- 250 g dextrose

[a] Numbers rounded for even calculations.

Complications of Parenteral Nutrition

Complications associated with PN fall into four general categories: infectious, mechanical, metabolic, and GI. Infectious complications are most often related to catheter and aseptic technique. Refeeding syndrome is the metabolic and physiologic consequence of depletion, repletion, compartmental shifts, and interrelationships of phosphorus, potassium, magnesium, glucose metabolism, vitamin deficiency, and fluid resuscitation. It is a serious complication resulting from overzealous nutritional resuscitation of the severely malnourished patient, which can result in sudden decompensation and death. Box 20.7 on page 372 provides examples of complications from the four categories. Additional information about acute and long-term complications may be found in the second edition of the *Academy of Nutrition and Dietetics Pocket Guide to Parenteral Nutrition*.[19]

BOX 20.7

Potential Mechanical, Metabolic, and Gastrointestinal Complications of Parenteral Nutrition

Mechanical

Pneumothorax

Hemothorax

Subclavian artery injury or thrombosis

Catheter occlusion

Metabolic

Hyperglycemia[a]

Hypoglycemia[b]

Electrolyte and fluid disorders related to shifts in electrolytes and fluid that may occur from movement between intracellular and extracellular spaces

Hypertriglyceridemia[c]

Acid-base disorders

Refeeding syndrome

Gastrointestinal

Hepatic steatosis

Cholestasis

[a] *May be related to severe stress, trauma, corticosteroid therapy, overfeeding, or diabetes.*
[b] *Related to the administration of insulin.*
[c] *May be due to overfeeding or administration of intravenous lipid emulsion.*

Summary

Parenteral nutrition can be a useful and life-sustaining therapy when a patient's GI tract is dysfunctional. Nutrition assessment, nutrition monitoring, and evaluation of the patient receiving PN are essential to ensuring the safe and efficacious use of PN therapy. Registered dietitian nutritionists are an integral part of nutrition care for patients on PN therapy.

References

1. Academy of Nutrition and Dietetics. Adult Nutrition Care Manual. Parenteral nutrition. 2021. Accessed November 15, 2020. www.nutritioncaremanual.org/topic\.cfm?ncm_toc_id=272589
2. Worthington P, Balint J, Bechtold M, et al. When is parenteral nutrition appropriate? *JPEN J Parenter Enteral Nutr*. 2017;41(3):324-377. doi:10.1177/0148607117695251
3. Academy of Nutrition and Dietetics. 2012 Critical Illness (CI) Evidence-Based Nutrition Practice Guideline. 2012. Accessed November 15, 2020. www.andeal.org/topic.cfm?menu=4800
4. Critical Care Nutrition. Systematic reviews 2018. 2018. Accessed November 11, 2020. www.criticalcarenutrition.com/resources/cpgs/past-guidelines/2018
5. Compher C, Bingham AL, McCall M, et al. Guidelines for the provision of nutrition support therapy in the adult critically ill patient: The American Society for Parenteral and Enteral Nutrition. *JPEN J Parenter Enteral Nutr*. 2022;46(1):12-41.
6. McClave SA, Taylor BE, Martindale RG, et al. Guidelines for the provision and assessment of nutrition support therapy in the adult critically ill patient: Society of Critical Care Medicine (SCCM) and American Society for Parenteral and Enteral Nutrition (A.S.P.E.N.). *JPEN J Parenter Enteral Nutr*. 2016;40(2):159-211. doi:10.1177/0148607109335234

7. Mirtallo J, Canada T, Johnson D, et al. Safe practices for parenteral nutrition. *JPEN J Parenter Enteral Nutr.* 2004;28(suppl):S39-S70. doi:10.1177/0148607104028006s39

8. Boullata JI, Gibert K, Sacks G, et al. A.S.P.E.N. clinical guidelines: parenteral nutrition ordering, order review, compounding, labeling, and dispensing. *JPEN J Parenter Enteral Nutr.* 2014;38(3):334-377. doi:10.1177/0148607114521833

9. Parenteral nutrients and formulations. In: Charney P, ed. *Pocket Guide to Parenteral Nutrition.* 2nd ed. Academy of Nutrition and Dietetics; 2019:66-99.

10. Rosmarin D, Wardlaw G, Mirtallo J. Hyperglycemia associated with high, continuous infusion rates of total parenteral nutrition. *Nutr Clin Pract.* 1996;11(4):151-156. doi:10.1177/0115426596011004151

11. ASPEN Board of Directors and the Clinical Guidelines Task Force. Guidelines for the use of parenteral and enteral nutrition in adult and pediatric patients. *JPEN J Parenter Enteral Nutr.* 2002;26(1 suppl):1SA-138SA.

12. Jeejeebhoy K. Zinc: an essential trace element for parenteral nutrition. *Gastroenterology.* 2009;137(suppl):S7-S12. doi:10.1053/j.gastro.2009.08.014

13. Ayers P, Adams S, Boullata J, et al. ASPEN parenteral nutrition safety consensus recommendations. *JPEN J Parenter Enteral Nutr.* 2014;38(3):296-333. doi:10.1177/0148607113511992

14. Infuvite. Package insert. Sab-Pharma, Inc. Accessed July 19, 2022. www.accessdata.fda.gov/drugsatfda_docs/label/2004/21163s011lbl.pdf

15. MVI-12. Package insert. AstraZeneca. Accessed July 19, 2022. www.accessdata.fda.gov/drugsatfda_docs/label/2004/08809scf052_mvi-12_lbl.pdf

16. Multitrace-4 Concentrate. Prescribing information. American Regent, Inc. Accessed July 22, 2022. www.drugs.com/pro/multitrace-4-concentrate.html

17. Tralement. Prescribing information. American Regent, Inc. Accessed July 22, 2022. www.accessdata.fda.gov/drugsatfda_docs/label/2020/209376s000lbl.pdf

18. Lefton J, Figueiroa S, Betzold A. The basics of macronutrients in parenteral nutrition. *Support Line.* 2018;40(1):2-9.

19. Charney P, ed. *Pocket Guide to Parenteral Nutrition.* 2nd ed. Academy of Nutrition and Dietetics; 2019.

21

Pediatric Enteral and Parenteral Nutrition

Jenifer L. Thompson, MS, RD, CSP
Tiffani L. Hays, MS, RD, LDN
Stephanie Merlino Barr, MS, RDN, LD

KEY POINTS

- When human milk is not available for infant feeding, enteral nutrition should be initiated, taking into consideration such factors as the infant's age, clinical condition, and possible food allergies or intolerances.
- For pediatric patients who cannot meet their nutritional needs orally, as evidenced by poor weight gain, decreased linear growth, or other signs of malnutrition, enteral nutrition is indicated; age, weight, and clinical condition of the child are factors to consider.
- When enteral nutrition is not sufficient or has been unsuccessful in a pediatric patient, parenteral nutrition should be initiated, while ensuring appropriate growth and avoiding deficiencies.

Introduction

Many pediatric patients with gastrointestinal (GI) disease require nutrition support in the form of enteral nutrition (EN) or parenteral nutrition (PN). This chapter focuses on the use of such interventions in pediatric patients and the unique challenges of nutrition support for children. See Chapter 19 for more information on EN and Chapter 20 for more information on PN.

Pediatric Enteral Nutrition

Enteral nutrition is the delivery, via oral administration or feeding tube, of liquid nutrition to the GI tract. Compared with PN, EN is a more physiologic approach to delivering nutrition support—one that more effectively preserves the integrity and function of the GI tract,[1,2] reduces the risk of infectious complications,[3] requires fewer resources to administer,[4] and ultimately incurs lower medical costs.[5,6] If the gut is functioning, it should be used in the digestive process. For these reasons, when treating pediatric patients, EN is typically the preferred delivery method of nutrition support.[7]

For patients who cannot meet their nutrient needs via oral intake, EN delivery via feeding tube may be indicated.[8] Indications may include: clinical conditions with increased energy requirements, an anatomic interference with the ability to safely consume orally, or an altered metabolism or absorption function that necessitates the specialized delivery of nutrients. EN may also be beneficial in pediatric patients who show signs of malnutrition, including poor weight gain and decreased linear growth. Box 21.1 lists indications and contraindications for EN in the pediatric population.[9,10]

Routes and Methods of Delivery

EN tube feedings can be administered by several routes—via nasogastric, orogastric, gastrostomy, nasoduodenal, nasojejunal, gastrojejunostomy, or jejunostomy tube. Feedings can be continuous, intermittent (bolus), or a combination of the two, depending on the patient's

BOX 21.1

Selected Indications and Contraindications for Enteral Nutrition in Children[9,10]

Potential indications

Conditions resulting in inadequate oral intake:

- prematurity
- congenital abnormalities (eg, cleft palate, tracheoesophageal fistula)
- critical illness (eg, mechanical ventilation, traumatic brain injury)
- psychological disorders (eg, anorexia nervosa, avoidant/restrictive food intake disorder)

Feeding disorders with concern for safety of oral feeding:

- swallowing disorders (eg, dysphagia)
- neurological disorders (eg, spinal muscular atrophy type I, cerebral palsy)

Conditions affecting typical digestion and absorption:

- cystic fibrosis
- short bowel syndrome
- inflammatory bowel disease

Conditions with excessive metabolic demands:

- burns
- congenital heart disease
- bronchopulmonary dysplasia
- sepsis

Growth failure or malnutrition

Potential contraindications

Compromised gut perfusion (eg, hemodynamic instability requiring increased vasopressor support, therapeutic hypothermia)

Congenital disease states affecting bowel anatomy and function:

- intestinal atresia
- gastroschisis
- omphalocele
- severe Hirschsprung disease

Acquired disease states affecting bowel anatomy and function:

- necrotizing enterocolitis
- short bowel syndrome

Other disease states that may require parenteral nutrition support:

- bowel obstruction
- severe inflammatory bowel disease
- high-output fistula or intractable diarrhea
- severe thrombocytopenia and mucositis in patients with cancer
- chylothorax

feeding tolerance, the chosen EN route, and the patient's level of GI function.[11] See Chapter 19 for additional information on enteral feeding routes and their advantages and disadvantages.

In considering the method of EN administration, bolus or continuous feeds are possible approaches. Bolus feeds are often preferred, if tolerated, because they provide a better quality of life and most closely resemble the typical physiology of digestion. However, the use of continuous feeds is often considered for specific disease states or when bolus feeds are not tolerated.

In preterm infants, continuous feeds are sometimes considered for their potential for improving feed tolerance and nutrient absorption. However, bolus feeds, as compared to continuous feeds, have been shown to increase splanchnic oxygenation, a measurement associated with improved tolerance to early enteral feeding.[12,13] An additional, yet important, consideration is that the use of continuous feeds when administering human milk (biological parent's own milk or donor human milk) can be problematic because of the substantial fat, calcium, and phosphorus losses that occur.[14] The published literature, while limited, suggests that bolus feeds are appropriate for the clinically stable premature infant.[15]

Strategies for feeding infants with short bowel syndrome–associated intestinal failure vary at the institutional level, with a need for further research to help develop evidence-based approaches to this complex patient population.[16]

Similarly, in patients with gastrostomy tubes, methods of feeding administration are often done based on clinical expertise rather than evidence-based best practices. Limited research exists on comparing benefits and complications in stable pediatric patients with gastrostomy tubes, but the available literature suggests that both methods are comparable in these regards.[17,18]

In children who are critically ill, there is a dearth of evidence to support an ideal method of EN delivery. In one randomized trial of pediatric patients receiving mechanical ventilation, bolus feeds resulted in higher nutrition delivery and a faster time to goal EN volume, with no safety concerns, as compared to a group receiving continuous feeds.[19]

Initiation, Advancement, and Weaning

Patient age, clinical condition, and route of feeding delivery affect EN initiation and advancement. Simultaneous increases in feeding rate and formula concentration are typically not recommended. See Table 21.1 for an overview of suggested feeding initiation and advancements.[20,21] Goal rates of enteral feed administration should take into account the patient's individual fluid and energy requirements, and a product that meets the individual's macronutrient and micronutrient requirements should be used.

Termination of EN support is similarly patient-specific, with the type of tube, length of time before tube-feed weaning, and complexity of the medical course playing major roles in the length of the EN wean.[22] If oral feeds are not achievable or are not expected to be achieved in a 2- to 3-month window, a gastrostomy tube should be considered.[23,24] However, guidelines outlining best practices are lacking for the transition from nasogastric to gastrostomy feeding; therefore, there is often large variability in this practice.[25]

For premature infants, the suck-swallow-breathe coordination that allows for oral feeding does not develop until around 32 to 34 weeks' gestation; termination of EN support in this population does not occur until oral feeds are feasible and well established. Though patients in the neonatal intensive care unit with feeding dysfunction can be discharged with a nasogastric tube, this practice requires close outpatient follow-up and extensive training of primary care providers to ensure the safety of feedings.[26,27]

Enteral Nutrition Selection

Human Milk

The World Health Organization and the American Academy of Pediatrics recommend that human milk be the sole nutrition source for the first 6 months of an infant's life and that it continue for 1 year or longer, as solid and complementary foods are introduced.[28,29] This approach has the following advantages[29]:

- Human milk has a human-specific nutrient composition with maximized bioavailability of macronutrients and micronutrients.
- Human milk meets nutritional requirements to support rapid growth and neurodevelopment in healthy, term infants.

TABLE 21.1 Initiation and Advancement of Enteral Nutrition in Children[20,21]

Age of patient	Initiation rates and volumes	Advancement rates
Continuous feeding		
Preterm infant	0.5-1.0 mL/kg/h	10-25 mL/kg/d
Full-term neonate (0-12 mo)	1-2 mL/kg/h	0.5-1.0 mL/kg/h Increase every 4-24 h
Age 1-6 y	1-2 mL/kg/h	0.5-1.0 mL/kg/h Increase every 4-12 h
Age 7-13 y	1-2 mL/kg/h	1 mL/kg/h Increase every 4-12 h
Bolus feeding		
Preterm infant	2-4 mL/kg/feed	2-4 mL/feed
Full-term neonate (0-12 mo)	10-15 mL/kg every 2-4 h	10-30 mL/feed
Age 1-6 y	5-10 mL/kg every 3-4 h	30-45 mL/feed
Age 7-13 y	90-120 mL every 3-4 h	60-90 mL/feed

- Feeding with human milk is associated with reduced risk of respiratory tract infections and reduced incidence of otitis media.
- Feeding with human milk is associated with reduced incidence of GI tract infections.[30]
- Feeding with human milk is associated with decreased incidence of necrotizing enterocolitis.

Human milk does not meet infant vitamin D or iron requirements; thus, all infants solely fed human milk require 400 IU vitamin D supplementation per day to promote bone health and prevent rickets.[31] Iron supplementation of 1 mg per kilogram of body weight per day should be provided at 4 months until iron-containing foods are started at 6 months of age to prevent iron deficiency and iron-deficiency anemia.[32]

Although human milk consumption is associated with numerous benefits, it is not a viable option for all infants. Box 21.2 on page 378 reviews breastfeeding contraindications and considerations.[33] Human milk may also not meet the nutritional requirements of some infants, including very low-birth weight infants. Infants with inborn errors of metabolism, such as phenylketonuria, require a combination of human milk feeds and phenylalanine-free formula in order to maintain healthy serum amino acid levels. Considerations of infant and lactating-parent disease states must be considered when developing an infant feeding plan with human milk.

BOX 21.2

Contraindications and Considerations in Human Milk Use[33]

Can direct breastfeeding occur?

No

Can expressed human milk be provided?

No

Clinical scenarios

Infant with classic galactosemia

Lactating parent infected with HIV (in the United States)

Lactating parent infected with human T-cell lymphotropic virus type 1 or type 2

Lactating parent with active illicit street drug use, not enrolled in a treatment program

Lactating parent with suspected or confirmed Ebola virus

Can direct breastfeeding occur?

No (temporarily)

Can expressed human milk be provided?

No (temporarily)

Clinical scenarios

Lactating parent infected with untreated brucellosis

Lactating parent taking certain medications deemed incompatible with breastfeeding

Lactating parent undergoing diagnostic imaging with radiopharmaceuticals

Can direct breastfeeding occur?

No (temporarily)

Can expressed human milk be provided?

Yes

Clinical scenarios

Lactating parent with untreated, active tuberculosis

Lactating parent with active varicella

Donor Human Milk

In recent years, the use of donor human milk has become a key EN option for premature infants and other high-risk infants when a biological parent's own milk is not available. The primary clinical benefit of donor human milk is that it may help in the prevention of necrotizing enterocolitis in very low-birth weight infants (born weighing less than 1,500 g). Donor milk may help reduce necrotizing enterocolitis in infants with congenital heart disease, although available literature only demonstrates an association rather than a causal relationship.[34] Donor human milk may be beneficial for infants with gastroschisis or intestinal atresia, with one study showing an association of a decreased number of central-line days and a shorter length of hospital stay when a biological parent's own milk was supplemented with donor milk rather than infant formula.[35] It is critical to note that human milk from a donor does not provide as great a benefit as milk from the biological parent. Lactation support should be provided to families in order to support the provision of ideal infant nutrition. The use of donor milk is typically contained to preterm infants in neonatal intensive care units, although policies exist at the hospital level for identifying eligible populations and length of use.

The Human Milk Banking Association of North America (HMBANA) is a nonprofit organization that has established processes and practices designed to provide safe donor human milk. Donor milk should be sourced from milk banks that employ HMBANA processes, including product pasteurization and sterilization and donor screening. Individual states in the United States have designated donor human milk as a human tissue and have separate laws and regulations regarding its handling and distribution. The US Food and Drug Administration (FDA) has not been involved in the establishment of HMBANA guidelines or state-level standards.

The use of unpasteurized or unsterilized donor human milk obtained from the internet or informal sharing is highly discouraged due to the lack of regulation and may unintentionally expose infants to medications and infectious contaminants.[6]

Infant Formula

Infant formulas are a necessary and life-saving tool for infants unable to receive human milk. Infant-formula manufacturers offer products with adequate nutrition to support infant growth and development. Components of infant formula are synthetically replicated based on human-milk research, although the ingredients are not identical to those in human milk. Compared with formula, human milk yields a higher bioavailability of many nutrients; therefore, most formulas are manufactured with a higher nutrient concentration to supply comparable nourishment to growing infants.

Optimal growth and development requirements for infants from birth to 1 year of age serve as the basis for quality-control and nutrient-level standards in the manufacture of infant formula. In the United States, nutrient-level standards for infant formula are set by the FDA, and the quality-control standards for all infant formulas are dictated by the Infant Formula Act, which was enacted in 1980 and amended in 1986.[36]

Preparation of Infant Formulas

Infant formulas are manufactured in ready-to-feed, concentrate, and powder forms. To resemble the approximate energy content provided in human breast milk, standard dilution and preparation of formula (see Box 21.3 on page 380) will yield 20 kcal/oz (0.67 kcal/mL). In a hospital setting, best practices for formula preparation should be followed.[37]

BOX 21.3

Standard Infant Formula Preparation[a]

Energy yield

20 kcal/oz (0.67 kcal/mL)

Preparation

Ready-to-feed

No preparation needed

Concentrate

1:1 dilution (1 oz concentrate + 1 oz water)

Powder

At home: 2 oz water + 1 scoop[b] powder

In hospital: use gram scale to measure powder

[a] Most term-infant formulas.
[b] Use only the scoop included in the formula container, packed per manufacturer specifications.

If a higher energy concentration is clinically indicated (eg, in infants with elevated metabolic needs or strict fluid restrictions), alternative recipes from the formula's manufacturer or a dietitian can be utilized. Increased formula concentrations result in increased renal solute load and osmolality; concentrations that exceed 27 kcal/oz (0.9 kcal/mL) are generally not recommended unless modular fat, modular carbohydrate, or both are added to the formula.[8]

Types of Infant Formulas

Cow's Milk–Based Formulas

Standard cow's milk–based formulas meet the nutritional requirements of healthy, full-term infants from birth to 1 year of age. The protein sources of these formulas consist of casein and whey from nonfat cow's milk. The carbohydrate and fat in cow's milk–based infant formulas are provided through lactose and vegetable oil, respectively. Additionally, because they are fortified with iron, standard cow's milk–based formulas assist in the prevention of iron-deficiency anemia in newborns.

These formulas may also come in organic and lactose-free options. For a formula to be certified and labeled as organic, its ingredients must meet regulations established by the US Department of Agriculture; specifically, production processes must have been free of certain types of pesticides, antibiotics, and growth hormones.

It is not possible to guarantee that any cow's milk–based formula is free of all galactose. For this reason, infants with galactosemia should not be fed these formulas, including low-lactose and lactose-free extensively hydrolyzed protein formulas. Infants with lactose intolerance may consume lactose-free formula; however, the diagnosis of congenital lactase deficiency in infants is extremely rare. Secondary lactase deficiency may occur temporarily and is typically a result of an acute GI illness.

Soy-Based Formulas

Soy-based infant formulas are appropriate for infants with galactosemia and as an option for infants whose caregivers prefer to use a vegetarian product. The high incidence of cross-reactivity between soy and cow's milk proteins (10%–42%) suggests a different infant formula alternative is preferred in the management of cow's milk protein allergy.[38-40] Soy protein is of lower biological value compared with casein, but soybeans nevertheless yield a high-quality protein. Soy formulas are fortified with L-methionine and taurine to improve the biological value and enhance the amino acid profile of soy-based formulas. Sucrose, corn syrup solids, and maltodextrin are carbohydrate sources used in soy-based infant formulas. The phytic acid present in soy protein isolate decreases the bioavailability of phosphate, zinc, calcium, and iron. Therefore, these minerals are supplemented in soy formulas.[41]

For infants with galactosemia, premature infants who are born weighing less than 1,800 g or infants with renal failure, soy formulas are not considered appropriate because of their elevated aluminum content, which creates the potential for toxicity and increased risk of metabolic bone disease.[42]

Protein-Modified Formulas

Altered protein formulas, which include partially and extensively hydrolyzed casein and/ or whey formulas and free amino acid–based (elemental) formula, have been developed to meet the needs of infants with severe food allergies (eg, cow's milk protein allergy) or malabsorption. See Box 21.4 for an overview of the different product types.

BOX 21.4

Types of Protein-Modified Infant Formulas

Partially hydrolyzed

Protein size: peptides

Not hypoallergenic

Use clinical judgment for indication to begin use

Does not include medium-chain triglycerides (MCTs)

Inexpensive

Extensively hydrolyzed

Protein size: dipeptides and tripeptides and amino acids

Hypoallergenic

Indicated for intact cow's milk or soy protein sensitivity, severe food allergies, and fat malabsorption

May include MCTs

Moderately expensive

Free amino acid (elemental)

Protein size: free amino acids

Hypoallergenic

Indicated for cow's milk or soy protein sensitivity, gastrointestinal impairment, sensitivity to extensively hydrolyzed proteins, severe food allergies, and fat malabsorption

May include MCTs

Expensive

Partially hydrolyzed cow's milk protein formulas contain reduced oligopeptides with a molecular weight of less than 5,000 Da. These formulas are not hypoallergenic and are not indicated for the treatment of cow's milk protein allergy. Although it was previously believed that these formulas reduced the risk of atopic dermatitis, this claim is no longer supported in the published clinical guidelines.[43] Partially hydrolyzed cow's milk protein formulas are now typically marketed with claims that they improve formula tolerance, promote softer stools, reduce infant fussiness, and reduce infant crying; however, these benefits have not been consistently demonstrated in the published literature.[44]

Extensively hydrolyzed cow's milk protein formulas contain only peptides with a molecular weight of less than 3,000 Da. The available extensively hydrolyzed cow's milk protein formulas have slight variations in their macronutrient composition, with varying amounts of fat from medium-chain triglycerides and differing sources of carbohydrates (maltodextrin, corn syrup solids, or sugar). All extensively hydrolyzed formulas are lactose-free and considered hypoallergenic; therefore, they are appropriate for most infants with cow's milk protein allergy.

Free amino acid–based, or elemental, formulas are indicated for infants with severe food allergies that are not managed by extensively hydrolyzed protein formulas or nutrient malabsorption. These formulas are peptide-free and contain a mixture of essential and non-essential amino acids. Due to their formulation, elemental formulas are expensive and have a higher osmolarity compared to all other formulas. Elemental formulas do not meet the nutrient requirements of premature infants and, therefore, often require supplementation of key nutrients, specifically calcium, phosphorus, and vitamin D, to prevent metabolic bone disease of prematurity.[45]

Specialized Infant Formulas

Many specialized formulas have been developed for use in patients with certain medical conditions and disease states. For example:

- Formulas with increased levels of protein, calcium, and phosphate are used in premature infants to optimize growth and bone mineralization.
- Reduced-fat or modified-fat formulas may be used in infants with chylothorax, rare lipid metabolism disorders, or lymphatic transport disorders; however, when these formulas are administered, the patients require careful monitoring to ensure that their essential fatty acid requirements are met.
- Specially composed formulas are often created for patients with specific inborn errors of metabolism to meet the requirements of each specific diagnosis and achieve a biochemical balance.
- A combination of specialized formula or human milk plus supplements and medications is often used in infants with renal disease who require EN that maintains normative biochemical values and appropriate growth.

Recent Innovations in Infant Formulas

Research is ongoing, and new developments continually improve the ability of infant formulas to mimic both the nutrient content and the function of human milk in infant development. All additives in infant formula have been deemed safe; however, studies of the long-term clinical benefits of additives in infant formulas continue, and their inclusion in formulas varies by company and product composition (see Box 21.5).[46-51]

BOX 21.5

Infant Formula
Additives[46-51]

Docosahexaenoic acid and arachidonic acid

Amount and type added	Variable; amount similar to human milk
Potential benefits	Plays a role in cognitive and visual function; increased benefit seen with preterm infants

Human milk oligosaccharides

Amount and type added	Variable, but most commonly 2'-fucosyllactose (2'-FL); not human milk derived
Potential benefits	Plays a role in immune system development and function

Nucleotides

Amount and type added	Variable; amount similar to human milk
Potential benefits	DNA and RNA synthesis

Prebiotics

Amount and type added	Variable
Potential benefits	Increased concentration of bifidobacteria

Probiotics

Amount and type added	Variable
Potential benefits	Promotes adequate growth
	Improvement in infectious diarrhea

Follow-Up Formulas

For infants transitioning to solid foods—typically from age 9 to 10 months through 24 months—follow-up formulas, also called *toddler formulas* or *next-step formulas*, are available for use. These formulas contain slightly more protein, iron, vitamin C, vitamin E, and zinc than standard full-term infant formula. In general, these products cost less than standard infant formulas but substantially more than whole cow's milk. There is no evidence of improved growth or development with the use of a follow-up formula compared to whole cow's milk; thus, these products are not routinely recommended.[52]

Pediatric Formulas

Pediatric formulas exist for patients who require EN support after the first year of life (or for preterm infants, after 12 months corrected age). These formulas are available in cow's milk–based, plant protein–based, partially hydrolyzed protein, and free amino acid formulations. Their nutrient contents meet the Dietary Reference Intakes (DRIs) for children aged

1 to 13 years in volumes of 1,000 mL/d to 1,500 mL/d. The standard energy concentration of pediatric formulas is 30 kcal/oz (1 kcal/mL); the typical protein load is 30 g/L.

Adolescents require specialized attention in their EN support administration, as most pediatric enteral products are designed to provide appropriate nutrition for children aged 1 to 13 years. Adult enteral formulas may be used, but careful monitoring of nutrient levels to ensure all DRIs are met is essential, as these products may not meet the elevated protein or micronutrient requirements of adolescents. For example, individuals with inflammatory bowel disease often have negative calcium imbalance and are at risk for bone demineralization; the use of an enteral product that supports an adolescent's daily calcium requirement of 1,300 mg and helps correct for any related deficiencies is critical for this population.[53]

Blenderized Formulas

Blenderized formulas, both homemade and commercially available, have increased in usage and in patient and caregiver preference. These formulas are typically only recommended for children older than 1 year of age and may be used in response to a patient's or caregiver's desire for a "more normal" mode of feeding when EN is required. Additionally, blenderized formulas may be used in an attempt to improve some GI symptoms including malabsorption, reflux, persistent emesis, and retching. These products are generally well tolerated and associated with clinical improvement in some upper GI symptoms.[54] The decision to use a homemade or commercial blenderized formula in gastrostomy tube feedings should be discussed with the patient's provider and registered dietitian nutritionist, as some patients may not be appropriate candidates for this modality of EN.[54,55] Candidates for blenderized tube feedings should have at least a 14-French gastrostomy tube, established tolerance to bolus feedings, and caregivers with adequate resources (eg, time, clean water supply, a refrigerator).[56] It is less feasible to use blenderized formulas with a gastrojejunostomy or jejunostomy tube because of the propensity for these formulas to clog feeding tubes when administered at a slow, continuous rate. It should be noted that micronutrient sufficiency must be monitored in homemade formulas, particularly in children with chronic GI conditions.

Pediatric Parenteral Nutrition

Parenteral nutrition is the intravenous administration of nutrients, including dextrose, amino acids, intravenous lipid emulsions (ILEs), vitamins, and minerals. Central venous PN is delivered into a large-diameter vein, usually the superior vena cava. Peripheral PN is delivered into a peripheral vein, usually in the hand or forearm. Peripheral PN is typically only used when the patient is expected to require PN for a short amount of time.

PN should only be considered when EN is not a viable option for nutrition support, when EN has failed, or when EN alone fails to meet the patient's nutrition needs. As is the case when treating adult patients, deliberation regarding whether to use PN in pediatric patients must weigh the risks associated with PN (eg, nosocomial infections, also called health care–associated infections) against the gravity of the development and consequences of malnutrition and nutrient deficiencies.

Age, disease state, and current nutritional status inform the decision as to when it is appropriate to begin PN administration in pediatric patients (see Box 21.6).[57,58] Because of the limited fat and protein stores in preterm and term infants and their additional energy needs for growth, earlier administration of PN is appropriate in these patients. Box 21.7 lists the indications and contraindications for PN in pediatric patients.[59-67] There are very few absolute indications for PN administration, as most patients will tolerate some level of EN support.

BOX 21.6

Timeline for Initiating Parenteral Nutrition in Pediatric Patients[57,58]

Patient age or nutritional status	When parenteral nutrition should be initiated
Preterm infants	Start parenteral nutrition immediately
	Start full parenteral nutrition by day 1 to 3 of life
Term infants	Within 3 days if nothing by mouth
Undernourished child	Within 3 to 5 days
Well-nourished child	Within 5 to 7 days

BOX 21.7

Indications and Contraindications for Parenteral Nutrition in Infants and Children[59-67]

Potential indications

Gastrointestinal (GI) obstruction

Severe gut injury and congenital GI tract anomalies, which may include intestinal atresia, gastroschisis, ileus, intestinal perforation, mucositis, necrotizing enterocolitis, omphalocele, and short bowel syndrome

Preterm birth (less than 32 weeks' gestation) or very low birth weight

Potentially compromised gut perfusion, severe sepsis, hemodynamic instability or use of vasopressors, and extracorporeal membrane oxygenation

Severe pulmonary disease or cystic fibrosis

Congenital heart disease

Chylothorax

Renal disease on peritoneal dialysis

Diaphragmatic hernia

Severe acute pancreatitis

Severe inflammatory bowel disease

High-output fistula

Anorexia nervosa

Potential contraindications

Anticipated need for nutrition support for 7 days or less in well-nourished children aged more than 1 month

Lack of vascular access

Fungal line infection

End-of-life care (parenteral nutrition is an aggressive therapy and should be considered by an interdisciplinary team that includes a clinical ethicist, the patient, the family, and their care team)

Egg allergy in patients requiring intravenous lipid emulsion (ILE), which requires administration of test dose of ILE; soy allergy may also be a contraindication with some multicomponent ILEs

Administration

PN is typically infused continuously over a 24-hour period. Lipid infusion rate should not exceed 0.15 g/kg of body weight per hour, which allows for varying infusion time depending on the dosage.

Cyclic PN, or intermittent delivery in less than 24 hours, may be considered for patients on long-term PN or home PN. Cyclic PN allows for time off the infusion, may help lessen the risk of PN-associated cholestasis (PNAC), and can allow for the administration of medications that are incompatible with PN. Infants who receive PN but not EN should not be disconnected from PN feeding for more than 4 hours because of the risk of hypoglycemia and fluid deficits. Tapering of PN rates, when cycling, is necessary in infants to prevent hypoglycemia. Cyclic PN should be considered only if the patient has a stable fluid and electrolyte balance. Blood glucose levels should be monitored at the peak infusion rate and 1 hour after infusion and should be checked again with any increase in the rate of administration if the hours are further compressed, to monitor for hypoglycemia. See Chapter 22 for additional information on PN in the home setting.

Selecting the Appropriate Solution

When selecting the appropriate PN solution, vascular access is the first criterion to consider. In most children, adequate PN delivery requires central access; if the need for PN support is projected to be longer than 7 days, central access should be attempted. To minimize the risk of infiltration and phlebitis, the osmolarity of peripheral solutions should typically not exceed 900 mOsm per kilogram of solution.[68,69]

In the pediatric population, 2-in-1 PN solutions—containing the carbohydrate requirement (dextrose) and the protein requirement (amino acids) together in one solution, along with micronutrients—are typically used, with fat requirement (ILE) delivered separately. Separation of these nutrients enhances the stability and compatibility of the solution. Fluid allowance, other infusions, estimated energy and nutrient needs, electrolyte requirements, and advancement of nutrients according to patient tolerance are other factors that must be considered when determining which PN solution to use (see Table 21.2).[70]

TABLE 21.2 General Recommendations for Advancement of Parenteral Nutrients in Children[70]

Nutrient		Premature infants	Term infants	Children (1-10 y)	Adolescents
Dextrose (mg/kg/min)	Begin	6-8	6-8	3-6	2.5-3.0
	Advance	1.4-1.7	3.5	2-3	1-2
	Goal	10-14 (max 14-18)	10-14 (max 14-18)	8-10	5-6
Amino acids (g/kg/d)	Begin	3-4	2.5-3.0	1.5-2.5	0.8-2.0
	Goal	3-4	2.5-3.0	1.5-2.5	0.8-2.0
Lipids (g/kg/d)	Begin	0.5-1.0	0.5-1.0	1-2	1
	Advance	0.5-1.0	0.5-1.0	0.5-1.0	1
	Goal	3 (max 0.15 g/kg/h)	2.5-3.0 (max 0.15 g/kg/h)	2.0-2.5	1-2

Fluid Allowance

To determine the volume allotted for PN, subtract the volume of all other necessary infusions from the patient's total fluid allowance. Concentrating other infusions administered to the patient may be needed to maximize PN volume. See the section on fluid restriction under "Special Considerations" for more information.

Energy Requirements

Indirect calorimetry is the recommended and most precise mode of determining energy needs. However, the equipment needed is expensive and not readily available; therefore, appropriate predictive equations that take into account the patient's age, growth, and status should be used to estimate goal energy requirements. Guidelines from the American Society for Parenteral and Enteral Nutrition (ASPEN) recommend using the Schofield or World Health Organization equations, without the addition of stress factors.[70] Estimated energy requirements for patients on PN are often 5% to 10% lower than estimates for those on EN because patients on PN do not expend energy on digestion and absorption.

Protein Requirements

The protein goal for non–critically ill pediatric patients receiving PN is based on the DRI for protein, which is determined by age, growth, activity, and injury factors, as well as adjustments for known or suspected protein losses. Preventing the loss of lean body mass and promoting healing and growth in the pediatric patient are the ultimate goals of protein delivery. See Table 21.2 for full details of protein (amino acid) initiation and goal administration.[70]

For infants receiving PN, specialized pediatric amino acid solutions that more closely mimic the amino acid profile of breast milk should be used. These pediatric solutions provide greater concentrations of conditionally essential amino acids for infants (including arginine, glycine, proline, tyrosine, glutamine, and cysteine) and have a lower pH, which allows for improved calcium and phosphorus solubility.[71]

Fat Requirements

Fat generally provides 30% to 40% of total energy in PN. Essential fatty acid deficiency can develop in children within 1 to 3 weeks; therefore, providing ILE during PN support is essential. To provide sufficient essential fatty acids, between 2% and 4% of the total energy should come from long-chain fatty acids (ie, long-chain triglycerides) delivered as 0.5 to 1 g fat per kilogram of body weight per day when using a soy-based ILE.[70] Multicomponent ILEs require larger doses to meet essential fatty acid requirements.

While monitoring the patient for hypertriglyceridemia, the practitioner should initiate ILE administration at 0.5 to 1 g/kg/d and advance by 0.5 to 1 g/kg/d as tolerated until the goal for fat intake is reached. See Table 21.2 for full details regarding goals.[70]

There are risks associated with the administration of ILE, including a small risk of an allergic response to ILE in patients with egg and soy allergies; therefore, providers should consider administering a test dose per the product package insert before initiating ILE in this patient population.[72] Long-term administration of ILE increases the risk of developing PNAC and may be mitigated by the use of alternative ILEs.[73,74] Multicomponent ILEs, though not approved for use in pediatric patients in the United States, are frequently used clinically for the prevention and treatment of PNAC.

Carbohydrate Requirements

To maintain euglycemia in neonates and to meet all pediatric patients' energy needs while avoiding ketosis, carbohydrate delivery is required. When initiating carbohydrate (dextrose) delivery, the glucose infusion rate (GIR) should match or be slightly higher than the GIR of the current intravenous fluids. In neonates, the GIR may be increased by 1 to 2 mg per kilogram of body weight per minute each day; in children, the dextrose concentration may be increased by 1 to 3 mg/kg/min each day, as tolerated, until the goals for carbohydrate and total energy intake are reached. Patients should be monitored for hyperglycemia until goal dextrose concentration is reached (see Table 21.2).[70] Insulin may be needed to maintain blood glucose concentration at or below 140 to 180 mg/dL in patients with critical illness while meeting minimum GIR requirements.[75]

Vitamin Requirements

All patients on PN should receive daily parenteral multivitamins provided in doses based on the patient's weight using manufacturer recommendations.[76] Pediatric parenteral multivitamins should be used, but shortages can and do occur. In these instances, pediatric parenteral multivitamins should be reserved for infants weighing less than 2.5 kg or who are less than 36 weeks postmenstrual age (gestational age plus chronological age). When severe renal or hepatic dysfunction or excessive GI losses are present, or if the patient is on long-term PN, modifications to vitamin administration should be considered.[77]

Trace Element Requirements

Parenteral trace elements should be delivered daily to all pediatric patients receiving PN.[76,78] The solution should be pediatric-designated to facilitate appropriate dosing levels in minimum volumes. Modifications to trace element administration may be considered when a patient has severe renal or hepatic dysfunction, excessive GI losses, or is on long-term PN.[77] Concerns for contaminants of trace elements with manganese and chromium have been well documented, and their exclusion in PN composition should be considered, particularly for patients receiving long-term PN.[79] Iron infusions should be considered for patients on long-term PN and those who are unable to receive sufficient iron enterally.

Electrolyte Requirements

Daily monitoring of electrolytes and any necessary related adjustments to PN should continue as needed until the patient's electrolyte levels are stable. Consideration of acid-base balance is also necessary when determining electrolyte administration in PN. Once the patient's electrolyte levels are stable, they should be monitored weekly.

Medications

Some medications are incompatible with PN solutions, ILE solutions, or both, but some common medications (eg, famotidine and insulin) may be added to the PN solution during compounding. Pharmacy departments should be able to provide information about solution-medication compatibility. Once a medication is added to the PN solution, all previous orders for that medication should be discontinued.

Patient Monitoring

When caring for a patient receiving PN, it is essential to monitor their blood chemistry and metabolic panels. Before initiating PN, practitioners should document baseline measurements of magnesium, phosphorus, and triglyceride levels and obtain a basic metabolic panel to aid in customizing the initial prescription to best fit a patient's needs. Table 21.3 provides an overview of suggested laboratory monitoring for patients on PN.[70]

TABLE 21.3 General Recommendations for Laboratory Monitoring of Pediatric Patients on Parenteral Nutrition[70]

Laboratory test	Frequency while advancing to goal PN	Frequency at goal PN with stable, normal electrolytes and acid-base status	Frequency with long-term PN (>3 wk) with stable, normal electrolytes and acid-base status
Basic metabolic panel	Daily	Weekly	Weekly
Serum phosphorus	Daily	Weekly	Weekly
Triglycerides	Daily	Weekly	Weekly
Liver function	Every 1-2 wk	Every 1-2 wk	Every 2 wk
Vitamins and trace minerals	N/A	N/A	Every 3-12 mo

N/A = not applicable | PN = parenteral nutrition

In hospitalized pediatric patients receiving PN, progress toward goals established during the Nutrition Care Process should be evaluated at least weekly, and more frequently depending on clinical status and nutritional risk level. In addition to laboratory monitoring, assessments should include the evaluation of growth trends; input and output data; clinical signs and symptoms of PN intolerance, fluid status, nutrient excess, or nutrient deficiency; and any changes in GI function or medication administration. Laboratory test results and any recommended changes to the nutrition support plan based on those values should be documented.[24,77]

Special Considerations

Acute risks and complications of PN in children mimic those seen in adults (see Chapter 20); however, PNAC—a potentially life-threatening complication of long-term PN administration—is more common in children. Because of the risks associated with PN, practitioners must continually monitor these patients' vital signs, electrolytes, and liver function tests for the duration of PN administration (see the section on patient monitoring).

Parenteral Nutrition–Associated Cholestasis

PNAC is a condition of impaired bile secretion. The first sign of PNAC is an increased level of conjugated bilirubin (concentration >2 mg/dL) after PN has been administered for at least 2 weeks, potentially followed by elevated levels of aminotransferase. Pediatric patients receiving prolonged PN are more likely than adult patients to develop PNAC and resulting liver failure.[80] Lack of enteral feedings, sepsis, length of remaining bowel, prematurity, and low birth weight are other clinical factors that have been associated with PNAC.[81-84] Other factors specific to PN administration associated with the development of PNAC include total energy (in particular, overfeeding), amino acid dose, taurine deficiency, PN contaminants (including aluminum, manganese, and chromium), ILE dose and source, and continuous vs cyclic infusion.[79,85-92] Multicomponent ILEs are now available for off-label use in pediatric patients and can be considered for the prevention and treatment of PNAC; fish oil–based ILE may be used to treat PNAC.[93,94] Box 21.8 on page 390 provides recommendations for minimizing PNAC.[79,85-95]

BOX 21.8

Recommendations for Reducing the Risk of Parenteral Nutrition–Associated Cholestasis[a,79,85-95]

[a] In patients expected to need PN for 3 months or longer

Initiate trophic enteral feeds as soon as medically feasible, and advance enteral feedings as often as is tolerated, including the patient's ability to maintain fluid and electrolyte balance.

Advance dextrose as tolerated to goal energy without overfeeding.

Use appropriate amino acid solutions for infants aged less than 1 year and aggressively titrate parenteral protein as enteral protein increases to the minimum needed to maintain protein status and growth.

Consider limiting soy-based intravenous lipid emulsion (ILE) to 1 g/kg/d, or consider using a multicomponent ILE with higher concentrations of omega-3 fatty acids.

Once a patient is clinically stable and growing well, consider cyclic parenteral nutrition (PN) to give the patient a break from the infusion.

Supplement carnitine in preterm infants receiving PN to ensure adequate lipid clearance.

Dialysis

Electrolyte, protein, and energy exchange must be accounted for when determining PN prescriptions for pediatric patients receiving renal replacement therapy. PN considerations for these patients depend on the route of dialysis (see Box 21.9).[55,96-99] Supplementation of carnitine in PN in this population is a topic of ongoing research. Recent evidence demonstrates that children on continuous renal replacement therapy can become carnitine deficient within 1 week; parenteral supplementation of carnitine at a dose of 20 mg/kg/d may be beneficial in preventing deficiency and improving myocardial strain in this population.[97,98]

Fluid Restriction

Given the osmolarity limitations of peripheral lines, nutrient delivery is often severely limited in pediatric patients who require fluid restriction and have peripheral line access. To concentrate nutrients for PN administration, central venous access is required, and nutrient levels must be increased proportionately, as tolerated by the patient. Typically, PN solutions delivered by a central line can provide at least 1 kcal/mL. In cases of prolonged fluid restriction, clinicians should consider concentrating other intravenous fluids and medications in order to meet the patient's overall nutrition goals.

Hyperammonemia

Hyperammonemia may occur in pediatric patients with liver failure and metabolic diseases. In cases of hepatic encephalopathy, specialized amino acid solutions with elevated levels of branched-chain amino acids may be considered in order to decrease the flow of aromatic amino acids across the blood-brain barrier; however, available evidence does not show a conclusive benefit to this therapy in the pediatric population.[100] Patients with inborn errors of metabolism may require customized solutions that limit the intake of specific amino acids. For patients with hyperammonemia, PN solutions need to provide sufficient energy and protein in order to avoid catabolism and the subsequent release of ammonia from muscle breakdown.

Hyperglycemia

The risk of hyperglycemia is increased in pediatric patients on PN support who are under stress or receiving steroid treatment. Gradually increasing the GIR minimizes the risk of hyperglycemia. If hyperglycemia persists, insulin administration may be indicated to

BOX 21.9

Parenteral Nutrition Modifications for Pediatric Patients on Dialysis[55,96-99]

Fluids

Predialysis	Match urine output
Hemodialysis	Ultrafiltration + urine output + insensible losses
Peritoneal dialysis	Fluid restriction normally not needed

Energy

Predialysis	Dietary Reference Intake (DRI) + catch-up growth
Hemodialysis	Based on clinical status
Peritoneal dialysis	Account for energy absorbed from dialysate (roughly 7–10 kcal/kg/d)

Protein

Predialysis	DRI
Hemodialysis	DRI + 0.1 g/kg/d
Peritoneal dialysis	DRI + 0.15 to 0.3 g/kg/d

Electrolytes

Predialysis	Restrict parenteral nutrition (PN) according to blood chemistries
Hemodialysis	Discuss with renal team before adjusting in PN
Peritoneal dialysis	Discuss with renal team before adjusting in PN

Micronutrients

Hemodialysis	Increased risk of thiamin, pyridoxine, folate, vitamin C, zinc, and selenium deficiencies; monitor and ensure these micronutrients are included in PN, particularly for PN-dependent patients
Peritoneal dialysis	Increased risk of pyridoxine, folate, and vitamin C deficiencies; monitor and ensure these micronutrients are included in PN, particularly for PN-dependent patients

maintain goal nutrient delivery while controlling blood glucose levels. However, administration of insulin to maintain tight glucose control increases the risk for hypoglycemia; therefore, blood glucose levels should be monitored cautiously in these situations.[101] Clinical guidelines issued in 2009 by ASPEN for nutrition support of critically ill children state that "aggressive glycemic control cannot be recommended as yet in the critically ill child."[102] Although more recent studies have investigated hyperglycemia protocols used in the pediatric intensive care unit, the ASPEN guidelines published in 2017 did not offer any additional guidance around glycemic control.[70,101-107] In general, these studies in critically ill pediatric patients have not demonstrated improved outcomes with tight glycemic control, and hypoglycemic events continue to be substantially higher in tight-glycemic-control groups. However, one author has suggested that evidence supports tight glycemic control for patients primarily being fed via PN.[107] When administering insulin to patients receiving PN, practitioners should prioritize defining a plan for replacing intravenous glucose or discontinuing insulin (or both) if PN is suddenly discontinued for any reason.

Hypertriglyceridemia

Patients with hepatic dysfunction related to prematurity, prolonged PN exposure, or disease states may also commonly experience hypertriglyceridemia. Monitoring triglyceride levels as ILE is gradually increased will help mitigate hypertriglyceridemia (see Table 21.4).[24,94] If ILE is held or severely restricted for an extended period of time and no other source of long-chain fatty acids is provided, the patient becomes at risk for essential fatty acid deficiency. When using a soy-based ILE, a dose of approximately 0.5 g/kg/d is necessary to prevent this deficiency; multicomponent ILEs have higher daily dosage requirements to meet essential fatty acid requirements. Deficiency may develop within 1 to 3 weeks in infants and very young children and should be monitored by checking the triene-to-tetraene ratio; a ratio of more than 0.2:0.4 is suggestive of essential fatty acid deficiency.

TABLE 21.4 Intravenous Lipid Emulsion Modifications Based on Triglyceride Levels[24,94]

Patient population	TG level, mg/dL	Modification to ILE
Infants	<250-265	Continue to advance ILE to goal
	>250-265	Reduce ILE and recheck TG level
Older children	<300-400	Continue to advance ILE to goal
	>300-400	Reduce ILE and recheck TG level

ILE = intravenous lipid emulsion | TG = triglyceride

Metabolic Bone Disease of Prematurity

Neonates who receive long-term PN support commonly develop osteopenia or metabolic bone disease of prematurity. Specialized amino acid solutions for infants have been developed to maximize solubility and allow for increased calcium and phosphorus delivery. Other components of PN that can influence the solubility of calcium and phosphorus are the pH of the solution, dextrose and amino acid concentrations, the ratio of calcium to phosphorus, and the addition of cysteine to the solution. Vitamin D, serum phosphorus, and alkaline phosphatase levels should be monitored, with supplementation of calcium, phosphorus, and vitamin D given as needed.

Refeeding Syndrome

There is a risk of refeeding syndrome when specialized nutrition support is initiated in acutely or severely malnourished pediatric patients. Potentially fatal hypophosphatemia, hypokalemia, and hypomagnesemia result from providing substrate that creates adenosine triphosphate and drives these anions into the cells. When overfeeding with carbohydrates occurs, an increase in the serum glucose level results in an increase in insulin secretion, which drives electrolytes intracellularly, causing critically low serum phosphorus and potassium levels.[108] Thus, initiation of nutrition support must be done cautiously for patients at risk for refeeding syndrome. The ASPEN 2020 consensus recommendations regarding the approach to avoidance and treatment of refeeding syndrome in at-risk pediatric patients are summarized in Box 21.10.[108]

ASPEN[a] Recommendations for Avoidance and Treatment of Refeeding Syndrome in At-Risk Pediatric Patients[108]

Carbohydrate

Initiate nutrition support with a glucose infusion rate (GIR) of 4 to 6 mg/kg/min and advance by 1 to 2 mg/kg/min as tolerated based on blood glucose levels. GIR should be advanced to a maximum of 15 to 18 mg/kg/min.

Consider dextrose input from all intravenous (IV) solutions (eg, medications, parenteral nutrition [PN]) when advancing to the above goal.

If the patient has already received IV dextrose or medications in a dextrose solution for several days, has stable electrolytes, and is asymptomatic, then energy from nutrition may be reintroduced at a higher rate than recommended above.

Electrolytes

Check serum potassium, magnesium, and phosphorus levels before initiating nutrition support.

Monitor electrolytes at least every 12 hours in high-risk patients.

Replete low electrolytes based on established standards of care.

If electrolytes become difficult to correct or drop precipitously during nutrition initiation, decrease kilocalories per gram of dextrose by 50% and advance the dextrose by approximately 33% of goal every 1 to 2 days based on clinical presentation.

Recommendations may be changed based on clinical judgment. Cessation of nutrition support may be considered when electrolytes are severely low or dropping precipitously.

Thiamin

Administer thiamin at a dose of 2 mg/kg to a maximum of 100 to 200 mg/d before feeding commences or before initiation of dextrose-containing IV fluids for high-risk patients.

Continue thiamin supplementation for at least 5 to 7 days. Patients with severe starvation, chronic alcoholism, or high risk for thiamin deficiency may require longer supplementation.

Thiamin levels do not need to be routinely monitored.

Other vitamins

Add a multivitamin to PN daily, unless contraindicated, for as long as PN is provided.

In patients receiving enteral nutrition support, give a multivitamin daily for at least 10 days based on clinical status.

[a] ASPEN = American Society for Parenteral and Enteral Nutrition

Close monitoring is necessary in patients at high risk for refeeding syndrome. ASPEN recommends monitoring vital signs every 4 hours in the first 24 hours after initiation of nutrition support. Daily weights should be monitored, along with intake and output. Individualized nutrition goals should be set daily until the patient is stable; once the patient is stable, institutional standards of care should be practiced.[108]

Transitioning to Enteral Feeds

To support growth and development in pediatric patients and neonates on long-term PN, it is necessary to maintain an adequate provision of parenteral nutrients during the transition to enteral feedings. Decreases in the parenteral provision of energy, protein, or fluid should only occur in conjunction with increases in enteral nutrients. Practitioners must strive to match macronutrient provision during the transition, as 1 mL of PN may contain substantially different amounts of nutrients from 1 mL of formula or tube feeding. PN nutrients may need to be concentrated during the transition in order to maintain the goal nutrient provision within a patient's fluid allotment. Providing micronutrients throughout the transition to enteral feedings is also worth consideration, as a patient's requirements may increase due to malabsorption. To maintain electrolyte stability and patient growth, patients with severe malabsorption who are transitioning to enteral feedings may need increased nutrients enterally. As a result, additional monitoring for vitamin and mineral deficiencies during the transition off PN becomes important.

Summary

When human milk is not available for infant feeding, clinicians should carefully consider which enteral formula to choose, taking into account factors such as the infant's age, clinical condition, and possible food allergies or intolerances. Efforts by manufacturers to continually improve the quality of formulas—especially their ability to mimic the components of human milk to promote adequate development—are ongoing. For patients older than 12 months, pediatric formulas that meet the nutrient needs of older children and younger adolescents are available.

For pediatric patients who cannot meet their nutritional needs orally, as evidenced by poor weight gain, decreased linear growth, or other signs of malnutrition, EN is indicated. Inadequate intake may be due to a disease state that is causing elevated energy needs, anatomic anomalies that interfere with adequate oral consumption, or the need to be fed a specialized nutrition therapy best delivered via a tube. Pediatric patients require a different approach to EN initiation and advancement compared with adults receiving EN support. The age, weight, and clinical condition of the child are major considerations in initiation and advancement decisions. Simultaneous increases in the feeding rate and concentration are not recommended.

When EN is not sufficient or has been unsuccessful in a pediatric patient, PN should be considered. Indications for PN in most pediatric patients (with the exception of neonates) are similar to those in adult patients. Delivery of adequate PN in children usually requires central access. Goals for PN nutrient levels are often substantially higher for pediatric patients than the estimated needs of adult patients. Amino acid solutions that specifically meet pediatric protein needs deliver conditionally essential amino acids for infants and increase the solubility of calcium and phosphorus. To improve the PN solution's stability and compatibility, ILE is generally provided as a 2-in-1 solution. Pediatric patients have an elevated risk of developing PNAC, metabolic bone disease of prematurity, and hyper-triglyceridemia. Careful assessment of the risks and benefits of nutrition support must be made, while ensuring appropriate growth and avoidance of deficiencies in the pediatric population.

References

1. Pierre JF. Gastrointestinal immune and microbiome changes during parenteral nutrition. *Am J Physiol Gastrointest Liver Physiol*. 2017;312(3):G246-G256. doi:10.1152/ajpgi.00321.2016

2. Schörghuber M, Fruhwald S. Effects of enteral nutrition on gastrointestinal function in patients who are critically ill. *Lancet Gastroenterol Hepatol*. 2018;3(4):281-287. doi:10.1016/S2468-1253(18)30036-0

3. van Puffelen E, Hulst JM, Vanhorebeek I, et al. Outcomes of delaying parenteral nutrition for 1 week vs initiation within 24 hours among undernourished children in pediatric intensive care: a subanalysis of the PEPaNIC randomized clinical trial. *JAMA Netw Open*. 2018;1(5):e182668. doi:10.1001/jamanetworkopen.2018.2668

4. Boitano M, Bojak S, McCloskey S, McCaul DS, McDonough M. Improving the safety and effectiveness of parenteral nutrition: results of a quality improvement collaboration. *Nutr Clin Pract*. 2010;25(6):663-71. doi:10.1177/0884533610385349

5. Yang M, Chen PY, Gong ST, et al. Cost-effectiveness analysis of an enteral nutrition protocol for children with common gastrointestinal diseases in China: good start but still a long way to go. *JPEN J Parenter Enteral Nutr*. 2014;38(2 suppl):72S-6S. doi:10.1177/0148607114550002

6. van Puffelen E, Polinder S, Vanhorebeek I, et al. Cost-effectiveness study of early versus late parenteral nutrition in critically ill children (PEPaNIC): preplanned secondary analysis of a multicentre randomised controlled trial. *Crit Care*. 2018;22(1):4. doi:10.1186/s13054-017-1936-2

7. Mehta NM, Skillman HE, Irving SY, et al. Guidelines for the provision and assessment of nutrition support therapy in the pediatric critically ill patient: Society of Critical Care Medicine and American Society for Parenteral and Enteral Nutrition. *JPEN J Parenter Enteral Nutr*. 2017;41(5):706-742. doi:10.1177/0148607117711387

8. Green-Corkins K, Beck A. Infant formulas and complementary feeding. In: Corkins MR, ed. *The ASPEN Pediatric Nutrition Support Core Curriculum*. 2nd ed. American Society for Parenteral and Enteral Nutrition; 2015:169-185.

9. Corkins M, ed. *The ASPEN Pediatric Nutrition Support Core Curriculum*. 2nd ed. American Society for Parenteral and Enteral Nutrition; 2015.

10. Braegger C, Decsi T, Dias J, et al; ESPGHAN Committee on Nutrition. Practical approach to paediatric enteral nutrition: a comment by the ESPGHAN Committee on Nutrition. *J Ped Gastroenterol Nutr*. 2010;51(1):110-122. doi:10.1097/MPG.0b013e3181d336d2

11. Academy of Nutrition and Dietetics. Pediatric Nutrition Care Manual. Nutrition support: pediatric enteral nutrition support-general guidance-delivery. 2021. Accessed July 2, 2021. www.nutritioncaremanual.org/topic.cfm?ncm_category_id=13&lv1=145089&lv2=145297&lv3=255500&ncm_toc_id=270847&ncm_heading=&

12. Bozzetti V, Paterlini G, De Lorenzo P, Gazzolo D, Valsecchi MG, Tagliabue PE. Impact of continuous vs bolus feeding on splanchnic perfusion in very low birth weight infants: a randomized trial. *J Pediatr*. 2016;176:86-92.e2. doi:10.1016/j.jpeds.2016.05.031

13. Dani C, Pratesi S, Barp J, et al. Near-infrared spectroscopy measurements of splanchnic tissue oxygenation during continuous versus intermittent feeding method in preterm infants. *J Pediatr Gastroenterol Nutr*. 2013;56(6):652-656. doi:10.1097/MPG.0b013e318287e9d7

14. Rogers SP, Hicks PD, Hamzo M, Veit LE, Abrams SA. Continuous feedings of fortified human milk lead to nutrient losses of fat, calcium and phosphorous. *Nutrients*. 2010;2(3):230-240. doi:10.3390/nu2030240

15. Wang Y, Zhu W, Luo BR. Continuous feeding versus intermittent bolus feeding for premature infants with low birth weight: a meta-analysis of randomized controlled trials. *Eur J Clin Nutr*. 2020;74(5):775-783. doi:10.1038/s41430-019-0522-x

16. Verlato G, Hill S, Jonkers C, et al; European Reference Network on Rare and Inherited Congenital Anomalies (ERNICA). Results of an international survey on feeding management in infants with short bowel syndrome-associated intestinal failure (SBS-IF). *J Pediatr Gastroenterol Nutr.* 2021;73(5):647-653. doi:10.1097/MPG.0000000000003269

17. Bruch S, Paige T, Saez K, et al. Bolus versus continuous feeding regimens post gastrostomy tube placement in children. *J Pediatr Surg.* 2021;56(4):717-720. doi:10.1016/j.jpedsurg.2020.09.004

18. Mahoney LB, Liu E, Rosen R. Continuous feedings are not associated with lower rates of gastroesophageal reflux when compared with bolus feedings. *J Pediatr Gastroenterol Nutr.* 2019;69(6):678-681. doi:10.1097/MPG.0000000000002464

19. Brown AM, Fisher E, Forbes ML. Bolus vs continuous nasogastric feeds in mechanically ventilated pediatric patients: a pilot study. *JPEN J Parenter Enteral Nutr.* 2019;43(6):750-758. doi:10.1002/jpen.1495

20. Courtney E, Grunko A, McCarthy T. Enteral nutrition. In: Hendricks KM, Duggan C, eds. *Manual of Pediatric Nutrition.* BC Decker; 2005:252-316.

21. Nevin-Folino N, Miller M. Enteral nutrition. In: Samour PQ, Helm KK, Lang CE, eds. *Handbook of Pediatric Nutrition.* Jones and Bartlett; 2004:513-549.

22. Lively EJ, McAllister S, Doeltgen SH. Variables impacting the time taken to wean children from enteral tube feeding to oral intake. *J Pediatr Gastroenterol Nutr.* 2019;68(6):880-886. doi:10.1097/MPG.0000000000002330

23. Sapsford A, Smith C. Enteral nutrition. In: Groh-Wargo S, Thompson M, Cox JH, eds. *Pocket Guide to Neonatal Nutrition.* 2nd ed. Academy of Nutrition and Dietetics; 2016:76-125.

24. ASPEN Board of Directors and the Clinical Guidelines Task Force. Guidelines for the use of parenteral and enteral nutrition in adult and pediatric patients. *JPEN J Parenter Enteral Nutr.* 2002;26(1 suppl):1SA-138SA.

25. Abdelhadi RA, Rempel G, Sevilla W, et al; ASPEN Enteral Nutrition Task Force Pediatric Work Group. Transitioning from nasogastric feeding tube to gastrostomy tube in pediatric patients: a survey on decision-making and practice. *Nutr Clin Pract.* 2021;36(3):654-664. doi:10.1002/ncp.10603

26. Ermarth A, Thomas D, Ling CY, Cardullo A, White BR. Effective tube weaning and predictive clinical characteristics of NICU patients with feeding dysfunction. *JPEN J Parenter Enteral Nutr.* 2020;44(5):920-927. doi:10.1002/jpen.1717

27. White BR, Ermarth A, Thomas D, Arguinchona O, Presson AP, Ling CY. Creation of a standard model for tube feeding at neonatal intensive care unit discharge. *JPEN J Parenter Enteral Nutr.* 2020;44(3):491-499. doi:10.1002/jpen.1718

28. World Health Organization. Breastfeeding. Accessed October 27, 2021. www.who.int/health-topics/breastfeeding#tab=tab_2

29. American Academy of Pediatrics. Policy statement: breastfeeding and the use of human milk. *Pediatrics.* 2022;150(1):e2022057988. doi:10.1542/peds.2022-057988

30. Plenge-Bönig A, Soto-Ramirez N, Karmaus W, Petersen G, Davis S, Forster J. Breastfeeding protects against acute gastroenteritis due to rotavirus in infants. *Eur J Pediatr.* 2010;169(12):1471-1476. doi:10.1007/s00431-010-1245-0

31. Wagner CL, Greer FR; American Academy of Pediatrics Section on Breastfeeding; American Academy of Pediatrics Committee on Nutrition. Prevention of rickets and vitamin D deficiency in infants, children, and adolescents. *Pediatrics.* 2008;122(5):1142-1152. doi:10.1542/peds.2008-1862

32. Baker RD, Greer FR; Committee on Nutrition American Academy of Pediatrics. Diagnosis and prevention of iron deficiency and iron-deficiency anemia in infants and young children (0-3 years of age). *Pediatrics.* 2010;126(5):1040-1050. doi:10.1542/peds.2010-2576

33. Contraindications to Breastfeeding or Feeding Expressed Breast Milk to Infants. Centers for Disease Control and Prevention. Updated 2021. Accessed October 27, 2021. www.cdc.gov/breastfeeding/breastfeeding-special-circumstances/contraindications-to-breastfeeding.html

34. Cognata A, Kataria-Hale J, Griffiths P, et al. Human milk use in the preoperative period is associated with a lower risk for necrotizing enterocolitis in neonates with complex congenital heart disease. *J Pediatr.* 2019;215:11-16.e2. doi:10.1016/j.jpeds.2019.08.009

35. Hoban R, Khatri S, Patel A, Unger SL. Supplementation of mother's own milk with donor milk in infants with gastroschisis or intestinal atresia: a retrospective study. *Nutrients.* 2020;12(2):589. doi:10.3390/nu12020589

36. Regulations and Information on the Manufacture and Distribution of Infant Formula. US Food and Drug Administration. Accessed October 27, 2021. www.fda.gov/food/infant-formula-guidance-documents-regulatory-information/regulations-and-information-manufacture-and-distribution-infant-formula

37. Steele C, Collins E, eds. *Infant and Pediatric Feedings: Guidelines for Preparation of Human Milk and Formula in Health Care Facilities.* 3rd ed. Academy of Nutrition and Dietetics; 2019.

38. Kattan JD, Cocco RR, Järvinen KM. Milk and soy allergy. *Pediatr Clin North Am.* 2011;58(2):407-426, x. doi:10.1016/j.pcl.2011.02.005

39. Klemola T, Vanto T, Juntunen-Backmanm K, Kalimo K, Korpela R, Varjonen E. Allergy to soy formula and to extensively hydrolyzed whey formula in infants with cow's milk allergy: a prospective, randomized study with a follow-up to the age of 2 years. *J Pediatr.* 2002;140(2):219-224. doi:10.1067/mpd.2002.121935

40. Sicherer SH, Eigenmann PA, Sampson HA. Clinical features of food protein-induced enterocolitis syndrome. *J Pediatr.* 1998;133(2):175-176. doi:10.1016/s0022-3476(98)70222-7

41. Chang T, Kleinman R. Standard and specialized enteral formulas. In: Walker WA, Watkins JB, Duggan C, eds. *Nutrition in Pediatrics.* BC Decker; 2003:935-944.

42. Bhatia J, Greer F; American Academy of Pediatrics Committee on Nutrition. Use of soy protein-based formulas in infant feeding. *Pediatrics*. 2008;121(5):1062-1068. doi:10.1542/peds.2008-0564

43. Greer FR, Sicherer SH, Burks AW; Committee on Nutrition; Section on Allergy and Immunology. The effects of early nutritional interventions on the development of atopic disease in infants and children: the role of maternal dietary restriction, breastfeeding, hydrolyzed formulas, and timing of introduction of allergenic complementary foods. *Pediatrics*. 2019;143(4):e20190281. doi:10.1542/peds.2019-0281

44. Picaud JC, Pajek B, Arciszewska M, et al. An infant formula with partially hydrolyzed whey protein supports adequate growth and is safe and well-tolerated in healthy, term infants: a randomized, double-blind, equivalence trial. *Nutrients*. 2020;13;12(7):2072. doi:10.3390/nu12072072

45. Abrams SA; Committee on Nutrition. Calcium and vitamin D requirements of enterally fed preterm infants. *Pediatrics*. 2013;131(5):e1676-1683. doi:10.1542/peds.2013-0420

46. Vannice G, Rasmussen H. Position of the Academy of Nutrition and Dietetics: dietary fatty acids for healthy adults. *J Acad Nutr Diet*. 2014;114:136-153. doi:10.1016/j.jand.2013.11.001

47. Rao S, Srinivasjois R, Patole S. Prebiotic supplementation in full-term neonates: a systemic review of randomized controlled trials. *Arch Pediatr Adolesc Med*. 2009;163:755-764. doi:10.1001/archpediatrics.2009.94

48. Saavedra JM, Abi-Hanna A, Moore N, Yolken RH. Long-term consumption of infant formulas containing live probiotic bacteria: tolerance and safety. *Am J Clin Nutr*. 2004;79:261-267. doi:10.1093/ajcn/79.2.261

49. Guandalini S. Probiotics for children with diarrhea: an update. *J Clin Gastroenterol*. 2008;42(suppl):S53-S57. doi:10.1097/MCG.0b013e3181674087

50. Goehring KC, Marriage BJ, Oliver JS, Wilder JA, Barrett EG, Buck RH. Similar to those who are breastfed, infants fed a formula containing 2'-fucosyllactose have lower inflammatory cytokines in a randomized controlled trial. *J Nutr*. 2016;146(12):2559-2566. doi:10.3945/jn.116.236919

51. Puccio G, Alliet P, Cajozzo C, et al. Effects of infant formula with human milk oligosaccharides on growth and morbidity: a randomized multicenter trial. *J Pediatr Gastroenterol Nutr*. 2017;64(4):624-631. doi:10.1097/MPG.0000000000001520

52. O'Connor NR. Infant formula. *Am Fam Physician*. 2009;1;79(7):565-570.

53. van Hogezand RA, Hamdy NA. Skeletal morbidity in inflammatory bowel disease. *Scand J Gastroenterol Suppl*. 2006;(243):59-64. doi:10.1080/00365520600664276

54. Batsis I, Davis L, Prichett L, et al. Efficacy and tolerance of blended diets in children receiving gastrostomy feeds. *Nutr Clin Pract*. 2020;35(2):282-288. doi:10.1002/ncp.10406

55. Carter H, Johnson K, Johnson T, Sprulock A. Blended tube feeding prevalence, efficacy, and safety: what does the literature say? *J Am Assoc Nurse Pract*. 2018;30:150-157. doi:10.1097/JXX.0000000000000009

56. Escuro AA. Blenderized tube feeding: suggested guidelines to clinicians. Nutrition Issues in Gastroenterology, Series #136. Accessed October 27, 2021. https://med.virginia.edu/ginutrition/wp-content/uploads/sites/199/2014/06/Parrish-Dec-14.pdf

57. Worthington P, Balint J, Bechtold M, et al. When is parenteral nutrition appropriate? *JPEN J Parenter Enteral Nutr*. 2017;41(3):324-377. doi:10.1177/0148607117695251

58. Jimenez L, Mehta NM, Duggan CP. Timing of the initiation of parenteral nutrition in critically ill children. *Curr Opin Clin Nutr Metab Care*. 2017;20(3):227-231. doi:10.1097/MCO.0000000000000369

59. Axelrod D, Kazmerski K, Iyer K. Pediatric enteral nutrition. *JPEN J Parenter Enteral Nutr*. 2006;30(1 suppl):S21-S26. doi:10.1177/01486071060300S1S21

60. Samour PQ, King K. *Handbook of Pediatric Nutrition*. 3rd ed. Helm Publishing; 2005.

61. Watkins JB, Walker W, Duggan C. *Nutrition in Pediatrics: Basic Science and Clinical Applications*. 3rd ed. BC Decker; 2003.

62. Abad-Sinden A, Sutphen J. Nutrition management of pediatric short bowel syndrome. *Pract Gastroenterol*. 2003;12:28-48.

63. Serrano M, Schmidt-Sommerfeld E. Nutrition support of infants with short bowel syndrome. *Nutrition*. 2002;18:966-970. doi:10.1016/s0899-9007(02)00986-3

64. Okada A. Clinical indications of parenteral and enteral nutrition support in pediatric patients. *Nutrition*. 1998;14(1):116-118. doi:10.1016/s0899-9007(97)00227-x

65. Puntis JW. Nutritional support in the premature newborn. *Postgrad Med J*. 2006;82:192-198. doi:10.1136/pgmj.2005.038109

66. Groh-Wargo S, Thompson M, Cox J, eds. *Nutritional Care for High-Risk Newborns, Revised*. 3rd ed. Precept Press; 2000.

67. Pettignano R, Heard M, Hart M, Davis R. Total enteral nutrition versus total parenteral nutrition during pediatric extracorporeal membrane oxygenation. *Crit Care Med*. 1998;26(2):358-363. doi:10.1097/00003246-199802000-00041

68. Boullata JI, Gilbert K, Sacks G, et al; American Society for Parenteral and Enteral Nutrition. ASPEN clinical guidelines: parenteral nutrition ordering, order review, compounding, labeling, and dispensing. *JPEN J Parenter Enteral Nutr*. 2014;38(3):334-377. doi:10.1177/0148607114521833

69. Hartman C, Shamir R, Simchowitz V, Lohner S, Cai W, Decsi T; ESPGHAN/ESPEN/ESPR/CSPEN Working Group on Pediatric Parenteral Nutrition. ESPGHAN/ESPEN/ESPR/CSPEN guidelines on pediatric parenteral nutrition: complications. *Clin Nutr*. 2018;37(6 pt B):2418-2429. doi:10.1016/j.clnu.2018.06.956

70. Crill C, Gura K. Parenteral nutrition support. In: Corkins M, ed. *The ASPEN Pediatric Nutrition Support Core Curriculum. 2nd ed.* American Society for Parenteral and Enteral Nutrition; 2015:593-614.

71. van Goudoever JB, Carnielli V, Darmaun D, Sainz de Pipaon M; ESPGHAN/ESPEN/ESPR/CSPEN Working Group on Pediatric Parenteral Nutrition. ESPGHAN/ESPEN/ESPR/CSPEN guidelines on pediatric parenteral nutrition: amino acids. *Clin Nutr*. 2018;37(6 pt B):2315-2323. doi:10.1016/j.clnu.2018.06.945

72. Lunn M, Fausnight T. Hypersensitivity to total parenteral nutrition fat-emulsion component in an egg-allergic child. *Pediatr*. 2011;128(4):e1025-e1028. doi:10.1542/peds.2010-2771

73. Kapoor V, Glover R, Malviya M. Alternative lipid emulsions versus pure soy oil based lipid emulsions for parenterally fed preterm infants. *Cochrane Database Syst Rev*. 2015;2015(12):CD009172. doi:10.1002/14651858.CD009172.pub2

74. Chang M, Puder M, Gura K. The use of fish oil lipid emulsion in the treatment of intestinal failure associated liver disease (IFALD). *Nutrients.* 2012:4:1828-1850. doi:10.3390/nu4121828

75. Agus M, Braithwaite SS, Deutschman C, et al. Guidelines for the use of an insulin infusion for the management of hyperglycemia in critically ill patients. *Crit Care Med*. 2012;40(12):3251-3276. doi:10.1097/CCM.0b013e3182653269

76. Ayers P, Adams S, Boullata J, et al; American Society for Parenteral and Enteral Nutrition. ASPEN parenteral nutrition safety consensus recommendations. *JPEN J Parenter Enteral Nutr*. 2014;38(3):296-333. doi:10.1177/0148607113511992

77. Wessel J, Balint J, Crill C, Klotz K; American Society for Parenteral and Enteral Nutrition; Task Force on Standards for Specialized Nutrition Support for Hospitalized Pediatric Patients. Standards for specialized nutrition support: hospitalized pediatric patients. *Nutr Clin Pract*. 2005;20(3):103-116. doi:10.1177/0115426505020001103

78. Hardy G, Wong T, Morrissey H, et al. Parenteral provision of micronutrients to pediatric patients: an international expert consensus paper. *JPEN J Parenter Enteral Nutr*. 2020;44(suppl 2):S5-S23. doi:10.1002/jpen.1990

79. Srikrishnaraj A, Chambers K, South C, et al. Trace elements' contamination of pediatric parenteral nutrition solutions in Canada: a cause for concern. *JPEN J Parenter Enteral Nutr*. 2021;45(2):347-356. doi:10.1002/jpen.1836

80. Kumpf VJ. Parenteral nutrition-associated liver disease in adult and pediatric patients. *Nutr Clin Pract*. 2006;21:279-290. doi:10.1177/0115426506021003279

81. Kelly DA. Liver complications of pediatric parenteral nutrition: epidemiology. *Nutrition*. 1998;14:153-157. doi:10.1016/s0899-9007(97)00232-3

82. Wolf A, Pohlandt F. Bacterial infection: the main cause of acute cholestasis in newborn infants receiving short-term parenteral nutrition. *J Pediatr Gastroenterol Nutr*. 1989;8:297-303.

83. Chung C, Buchman AL. Postoperative jaundice and total parenteral nutrition-associated hepatic dysfunction. *Clin Liver Dis*. 2002;6:1067-1084. doi:10.1016/s1089-3261(02)00057-0

84. Cavicchi M, Beau P, Crenn P, Degott C, Messing B. Prevalence of liver disease and contributing factors in patients receiving home parenteral nutrition for permanent intestinal failure. *Ann Intern Med*. 2000;132:525-532. doi:10.7326/0003-4819-132-7-200004040-00003

85. Spencer AU, Yu S, Tracy TF, et al. Parenteral nutrition-associated cholestasis in neonates: multivariate analysis of the potential protective effect of taurine. *JPEN J Parenter Enteral Nutr*. 2005;29:337-344. doi:10.1177/0148607105029005337

86. Chung PH, Wong KK, Wong RM, et al. Clinical experience in managing pediatric patients with ultra-short bowel syndrome using omega-3 fatty acids. *Eur J Pediatr Surg*. 2010;20:139-142. doi:10.1055/s-0029-1238283

87. de Meijer VE, Gura KM, Le HD, Meisel JA, Puder M. Fish oil-based lipid emulsions prevent and reverse parenteral nutrition-associated liver disease: the Boston experience. *JPEN J Parenter Enteral Nutr*. 2009;33:541-547. doi:10.1177/0148607109332773

88. Diamond IR, Steresca A, Pencharz PB, Kim JH, Wales PN. Changing the paradigm: Omegaven for the treatment of liver failure in pediatric short bowel syndrome. *J Pediatr Gastroenterol Nutr*. 2009;48:209-215. doi:10.1097/MPG.0b013e318182c8f6

89. Gura KM, Lee S, Valim C, et al. Safety and efficacy of a fish-oil based fat emulsion in the treatment of parenteral nutrition-associated liver disease. *Pediatrics*. 2008;121:e678-e686. doi:10.1542/peds.2007-2248

90. Lee S, Valim C, Johnston P, Le HD, et al. Impact of fish oil-based lipid emulsion on serum triglyceride, bilirubin, and albumin levels in children with parenteral nutrition-associated liver disease. *Pediatr Res*. 2009;66(6):698-703. doi:10.1203/PDR.0b013e3181bbdf2b

91. Blaiche IF, Khalidi N. Parenteral nutrition-associated liver complications in children. *Pharmacotherapy*. 2002;22:188-211. doi:10.1592/phco.22.3.188.33553

92. Hwang TL, Lue MC, Chen LL. Early use of cyclic TPN prevents further deterioration of liver functions for the TPN patients with impaired liver function. *Hepatogastroenterology*. 2000;47:1347-1350.

93. Park HW, Lee NM, Kim JH, Kim KS, Kim SN. Parenteral fish oil-containing lipid emulsions may reverse parenteral nutrition-associated cholestasis in neonates: a systematic review and meta-analysis. *J Nutr*. 2015;145(2):277-283. doi:10.3945/jn.114.204974

94. Lapillonne A, Fidler Mis N, Goulet O, van den Akker CHP, Wu J, Koletzko B; ESPGHAN/ESPEN/ESPR/CSPEN Working Group on Pediatric Parenteral Nutrition. ESPGHAN/ESPEN/ESPR/CSPEN guidelines on pediatric parenteral nutrition: lipids. *Clin Nutr*. 2018;37(6 pt B):2324-2336. doi:10.1016/j.clnu.2018.06.946

95. Crill CM, Storm MC, Christensen ML, Hankins CT, Bruce Jenkins M, Helms RA. Carnitine supplementation in premature neonates: effect on plasma and red blood cell total carnitine concentrations, nutrition parameters and morbidity. *Clin Nutr*. 2006;25(6):886-896 doi:10.1016/j.clnu.2006.05.002

96. Nelms C, Juarez M, Warady B. Renal Disease. In: Corkins M, ed. *The ASPEN Pediatric Nutrition Support Core Curriculum*. 2nd ed. American Society for Parenteral and Enteral Nutrition; 2015:374.

97. Sgambat K, Moudgil A. Carnitine deficiency in children receiving continuous renal replacement therapy. *Hemodial Int*. 2016;20(1):63-67. doi:10.1111/hdi.12341

98. Sgambat K, Clauss S, Moudgil A. Effect of levocarnitine supplementation on myocardial strain in children with acute kidney injury receiving continuous kidney replacement therapy: a pilot study. *Pediatr Nephrol*. 2021;36(6):1607-1616. doi:10.1007/s00467-020-04862-3

99. Harshman LA, Lee-Son K, Jetton JG. Vitamin and trace element deficiencies in the pediatric dialysis patient. *Pediatr Nephrol*. 2018;33(7):1133-1143. doi:10.1007/s00467-017-3751-z

100. Ooi PH, Gilmour SM, Yap J, Mager DR. Effects of branched chain amino acid supplementation on patient care outcomes in adults and children with liver cirrhosis: a systematic review. *Clin Nutr ESPEN*. 2018;28:41-51. doi:10.1016/j.clnesp

101. Srinivasan V, Spinella PC, Drott HR, et al. Association of timing, duration, and intensity of hyperglycemia with intensive care unit mortality in critically ill children. *Pediatr Crit Care Med*. 2004;5(4):329-336. doi:10.1097/01.pcc.0000128607.68261.7c

102. Mehta NM, Compher C, A.S.P.E.N. Board of Directors. A.S.P.E.N. clinical guidelines: nutrition support of the critically ill child. *JPEN J Parenter Enteral Nutr*. 2009;33:260-276. doi:10.1177/0148607109333114

103. Vlasselaers D, Milants I, Desmet L, et al. Intensive insulin therapy for patients in paediatric intensive care: a prospective, randomized controlled study. *Lancet*. 2009;373:547-556. doi:10.1016/S0140-6736(09)60044-1

104. Agus M, Wypij E, Hirshberg V, et al. Tight glycemic control in critically ill children. *New Engl J Med*. 2017;376(8):729-741. doi:10.1056/NEJMoa1612348

105. Chen L, Li T, Fang F, Zhang Y, Faramand A. Tight glycemic control in critically ill pediatric patients: a systematic review and meta-analysis. *Crit Care*. 2018;22:57-68. doi:10.1186/s13054-018-1976-2

106. Faustino E, Hirshberg E, Asara L, et al. Short-term adverse outcomes associated with hypoglycemia in critically ill children. *Pediatr Crit Care*. 2019:47(5):706-712. doi:10.1097/CCM.0000000000003699

107. Srinivasan V. Nutrition support and tight glucose control in critically ill children: food for thought. *Front Pediatr*. 2018;6:1-8. doi:10.3389/ped.2018.00340

108. da Silva JSV, Seres DS, Sabino K, et al; Parenteral Nutrition Safety and Clinical Practice Committees, American Society for Parenteral and Enteral Nutrition. ASPEN consensus recommendations for refeeding syndrome. *Nutr Clin Pract*. 2020;35(2):178-195. doi:10.1002/ncp.10474

22

Home Parenteral and Enteral Nutrition

Therese Berry, MS, RDN, LD, CNSC
Mark DeLegge, MD

KEY POINTS

- Home parenteral and enteral nutrition support is appropriate for patients who no longer require acute care but still need nutrition support because of their underlying gastrointestinal dysfunction.
- Providing complete and careful instruction to patients in the discharge and initiation stages, assisting with the selection of an appropriate home care provider, and helping with the reimbursement process are all essential for success.
- Regular follow up is necessary to assess patients' nutritional and health status, quality of life, and risk for complications. Patients should be transitioned off home parenteral and enteral nutrition whenever possible.

Introduction

Home parenteral and enteral nutrition (HPEN) support is appropriate for patients who no longer require acute care but still require nutrition support because of their underlying gastrointestinal (GI) dysfunction.[1] The goals of HPEN are to promote nutritional rehabilitation, avoid therapy-related complications associated with specialized nutrition support, minimize therapy dependence, and improve the patient's quality of life. Refer to Chapters 19, 20, and 21 for additional information about enteral, parenteral, and pediatric nutrition support, respectively.

Hospital Discharge Considerations for Home Parenteral and Enteral Nutrition

Selecting a Home Care Provider

When transitioning a patient from a hospital or rehabilitation facility to the home for HPEN therapy, it is important to recognize that both the patient management and therapy goals for home nutrition support are substantially different from those in the acute-care setting (see Box 22.1).[1,2] To facilitate a smooth discharge, the patient and hospital personnel should evaluate objective qualitative and quantitative information and select a home care provider that has experience with similar patients, has data demonstrating achievement of positive clinical outcomes, and otherwise meets the needs of the specific individual (see Box 22.2 on page 402).[2] Once selected, the home care provider then assists with the evaluation of the patient and their specific individual needs to determine whether the patient is an appropriate candidate for HPEN (see Box 22.3 on page 402).[1,3]

Selecting a Home Nutrition Support Device

Before discharge, the physician and other members of the nutrition support team must select the appropriate access device for the patient who requires HPEN.

BOX 22.1

Differences in Care Management Between Acute and Home Care[1,2]

	Acute care	Home care
Individual referred to as	Patient	Consumer
Management type	Crisis management to stabilize the patient	Long-term management to promote quality of life
Therapy goals	Nutrition maintenance by the best-tolerated route	Nutritional repletion and transition to the most physiologic therapy
Potential complications	Infectious or mechanical complications involving the catheter or tube Metabolic complications Gastrointestinal (GI) intolerance	Infectious or mechanical complications involving the catheter or tube Metabolic complications GI intolerance Long-term parenteral nutrition issues: metabolic bone disease, liver dysfunction, micronutrient abnormalities Therapy nonadherence Difficulty coping Psychological complications Impaired quality of life
Therapy provision	Dependent and managed by clinicians	Independent and managed by consumer and caregiver with periodic oversight by clinicians
Reimbursement	Generally covered as part of the bed day rate	Variable coverage depending on the insurance plan and insurer
Provider	Hospital to which the patient is admitted	Choice of a variety of local, regional, and national home-infusion and durable medical equipment providers
Environment	Tightly controlled and managed by clinicians	Must meet basic safety and compliance criteria, with periodic practitioner monitoring

For patients who require home enteral nutrition (HEN), device selection criteria include the intended length of therapy and the patient's current GI anatomy.[4] Common HEN devices include percutaneous endoscopic gastrostomy, percutaneous endoscopic jejunostomy, and gastrojejunostomy tubes. Low-profile devices are often used for pediatric patients and ambulatory adults.

For patients requiring home parenteral nutrition (HPN), the goal is to assess the type of central venous access device and to implement strategies to produce the lowest occurrence of infectious and mechanical complications. Device selection criteria include the intended length of therapy, other intravenous needs of the patient, the patient's vascular history, caregiver

BOX 22.2

Factors in Selecting a Home Parenteral and Enteral Nutrition Provider[2]

Consideration	Types of data to evaluate
Patient population served	Patient demographics (eg, patient age, gender, primary and secondary diagnoses, average length of therapy, concurrent therapies, and geographic location)
	Experience with the ordering physician and insurance provider
Clinical outcomes	Rehospitalization rate
	Rates of catheter complications (catheter sepsis, exit-site infection, thrombus, occlusion, and mechanical issues)
	Patient satisfaction with care and services
	Reasons for discharge
	Complications associated with therapy provision
General profile	Size and geographic coverage
	Years in operation
	Accreditation status
Availability and services	24-hour availability
	Ability to troubleshoot pump or therapy complications
	Proximity to patient
	Ability to accommodate patient work or travel schedule
	Knowledge to reinforce patient teaching
	Patient monitoring and nursing care
	Availability of registered dietitian nutritionists with nutrition support expertise
	Policies and procedures to continue care in pandemic or other emergent situations, such as COVID-19
Reimbursement and payment policies	Private insurance contracts
	Reimbursement by public payers (eg, Medicare)
	Indigent care policy

BOX 22.3

Patient Criteria for Home Nutrition Support[1,3]

Hemodynamic and clinical stability

Long-term intravenous or enteral access established

Physical and emotional ability to cope with home therapy

Presence of a capable and willing care partner

Consent to home therapy

Willingness to comply with home therapy

Safe and adequate home environment: refrigeration, electricity, clean water supply, access to a telephone, storage space, clean workspace for therapy preparation, safety issues identified and resolved

Adequate insurance coverage for prescribed therapy

availability, patient preference, and formulation osmolarity. Common central venous access devices are tunneled catheters (Hickman, Broviac), implantable ports, and peripherally inserted central catheters (PICCs). A PICC is often used if the duration of therapy is uncertain or expected to be less than 2 to 3 months.[5,6] Broviac catheters are usually reserved for pediatric patients. Box 22.4 summarizes considerations for selecting the appropriate device.[1,6]

The central venous access device should have the fewest number of lumens needed for the patient's therapy. This lowers the risk for central line–associated blood stream infections, reduces the number of manipulations for catheter flushing, and requires less maintenance for patients and caregivers.[5] A PICC line may require an extension set if the patient is hooking up and disconnecting their own PN.

BOX 22.4

Considerations for Selecting a Central Venous Access Device[1,6]

The location of the central venous access device should be easily visualized and accessible for self-caring patients.

Tunneled or implanted devices are preferred for long-term use.

Right-sided venous access is preferred to reduce the risk of thrombosis.

The catheter tip should be in the lower third of the superior vena cava and the atriocaval junction.

Predischarge and Postdischarge Education

Teach-back education with the patient and the caregiver before discharge from the hospital builds patient independence and promotes the provision of safe and effective therapy. During predischarge education, valuable information about safety, therapy administration, and supply management is imparted to the patient; questions from the patient are answered; any misconceptions are corrected; and, ideally, all the patient's fears about HPEN are alleviated or diminished. Topics to cover in predischarge education include the following[7]:

- rationale for HPEN prescription
- anticipated length of therapy
- pumps, equipment, and procedures
- the enteral or parenteral access device and its care
- aseptic (sterile) techniques necessary for safe therapy administration
- nutritional formulations and additives and their storage and preparation
- precautions to prevent and treat complications (self-monitoring)
- development of an emergency plan
- contact information, whom to call, and when to call

The patient's and caregiver's learning needs, capabilities, and readiness to learn should be assessed before education begins, and the teaching techniques and materials should then be tailored to the individual. A combination of written, verbal, and demonstration techniques can be used in patient education. The patient should be taught with the equipment and supplies that will be used in the home setting.

Patient and caregiver education should continue after discharge as well, with the goal being for the patient or caregiver to be able to demonstrate that they can safely and effectively administer feedings and medications, care for the access device, and, if applicable, use a pump. Home health providers need to be available for the first hookup and first disconnect of PN. Typically, patients and caregivers are deemed independent after two to three home health visits once they can demonstrate proper procedures for administering enteral feeds or, in the case of PN, proper procedures for hooking up and disconnecting, flushing the catheter, and using the pump.

If a patient is having frequent complications with either EN or PN, the home health provider may need to reeducate and reassess the patient's or caregiver's technique to ensure that proper procedures are followed going forward.

Discharge Orders

Before discharge, physician orders for the HPEN therapy are received and reviewed by the home care clinicians to ensure the orders are appropriate for the individual patient's needs and to make therapy administration as easy as possible (see Box 22.5).[1,7,8] At this time, the insurance coverage for the prescribed therapy should be verified.

BOX 22.5

Information Included on Physician Discharge Orders for Home Parenteral and Enteral Nutrition[1,7,8]

Information for all patients

- Basic physician information (name, contact information, and other vital details)
- Patient name, age, gender, and other relevant demographic or general health data
- Medication profile
- Allergy history
- Home parenteral and enteral nutrition therapy prescription
- Reason for therapy, including International Statistical Classification of Diseases and Related Health Problems, 11th revision (ICD-11) code or codes
- Insurance policy information
- Monitoring parameters, including laboratory orders and frequency

Information specific to the enteral prescription

- Product name
- Number of cans per day or dosage
- Formula rate and duration
- Days per week to infuse, if less than daily
- Method of administration (bolus, intermittent, continuous)
- Tube type, French size, and placement
- Pump choice
- Flushing regimen

Information specific to the parenteral prescription

- Catheter type, number of lumens, and flushing protocol
- Macronutrient content
- Specialty amino acid or lipid product specifications, as needed
- Volume and infusion schedule
- Electrolyte content
- Additives (eg, multivitamin, trace elements, insulin, H_2 blocker, heparin)

Formula Selection

Enteral Formulas

Factors to consider when choosing an enteral formula for use in HEN include the patient's current GI anatomy and digestive capability, nutrient and fluid requirements, and any disease-specific considerations, such as nutrients that may be malabsorbed and any GI motility issues. Another consideration is whether the formula selected is available from the home care provider, or if there is a comparable product available for home use.[4,7]

When preparing to do home education, the nutrition support team should also evaluate the consumer's schedule at home (work, family care, and medical treatment schedule) in order to develop a prescription that promotes both adherence to therapy and quality of life. Box 22.6 lists components of teaching about HEN.[8,9]

Blenderized Tube Feeding

Food-based blenderized tube feeding (BTF) is growing in popularity. Interest may be due to the financial challenges of obtaining commercial formulas, food or preservative allergies, intolerance to tube feeding, or a desire for fiber or phytonutrients that are not found in commercial products. Consumers on HEN and their caregivers may feel that BTF brings back the joy of cooking or see the preparation as an act of love.[9-12] Some may use BTF formulas occasionally, along with a commercially prepared formula, and some will use BTF preparations exclusively. Consumers and caregivers need to adhere to food safety guidelines, such as proper handwashing, thorough washing of produce, and general safe food preparation

BOX 22.6

Components of Teaching Patients About Home Enteral Nutrition[8,9]

Establish enteral nutrition tolerance before the patient is discharged from the acute care facility.

Review with the patient or caregiver the reason for home enteral nutrition.

Review the feeding plan: formula name, volume to administer, administration type (bolus, gravity, pump), timing of feeding, and frequency and volume of water flushes.

Have the patient or caregiver demonstrate competency in enteral administration.

Review the appropriate delivery of enteral medications. (American Society for Parenteral and Enteral Nutrition [ASPEN] recommends flushing the tube with 15 mL water before, between, and after medication administration.)

Review correct body positioning for during and after feeding.

Educate the patient or caregiver about infection prevention measures: proper handwashing; disinfection of the surrounding surfaces that supplies will touch; and cleaning of formula containers, pump sets, tubing, feeding tube, extension sets, and pumps.

Review refrigeration and temperature recommendations, the mixing of formula, and how to add modulars, if indicated.

Show the patient or caregiver how to care for the tube and stoma site.

Provide contact information for reporting adverse effects, such as diarrhea, abdominal distension, bloating, and constipation.

Explain the need for adequate hydration via tube (or by mouth).

practices for cooked foods. A high-speed blender is required for BTF preparation. Popular items to blend include sweet potatoes, bananas, avocados, quinoa, oatmeal, nuts, nut butters, chicken, yogurt, various milks (cow, nut), broths, and coconut water. The hang time for BTF formulas should not exceed 2 hours; the unused portion can be refrigerated for 24 hours.[8-12] A 2019 study of a BTF formula using whole foods found that the total bacterial count was within acceptable limits when measured at 0, 2, and 4 hours after the formula was prepared.[13] Samples were measured for growth of *Staphylococcus aureus*, coliform bacteria, and *Escherichia coli*.

A 14-French or larger tube is needed to administer BTF. Preferably, the intact nutrients are delivered into the stomach, typically as a bolus feed. A registered dietitian nutritionist (RDN) should review the BTF composition to ensure it meets 100% of the Dietary Reference Intakes. Food-based commercial products are also available.[10,12] Because of the rise in use of BTF, it is important for nutrition support teams and RDNs to be informed about and competent in blenderized feedings to be able to support their patients.[14]

Parenteral Formulations

Most home care providers have the ability to customize an HPN formulation to the patient's unique needs. The following can usually be customized to the individual patient:

- energy and nutrient content of the formulation (eg, depending on whether the formulation is intended to replete nutrient stores or promote weight loss)
- electrolyte content of the formulation (vs premixed PN formulations)
- compatibility and stability guidelines related to the weekly compounding regimen
- cycling of HPN (which can allow for activities of daily living and reduce stress)
- adjustments to the formulation for increased GI losses
- the use of HPN as a supplement to oral nutrition or EN
- drug additives (eg, H_2 receptor blockers and insulin)

Before the initiation of home care therapy, the RDN should conduct an assessment to confirm that the appropriate macronutrients are being provided (avoiding any overfeeding or underfeeding) and the safe range for electrolytes. The appropriate volume of formulation, based on the patient's weight, GI losses, and any underlying diseases (eg, congestive heart failure or liver disease) should also be confirmed as well as the formulation stability and the need for any product substitutions and related approvals (to be discussed with the prescriber) before obtaining the final order.

Intravenous Lipid Emulsion

Several intravenous lipid emulsion (ILE) products are available in the United States (Table 22.1).[15-18] Intralipid and Nutrilipid are 100% soybean oil–based lipid emulsions. Soybean oil is rich in linoleic acid, an omega-6 fatty acid that promotes the production of proinflammatory eicosanoids that increase oxidative stress and systemic inflammation.[15] However, the same fatty acid is necessary for preventing essential fatty acid deficiency. Soybean oil ILEs have been associated with intestinal failure–associated liver disease in pediatric and adult patients.

Clinolipid is 80% olive oil, which is rich in oleic acid, an omega-9 fatty acid that is monounsaturated and is considered immune neutral. The other 20% is soybean oil, to meet essential fatty acid requirements.[16] Clinolipid can be considered when the prescriber wants to minimize the use of a soybean oil ILE. Clinolipid should be given daily to patients with no oral or enteral soy-fat intake.

SMOFlipid contains soybean oil (30%), medium-chain triglyceride oil (30%), olive oil (25%), and fish oil (15%). SMOFlipid contains a lesser amount of omega-6 fatty acid than

100% soybean oil ILEs and is considered less inflammatory.[17] SMOFlipid can also be considered when the prescriber wants to minimize the use of a soybean oil ILE. The recommended dosing for adults is 1 to 2 g/kg of body weight per day, as it contains less linoleic acid and α-linolenic acid than 100% soybean oil ILE. SMOFlipid should be given daily to patients with no oral or enteral soy-fat intake.[17]

Omegaven is a 100% fish oil–based ILE. The US Food and Drug Administration (FDA) has approved Omegaven for use in pediatric patients to provide energy and fatty acids in those with parenteral nutrition–associated cholestasis and a direct bilirubin level above 2 mg/dL. It is not indicated for the prevention of parenteral nutrition–associated cholestasis. Omegaven may be administered in conjunction with a soybean oil ILE to meet essential fatty acid requirements.[15] The recommended and maximum dosing for Omegaven is 1 g/kg/d.[18] It should be administered until the patient's direct bilirubin level is less than 2 mg/dL, or until the patient no longer requires PN.

TABLE 22.1 Intravenous Lipid Emulsions[15-18]

	Intralipid; Nutrilipid	Clinolipid	SMOFlipid	Omegaven
Manufacturer	Fresenius Kabi; B. Braun	Baxter	Fresenius Kabi	Fresenius Kabi
Oil source	100% soybean oil	80% olive oil, 20% soybean oil	30% soybean oil, 30% MCT oil, 25% olive oil, 15% fish oil	100% fish oil
Considerations	Source of energy and EFAs	Source of energy and EFAs; can be considered when the prescriber wants to minimize use of soybean oil ILE	Source of energy and EFAs; can be considered when the prescriber wants to minimize use of soybean oil ILE	Indicated in pediatric patients to provide energy and EFAs in those with PNAC
Dosing[a]	Adults: <1 g/kg/d in stable, long-term patients	1.0-1.5 g/kg/d, not to exceed 2.5 g/kg/d	Adults: 1-2 g/kg/d, not to exceed 2.5 g/kg/d or 60% of energy	Recommended and maximum: 1 g/kg/d in pediatrics

EFA = essential fatty acid | ILE = intravenous lipid emulsion | MCT = medium-chain triglyceride | PNAC = parenteral nutrition–associated cholestasis
[a] Dosing amounts based on kilograms of body weight

Financial Reimbursement

Before the patient is discharged from the hospital or rehabilitation facility, an RDN based in the facility should work with the discharge case manager and the selected home care provider to ensure reimbursement of HPEN. The home care provider may also be able to assist in guiding the discharge team to the required documentation to obtain insurance authorization.

Medicare Coverage

In October 2020, the Centers for Medicare & Medicaid Services announced the retirement of the local coverage determinations for PN,[19] which had been in effect since 1984. The new coverage criteria went into effect November 12, 2020. The new guidelines remove outdated barriers for Medicare beneficiaries who need life-sustaining therapy. Situations G and H are no longer used for PN. It is now appropriate to use a combination of objective evidence and physician progress notes to "paint the picture" that supports the patient's clinical situation. The new coverage criteria pertain to all four Durable Medical Equipment Medicare Administrative Contractor jurisdictions.[19]

The following language remains the same[19]:

Parenteral nutrition is considered reasonable and necessary for a patient with severe pathology of the alimentary tract which does not allow absorption of sufficient nutrients to maintain weight and strength commensurate with the patient's general condition.

Enteral nutrition is considered reasonable and necessary for a patient with a functioning gastrointestinal tract who, due to pathology or non-function of the structures that normally permit food to reach the digestive tract, cannot maintain weight and strength commensurate with his or her general condition.

There is no coverage for oral supplements or tube feed lasting less than 90 days.[19] Common conditions that qualify for Medicare coverage of HEN include oral, esophageal, gastric, or proximal small bowel obstruction; severe dysphagia; Crohn's disease or pancreatitis, when intact nutrients are malabsorbed; severe intestinal motility disorders; and cystic fibrosis. Documentation required for Medicare coverage is summarized in Box 22.7.[19]

Medicare will *not* bear the cost of coverage in the following circumstances: when HPEN is used as a supplement to another route of nutrition support, when HPEN is required because the patient refuses to take adequate nutrition (psychological or anorexia due to medication), or when HPEN therapy is required for less than 90 days.[9,19]

Medicaid Coverage

Medicaid coverage for HPEN varies from state to state. Refer to individual state policies for details. Some plans require authorization.

Private Payers

Most commercial insurers will pay for HPN with documentation of medical necessity and a physician's prescription. Some commercial insurers require a member to use Medicare criteria for coverage to demonstrate the medical necessity of HPN. In some cases, prior authorization of HPN services is required; however, it is not a guarantee of payment.

Commercial insurance coverage for HEN is variable. HEN coverage may be covered under the pharmacy benefit, as is HPN, or it may be covered under the durable medical equipment benefit. Under some plans, only HEN supplies and equipment may be covered, leaving the patient to pay out-of-pocket for formula.

Initiation of Parenteral and Enteral Nutrition in the Home

For a subset of patients, initiation of EN or PN can occur in the home, which allows the patient to avoid hospitalization. Considerations for the safe initiation of HPEN include the following[1]:

- The patient was recently examined by the prescribing physician.
- The patient is clinically stable (eg, no congestive heart failure, renal failure, poorly controlled diabetes, or substance abuse).
- The access device is established and appropriate for formula.
- Baseline laboratory values (ie, comprehensive metabolic panel, complete blood count, phosphorus, and magnesium) indicate metabolic stability.
- The home environment and care partner are suitable.
- The patient consents to therapy.

BOX 22.7

Documentation Required for Medicare Coverage of Home Enteral Nutrition and Home Parenteral Nutrition[19]

The following is required for Medicare coverage of enteral nutrition (EN):

- documentation supporting that EN is needed for at least 90 days and a physician-written order or prescription
- sufficient medical documentation (hospital records, physician clinical findings) to permit an independent conclusion to be drawn that the patient's medical condition meets Medicare criteria and is medically necessary
- written medical justification for pumps (eg, jejunostomy tube or malabsorption diagnosis, blood glucose fluctuations) and for specific nutrients (elemental or disease-specific formulas)
- additional documentation in cases of EN of less than 750 kcal/d or more than 2,000 kcal/d

The following is required for Medicare coverage of parenteral nutrition (PN):

- documentation supporting that total PN is needed for at least 90 days ("indefinite" is acceptable as lifetime), and a note from the prescriber dated within the last 30 days
- documentation that the patient has a condition involving the small bowel or its exocrine glands that impairs absorption or a motility disorder that impairs the ability of nutrients to be transported through the gastrointestinal tract
- standard written order and Durable Medical Equipment Information Form; proof of delivery
- additional documentation to support formulations providing less than 20 kcal/kg of body weight per day or more than 35 kcal/kg/d; dextrose less than 10% final concentration; amino acids less than 0.8 g/kg/d or more than 1.5 g/kg/d; and lipids more than 50 g/d

Examples of supportive documentation for home parenteral nutrition may include:

- objective test results confirming the diagnosis (see Box 22.8)
- a nutrition assessment: diet and weight history
- laboratory test results from within the last 7 days
- medication list demonstrating prokinetic use or failure
- documentation of a failed tube-feed trial, documentation explaining why placement of a small bowel feeding tube is contraindicated, or documentation of another reason why tube feeding is not warranted

Appropriate candidates for HEN initiation are those who have a gastric or jejunal feeding tube placed in an endoscopy suite, radiology suite, or other outpatient setting and who are not severely debilitated by malnutrition or comorbid disease. Appropriate candidates for initiation of HPN include the following: patients who have attempted enteral feedings without success; patients who have GI diseases without excessive GI fluid or nutrient losses; or patients with an oncology diagnosis and an inability to tube feed.

Patients who are severely malnourished, pediatric patients, pregnant women, and those with severe electrolyte abnormalities are exceptions and should have HPEN initiated in the hospital setting, where vital signs and laboratory values can be monitored more frequently.[20]

Malabsorption; short bowel syndrome

Operative report; small bowel follow-through (SBFT); fecal fat test (Sudan stain); d-xylose absorption; serum citrulline; small bowel biopsy; physician progress note documenting that diarrhea or high ostomy output is associated with weight loss or dehydration or electrolyte imbalance

Dysmotility

Gastric emptying test; motility-monitoring "smart" capsule; SBFT; enterography; abdominal film showing dilated small bowel with physician progress note stating results are consistent with small bowel dysmotility; prokinetic medications trialed (or statement of why they cannot be used)

If patient is on narcotics, physician must address why patient cannot be off them

Intestinal obstruction

Imaging to confirm obstruction; physician progress note stating patient is not a candidate for surgical correction of obstruction

Nonfunctioning small bowel; inability to feed via gastrointestinal (GI) tract

Physician progress note detailing why the small bowel cannot be used for tube feeds, including description of tube feed trials or attempts made to place a tube, and stating that the patient is intolerant to oral intake and can only be fed with parenteral nutrition; imaging to support the case (ie, operative report showing failed tube placement, computed tomography [CT] scan showing carcinomatosis)

GI tract fistula requiring bowel rest and minimal oral intake for 90 days or more

Imaging confirming the fistula or wound care notes describing the location of the fistula and drainage or output as stool, food, or succus

Regional enteritis of intestine requiring bowel rest and minimal oral intake for 90 days or more

Endoscopy, magnetic resonance enterography, or other objective report showing active enteritis

Pancreatitis with or without pseudocyst requiring bowel rest and minimal oral intake for 90 days or more

CT scan or laboratory test results (amylase, lipase) showing pancreatitis

Refeeding Syndrome in Home Parenteral and Enteral Nutrition

Refeeding syndrome is a concern more commonly related to the initiation of HPEN. This can occur in the hospital setting as well as in the home. Patients who only received a few days of EN or PN as an inpatient or who have not been ramped up to their goal nutrition prior to discharge from the hospital can be at risk for refeeding syndrome after discharge to home as well.

With proper evaluation and management, refeeding syndrome can be prevented, but there are no universally accepted recommendations. Management includes checking baseline electrolytes and rehydrating the patient with fluid and electrolytes before initiating HPEN, as needed, to normalize blood chemistry. Thiamin should be supplemented when giving nutrients for the first 5 to 7 days or longer.[20] HPN initiation should start with 15 to 20 kcal/kg/d and advance by 200 to 300 kcal every 1 to 3 days.[21] The total fluid volume should be moderate and be low in carbohydrate content, with no more than 100 to 150 g dextrose or no greater than 50% of estimated carbohydrate needs. The PN should be compounded with optimal potassium, phosphorus, and magnesium content. Gradual advancement of the energy content of the PN formulation over 7 to 10 days to goal is ideal. Starting HEN at a volume of 25% of estimated needs may be indicated to prevent the negative sequelae of refeeding syndrome. The enteral formula can be advanced over 3 to 5 days to goal. Vital signs and electrolytes should be monitored closely.[4]

Continuation of Care in Home Parenteral and Enteral Nutrition

Ultimately, the goal of HPEN is to promote nutritional rehabilitation and quality of life through the prevention of therapy-related complications (Box 22.9)[7-9,14,20-24] and reduction of HPEN dependency. To achieve these goals, ongoing nutrition assessment and monitoring are required (see Box 22.10 on page 414),[2,24] and consumer education must be provided periodically.

For both HPN and HEN, ongoing assessment should include the following:

- creating measurable goals, such as achieving goal weight, adequate fluid balance, stable glucose and electrolytes, and achieving an HPEN schedule that accommodates the patient's lifestyle
- determining whether the patient is meeting those goals, and if not, determining why not
- assessing for therapy adherence and conveying any nonadherence issues to the prescriber
- evaluating for tolerance to any formula substitutions (eg, substitutions because of national drug component shortages)
- obtaining any notes from hospital or clinic visits for the home care records
- determining whether the patient is clinically stable enough to recommend reduced laboratory monitoring (ie, weekly, then every other week, then once monthly)

BOX 22.9

Complications of Home Parenteral and Enteral Nutrition[7-9,14,20-24]

Mechanical—enteral nutrition (EN)

Complication	Symptoms	Intervention
Damage	Visible break or crack in feeding tube	Clamp the tube between the damaged area and the stoma. Replace tube.
	Leaking from the feeding tube	Check and reinforce all connections.
	Burning or discomfort at stoma site	Avoid tension on feeding tube. Never use force to irrigate.

Box continues

BOX 22.9 (CONTINUED)

Complication	Symptoms	Intervention
Occlusion	Inability to infuse formula	Check flow control clamps. Check feeding tube for kinks or obstructions.
	Inability to irrigate feeding tube	Flush feeding tube with warm water as prescribed and before and after medications.
	Pump alarming occlusions	Check pump for malfunction. Secure the administration set to prevent kinks and accidental disconnection.
Tube dislodgement	Coughing, gagging, dyspnea, cyanosis	Assess location of distal tip of feeding tube before each feeding.
	Bloating, pain, or fullness	Elevate head of bed at least 30 degrees to avoid coughing and vomiting, which can dislodge tube.
	Leakage of formula around feeding tube	Secure feeding tube to prevent pulling or tension on stoma. Evaluate for infection or need for tube replacement.
Aspiration	Paroxysmal coughing, fever, chills, dyspnea, wheezing	Seek medical attention at a medical facility.

Mechanical—parenteral nutrition (PN)

Complication	Symptoms	Intervention
Clotting or blockage of catheter	Resistance or inability to infuse PN Unable to flush the catheter	Check that clamps are open. Assess need to declot catheter with tissue plasminogen activator.
Air embolism	Coughing, shortness of breath, chest pain	Clamp catheter immediately. Have patient lie on left side. Seek medical attention.
Thrombosis	Swelling of arm, shoulder, neck, or face accompanied by eye tearing or runny nose	Hold PN infusion. Seek immediate medical attention.
Catheter dislodgement	Pain or discomfort in neck or chest, especially when infusing	Hold PN infusion. Confirm catheter tip placement by x-ray. Seek medical attention.
Catheter breakage	Blood or fluids leaking from catheter	Clamp catheter between the patient and breakage. Pursue catheter repair or replacement.

Infectious—EN

Complication	Symptoms	Intervention
Local infection	Redness, swelling, tenderness at stoma site	Increase frequency of feeding tube changes. Obtain order for topical antibiotic treatment if indicated. Reinforce good handwashing practices.

Box continues

BOX 22.9 (CONTINUED)

Complication	Symptoms	Intervention
Feeding tube–related systemic sepsis	Fever, chills, malaise, diaphoresis	Seek medical attention at medical facility.

Infectious—PN

Complication	Symptoms	Intervention
Exit-site infection	Redness, swelling, tenderness, drainage at exit site	Contact managing physician for antibiotic treatment for catheter salvage.
Tunnel infection	Redness, swelling, tenderness along the catheter track	Remove and replace catheter. Prescribe intravenous (IV) antibiotics.
IV catheter systemic infection	Fever, chills, malaise, diaphoresis; leukocytosis; positive blood cultures	Stop PN infusion. Seek medical attention.

Metabolic—EN

Complication	Symptoms	Intervention
Diarrhea	Frequent loose, watery stools	Gradually increase feedings to goal rate. Use fiber-containing formula. Use antidiarrheals as appropriate. Decrease the amount of formula taken at one time. Use room-temperature formula. Consider lower-osmolality formula.
Constipation	Infrequent or hard stools, bloating, distension	Provide adequate water flushes. Use fiber-containing formula. Use stool softeners and laxatives as appropriate. Recommend exercise, if patient is able.
Vomiting and abdominal distension	Increased gastric residual, bloating, abdominal pain	Decrease flow rate or discontinue feeding. Reinitiate gradually. Administer antiemetics or antigas medications as appropriate.
Refeeding syndrome	Hypophosphatemia, hypokalemia, hypomagnesemia, shortness of breath, muscle spasms, pulmonary congestion	Initiate feeding gradually. Monitor serum electrolytes closely and replete as necessary. Gradually increase feedings to goal fluid requirement.

Metabolic—PN

Complication	Symptoms	Intervention
Hypoglycemia	Symptomatic low blood glucose	Increase to a 2-hour tapering down at end of cycle. Decrease insulin. Closely monitor blood glucose levels.
Hyperglycemia	Blood glucose >140 mg/dL	Rule out infection. Ensure dextrose content is not excessive. Administer insulin if required. Ensure accurate fluid volume delivery. Lengthen infusion period.

Box continues

BOX 22.9 (CONTINUED)

Complication	Symptoms	Intervention
Electrolyte abnormalities	Sodium, potassium, chloride, phosphorus, magnesium levels above or below laboratory reference ranges, with or without clinical symptomology	Identify and treat the underlying cause for increase or decrease of the electrolyte(s). Monitor intake and output. Replete or withhold individual electrolytes as indicated.
Dehydration (intra-vascular reduction of fluid volume)	Thirst, weight loss, and dry mucous membranes	Monitor intake and output. Assess and treat underlying cause. Replete fluids as indicated.
Fluid retention (intra-vascular or third spacing of fluids)	Weight gain or edema	Monitor intake and output. Assess and treat underlying cause. Withhold or reduce fluids as indicated.
Liver dysfunction	Elevated liver function test values or total bilirubin, jaundice, hepatomegaly	Avoid overfeeding beyond total energy. Keep soy lipid content <1 g/kg/d. Consider alternative intravenous lipid emulsion (ILE) containing less soybean oil. Cycle PN. Initiate oral or enteral feedings if possible.
Essential fatty acid deficiency	Dermatitis, alopecia	Provide a minimum of 500 mL 20% soybean oil ILE weekly to prevent deficiency.
Micronutrient deficiency or toxicity	Changes in skin, hair, or nails; altered taste; poor wound healing; anemia	Periodically monitor clinical symptoms and micronutrient levels. Adjust dose based on results.
Refeeding syndrome	Hypophosphatemia, hypokalemia, hypomagnesemia, shortness of breath, muscle spasms, pulmonary congestion	Initiate feeding gradually. Monitor serum electrolytes closely, and replete as necessary. Provide thiamin supplementation for the first 5 to 7 days of refeeding. Gradually increase to goal fluid requirement.

BOX 22.10

Monitoring Parameters for Home Parenteral and Enteral Nutrition[2,24]

Current weight and progress toward goal weight

Completion of pediatric growth charts

Vital signs and history of fever

Hydration status

Gastrointestinal, metabolic, or comorbid disease–related complications

Equipment and supply issues

Patient adherence to therapy

Medication changes

Tube and stoma site assessment or vascular access device assessment (redness, drainage, or tube patency)

Insurance changes

Quality-of-life measure—functional performance status

Ongoing Nutrition Assessment and Monitoring of Home Parenteral Nutrition

It is important to have a knowledgeable home care team that is multidisciplinary.[9] The RDN can provide initial and periodic follow-up nutrition assessment via phone, outpatient clinic visit, or home visit. Virtual visits using software for face-to-face evaluations are becoming more common. Assessment parameters in home care are similar to those in the acute care setting; however, there are a few unique considerations. In the home setting, patients should be assessed for physical activity, quality of life, bowel adaptation and the associated potential for transition to oral nutrition or EN, and the potential for complications related to long-term therapy (eg, liver dysfunction, metabolic bone disease, and micronutrient deficiency and toxicity). The RDN's assessment should evaluate the HPN consumer's ability to carry out essential activities of daily living, including physical activity, self-care and care for other family members, travel for medical reasons or pleasure, managing household chores or maintenance, and obtaining required medical treatments and procedures for treatment of the underlying disease. Self-care activities may include ostomy care, wound care, and administration of multiple oral or intravenous medications.

Follow-up assessments should be scheduled as needed in accordance with patient acuity, plan-of-care goals, frequency of laboratory testing (see Box 22.11),[23] and the individual's response to therapy (see Box 22.10). Formulation and supply needs should be reviewed regularly to help determine patient adherence to the therapy prescription and the need for additional education.

BOX 22.11

Laboratory Monitoring of Home Parenteral Nutrition Consumers[23]

Test	Monitoring frequency[a]
Electrolytes, blood glucose, potassium, chloride, bicarbonate, glucose, blood urea nitrogen (BUN), creatinine, calcium, phosphorus, magnesium	Weekly until stable, then monthly for 3 months, then every other month if stable
Complete blood count (CBC), platelets	Baseline; monthly for 3 months, then every other month
Triglycerides	Baseline; monthly for 3 months, then every other month if stable
Aspartate aminotransferase (AST), alanine aminotransferase (ALT), alkaline phosphatase (ALP), total bilirubin, prothrombin time (PT), international normalized ratio (INR)	Baseline; monthly for 3 months, then every 3 to 6 months
Albumin	Baseline; monthly for 3 months, then every 3 to 6 months
Vitamins, minerals, trace elements Carnitine (in pediatric patients)	Targeted measurement based on clinical signs and symptoms or ordering physician standard of care
Iron studies	Baseline, at 3 months, and then every 6 months or if clinical evidence suggests deficit or toxicity

[a] May be adapted to fit consumer's needs.

Micronutrient Monitoring in Home Parenteral Nutrition

Micronutrient assessment should be done every 6 to 12 months in patients on long-term HPN.[23] Trace elements can be adjusted in the PN formulation to address any deficiencies or toxicities. Factors to consider include the following[23]:

- deficiency or toxicity at start of care
- increased fluid losses due to fistula, high-output ostomy or diarrhea; or increased needs for wound healing, or chronic inflammation
- alterations in excretion as a result of liver failure or chronic kidney disease
- trace element contamination from individual PN components
- improvement in oral or enteral absorption, which may reduce the PN requirement

When changes are made to the micronutrient provision in the PN formulation, it is important to monitor the levels and associated clinical symptoms to ensure the change is appropriate and to avoid any unintended deficiency or toxicity states. For example, copper and manganese are excreted in the bile and can become elevated in patients with an elevated bilirubin level.

Tralement in Home Parenteral Nutrition

Tralement (produced by American Regent) is the first and only FDA-approved multiple trace element injection for PN.[25] It was approved by the FDA in July 2020 for use in adult and pediatric patients weighing more than 10 kg (22 lb) as a source of zinc, copper, selenium, and manganese for PN. Tralement aligns with dosage recommendations for trace element supplementation in adults (see Table 22.2).[25,26] It is free of preservatives, and the vial closure is not made with natural rubber latex.[25] It is stable for up to 9 days when added to the PN admixture and refrigerated.

The dose is 1 mL/d in patients weighing more than 50 kg (110 lb). One milliliter contains 3 mg zinc, 0.3 mg copper, 55 mcg manganese, and 60 mcg selenium.[25] American Regent's previous multiple trace element preparation, Multitrace-5 Concentrate, has been discontinued. Tralement is not an equivalent product to Multitrace-5 Concentrate.

TABLE 22.2 Comparison of ASPEN[a] Dosage Recommendations for Parenteral Trace Element Supplementation in Adults vs Tralement[25,26]

Trace element	ASPEN daily requirements for parental nutrition trace elements in adults	Tralement (1 mL)
Chromium	<10 mcg	0 mcg
Copper	0.3-0.5 mg	0.3 mg
Manganese	55 mcg	55 mcg
Selenium	60-100 mcg	60 mcg
Zinc	3-5 mg	3 mg

[a] ASPEN = American Society for Parenteral and Enteral Nutrition

Parenteral Nutrition Shortages in the Home Setting

Consumers on HPN can be vulnerable during a PN drug component shortage, as these individuals are not monitored as closely as hospitalized patients. The prescriber and home care company should work together to ensure consumer safety and conservation of the product.[2] Critical components should be reserved for pediatric consumers or high-risk adult consumers. It is good practice to assess and routinely reassess a patient's need for PN and the ability to use the oral or enteral route to meet nutrition needs whenever feasible. The home care provider must have a plan in place to communicate to consumers and clinicians when a shortage is resolved and it is appropriate to return to full dosing.[2,27] Resources for information on drug shortages are provided in Box 22.12.[2,24,27]

BOX 22.12

Resources for Information on Drug Shortages[2,24,27]

American Society for Parenteral and Enteral Nutrition

Guidelines for managing drug shortages

www.nutritioncare.org/PNResources/

US Food and Drug Administration

Drug shortage information

www.fda.gov/drugs/drug-safety-and-availability/drug-shortages

American Society of Health-System Pharmacists

Information on drug shortages and supply updates

www.ashp.org/Drug-shortages/Current-Shortages

Institute for Safe Medication Practices

For reporting medication errors

www.ISMP.org/report-error/merp

Ongoing Nutrition Assessment and Monitoring of Home Enteral Nutrition

Consumers on HEN generally require less frequent monitoring than HPN consumers. However, periodic follow-up should be completed to review the individual's response to therapy and evaluate whether nutrition goals are being met. Following are reasons why an HPN consumer may require more frequent monitoring:

- use of a jejunostomy tube
- use of a condition-specific formula
- significant malabsorptive disease
- risk for refeeding syndrome
- significant malnutrition
- evidence of a micronutrient deficiency
- glucose intolerance
- a history of complications requiring a hospital admission
- associated significant renal, cardiac, or pulmonary disease

Ongoing Education and Consumer Quality of Life

Ongoing education about disease process and therapy helps HPEN consumers maintain a desired quality of life, particularly if they are expected to require HPEN for years or for life. The education and support needs of HPEN consumers with chronic intestinal failure differ from those of short-term HPEN consumers. The burden of the underlying disease in individuals with chronic intestinal failure plays a primary role in determining quality of life while on HPEN.[28] In addition to the need for education to prevent potential long-term complications of HPEN therapy, long-term consumers face insurance coverage challenges and coping issues that differ from those of the short-term consumer.

Consumers and caregivers need to be trained to find social activities outside of mealtimes. They also need support to manage emotional needs, guilt, and social embarrassment that can come from dependence on long-term HPEN support. Assessing quality of life should be a part of routine care provided by clinicians (see Box 22.13).[2,29,30] The Oley Foundation provides support to HPEN consumers and caregivers. Their goal is "striving to enrich the lives of those living with home intravenous nutrition and tube feeding through education, advocacy and networking."

BOX 22.13

Factors Affecting
Qualify of
Life in Home
Parenteral and
Enteral Nutrition
Consumers[2,29,30]

Sleep disturbances

Frequent urination

Fear or anxiety related to complications of nutrition therapy

Management of a chronic medical condition along with nutrition therapy

Inability to eat

Change in spouse, family, friend, or work relationship roles

Effect on autonomy, self-esteem, socialization

Role of food in social situations

Use of food as a means of social and emotional coping

Frequency of central-line infections

Limitations from underlying disease state (particularly if gastrointestinal symptoms and diarrhea are present)

Transitioning Off Home Parenteral or Enteral Nutrition

Consumers should be transitioned off HPEN when they are able to tolerate at least 75% to 80% of oral or enteral (for HPN consumers) nutrition. Factors to consider when weaning someone from nutrition support include the following[31]:

- current GI anatomy, including length of remaining small bowel (resections of the proximal bowel are generally better tolerated than ileal resection); presence of residual disease in the remnant bowel; presence of ileocecal valve; and continuity of colon (because of its role in fluid and nutrient absorption)
- enteral intake vs output: intake should be at least 1 L/d greater than output
- urine output: should be greater than 1,000 mL/d
- weight: should be stable or near target
- goal of nutrition therapy: reduction vs complete elimination of PN and transition to oral or enteral nutrition

The potential for bowel adaptation and intestinal rehabilitation efforts should be assessed. The integrity and location of the remaining bowel is important to consider. Patients have better absorption with an intact ileum vs jejunum. Evaluation of weight, intake and output records, and laboratory data (including electrolytes and blood glucose levels) are also necessary to ensure adequate hydration during the transition process.[31] A multipronged approach is used in the weaning process, including diet, oral rehydration solutions, EN, and appropriate medications. For more in-depth discussion on short bowel syndrome, refer to Chapter 4.

Consumers can be weaned from HEN by gradually eliminating intermittent or bolus feedings or by decreasing the infusion period of a continuous feeding based on the patient's tolerance to oral intake. HPN can be reduced by decreasing the daily volume and energy content, or by reducing the number of infusion days as warranted by the individual's oral or enteral intake.

After a consumer has fully transitioned to a new form of nutrition, timely evaluation of their hydration (intake and output, and daily and weekly weights), electrolyte status (potassium, magnesium, and others that may require oral supplementation), and vitamin and mineral status (serum levels for those being specifically supplemented) should occur to determine tolerance.[32]

Therapy Nonadherence

Nonadherence in the home setting can be challenging. It can affect the consumer's ability to meet nutrition goals, lead to associated complications, and contribute to waste of health care resources (see Box 22.14).[2] Individuals may have difficulty adhering to HPEN for many reasons during the transition to a new nutrition regimen, all of which should be evaluated and addressed by the home care provider.[33] The consumer and caregiver should demonstrate a clear understanding of the path forward and potential resources that will be required. Home visits provide psychological support and can address technical issues that may be a barrier to therapy compliance.[30]

BOX 22.14

Therapy Nonadherence: Types, Reasons, and Indications[2]

Types of nonadherence

Intake of restricted foods

Medication nonadherence affecting home enteral nutrition (HEN) or home parenteral nutrition (HPN)

Missed HEN or HPN infusions

Refusal of blood draws for laboratory testing

Failure to show for appointments

Poor phone-call follow-up

Reasons for nonadherence

Anxiety or fear

Depression

Lack of support (health care team or emotional)

Inability to perform tasks (shopping, cooking)

Poor understanding (of new prescription or rationale)

Indications of nonadherence

Discrepancy in HPN bag counts

Excessive quantities of unused supplies

Unexpected abnormalities in laboratory tests

Excessive weight loss or gain

Failure to meet nutrition goals

Summary

HPEN provides nutrition support for patients whose GI dysfunction prevents sufficient intake of energy and nutrients from oral intake. For HPEN to succeed, clinicians must provide careful instruction to patients in the discharge and initiation stages, assist them to select an appropriate home care provider, and help them obtain reimbursement. Regular follow-up is needed to assess the nutritional and health status, quality of life, and risk for complications in the HPEN consumer. Individuals should be transitioned off HPEN whenever possible. Those who must remain on HPEN for the long term will require ongoing education and monitoring to ensure that their nutrition care plan remains adequate and appropriate.

References

1. Pironi L, Boeykens K, Bozzetti F, et al. ESPEN guideline on home parenteral nutrition. *Clinical Nutrition*. 2020;39(6):1645-1666.
2. Kumpf V. Challenges and obstacle of long-term home parenteral nutrition. *Nutr Clin Pract*. 2019;34(2):196-203.
3. Pironi L, Steiger E, Brandt C, et al. Home parenteral nutrition provision modalities for chronic intestinal failure in adult patients: an international survey. *Clinical Nutrition*. 2020;30(2):585-591.
4. Bankhead R, Boullata J, Brantley S, et al; A.S.P.E.N. Board of Directors. Enteral nutrition practice recommendations. *JPEN J Parenter Enteral Nutr*. 2009;33(2):122-167.
5. Kovacevich D, Corrigan M, Ross VM, McKeever L, Hall A, Braunschweig C. American Society for Parenteral and Enteral Nutrition guidelines for the selection and care of central venous access devices for adult home parenteral nutrition administration. *JPEN J Parenter Enteral Nutr*. 2019;43(1):15-31.
6. Dibb M, Lal S. Home parenteral nutrition: vascular access and related complications. *Nutr Clin Pract*. 2017;32(6):769-776.
7. Englert M. Components of a successful home enteral teaching program. *Support Line*. 2017;39(1):3-6.
8. Hall BT, Blaseg K, Wessel K, Englehart M. Home enteral nutrition complications: a nutrition support clinic experience. *Support Line*. 2017;39(1):7-11.
9. Anderson M. Management of adult home enteral nutrition. *Support Line*. 2018;40(5):16-22.
10. Martin K, Gardner G. Home enteral nutrition: updates, trends, and challenges. *Nutr Clin Pract*. 2017;32(6):712-721.
11. Epp L, Lammert L, Vallumsetla N, Hurt R, Mundi M. Use of blenderized tube feeding in adult and pediatric home enteral nutrition patients. *Nutr Clin Pract*. 2017;32(2):201-205.
12. Fessler T. Home tube feeding with blenderized foods. *Oley Lifeline Letter*. November/December 2014.
13. Johnson TW, Milton DL, Johnson K, et al. Comparison of microbial growth between commercial formula and blenderized food for tube feeding. *Nutr Clin Pract*. 2019;34(2)257-263.
14. Johnson T, Seegmiller S, Epp L, Mundi M. Addressing frequent issues of home enteral nutrition patients. *Nutr Clin Pract*. 2019;34(2):186-195.
15. Gramlich L, Ireton-Jones C, Miles J, Morrison M, Pontes-Arruda A. Essential fatty acid requirements and intravenous lipid emulsions. *JPEN J Parenter Enteral Nutr*. 2019;43(6):697-707.
16. Clinolipid. Baxter. Accessed September 4, 2020. www.baxter.com
17. SMOFlipid. Package insert. Fresenius Kabi; 2016. Accessed July 8, 2020. http://editor.fresenius-kabi.us/PIs/US-PH-Smoflipid-FK-451418-05-2016-PI.pdf
18. Omegaven. Fresenius Kabi. Accessed July 8, 2020. www.fresenius-kabi.com/us/
19. Parenteral nutrition. Article A58836. Centers for Medicare & Medicaid Services Medicare Coverage Database. September 5, 2020. Accessed November 3, 2021. www.cms.gov/medicare-coverage-database/view/article.aspx?articleid=58836
20. da Silva J, Seres D, Sabino K, Adams S, Berdahl G. ASPEN consensus recommendations for refeeding syndrome. *Nutr Clin Prac*. 2020;35(2):178-195.

21. McCray S, Rees Parrish C. Refeeding the malnourished patient: lessons learned. *Practical Gastroenterology*. September 2016:56-66.

22. Hamilton C, Austin T, Seidner D. Essential fatty acid deficiency in human adults during parenteral nutrition. *Nutr Clin Prac*. 2006;21(4):387-394.

23. Blaauw R, Osland E, Siriam K, Ali A, Allard J. Parenteral provision of micronutrients to adult patients: an expert consensus paper. *JPEN J Parenter Enteral Nutr*. 2019;43(1):S5-S23.

24. Schauer L, Kruse L, Corrigan M. Managing complications in adult home parenteral nutrition patients: an update. *Support Line*. 2019;42(3)4-13.

25. Tralement. Package insert. American Regent; 2020. Accessed February 15, 2021. https://americanregent .com/media/2998/tralement_prescribinginformation _commercialinsert_16jul2020.pdf

26. American Society for Parenteral and Enteral Nutrition. Appropriate dosing for parenteral nutrition: ASPEN recommendations. ASPEN. November 17, 2020. Accessed February 22, 2022. www.nutritioncare.org /uploadedFiles/Documents/Guidelines_and_Clinical _Resources/PN%20Dosing%201-Sheet-Final.pdf

27. American Society for Parenteral and Enteral Nutrition. Parenteral nutrition resources. ASPEN. Accessed September 8, 2020. www.nutritioncare.org/PNResources/

28. Baxter J, Fayers P, Bozzetti F, et al. An international study of the quality of life of adult patients treated with home parenteral nutrition. *Clinical Nutrition*. 2019;38(4):1788-1796.

29. Price J, Larsen S, Miller L, Smith H, Apps J, Weis Jo M. Clinical biopsychosocial reflection on coping with chronic illness and reliance upon nutrition support: an integrated healthcare approach. *Nutr Clin Pract*. 2019;34(2):220-225.

30. Jukic N, Gagliardi C, Fagnani D, Venturini C, Orlandoni P. Home enteral nutrition therapy: difficulties, satisfaction and support needs of caregivers assisting older patients. *Clin Nutr*. 2017;36(4):1062-1067.

31. Matarese L. Nutrition and fluid optimization for patients with short bowel syndrome. *JPEN J Parenter Enteral Nutr*. 2013;37(2):161-170.

32. Seidner D, Schwartz L, Winkler M, Jeejeebhoy K, Boullata J, Tappenden K. Increased intestinal absorption in the era of teduglutide and its impact on management strategies in patients with short bowel syndrome-associated intestinal failure. *JPEN J Parenter Enteral Nutr*. 2013;37(2):201-211.

33. Bond A, Teubner A, Willbraham L. A novel discharge pathway for patients with advanced cancer requiring home parenteral nutrition. *J Hum Nutr Diet*. 2019;32(4):492-500.

23

Drug–Nutrient Interactions With Gastrointestinal Drugs

Vanessa J. Kumpf, PharmD, BCNSP, FASPEN
Jane Gervasio, PharmD, BCNSP

KEY POINTS

- Drug–nutrient interactions are often underappreciated and pose a challenge to clinicians who care for patients who may be at risk.
- Nutrients have the potential to influence drug absorption and drug activity. Conversely, drugs have the potential to influence nutrient absorption and nutritional status.
- Such interactions can result in loss of medication activity, nutrient abnormalities, or other adverse effects. In some cases, the interaction may have a beneficial or intended therapeutic effect. When the potential for drug–nutrient interactions is recognized, it allows for appropriate interventions to improve patient outcomes.

Introduction

This chapter reviews several categories of gastrointestinal (GI) medications that can potentially interact with nutrients. Drug-nutrient interactions are often underappreciated and pose a challenge to clinicians who care for patients who may be at risk. Nutrients have the potential to influence drug absorption and drug activity.[1-3] Conversely, drugs have the potential to influence nutrient absorption and nutritional status. This chapter focuses on GI medications with the potential for drug–nutrient interactions that are considered clinically significant in that they have the potential to alter therapeutic response or compromise nutritional status. Some of these drug–nutrient interactions may have beneficial or intended therapeutic effects. Alternative therapies, including herbal supplements, are not included in this discussion. For each category of drug, we provide an overview of the potential for drug-nutrient interactions and offer recommendations for management of the interactions.

Antacids

The rate or extent of drug absorption (or both) may be altered by antacids because of their effects on GI transit time and because they bind or chelate to certain medications. Nutrients, at least theoretically, may be influenced in the same way. Antacids increase gastric pH, which may impair the absorption of nutrients requiring an acid environment, such as calcium and iron. Drugs in this category include aluminum-containing antacids (carbonate, hydroxide, phosphate), magnesium-containing antacids (carbonate, hydroxide, oxide, trisilicate), and sodium bicarbonate. A list of their potential nutrient interactions can be found in Box 23.1.[4]

Aluminum-containing antacids

Phosphate binding in the gastronintestinal tract leads to increased bone loss and increased urinary calcium loss. Hypophosphatemia may occur with prolonged administration or large doses of aluminum salts, especially in patients with inadequate dietary intake of phosphorus.

Magnesium-containing antacids

The laxative effect of magnesium-containing antacids can cause fluid and electrolyte imbalances.

Sodium bicarbonate

Urinary potassium losses are increased through physiologic effects on the kidneys.

Recommendations

Practitioners are recommended to administer antacids 1 to 2 hours apart from mineral supplements. Additionally, serum phosphate concentrations should be monitored in patients receiving chronic aluminum-containing antacid therapy.

Antidiarrheal Agents

The rate or extent of fluid and nutrient absorption (or both) may be altered by antidiarrheal agents because of effects on GI transit time. In patients with diarrhea caused by increased intestinal motility, antidiarrheal agents that slow intestinal transit time and increase contact time with the absorptive surface within the GI tract are expected to improve absorption of fluid and nutrients. Electrolyte losses, especially sodium, potassium, and magnesium, may be reduced with decreased stool output. The effect on electrolyte balance is difficult to predict because electrolyte losses can vary depending on the etiology, volume, and consistency of diarrhea. Drugs in this category include diphenoxylate, loperamide, and opium preparations (paregoric [camphorated opium tincture] and opium tincture deodorized). Diphenoxylate preparations are available in combination with atropine sulfate to reduce potential for abuse. The drug nutrient interactions of this combination are noted in Box 23.2.

BOX 23.2

Diphenoxylate Drug–Nutrient Interactions

Diphenoxylate plus atropine sulfate

Atropine sulfate can cause dryness of the mouth and thirst. This effect can be confused with dehydration and lead to excessive fluid intake. In patients with short bowel syndrome who are taking combination diphenoxylate and atropine sulfate for management of diarrhea, excessive intake of hypotonic or sugar-containing fluids can result in a paradoxical increase in stool output.

Recommendations

Experts recommend monitoring fluid and electrolyte balance in patients receiving antidiarrheal agents. Patients taking combination diphenoxylate and atropine sulfate should be provided with strategies for relieving dry mouth, such as gum chewing and proper dental hygiene.

Cathartics and Laxatives

All agents classified as cathartics or laxatives increase GI tract motility and reduce the time intestinal contents are in contact with the absorptive surface of the GI tract. Reduced absorption of drugs and nutrients may occur with rapid transit through the GI tract, although it is difficult to predict the exact effect. Drugs in this category include bulk-forming laxatives (malt soup extract, methylcellulose, psyllium hydrophilic mucilloid), stimulant laxatives (anthraquinone laxatives [senna preparations], bisacodyl, castor oil), hyperosmotic laxatives (glycerin, sorbitol), mineral oil, and saline laxatives. Box 23.3 lists the potential nutrient interactions for these medications.[5,6]

Recommendations

Bulk-Forming Laxatives

Some practitioners recommend at least a 3-hour separation period between drugs known to be bound by these agents and the bulk-forming laxative itself. This same separation period would be reasonable for vitamin and mineral supplements to avoid the potential for trapping nutrients within the gel matrix, although there are no studies documenting loss of vitamins and minerals with bulk-forming laxatives.

Stimulant Laxatives

Patients should use stimulant laxatives infrequently for self-care. Long-term use (eg, with chronic opiate use for pain management) should be under the supervision of a physician. Laxative use should be stopped or the dose or frequency reduced if stools are loose. Appropriate use and dosage adjustment of stimulant laxatives should limit adverse nutritional consequences. With long-standing laxative abuse, evaluation for systemic effects of malabsorption, protein-losing enteropathy, and colonic dysfunction may be appropriate.

Following are specific recommendations for bisacodyl:

- Tablets are enteric-coated, and the patient should not crush or chew them.
- Separate oral administration of bisacodyl from milk or antacid ingestion by at least 1 hour.

Mineral Oil

Practitioners should administer mineral oil on an empty stomach. Patients may use mineral oil without medical supervision for a maximum of 1 week.

Concomitant oral administration of mineral oil and fat-soluble multivitamins should be avoided when possible. Consider separating the administration of these agents by several hours to minimize the risk of interaction. Fat-soluble vitamin status should be monitored with chronic use of mineral oil over several months.

Saline Laxatives

Patients should limit use of saline laxatives to a single dose with infrequent intervals when used for self-care. Monitor appropriate serum electrolytes when multiple doses or frequent use of a saline laxative are ordered by the health care provider, and consider other laxative agents when frequent use or multiple doses are necessary.

BOX 23.3

Cathartic and Laxative Drug–Nutrient Interactions[5,6]

Bulk-forming laxatives

Chronic use of bulk-forming laxatives has been associated with reduced serum cholesterol concentrations. This is likely the result of cholesterol and bile acids being trapped within the gel matrix that is produced when bulk-forming laxatives mix with water. Substances trapped within the gel matrix are removed in the feces rather than absorbed.

Other nutrients present in the gastrointestinal (GI) tract could potentially be removed in the feces as well, although data for specific nutrient losses are lacking.

Stimulant laxatives

Electrolyte abnormalities—including hyponatremia, hypokalemia, and hypocalcemia—and malabsorption with protein-losing enteropathy may occur with chronic, long-term use of these drugs.

Hyperosmotic laxatives

Hyperosmotic laxatives are generally administered rectally and, as such, act low in the GI tract, where interference with nutrient absorption should be negligible.

If administered orally, reduced absorption of nutrients may occur because of rapid GI transit.

Infrequent use of hyperosmotic laxatives is unlikely to result in clinically relevant changes in nutrient absorption.

Mineral oil

Absorption of fat-soluble nutrients (vitamins A, D, E, K, and beta carotene) may be impaired with chronic use of mineral oil. Short-term, infrequent small doses are unlikely to have a clinically significant effect on fat-soluble vitamin status, although beta carotene serum concentrations may be reduced.[5]

Saline laxatives[6]

Electrolytes used in these laxatives can be absorbed and may result in serious, potentially life-threatening electrolyte abnormalities with excessive doses or prolonged periods of use.

Patients with poor renal function may be at increased risk of electrolyte abnormalities.

Hypermagnesemia can occur with magnesium-containing saline laxatives because approximately 15% to 20% of an orally administered dose is absorbed.

Hypertonic sodium phosphate laxatives can cause hyperphosphatemia with resultant hypocalcemia. The hypocalcemia results from precipitation of calcium-phosphate into soft tissue. Renal failure is a potential consequence of calcium-phosphate precipitation in the kidneys. Other systemic effects may also occur, depending on the tissues in which precipitation occurs.

Digestants

Agents classified as digestants provide pancreatic enzymes, primarily lipase with some amylase and protease, for the treatment of malabsorption resulting from pancreatic insufficiency. Enzyme replacement should improve absorption of fat-soluble vitamins when pancreatic insufficiency is the cause of malabsorption, when taken with food, and when the dose of enzymes is adequate. Drugs in this category include the following proprietary pancrelipase preparations: Creon (AbbVie, Inc), Enzadyne (Sterling Knight Pharmaceuticals LLC), Pancreaze (Vivus LLC), Pertzye (Digestive Care, Inc), Viokace (Aptalis Pharma, Inc), and Zenpep (Nestlé). See Chapter 8 for more information on pancreatic enzyme replacement therapy.

Antiemetics

Considerable nutrient depletion may occur when vomiting is frequent and prolonged because food intake and retention may be inadequate to meet nutritional requirements. Antiemetic agents, when effective, allow food to be retained for digestion and absorption. In addition, effective antiemetic therapy reduces the fluid and electrolyte losses associated with vomiting. Drugs in this category include antihistamines (dimenhydrinate, meclizine, prochlorperazine, trimethobenzamide), 5-HT$_3$ receptor antagonists (dolasetron, granisetron, ondansetron, palonosetron), and miscellaneous antiemetics (aprepitant, diphenidol, phenothiazine, promethazine, scopolamine). The potential nutrient interactions for these medications are listed in Box 23.4.[7,8]

Practitioners should monitor fluid and electrolyte balance in patients receiving antiemetic agents.

BOX 23.4

Antiemetic Drug–Nutrient Interactions[7,8]

Prochlorperazine and related drugs

Riboflavin excretion in the urine may be increased by drugs in the same class as prochlorperazine, including chlorpromazine and some tricyclic antidepressant drugs (eg, amitriptyline, imipramine). There are structural similarities between the phenothiazine ring and riboflavin that may be responsible for the interaction.[7,8]

Antiulcer Agents and Acid Suppressants

Drugs used to treat ulcers either suppress gastric acid production or reduce proteolytic enzyme (pepsin) production. Most antiulcer agents decrease gastric acid production.

Gastric acid plays an important role in the solubility of minerals, activation of proteolytic enzymes, and release of nutrients from foods. Drugs causing suppression of gastric acid may result in poor release of nutrients from food and thereby result in impaired nutrient absorption.

Minerals including calcium, magnesium, and iron are primarily absorbed in the proximal small bowel where there is an acidic environment. Solubility of these minerals decreases as pH increases, resulting in reduced absorption. Although the influence of altered acidity on dietary calcium absorption is unclear, its influence on iron absorption is well documented.

The more effective a drug is in suppressing gastric acid production, and the longer the duration of use, the greater the risk of drug–nutrient interactions resulting in clinically significant nutrient malabsorption. Drugs in this category include histamine H$_2$ antagonists (cimetidine, famotidine, nizatidine, ranitidine), proton pump inhibitors (esomeprazole, lansoprazole, omeprazole, pantoprazole, rabeprazole) and protectants (sucralfate [aluminum sucrose sulfate]). Antiulcer agents and acid suppressants that pose a risk for drug-nutrient interactions are listed in Box 23.5.[4,9-21]

BOX 23.5

Antiulcer Agent and Acid Suppressant Drug–Nutrient Interactions[4,9-21]

Histamine H$_2$ antagonists

Agents in this category suppress gastric acid production. Drug–nutrient interactions reported for one drug in this class are likely to be similar for all the drugs when the interaction results from reduced gastric acidity.

Vitamin B12 in foods is protein-bound and requires the acid milieu of the stomach for dissociation. Malabsorption of vitamin B12 from foods has been reported in patients receiving cimetidine, while absorption of unbound cobalamin from vitamin B12 supplements does not appear to be altered.[9-11] In a large, adult, community-based population, use of a histamine H$_2$ antagonist or proton pump inhibitor (PPI) for 2 years or more increased the risk of developing vitamin B12 deficiency (odds ratio, 1.25; 95% confidence interval, 1.17–1.34).[12]

Zinc absorption may be reduced after cimetidine administration, most likely as the result of reduced gastric acidity.[13] It is likely this interaction could occur with all H$_2$ antagonists.

Proton pump inhibitors (PPIs)

PPIs suppress gastric acid production. Drug–nutrient interactions reported for one PPI are likely to be similar for all PPIs when the interaction results from reduced gastric acidity.

Vitamin B12 absorption may be reduced with PPI therapy.[14-17] As noted for long-term use of H$_2$ antagonists, use of any PPI for 2 years or more increased the risk of vitamin B12 deficiency in a large, adult, community-based population. The effect of PPIs was greater than for histamine H$_2$ antagonists (odds ratio, 1.65 vs 1.25), and higher doses were associated with vitamin B12 deficiency to a greater extent than lower doses.[12]

Beta carotene (vitamin A) absorption seems to be reduced with omeprazole therapy. The results of a small study suggest that beta carotene absorption may be significantly reduced with relatively short-term (7 days) use of omeprazole at standard doses (20 mg, twice daily). All PPIs would likely have similar effects.[18]

Hypomagnesemia has been reported in patients receiving PPI therapy. Case reports describe severe hypomagnesemia with secondary hypoparathyroidism and severe hypomagnesemia with secondary hypocalcemic seizures following long-term PPI use.[19,20] Daily PPI use was associated with significantly lower serum magnesium concentrations and an increased risk of hypomagnesemia compared with no PPI use in a large group of hospitalized adult patients.[21]

Protectants

Protectants form a barrier between gastric acid and tissue. In addition, pepsin is inhibited.

The aluminum content of sucralfate (aluminum sucrose sulfate) is expected to cause the same interaction with phosphorus and calcium as noted with aluminum-containing antacids.[4] Phosphate binding in the gastrointestinal tract leads to increased bone loss and increased urinary calcium loss.

Recommendations

Histamine H$_2$ Antagonists and Proton Pump Inhibitors

Calcium citrate solubility is less dependent on an acid environment than other calcium salts; therefore, calcium citrate may be a better choice for a calcium supplement when a gastric acid–suppressing agent is used.

Practitioners should monitor serum vitamin B12 concentrations in patients receiving long-term gastric acid–suppressing medications. Unexplained macrocytosis or macrocytic anemia in these individuals should prompt testing for vitamin B12 deficiency. Routine use of a vitamin B12 supplement is recommended for patients aged 50 years and older who are taking gastric acid–suppressing medications.

Magnesium and iron may be better absorbed if taken with an acidic juice. Consider obtaining baseline and periodic serum magnesium concentrations when prolonged PPI administration is expected or when patients are receiving other medication capable of causing hypomagnesemia. If hypomagnesemia occurs, magnesium supplementation and PPI discontinuation may be required.

Protectants (Sucralfate)

Administer sucralfate 2 hours before or after drugs and mineral supplements known to bind to sucralfate. Risk factors for osteoporosis should be considered in patients receiving sucralfate for the long term, and bone density monitored accordingly.

Prokinetic Agents

Prokinetic agents stimulate upper GI motility and can potentially alter the absorption of nutrients by increasing the rate of transit through the stomach and small bowel. When used to treat nausea and vomiting, they may improve tolerance to dietary intake. Drugs in this category include metoclopramide and erythromycin. Prokinetic agents with the potential for drug–nutrient interactions are listed in Box 23.6.[22-25]

BOX 23.6

Prokinetic Agent Drug–Nutrient Interactions[22-25]

Metoclopramide

Fluid and sodium retention secondary to transient elevations in plasma aldosterone concentrations can occur. Plasma aldosterone concentrations appear to return to pretreatment levels with prolonged use.[22]

Erythromycin

The rate of gastric emptying is increased by erythromycin through effects on motilin. A relatively small dose is required for this effect, compared to the typical dose for effective antibiotic therapy.

Dose-related nausea, diarrhea, and anorexia are frequently reported, which may contribute to reduced dietary intake.

Reductions in commensal gastrointestinal (GI) flora, such as acidophilus and bifidobacteria, may occur. The commensal GI flora produce substantial quantities of several B vitamins and vitamin K, and this may be altered in patients receiving antibiotic therapy.[23-25]

Recommendations

Practitioners should use metoclopramide with caution in patients at risk for volume overload, such as those with cirrhosis or congestive heart failure. Patients who are taking erythromycin should be monitored for worsening GI symptoms, such as nausea, diarrhea, or anorexia. Consider the use of a probiotic in patients taking erythromycin.

Anti-Inflammatory Agents

Agents used to suppress inflammation in the GI tract are primarily aimed at control of inflammatory bowel disease. Sulfasalazine is a prodrug of 5-aminosalicylic acid (5-ASA) linked to sulfapyridine and is associated with a risk of folate depletion. Its potential for drug–nutrient interactions is described in Box 23.7.[26,27]

BOX 23.7

Sulfasalazine Drug–Nutrient Interactions[26,27]

Sulfasalazine inhibits folate transport and inhibits the pathway for conversion to active folate.[26,27] This effect can cause folate depletion and contribute to the megaloblastic anemia associated with sulfasalazine therapy.

Iron binds with sulfasalazine in the gastronintestinal tract and may decrease absorption of both.

Nausea, vomiting, and anorexia are frequently reported with sulfasalazine, which may contribute to reduced dietary intake.

Recommendations

Experts recommend 1 mg per day of folate for patients on sulfasalazine. During pregnancy, the recommended dose increases to 2 mg per day. Folate status should be monitored in patients taking sulfasalazine.

Experts recommend separating doses of iron by 2 hours before or after sulfasalazine administration. Consider the same for other 5-ASA agents, including mesalamine, olsalazine, and balsalazide.

Lipid-Regulating Drugs

Lipid-regulating drugs work within the GI tract to regulate lipid levels in the body and to treat bile acid malabsorption. Drugs in this category include cholestryramine, colestipol, colesevelam, and ezetimibe. The potential nutrient interactions for these medications are listed in Box 23.8 (see page 430).[28-31]

Recommendations

Cholestyramine and Colestipol

Periodic assessment of fat-soluble vitamins status is recommended with long-term use of cholestyramine and colestipol, including vitamin A, E, and D serum concentrations and international normalized ratio for assessment of vitamin K functional status. Supplementation of water-miscible (or parenteral) fat-soluble vitamins A, D, E, and K may be necessary in patients receiving long-term therapy. Parenteral administration of vitamin K may be appropriate for bleeding due to hypoprothrombinemia associated with vitamin K deficiency.

Monitor patients for folate deficiency and consider supplementation with folate, 5 mg per day, especially in children and patients otherwise at risk of folate deficiency. Administer dietary supplements at least 1 hour before or 4 to 6 hours after administration of cholestyramine or colestipol to minimize the risk of impaired absorption.

Colesevelam

Patients at risk for fat-soluble vitamin deficiency should be monitored for potential decline in vitamin status with long-term use of colesevelam.

Miscellaneous Gastrointestinal Drugs

Various other GI drugs have the potential for drug–nutrient interactions, including orlistat and teduglutide. Details are provided in Box 23.9.[32-35]

Recommendations

Orlistat

It is recommended to use a multivitamin containing the fat-soluble vitamins and to separate vitamin administration by 2 hours before or after the orlistat dose. Nonprescription forms of orlistat are intended for short-term use and, as such, should carry minimal risk of clinically significant vitamin deficiencies unless there are other risk factors for deficiency. Consider monitoring fat-soluble vitamin status in any patient using orlistat routinely for more than a few weeks.

Teduglutide

Monitor urine output, weight, BUN, serum creatinine, and serum electrolytes and minerals weekly upon initiation of teduglutide therapy. Monitor all concomitant oral medications for increased clinical response or evidence of toxicity, especially those with a narrow therapeutic index.[36]

Practitioners should consider the following with regard to parenteral nutrition and teduglutide[36]:

- Decrease overall parenteral fluid intake by increments of 10% to 20% if urine output exceeds baseline by 10% to 20%.
- Reduce parenteral energy intake by increments of 10% to 20% if body weight exceeds target weight.
- Reduce parenteral electrolyte or mineral intake and transition to oral supplementation as appropriate, based on serum electrolyte monitoring.
- Incorporate oral multivitamin supplementation when parenteral nutrition frequency is less than daily.

Summary

It is important for clinicians to recognize the potential for drug–nutrient interactions. Such interactions can result in the loss of medication activity, nutrient abnormalities, or other adverse effects. In some cases, the interaction may have a beneficial or intended therapeutic effect. When the potential for drug–nutrient interactions is recognized, it allows for appropriate interventions to improve patient outcomes.

References

1. American Society of Health-System Pharmacists. *AHFS Drug Information 2020*. American Society of Health-System Pharmacists; 2020.
2. Micromedex (electronic version). IBM Watson Health. Accessed February 20, 2021. www.micromedexsolutions.com
3. Boullata, JI, Armenti VT. *Handbook of Drug–Nutrient Interactions*. 2nd ed. Humana Press; 2010.
4. Spencer H, Lender M. Adverse effects of aluminum-containing antacids on mineral metabolism. *Gastroenterology*. 1979;76(3):603-606.
5. Clark JH, Russell GJ, Fitzgerald JK, Nagamori KE. Serum beta-carotene, retinol, and alpha-tocopherol levels during mineral oil therapy for constipation. *Am J Dis Child*. 1987;141(11):1210-1212. doi:10.1001/archpedi.1987.04460110080028

6. Xing JH, Soffer EE. Adverse effects of laxatives. *Dis Colon Rectum*. 2001;44(8):1201-1209. doi:10.1007/BF02234645

7. Pinto J, Huang YP, Pelliccione N, Rivlin RS. Cardiac sensitivity to the inhibitory effects of chlorpromazine, imipramine and amitriptyline upon formation of flavins. *Biochem Pharmacol*. 1982;31(21):3495-3499. doi:10.1016/0006-2952(82)90632-3

8. Bell IR, Edman JS, Morrow FD, et al. Brief communication: vitamin B1, B2, and B6 augmentation of tricyclic antidepressant treatment in geriatric depression with cognitive dysfunction. *J Am Coll Nutr*. 1992;11:159-163.

9. Streeter AM, Goulston KJ, Bathur FA, Hilmer RS, Crane GG, Pheils MT. Cimetidine and malabsorption of cobalamin. *Dig Dis Sci*. 1982;27(1):13-16. doi:10.1007/BF01308115

10. Steinberg WM, King CE, Toskes PP. Malabsorption of protein-bound cobalamin but not unbound cobalamin during cimetidine administration. *Dig Dis Sci*. 1980;25(3):188-191. doi:10.1007/BF01308137

11. Salom IL, Silvis SE, Doscherholmen A. Effect of cimetidine on the absorption of vitamin B12. *Scand J Gastroenterol*. 1982;17(1):129-131. doi:10.3109/00365528209181056

12. Lam JR, Schneider JL, Zhoa W, et al. Proton pump inhibitor and histamine 2 receptor antagonist use and vitamin B-12 deficiency. *JAMA*. 2013;310(22):2435-2442. doi:10.1001/jama.2013.280490

13. Sturniolo GC, Montino MC, Rossetto L, et al. Inhibition of gastric acid secretion reduces zinc absorption in man. *Am J Coll Nutr*. 1991;10(4):372-375. doi:10.1080/07315724.1991.10718165

14. Bradford GS, Taylor CT. Omeprazole and vitamin B12 deficiency. *Ann Pharmacother*. 1999;33(5):641-643.

15. Marcuard SP, Albernaz L, Khazanie PG. Omeprazole therapy causes malabsorption of cyanocobalamin (vitamin B12). *Ann Intern Med*. 1994;120(3):211-215. doi:10.7326/0003-4819-120-3-199402010-00006

16. King CE, Leibach J, Toskes PP. Clinically significant vitamin B12 deficiency secondary to malabsorption of protein-bound vitamin B12. *Dig Dis Sci*. 1979;24(5):397-402. doi:10.1007/BF01297127

17. Schenk BE, Festen HP, Kuipers EJ, Klinkenberg-Knol EC, Meuwissen SG. Effect of short-and long-term treatment with omeprazole on the absorption and serum levels of cobalamine. *Aliment Pharmacol Ther*. 1996;10(4):541-545. doi:10.1046/j.1365-2036.1996.27169000

18. Tang G, Serfaty-Lacrosniere C, Camilo ME, Russell RM. Gastric acidity influences the blood response to a beta-carotene dose in humans. *Am J Clin Nutr*. 1996;64:622-626.

19. Kuipers MT, Thang HD, Arntzenius AB. Hypomagnesaemia due to use of proton pump-inhibitors—a review. *Neth J Med* 2009;67(5):169-172.

20. Cundy T, Dissanayake A. Severe hypomagnesaemia in long-term users of proton-pump inhibitors. *Clin Endocrinol (Oxf)*. 2008;69(2):338-341. doi:10.1111/j.1365-2265.2008.03194

21. Gau JT, Yang YX, Chen R, Kao TC. Uses of proton pump inhibitors and hypomagnesemia. *Pharmacoepidemiol Drug Saf*. 2012;21(5):553-559. doi:10.1002/pds.3224

22. Brown RD, Wisgerhof M, Jiang N, Kao P, Hegstad R. Effect of metoclopramide on the secretion and metabolism of aldosterone in man. *J Clin Endocrinol Metab*. 1981;52(5):1014-1018. doi:10.1210/jcem-52-5-1014

23. Cummings JH, Macfarlane G. Role of intestinal bacteria in nutrient metabolism. *JPEN J Parenter Enteral Nutr*. 1997;21(6):357-366.

24. Deguchi Y, Takashi M, Masahiko M. Comparative studies on synthesis of water-soluble vitamins among human species of bifidobacteria. *Agric Biol Chem*. 1985;49(1):13-19. doi:10.1080/00021369.1985.10866683

25. Hill MJ. Intestinal flora and endogenous vitamin synthesis. *Eur J Cancer Prev*. 1997;6(suppl 1):S43-S45.

26. Sulfasalazine inhibits folate absorption. *Nutr Rev*. 1988;46:320-323. doi:10.1111/j.1753-4887.1988.tb05472.x

27. Jansen G, van der Heijden J, Oerlemans R, et al. Sulfasalazine is a potent inhibitor of the reduced folate carrier: implications for combination therapies with methotrexate in rheumatoid arthritis. *Arthritis Rheum*. 2004;50(7):2130-2139. doi:10.1002/art.20375

28. West RJ, Lloyd JK. The effect of cholestyramine on intestinal absorption. *Gut*. 1975;16(2):93-98. doi:10.1136/gut.16.2.93

29. Watkins DW, Khalafi R, Cassidy MM, Vahouny GV. Alterations in calcium, magnesium, iron, and zinc metabolism by dietary cholestyramine. *Dig Dis Sci*. 1985;30(5):477-482. doi:10.1007/BF01318182

30. Schwartz KB, Goldstein PD, Witztum JL, Schonfeld G. Fat-soluble vitamin concentrations in hypercholesterolemic children treated with colestipol. *Pediatrics*. 1980;65(2):243-250. doi:10.1542/peds.65.2.243

31. Tonstad S, Sivertsen M, Aksnes L, Ose L. Low dose colestipol in adolescents with familial hypercholesterolaemia. *Arch Dis Child*. 1996;74:157-160.

32. Zhi J, Melia AT, Koss-Twardy SG, Arora S, Patel IH. The effect of orlistat, an inhibitor of dietary fat absorption, on the pharmacokinetics of beta-carotene in healthy volunteers. *J Clin Pharmacol*. 1996;36(2):152-159. doi:10.1002/j.1552-4604.1996.tb04180.x

33. Finer N, James WP, Kopelman PG, Lean ME, Williams G. One-year treatment of obesity: a randomized, double-blind, placebo-controlled, multicenter study of orlistat, a gastrointestinal lipase inhibitor. *Int J Obes Relat Metab Disord*. 2000;24(3):306-313. doi:10.1038/sj.ijo.0801128

34. Jeppesen PB, Gilroy R, Pertkiewicz M, et al. Randomised placebo-controlled trial of teduglutide in reducing parenteral nutrition and/or intravenous fluid requirements in patients with short bowel syndrome. *Gut*. 2011;60(7):902-914. doi:10.1136/gut.2010.218271

35. Jeppesen PB, Pertkiewicz M, Messing B, et al. Teduglutide reduces need for parenteral support among patients with short bowel syndrome with intestinal failure. *Gastroenterology* 2012;143(6):1473-1481. doi:10.1053/j.gastro.2012.09.007

36. Seidner DL, Schwartz LK, Winkler MF, Jeejeebhoy K, Boullata JI, Tappenden KA. Increased intestinal absorption in the era of teduglutide and its impact on management strategies in patients with short bowel syndrome-associated intestinal failure. *JPEN J Parenter Enteral Nutr*. 2013;37(2):201-211. doi:10.1177/0148607112472906

CHAPTER

24

Nutraceutical Supplements

Alyssa M. Parian, MD
Berkeley Limketkai, MD, PhD
Gerard E. Mullin, MD, AGAF, FACG, FACN

KEY POINTS

- Approximately 50% of patients with digestive disorders in the United States use dietary supplements, also known as nutraceutical agents.
- Herbal agents have been well studied for their efficacy and potential toxicity in people with gastrointestinal conditions. Traditional Chinese medicines have been used for centuries in the Far East as first-line agents for gastrointestinal and other ailments; however, many carry a higher risk for potential toxicity.
- Natural anti-inflammatory products, such as *Boswellia serrata*, turmeric, ginger, fish oils, and vitamin D3, have all shown benefit in limited clinical trials for gastrointestinal inflammatory conditions. STW 5 and enteric-coated peppermint oil have been shown in multiple studies to improve symptom control in patients with irritable bowel syndrome.

Introduction

Nutraceutical supplements are products that are derived from food sources and used with the intent to provide a health benefit.[1] Use in patients with gastrointestinal (GI) disorders is widespread and continues to grow. The Council for Responsible Nutrition's 2021 Consumer Survey on Dietary Supplements found that 80% of Americans consumed dietary supplements, whereas a 2013 analysis of data from the National Health and Nutrition Examination Survey found that approximately 50% of Americans reported using supplements (based on 24-hour recall data).[2,3] A 2012 survey of individuals with a diagnosed GI condition in the past year found that 42% (5,629) of the 13,505 respondents used complementary and alternative medicine (CAM) in the past year, with herbals and dietary supplements being the most common modality. Of those using CAM to address a GI condition, more than 80% felt that it was helpful.[4] A 2017 review article estimated that 50% of patients with digestive disorders use nutraceutical supplements.[5] In the pediatric population, the use of CAM modalities appears to be high as well. In a 2019 study, CAM use for pediatric inflammatory bowel disease was as high as 84%.[6] With more than 90 million Americans diagnosed with a GI condition—and with many of these patients seeking expert advice from a registered dietitian nutritionist (RDN) about which supplements have the most potential to address their symptoms effectively—it is imperative that nutrition and health practitioners familiarize themselves with the evidence surrounding nutraceutical supplement use.

The vast majority of research for supplements used for GI and liver diseases has been conducted for only a small number of conditions—namely, irritable bowel syndrome (IBS), inflammatory bowel disease (IBD), and chronic liver disease. Further controlled clinical trials of the potential efficacy of natural supplementation in these and other GI and liver disorders are needed.

The most commonly used nutraceutical supplements today are discussed in this chapter. The list of supplements covered here is by no means a comprehensive one. Given the increased use of immune-modulating dietary supplements during the COVID-19 pandemic, the potential impact of nutraceuticals used for digestive diseases on COVID-19 is also included when pertinent.

Use of Supplements in Digestive Health and Disease

Although the nutraceutical supplement industry is growing in Europe, use of nutraceuticals for all digestive indications is seemingly more common in North America. The most popular form of alternative medicine for GI disorders is herbal therapy.[7] In patients with digestive disorders, nutraceutical use is most prevalent among those with IBD and IBS,[8] possibly because these disorders are chronic and refractory in nature.

Considering the widespread use of nutraceutical supplements among patients with GI and liver disorders, physicians and RDNs should become familiar with the potential benefits and risks of these products.[9] For example, many herbs have the potential for hepatotoxicity (see Box 24.1 on page 435).[10] Recent years have seen a growing number of accounts of hepatotoxicity from herbals and increased reporting of dietary supplement toxicity to poison control centers.[11,12] Hepatotoxicity is typically dose dependent, and some herbal preparations may have idiosyncratic reactions. Thus, it is imperative for RDNs to ask their clients about the use of potentially hepatotoxic products during nutrition assessments.

Herbal Therapies

Traditional Chinese Medicine

The Chinese literature contains numerous reports of the treatment of digestive and liver disease with herbal remedies; however, only the abstracts for these articles are available in English. In the treatment of IBD, studies have demonstrated that traditional Chinese medicine (TCM) was more effective than both placebo and conventional medical therapy for IBD.[13,14]

For liver disease, controlled studies using the TCM herbal preparation TJ-9 for chronic hepatitis C have established anti-inflammatory effects[15,16] and antifibrotic effects.[17] TCM is very popular among patients with IBS, and there is emerging evidence for its use in functional bowel diseases.[18] Tong xie yao fang (TXYF), a TCM prepared from four herbs, has been shown to be effective for the diarrhea subtype of IBS (IBS-D).[19,20] TXYF has been shown to help rebalance serotonin, mast cell mediators, and gut microbial ecology in patients with IBS-D.[20,21] Furthermore, TXYF has been shown to impart mucosal healing properties in animal models of IBS-D and even IBD.[22,23]

Some TCM products have been contaminated with heavy metals.[24] Clinicians should warn patients to exercise caution when pursuing TCM therapies that are not verified by an independent third party (such as the United States Pharmacopeia, indicated as USP on the product label).

Aloe vera

In patients with moderately active ulcerative colitis, 10 mL of oral *Aloe vera* gel twice a day for 4 weeks proved to have a higher clinical response than placebo in a randomized, double-blind, controlled study (47% vs 14%, P<.05).[25] *Aloe vera* gel has been shown to protect against dextran-induced colitis in animal models.[26] Although *Aloe vera* is used by many for peptic ulcers, Crohn's disease, and gastroesophageal reflux disease (GERD), there is a paucity of evidence for its effectiveness from randomized controlled trials in the literature.[27] For GERD, only one randomized controlled trial, involving 79 participants, demonstrated efficacy: when administered in a syrup containing 50 mg plant polysaccharide per day for 4 weeks, *Aloe vera* was safe and well tolerated, and it reduced the frequency of GERD symptoms; its efficacy was no different from 20 mg omeprazole or 150 mg ranitidine twice a day, with no adverse events requiring withdrawal.[28]

BOX 24.1

Herbal Preparations With Potential for Hepatotoxicity[10]

Herb	Type of liver injury
Atractylis gummifera	Acute hepatitis, fulminant liver failure
Callilepis laureola	Acute hepatitis, fulminant liver failure
Camphor	Necrolytic hepatitis
Cascara sagrada	Cholestatic hepatitis
Chaparral leaf, germander	Zone 3 necrosis, cirrhosis, cholestasis, chronic hepatitis
Crotalaria, heliotrope, *Senecio longilobus*, *Symphytum officinale* (pyrrolizidine alkaloids)	Sinusoidal obstruction syndrome (veno-occlusive disease)
Germander	Acute and chronic hepatitis, fulminant liver failure
Greater celandine	Chronic hepatitis, cholestasis, fibrosis
Impila	Acute hepatitis, fulminant liver failure
Isabgol	Giant cell hepatitis
Jin bu huan	Acute and chronic cholestatic hepatitis, microvesicular steatosis, fibrosis
Kava kava	Acute and chronic hepatitis, fulminant liver failure
Ma huang	Acute hepatitis, autoimmune hepatitis
Mistletoe	Chronic hepatitis
Margosa oil	Microvesicular steatosis, Reye syndrome, hepatic necrosis
Oil of cloves	Hepatic necrosis
Paeonia spp	Acute hepatitis, fulminant liver failure
Pennyroyal (squamit) oil	Zone 3 necrosis, microvesicular steatosis, fulminant liver failure
Sassafras	Hepatocarcinogen
Saw palmetto	Mild hepatitis
Shou-wu-pian	Acute hepatitis
TJ-8, Dai-saiko-to	Autoimmune hepatitis
TJ-9, Sho-saiko-to	Acute and chronic hepatitis
Usnic acid	Fulminant liver failure
Valerian	Mild hepatitis

The National Institute of Integrative Medicine in Australia conducted an open-label trial of a nutraceutical blend containing *Aloe vera*, curcumin, pectin, peppermint oil, slippery elm, and glutamine at a dose of 10 g/d for 4 weeks in 43 patients with functional GI symptoms.[29] Overall, over 3 months, the blend significantly improved GI symptoms and associated quality of life in patients while reducing intestinal permeability, improving the microbial profile, reducing the need for reflux medication, and enabling the consumption of previous food triggers.

Glycyrrhizin (Licorice Root)

Glycyrrhiza glabra (licorice root) has been used for centuries in traditional medicine to treat cough, bronchitis, gastritis, and liver inflammation. In the United States, it is available over the counter in liquid, powder, and pill forms.

A large number of components have been isolated from licorice; glycyrrhizic acid (glycyrrhizin) is the main biologically active component. Glycyrrhizin has antioxidant, immunosuppressive, and anti-inflammatory properties. It also enhances interferon production and stimulates the activity of natural killer cells.[30]

Clinical trials using intravenous glycyrrhizin have specifically involved the treatment of hepatitis C in patients who are refractory to or intolerant of interferon treatment.[31] Very few studies have shown enhanced antiviral effects with glycyrrhizin.

A comparative study found that oral licorice in combination with famotidine therapy could heal ulcers in rats as effectively as an H_2 blocker.[32] Glycyrrhizin has antiulcer properties through increased local concentration of prostaglandins that promote mucous secretion and cell proliferation in the stomach.[33]

Several studies have confirmed that licorice root has activity against *Helicobacter pylori*.[34] However, there is a paucity of clinical evidence to support its use for this purpose in clinical practice. In one randomized controlled trial, 107 patients with *H pylori* were evaluated for the efficacy of 150 mg glycyrrhizin daily vs placebo for 60 days to clear gastric infection as confirmed by the resolution of the presence of stool antigen.[35] On day 60, the results of *H pylori* stool antigen were negative in 28 (56%) of the patients treated with glycyrrhizin, whereas only 2 patients (4%) treated with placebo showed clearance of *H pylori*; the difference between the groups was statistically significant.[34] Despite the lack of evidence, many individuals with GERD use licorice root as first-line treatment.

The main side effects of glycyrrhizin treatment are fluid retention, hypernatremia, and hypokalemia due to its mineralocorticoid effect, which can lead to hypertension and provoke underlying cardiac events in some individuals.[36,37] Licorice root should be avoided in patients with cirrhosis, chronic liver disease, and congestive heart failure who are prone to fluid retention. Additionally, licorice root is contraindicated in pregnancy.

Silymarin (Milk Thistle)

Silymarin is the active ingredient extracted from *Silybum marianum* (also known as milk thistle) used by ancient physicians and herbalists to treat a variety of liver and gallbladder diseases. The main effects of silymarin are its membrane-stabilizing and antioxidant effects. It can help with liver cell regeneration, and it can decrease the inflammatory reaction and inhibit the fibrogenesis in the liver. These results support the administration of silymarin preparations in the treatment of chronic liver disease.

A large number of animal studies have reported that silymarin offers hepatoprotection against a diverse range of toxins, including acetaminophen, carbon tetrachloride, mushroom poisoning (phalloidin), radiation, iron overload, phenylhydrazine, alcohol, cold ischemia, and thioacetamide.[38] Silymarin works as an antioxidant by reducing free radical production, protecting against lipid peroxidation, stabilizing cell membranes, providing antifibrotic properties, and inhibiting nuclear factor κB (NF-κB) activation with favorable immuno-modulatory effects.[39,40]

In the United States, silymarin is one of the most commonly used CAM agents in the treatment of liver disease, in part because of its favorable safety profile. A 2018 systematic review concluded that the use of silymarin is reasonable as a supportive element in the therapy of *Amanita phalloides* poisoning and treatment of chronic liver disease.[41] Controlled trials of silymarin and, separately, the herbal preparation Liv-52 continue to explore the potential use of these hepatoprotective herbals in patients with alcoholic liver disease and noncirrhotic nonalcoholic steatohepatitis.[42,43]

Silymarin has been found to exhibit antiviral activities against several viruses, including the flaviviruses (hepatitis C virus and dengue virus), togaviruses (chikungunya virus and Mayaro virus), influenza virus, HIV, and hepatitis B virus.[44] Silymarin has the potential to be used as a therapeutic modality for viral hepatitis.[45-47]

Polyphenols

Polyphenols (a group of phytochemicals in food) are nonessential nutrients, which means that the possibility of polyphenol deficiency has not been identified in research. However, researchers have found polyphenols to be potentially immune-modulating and theorize that they may play a biologically active role.[48] Polyphenols modify immunity and inflammation, downregulate inflammatory mediators, inhibit transcription of NF-κB, and are prebiotic (ie, they help friendly bacteria thrive).

In studies of various polyphenols for their efficacy in treating colitis in animals, prophylactic and therapeutic effects were observed with resveratrol, epigallocatechin, curcumin, and quercetin, although quercetin was deemed the least effective.[48] Clinical studies of polyphenol use in the treatment of IBD in humans have been limited primarily to *Boswellia serrata* and *Curcuma longa*.

Boswellia serrata

The immune-modulating properties of *B serrata* (frankincense, a traditional Ayurvedic remedy and incense component) have been studied for their effect on IBD.[49] The mechanism of action is possibly related to a reduction in inflammatory cytokines as well as a reduction in leukotriene synthesis by way of the inhibition of 5-lipoxygenase (the key enzyme of leukotriene biosynthesis).[50] The preliminary results of a pilot trial conducted in India comparing the efficacy of gum resin from *B serrata* (350 mg three times daily) with sulfasalazine (1 g three times daily) for 6 weeks in moderately active ulcerative colitis found the remission rates in the *B serrata* group comparable to those for patients given conventional therapy (82% vs 75%, respectively); however, few details were made available.[50] In 2001, a randomized controlled trial version of this pilot trial was published that included 30 patients with active distal ulcerative colitis and showed an improvement in the rate of remission among the *B serrata* group, with a 70% remission rate in the 20 patients who took *B serrata* for 6 weeks and a remission rate of 40% in the 10 patients who took sulfasalazine.[51]

Another study compared the efficacy of the *B serrata* extract with mesalamine in treating active Crohn's disease. That 8-week, double-blind, randomized controlled trial, which was powered to show noninferiority, included 102 patients.[52] As in previous trials with 5-aminosalicylic acid (mesalamine) preparations, decreases in the mean Crohn's disease activity index were measured in both groups, and *B serrata* was well tolerated.[53,54]

A novel delivery system of *B serrata* (brand name Casperome) was tested in patients with ulcerative colitis in remission. After 4 weeks, there was a decrease in abdominal pain, blood in the stool, diarrhea, fatigue, anemia, and fecal calprotectin.[55] *B serrata* is also undergoing evaluation for its potential benefit for microscopic and collagenous colitis.[56] One study found a symptomatic benefit at dosages of 400 mg three times a day, over placebo (64% vs 44%, P=.04) for the treatment of active collagenous colitis over a 6-week period, although there was no change in the colonic histology.

Curcuma longa (Turmeric)

In vitro studies have demonstrated multiple immunomodulatory and anti-inflammatory properties in curcumin, the yellow pigment of turmeric (*Curcuma longa*), a key ingredient in curry powder.[57-60] When taken orally, curcumin benefited four of five patients with Crohn's disease and five of five patients with ulcerative proctitis in an uncontrolled trial.[61] The first study of curcumin's potential role in ulcerative colitis maintenance was a randomized, multicenter, double-blind, placebo-controlled trial conducted in Japan that included 89 patients with quiescent ulcerative colitis on 3 g mesalamine maintenance therapy.[62] Oral curcumin, 2 g/d, for 6 months decreased symptoms, incidence of flares, and endoscopic index scores compared to placebo. The results demonstrated that curcumin, when taken with mesalamine medication, maintained remission better than mesalamine alone. A double-blind, randomized controlled trial involving 50 participants with mild to moderate active ulcerative colitis in whom maximal mesalamine oral and enema therapy were unsuccessful, showed that 3 g curcumin taken orally (n=26) in combination with optimized mesalamine resulted in a 54% clinical remission rate in those with refractory mild to moderate disease compared to 0% in the placebo-plus-mesalamine arm (n=24) (P=.01).[63] Low-dose curcumin (450 mg/d) was ineffective in treating mild to moderate ulcerative colitis[64]; however, curcumin enemas yielded better clinical outcomes and improvement on endoscopy.[65] Another study assessed the efficacy and safety of a novel, hydrophilic, bioenhanced curcumin (n=34), as add-on therapy to standard mesalamine at 50 mg/d, vs placebo (n=35) in inducing clinical and endoscopic remission in patients with mild to moderately active ulcerative colitis. Clinical response at 6 weeks was significantly higher in the bioenhanced curcumin group (18 of 34 patients, or 52.9%) compared with placebo (5 of 35 patients, or 14.3%) (P=.001). Thus, curcumin is emerging as a "rising star" in the digestive health supplement industry.[66] A systematic review and meta-analysis by authors in Brazil confirm promising results for the use of curcumin as adjunctive therapy in IBD, but small sample sizes and publication bias are drawbacks.[67]

Curcumin is an important polyphenol to consider for SARS-CoV-2, the virus that causes COVID-19. Curcumin can exert its anti-inflammatory role mainly by preventing the activation of NLRP3 inflammasomes in COVID-19 and have antiviral activities.[68-70] Curcumin downregulates NF-κB signaling, interrupts interleukin-1β maturation, and reduces the secretion and release of interleukins. Collectively, these actions are the most prominent mechanisms of curcumin in modulating inflammasomes.[68] A 2020 review of phytochemicals and their influence on intracellular signaling mechanisms of action on NLRP3 inflammasome activation focused on sulforaphane, curcumin, and resveratrol.[69]

Curcumin also has known antiviral properties against HIV, herpes simplex virus, human papillomavirus, influenza virus, Zika virus, hepatitis viruses, and adenovirus, and potentially SARS-CoV-2.[71] SARS-CoV-2 is believed to gain access to human cells through angiotensin-converting enzyme 2 membrane receptors. Curcumin has been shown to bind to the same area, effectively creating an antagonizing effect and prohibiting SARS-CoV-2 from entering human cells.[71] These theories remain hypothetical through cellular work and have not yet been tested in human studies.

Cannabis sativa (Marijuana)

Cannabis sativa, commonly referred to as marijuana, is a Schedule I drug, making it illegal at the federal level; however, individual state laws are increasingly legalizing its use. Patient interest continues to grow in the use of marijuana for the treatment of multiple chronic illnesses, including IBD.

The most pharmacologically active ingredient in the plant *C sativa* is Δ-9-tetrahydrocannabinol, commonly known as THC, which acts on cannabinoid 1 and 2 receptors (CB1 and CB2) in the endocannabinoid system. Naturally produced endogenous cannabinoids (2-arachidonoylethanolamine and 2-arachidonoylgylcerol) bind with differing affinities to CB1 and CB2.

Although *C sativa* may have applications in a diverse spectrum of digestive disorders having chronic pain, poor quality of life, and disability in common, the most well-studied applications to date are for treatment of IBD.[72] In IBD, medical marijuana has the potential to improve control of pain, nausea, and anorexia, and may have anti-inflammatory properties.[73] Several studies have confirmed symptomatic improvement with *C sativa* use,[74] but objective data on endoscopic improvement is lacking. Younger patients and those with chronic abdominal pain were more likely to use marijuana.

A 2020 systematic review evaluated the safety and efficacy of *C sativa* in IBD. The review included five randomized controlled trials—three Crohn's disease studies and two ulcerative colitis studies—for a total of 185 participants.[75] Adverse events were more prevalent in the *C sativa* groups for both the Crohn's disease and ulcerative colitis studies. A Grading of Recommendations Assessment, Development, and Evaluation (GRADE) analysis of the studies found them to range in quality from very low to moderate. The authors of the review were unable to draw conclusions about the safety or effectiveness of *C sativa* and cannabinoids in adults with Crohn's disease and ulcerative colitis. The safety profile of marijuana is not well documented, but some associated adverse effects have been described. Neuropsychological side effects seem to be the most common and include anxiety, panic, and psychosis.

Emerging research suggests that nonpsychoactive phytocannabinoids, including cannabidiol, may be useful in the treatment of disorders and diseases of the GI tract such as IBD and IBS.[76]

Peppermint Oil

Peppermint oil has been evaluated in patients with IBS and was found to be beneficial in symptom relief.[77] The presumed mechanism of action is via calcium channel blockade—mediated smooth-muscle relaxation. There have been several systematic reviews, all showing positive benefit for adequate relief of abdominal pain, global IBS symptoms, and quality of life.[77,78] The number of patients needed to be treated by peppermint oil to achieve benefit is only two (ie, number need to treat [NNT]=2), whereas the prescription-strength antispasmodic hyoscyamine has an NNT of 8.[79]

STW 5 is a German-derived multiherb combination sold under the brand name Iberogast (Bayer) for gut rescue from dyspepsia and IBS that features peppermint oil as a main ingredient. A study involving 208 patients demonstrated the efficacy in IBS of using the herbal preparations STW 5 and STW 5-II.[80] STW 5 contains nine herbs: candytuft, chamomile, peppermint, caraway, licorice root, lemon balm, celandine, milk thistle, and angelica. STW 5-II contains six herbs: candytuft, chamomile, peppermint, caraway, licorice root, and lemon balm. Both formulations contain peppermint oil and chamomile, which act by relaxing intestinal smooth muscle.

Several studies have shown that STW 5 was superior to placebo for nonulcer dyspepsia.[81] STW 5 has evidence to support its use to improve functional dyspepsia and functional heartburn that are recalcitrant to proton pump inhibitors and even neuromodulators.[82] Clinicians are beginning to use STW 5 as an adjunctive treatment for gastroparesis, as evidence is emerging for its use as a prokinetic.[83]

Fish Oils

A wide range of health benefits from consuming essential omega-3 fatty acids—namely, the prevention and treatment of a multitude of diseases—has been supported in the literature.[84] Fish oil is abundant in omega-3 polyunsaturated fatty acids (PUFAs). Long-chain omega-3 PUFAs include eicosapentaenoic acid (EPA) and docosahexaenoic acid (DHA), which are found mainly in fatty fish. Short-chain omega-3 PUFAs, such as α-linolenic acid, are abundant in walnuts, chia seeds, and flax seeds, but they are a poor source of DHA and EPA as its conversion from α-linolenic acid is inefficient in humans and may be age-dependent.[85]

PUFAs have anti-inflammatory and immunoregulatory properties, both in the gut and systemically.[86] EFA downregulates the cyclooxygenase (COX) pathway (primarily COX-2) and inhibits the 5-lipoxygenase pathway, resulting in diminished proinflammatory leukotriene B_4.[87] EPA and DHA are substrates for the formation of novel protective mediators, termed *resolvins*, produced for termination of neutrophil infiltration, stimulation of the clearance of apoptotic cells by macrophages, and promotion of tissue remodeling and homeostasis.[88] A number of autoimmune diseases have been linked to the incomplete resolution of inflammatory byproducts, thus a deficiency of EPA or DHA could promote chronic inflammation on this basis.[89] Thus, the theory has advanced that relapse treatment or prevention for chronic inflammatory diseases could potentially benefit from omega-3 fatty acid supplementation.

In vivo and in vitro studies of omega-3 fatty acids in mice models have demonstrated effective prevention and treatment of colitis.[90,91] A dose of up to 3 g per day of EPA plus DHA has been determined to be safe for general consumption.[86,92]

Seven randomized controlled trials with a small overall number of study participants showed that fish oil induced remission in patients with active ulcerative colitis.[93-100] However, based on a Cochrane systematic review and a meta-analyses review, fish oils cannot be recommended as the only therapy for maintenance of ulcerative colitis.[100,101]

Three Cochrane meta-analyses have explored the potential efficacy of omega-3 PUFAs for the maintenance of remission in Crohn's disease.[100,102,103] The most recent (2014) was updated to include the two trials of Epanova (a proprietary prescription formulation of omega-3 carboxylic acids), whose outcomes were different from the four randomized controlled trials included in the previous version of the review. The primary outcome for the 2014 pooled meta-analysis was relapse at 12 months; six studies were included for a total of 1,039 participants.[102] Of patients in the omega-3 PUFA group, 39% relapsed at 12 months, compared with 47% of patients in the placebo group (relative risk, 0.77; 95% confidence interval, 0.61–0.98). The GRADE analysis rated the quality of the evidence as very low due to unexplained high heterogeneity (I^2=58%), publication bias, and a high or unknown risk of bias for randomization and concealed allocation in the four randomized controlled trials that preceded the Epanova trials.[104-107] Despite the confusing and contradictory data, there is very little downside to recommending fish oils to patients with Crohn's disease to be used in conjunction with medical therapy.

Other Nutraceuticals

Vitamin D

Vitamin D is a versatile, fat-soluble hormone that regulates calcium homeostasis, and research shows it plays a role in immune modulation, cell growth, and intercellular adhesion. Vitamin D, once converted to the active 1,25-dihydroxyvitamin D form, has endocrine and paracrine properties. The paracrine action of 1,25-dihydroxyvitamin D may be most important for immunity. Activated vitamin D augments innate cellular immunity against microbes, protects against bacterial and viral acute respiratory tract infections (including influenza), and regulates adaptive immune responses, such as those seen in the COVID-19–associated cytokine storm.[108,109] Vitamin D influences T-helper cell (Th) differentiation by its effect on antigen-presenting cells. Vitamin D is involved in antigen-presenting cell activity that modulates Th-cell differentiation into an effector cell with proinflammatory (Th1) or anti-inflammatory (Th2) properties; thus, modulation of antigen-presenting cells is crucial in initiating and maintaining adaptive immune response and self-tolerance. Vitamin D modulates adaptive immunity by suppressing Th1 and Th17 responses that are overactivated.[110,111] Vitamin D induces Th2 cytokines, such as interleukin-10, which counterbalance Th1 proinflammatory cytokines while increasing regulatory T cells (Tregs) and their activity.[112] By inducing Tregs and increasing their numbers, vitamin D harmonizes inflammatory responses that are uncontrolled in chronic IBD. In COVID-19, Th1 and Th17 cytokines are reportedly high, Th2 cytokines are reportedly low, and Tregs are reportedly low in number and dysfunctional in the setting of a cytokine storm.[113,114]

The highest prevalence of IBD is found in northern climates, including North America and northern Europe, where vitamin D from sunlight exposure is more limited than in southern regions.[115,116] Vitamin D deficiency is common in patients with a number of digestive disorders that are characterized by intestinal malabsorption of fat-soluble vitamins as well as in patients with chronic liver disease.[117] Its deficiency in chronic inflammatory diseases, such as IBD, has been linked to intestinal dysbiosis, decreased bone density, inflammation, and disease severity.

Patients with IBD, especially Crohn's disease, are known to have lower levels of vitamin D than the general population, and the reason for this is believed to be multifactorial: the deficit may be due to malabsorption from ongoing inflammation or surgical resection, low intake resulting from concomitant lactose intolerance, and sun avoidance secondary to disease severity or medication interactions.[118] A large cohort study on a subset of patients with IBD showed a lower incidence of Crohn's disease in participants with a higher predicted vitamin D level.[119] Low vitamin D levels have been associated with higher disease activity in both forms of IBD. Patients with Crohn's disease appear to have fewer flares and improved diseases activity scores with vitamin D supplementation.

A large prospective study of 3,217 patients (55% with Crohn's disease) supplemented patients with vitamin D to sufficient levels (30–50 ng/mL) and showed that normalization of plasma 25-hydroxyvitamin D levels was associated with a reduction in Crohn's disease-related surgery.[120] A subsequent double-blind, randomized controlled trial in Denmark assessed the relapse rate in 94 patients with Crohn's disease who were supplemented daily with 1,200 IU of vitamin D3 or placebo for 12 months.[121] Although the investigators showed a decrease in the rate of relapse among the vitamin D contingent compared to the placebo group (13% vs 29%), the difference was not statistically significant ($P=.06$). A different team of investigators from Denmark subsequently found that higher doses of vitamin D3 (10,000 IUs daily) (n=18) given to patients with Crohn's disease in remission decreased clinical relapse rates when compared to 1,000 IU daily (n=16) (0% vs 37.0%, $P=.049$).[122]

Although low levels of vitamin D have been epidemiologically linked to the development and higher activity of IBD, studies have yet to show firm causality proving vitamin D is an effective treatment for IBD. Low vitamin D levels may simply be a marker for more severe disease or truly render vulnerability. Randomized, prospective studies are needed to better evaluate the efficacy of vitamin D as an immunomodulatory agent. However, recent evidence suggests that vitamin D may be working in concert with the gut microbiota to modulate mucosal immunity in patients with IBD.[72] Because the risk of osteoporosis and vitamin D deficiency is higher in patients with IBD, every patient should be tested for 25-hydroxyvitamin D levels.[123] We know vitamin D is important for calcium absorption and in bone health; therefore, supplementation to adequate levels (>30 ng/mL) is recommended in all patients with IBD.

Zinc

Zinc is an essential micronutrient and functions as a coenzyme important for growth and development, protein and collagen synthesis, and wound healing. It is a micronutrient with an established role in robust and effective immune responses, including antiviral immunity and adaptive immune responses, such as antibody formation.[124] Older adults (65 years and older) are at increased risk of zinc deficiency. Zinc is important in the normal functioning of innate immune mediating cells, specifically macrophages and natural killer cells.[125] Patients with chronic diarrhea or malabsorptive disorders, including IBD, are frequently found to have low zinc levels.[126] There is a high incidence of diarrhea with SARS-CoV2 infection (seen in approximately 20% of patients), and these patients appear to be acutely zinc deficient.[127]

Preclinical data as well as human studies suggest that zinc deficiency may contribute to mucosal inflammation in patients with IBD.[128] In addition to the impact of zinc on immune function, studies involving both animal models of colitis and patients with Crohn's disease have demonstrated improvement in mucosal permeability with zinc supplementation.[129,130]

The Dietary Reference Intake for zinc is 8 mg/d for females and 11 mg/d for males.* Zinc sulphate in a dose of 220 mg orally (which contains 50 mg of elemental zinc) taken twice a day has been used as a standard adult oral replacement dose in patients with moderately low zinc levels. High levels of zinc can impede absorption of iron and copper, eventually leading to deficiency, which can masquerade as a progressive neurodegenerative process.[131] Thus, longer-term use of zinc should be monitored with regular serum zinc and copper levels.

Supplements for Inflammatory Bowel Disease

Many other nutraceutical supplements have been studied for the treatment of IBD, both Crohn's disease and ulcerative colitis, with some encouraging early data from both animal and human studies. Box 24.2 on pages 443 to 445 outlines herbal therapies that have limited data to date on efficacy but show some promise for the future.[132-156]

---

* Specific recommendations for transgender people were not provided.

BOX 24.2

Other Dietary Supplements for the Treatment of Inflammatory Bowel Disease[132-156]

Glutamine

Mechanism of action	Small amino acid that becomes essential in catabolic conditions, the main energy source for small intestinal enterocytes and an intracellular antioxidant
Evidence in treatment of inflammatory bowel disease (IBD)	Mice deficient in glutamine develop intestinal atrophy and increased gut permeability.[132] Patients who are critically ill on parental nutrition supplemented with glutamine had improved gut permeability and prevented intestinal atrophy.[133]
Side effects	When in excess in the colon: oxidative tissue injury and possible worsening colitis
Recommendation	Glutamine is not recommended for treatment of IBD.[134]

Aloe vera

Mechanism of action	Inhibits the production of reactive oxygen metabolites, eicosanoids, interleukin-6 (IL-6), and interleukin-8 (IL-8)[135]
Evidence in treatment of inflammatory bowel disease (IBD)	A randomized, double-blind trial in 44 patients with ulcerative colitis found 100 mg of oral *Aloe vera* gel improved clinical and histologic disease activity over placebo.[136]
Side effects	Diarrhea
Recommendation	It may have benefit in ulcerative colitis, has not been studied in Crohn's disease, and is not regulated by the US Food and Drug Administration.[137]

Andrographis paniculata (HMPL-004)

Mechanism of action	Decreases release of proinflammatory mediators such as nitric oxide, IL-6, prostaglandin E2, and leukotriene B4
Evidence in treatment of inflammatory bowel disease (IBD)	A paniculata inhibited colitis in rodent models.[138] At 1,200 mg/d, it was equivalent to mesalamine in clinical and endoscopy response and remission in 125 patients with ulcerative colitis.[139] Dosages of 1,800 mg/d had a higher rate of clinical response vs placebo in 224 patients with ulcerative colitis.[140]
Side effects	Possible loss of appetite, nausea, diarrhea, headache, elevation of liver enzymes
Recommendation	More studies of efficacy and toxicities are needed.

Box continues

BOX 24.2 (CONTINUED)

Artemisia absinthium (wormwood)

Mechanism of action	Suppresses tumor necrosis factor β (TNF-β) and other inflammation interleukins[141]
Evidence in treatment of inflammatory bowel disease (IBD)	Patients with Crohn's disease (n = 40) had higher rates of steroid reduction while on 1,500 mg/d vs placebo. Patients with Crohn's disease (n = 20) given 2,250 mg/d had decreased disease activity scores, serum TNF-α, and mood scores vs placebo.[141]
Side effects	Potential for neurotoxicity and seizures at very high dose
Recommendation	More studies are needed.

Tripterygium wilfordii

Mechanism of action	Traditional Chinese drug with anti-inflammatory, immune-modulating, and antiproliferative properties
Evidence in treatment of inflammatory bowel disease (IBD)	Patients with active Crohn's disease (n = 20) had a decrease in disease activity, endoscopic inflammation, and C-reactive protein (CRP).[142]
Side effects	Unknown
Recommendation	More studies are needed.

Mastic gum

Mechanism of action	Produced by trees endemic to Greek island of Chios; contains antioxidant substances, TNF-α inhibitor, and migration inhibitory factor stimulator
Evidence in treatment of inflammatory bowel disease (IBD)	Mastic gum significantly decreased Crohn's disease activity scores and plasma levels of IL-6 and CRP. Treatment of patients with Crohn's disease with mastic gum resulted in a reduction in TNF-α secretion.[143]
Side effects	Unknown
Recommendation	More studies are needed.

Box continues

BOX 24.2 (CONTINUED)

Triticum aestivum (wheat grass)

Mechanism of action	Antioxidant properties due to free-radical scavenging, and anti-inflammatory properties[144]
Evidence in treatment of inflammatory bowel disease (IBD)	Patients with ulcerative colitis (n = 23) had significant reduction in disease activity and rectal bleeding on 100 mL wheat grass juice vs placebo.[145]
Side effects	Nausea, constipation, mold contamination
Recommendation	More studies are needed.[146]

Xilei-san (XLS)

Mechanism of action	Mixture of eight natural Chinese herbs and minerals with anti-inflammatory effects
Evidence in treatment of inflammatory bowel disease (IBD)	Animal studies found decreased colitis when given XLS enemas.[147] Human studies found suppositories (0.1 g/d) given to 30 patients with ulcerative colitis proctitis resulted in improved clinical and endoscopic outcomes vs placebo.[148] Patients with ulcerative colitis proctitis (n = 35) treated with XLS enemas had equivalent response to treatment with dexamethasone, clinically and endoscopically.[149]
Side effects	No major side effects
Recommendation	It may be considered as an alternative or adjuvant therapy for ulcerative proctitis.[144]

Indigo naturalis (Qing-Dai)

Mechanism of action	Aryl hydrocarbon receptor ligand that induces interleukin-22 and promotes mucosal regeneration[150] Suppresses colinic oxidative stress and T helper 1 (Th1) and Th17 responses in mice with chemical colitis[151]
Evidence in treatment of inflammatory bowel disease (IBD)	Of 86 patients with active ulcerative colitis, those treated with *Indigo naturalis* had a five to six times higher clinical response rate, an eight to 12 times higher clinical remission rate, and a three to four times higher mucosal healing rate.[152]
Side effects	Elevated liver enzymes[153] Possible pulmonary arterial hypertension[154]
Recommendation	Further evaluation of side effects is needed.[155,156]

Summary

Many patients with digestive diseases try nutraceutical supplements to achieve better control of their illness. There is an abundance of clinical research demonstrating the efficacy of nutraceutical supplements in IBD and IBS. The mechanisms of action of these supplements include the downregulation of the inflammatory response, rebalancing the intestinal flora, and restoring proper gut immunity. TCM has been shown in limited trials to be effective, but study design and lack of reporting on toxicity are concerning. For IBD, *C longa*, *B serrata*, and fish oils have evidence, in some cases, noninferior to standard medical therapy in well-designed randomized controlled trials. For IBS, peppermint oil has been shown in several studies and a meta-analysis to be superior to placebo. In chronic liver disease, the use of silymarin and Liv-52 may provide benefit and has no known adverse effects.

Clinical trials are needed to explore the potential efficacy of natural approaches in combination with conventional therapy to achieve better outcomes in digestive disorders. Lastly, further education of physicians, RDNs, and other health care professionals about the potential risks and benefits of nutraceutical supplements is essential if we are to give well-informed advice to patients who are considering or already using alternative therapies for GI and liver diseases.

References

1. Kalra EK. Nutraceutical—definition and introduction. *AAPS PharmSci*. 2003; 5(3):E25. doi:10.1208/ps050325
2. Bailey RL, Gahche JJ, Miller PE, Thomas PR, Dwyer JT. Why US adults use dietary supplements. *JAMA Intern Med*. 2013;173(5):355-361.
3. Council for Responsible Nutrition. 2021 CRN consumer survey on dietary supplements. Accessed March 11, 2022. www.crnusa.org/2021survey
4. Dossett ML, Davis RB, Lembo AJ, Yeh GY. Complementary and alternative medicine use by US adults with gastrointestinal conditions: results from the 2012 National Health Interview Survey. *Am J Gastroenterol*. 2014;109(11):1705-1711.
5. Korzenik J, Koch AK, Langhorst J. Complementary and integrative gastroenterology. *Med Clin North Am*. 2017;101(5):943-954.
6. Phatak UP, Alper A, Pashankar DS. Complementary and alternative medicine use in children with inflammatory bowel disease. *J Pediatr Gastroenterol Nutr*. 2019;68(2):157-160.
7. Anheyer D, Frawley J, Koch AK, et al. Herbal medicines for gastrointestinal disorders in children and adolescents: a systematic review. *Pediatrics*. 2017;139(6):e20170062.
8. Salem AE, Singh R, Ayoub YK, Khairy AM, Mullin GE. The gut microbiome and irritable bowel syndrome: state of art review. *Arab J Gastroenterol*. 2018;19(3):136-141.
9. Korotkaya Y, Conner K, Lau J, et al. Use of dietary supplements in pediatric liver disease and transplantation. *J Pediatr Gastroenterol Nutr*. 2021;72(1):e10-e14. doi:10.1097/MPG.0000000000002922
10. Lee JY, Jun SA, Hong SS, Ahn YC, Lee DS, Son CG. Systematic review of adverse effects from herbal drugs reported in randomized controlled trials. *Phytother Res*. 2016;30(9):1412-1419.
11. Roytman MM, Poerzgen P, Navarro V. Botanicals and hepatotoxicity. *Clin Pharmacol Ther*. 2018;104(3):458-469.
12. Rao N, Spiller HA, Hodges NL, et al. An increase in dietary supplement exposures reported to US Poison Control Centers. *J Med Toxicol*. 2017;13(3):227-237.
13. Shang HX, Wang AQ, Bao CH, et al. Moxibustion combined with acupuncture increases tight junction protein expression in Crohn's disease patients. *World J Gastroenterol*. 2015;21(16):4986-4996.
14. Kou FS, Shi L, Li JX, et al. Clinical evaluation of traditional Chinese medicine on mild active ulcerative colitis: a multi-center, randomized, double-blind, controlled trial. *Medicine (Baltimore)*. 2020;99(35):e21903.

15. Kusunose M, Qiu B, Cui T, et al. Effect of Sho-saiko-to extract on hepatic inflammation and fibrosis in dimethylnitrosamine induced liver injury rats. *Biol Pharm Bull.* 2002;25(11):1417-1421.

16. Stickel F, Brinkhaus B, Krahmer N, Seitz HK, Hahn EG, Schuppan D. Antifibrotic properties of botanicals in chronic liver disease. *Hepatogastroenterology.* 2002;49(46):1102-1108.

17. Sakaida I, Hironaka K, Kimura T, Terai S, Yamasaki T, Okita K. Herbal medicine Sho-saiko-to (TJ-9) increases expression matrix metalloproteinases (MMPs) with reduced expression of tissue inhibitor of metalloproteinases (TIMPs) in rat stellate cell. *Life Sci.* 2004;74(18):2251-2263.

18. Ling W, Li Y, Jiang W, Sui Y, Zhao HL. Common mechanism of pathogenesis in gastrointestinal diseases implied by consistent efficacy of single Chinese medicine formula: a PRISMA-compliant systematic review and meta-analysis. *Medicine (Baltimore).* 2015;94(27):e1111.

19. Li YL, Yao CJ, Lei R, et al. Acupuncture combined with Tong-xie-yao-fang for diarrhea-type irritable bowel syndrome: a protocol for meta-analysis. *Medicine (Baltimore).* 2020;99(48):e23457.

20. Vitta S, Sayuk GS. Editorial: Tong-Xie-Yao-Fang (TXYF) for irritable bowel syndrome with diarrhoea (IBS-D)—ancient medicine meets modern study. *Aliment Pharmacol Ther.* 2018;48(4):485-486.

21. Ma X, Wang X, Kang N, et al. The effect of Tong-Xie-Yao-Fang on intestinal mucosal mast cells in postinfectious irritable bowel syndrome rats. *Evid Based Complement Alternat Med.* 2017;2017:9086034.

22. Gong SS, Fan YH, Wang SY, et al. Mucosa repair mechanisms of Tong-Xie-Yao-Fang mediated by CRH-R2 in murine, dextran sulfate sodium-induced colitis. *World J Gastroenterol.* 2018;24(16):1766-1778.

23. Hou Q, Huang Y, Zhu Z, et al. Tong-Xie-Yao-Fang improves intestinal permeability in diarrhoea-predominant irritable bowel syndrome rats by inhibiting the NF-κB and notch signalling pathways. *BMC Complement Altern Med.* 2019;19(1):337.

24. Liu R, Li X, Huang N, Fan M, Sun R. Toxicity of traditional Chinese medicine herbal and mineral products. *Adv Pharmacol.* 2020;87:301-346.

25. Langmead L, Feakins RM, Goldthorpe S, et al. Randomized, double-blind, placebo-controlled trial of oral *Aloe vera* gel for active ulcerative colitis. *Aliment Pharmacol Ther.* 2004;19(7):739-747.

26. Hassanshahi N, Masoumi SJ, Mehrabani D, Hashemi SS, Zare M. The healing effect of *Aloe vera* gel on acetic acid-induced ulcerative colitis in rat. *Middle East J Dig Dis.* 2020;12(3):154-161.

27. Sadoyu S, Rungruang C, Wattanavijitkul T, Sawangjit R, Thakkinstian A, Chaiyakunapruk N. *Aloe vera* and health outcomes: an umbrella review of systematic reviews and meta-analyses. *Phytother Res.* 2021;35(2):555-576.

28. Panahi Y, Khedmat H, Valizadegan G, Mohtashami R, Sahebkar A. Efficacy and safety of *Aloe vera* syrup for the treatment of gastroesophageal reflux disease: a pilot randomized positive-controlled trial. *J Tradit Chin Med.* 2015;35(6):632-636.

29. Ried K, Travica N, Dorairaj R, Sali A. Herbal formula improves upper and lower gastrointestinal symptoms and gut health in Australian adults with digestive disorders. *Nutr Res.* 2020;76:37-51.

30. Yoshikawa M, Matsui Y, Kawamoto H, et al. Effects of glycyrrhizin on immune-mediated cytotoxicity. *J Gastroenterol Hepatol.* 1997;12(3):243-248.

31. Suzuki H, Ohta Y, Takino T, et al. Effect of glycyrrhizin on biochemical tests in patients with chronic hepatitis—double blind trial. *Asian Med J.* 1984;26(7):423-438.

32. Aly AM, Al-Alousi L, Salem HA. Licorice: a possible anti-inflammatory and anti-ulcer drug. *AAPS PharmSciTech.* 2005;6(1):E74-E82.

33. Baker ME. Licorice and enzymes other than 11 beta-hydroxysteroid dehydrogenase: an evolutionary perspective. *Steroids.* 1994;59(2):136-141.

34. Fukai T, Marumo A, Kaitou K, Kanda T, Terada S, Nomura T. Anti-*Helicobacter pylori* flavonoids from licorice extract. *Life Sci.* 2002;71(12):1449-1463.

35. Puram S, Suh HC, Kim SU, et al. Effect of GutGard in the management of *Helicobacter pylori*: a randomized double blind placebo controlled study. *Evid Based Complement Alternat Med.* 2013;2013:263805.

36. Luis A, Domingues F, Pereira L. Metabolic changes after licorice consumption: a systematic review with meta-analysis and trial sequential analysis of clinical trials. *Phytomedicine.* 2018;39:17-24.

37. Ottenbacher R, Blehm J. An unusual case of licorice-induced hypertensive crisis. *S D Med.* 2015;68(8):346-347, 349.

38. Jacobs BP, Dennehy C, Ramirez G, Sapp J, Lawrence VA. Milk thistle for the treatment of liver disease: a systematic review and meta-analysis. *Am J Med.* 2002;113(6):506-515.

39. Dehmlow C, Erhard J, de Groot H. Inhibition of Kupffer cell functions as an explanation for the hepatoprotective properties of silibinin. *Hepatology.* 1996;23(4):749-754.

40. Manna SK, Mukhopadhyay A, Van NT, Aggarwal BB. Silymarin suppresses TNF-induced activation of NF-κB, c-Jun N-terminal kinase, and apoptosis. *J Immunol.* 1999;163(12):6800-6809.

41. Ye Y, Liu Z. Management of *Amanita phalloides* poisoning: a literature review and update. *J Crit Care.* 2018;46:17-22.

42. Milosevic N, Milanovic M, Turkulov V, Medic-Stojanoska M, Abenavoli L, Milic N. May patients with alcohol liver disease benefit from herbal medicines? *Rev Recent Clin Trials.* 2016;11(3):227-237.

43. Saha P, Talukdar AD, Nath R, et al. Role of natural phenolics in hepatoprotection: a mechanistic review and analysis of regulatory network of associated genes. *Front Pharmacol.* 2019;10:509.

44. Liu CH, Jassey A, Hsu HY, Lin LT. Antiviral activities of silymarin and derivatives. *Molecules.* 2019;24(8):1552.

45. Rendina M, D'Amato M, Castellaneta A, et al. Antiviral activity and safety profile of silibinin in HCV patients with advanced fibrosis after liver transplantation: a randomized clinical trial. *Transpl Int.* 2014;27(7):696-704.

46. Marino Z, Crespo G, D'Amato M, et al. Intravenous silibinin monotherapy shows significant antiviral activity in HCV-infected patients in the peri-transplantation period. *J Hepatol.* 2013;58(3):415-420.

47. Reddy KR, Belle SH, Fried MW, et al. Rationale, challenges, and participants in a phase II trial of a botanical product for chronic hepatitis C. *Clin Trials.* 2012;9(1):102-112.

48. Shapiro H, Singer P, Halpern Z, Bruck R. Polyphenols in the treatment of inflammatory bowel disease and acute pancreatitis. *Gut.* 2007;56(3):426-435.

49. Ammon HP. Boswellic acids in chronic inflammatory diseases. *Planta Med.* 2006;72(12):1100-1116.

50. Gupta I, Parihar A, Malhotra P, et al. Effects of *Boswellia serrata* gum resin in patients with ulcerative colitis. *Eur J Med Res.* 1997;2(1):37-43.

51. Gupta I, Parihar A, Malhotra P, et al. Effects of gum resin of *Boswellia serrata* in patients with chronic colitis. *Planta medica.* 2001;67(5):391-395.

52. Gerhardt H, Seifert F, Buvari P, Vogelsang H, Repges R. [Therapy of active Crohn disease with *Boswellia serrata* extract H 15]. *Z Gastroenterol.* 2001;39(1):11-17.

53. Hanauer SB. The case for using 5-aminosaliciclates in Crohn's disease: pro. *Inflamm Bowel Dis.* 2005;11(6):609-612.

54. Hanauer SB. Supplemental evidence. *Nat Clin Pract Gastroenterol Hepatol.* 2005;2(9):375.

55. Pellegrini L, Milano E, Franceschi F, et al. Managing ulcerative colitis in remission phase: usefulness of Casperome, an innovative lecithin-based delivery system of *Boswellia serrata* extract. *Eur Rev Med Pharmacol Sci.* 2016;20(12):2695-2700.

56. Chande N, MacDonald JK, McDonald JW. Interventions for treating microscopic colitis: a Cochrane Inflammatory Bowel Disease and Functional Bowel Disorders Review Group systematic review of randomized trials. *Am J Gastroenterol.* 2009;104(1):235-241; quiz 234, 242.

57. Gautam SC, Gao X, Dulchavsky S. Immunomodulation by curcumin. *Adv Exp Med Biol.* 2007;595:321-341.

58. Camacho-Barquero L, Villegas I, Sanchez-Calvo JM, et al. Curcumin, a *Curcuma longa* constituent, acts on MAPK p38 pathway modulating COX-2 and iNOS expression in chronic experimental colitis. *Int Immunopharmacol.* 2007;7(3):333-342.

59. Kurup VP, Barrios CS, Raju R, Johnson BD, Levy MB, Fink JN. Immune response modulation by curcumin in a latex allergy model. *Clin Mol Allergy.* 2007;5:1.

60. Sharma S, Chopra K, Kulkarni SK, Agrewala JN. Resveratrol and curcumin suppress immune response through CD28/CTLA-4 and CD80 co-stimulatory pathway. *Clin Exp Immunol.* 2007;147(1):155-163.

61. Holt PR, Katz S, Kirshoff R. Curcumin therapy in inflammatory bowel disease: a pilot study. *Dig Dis Sci.* 2005;50(11):2191-2193.

62. Hanai H, Iida T, Takeuchi K, et al. Curcumin maintenance therapy for ulcerative colitis: randomized, multicenter, double-blind, placebo-controlled trial. *Clin Gastroenterol Hepatol.* 2006;4(12):1502-1506.

63. Lang A, Salomon N, Wu JC, et al. Curcumin in combination with mesalamine induces remission in patients with mild-to-moderate ulcerative colitis in a randomized controlled trial. *Clin Gastroenterol Hepatol.* 2015;13(8):1444-1449.e1. doi:10.1016/j.cgh.2015.02.019

64. Kedia S, Bhatia V, Thareja S, et al. Low dose oral curcumin is not effective in induction of remission in mild to moderate ulcerative colitis: Results from a randomized double blind placebo controlled trial. *World J Gastrointest Pharmacol Ther.* 2017;8(2):147-154. doi:10.4292/wjgpt.v8.i2.147

65. Singla V, Pratap Mouli V, Garg SK, et al. Induction with NCB-02 (curcumin) enema for mild-to-moderate distal ulcerative colitis—a randomized, placebo-controlled, pilot study. *J Crohns Colitis.* 2014;8(3):208-214.

66. Hanai H, Sugimoto K. Curcumin has bright prospects for the treatment of inflammatory bowel disease. *Curr Pharm Des.* 2009;15(18):2087-2094.

67. Goulart RA, Barbalho SM, Lima VM, et al. Effects of the use of curcumin on ulcerative colitis and Crohn's disease: a systematic review. *J Med Food.* 2021;24(7):675-685. doi:10.1089/jmf.2020.0129

68. Hasanzadeh S, Read MI, Bland AR, Majeed M, Jamialahmadi T, Sahebkar A. Curcumin: an inflammasome silencer. *Pharmacol Res.* 2020;159:104921.

69. Olcum M, Tastan B, Ercan I, Eltutan IB, Genc S. Inhibitory effects of phytochemicals on NLRP3 inflammasome activation: a review. *Phytomedicine.* 2020;75:153238.

70. Rajagopal K, Varakumar P, Baliwada A, Byran G. Activity of phytochemical constituents of *Curcuma longa* (turmeric) and *Andrographis paniculata* against coronavirus (COVID-19): an in silico approach. *Futur J Pharm Sci.* 2020;6(1):104.

71. Praditya D, Kirchhoff L, Bruning J, Rachmawati H, Steinmann J, Steinmann E. Anti-infective properties of the golden spice curcumin. *Front Microbiol.* 2019;10:912.

72. Cohen L, Neuman MG. Cannabis and the gastrointestinal tract. *J Pharm Pharm Sci.* 2020;23:301-313.

73. Desmarais A, Smiddy S, Reddy S, El-Dallal M, Erlich J, Feuerstein JD. Evidence supporting the benefits of marijuana for Crohn's disease and ulcerative colitis is extremely limited: a meta-analysis of the literature. *Ann Gastroenterol.* 2020;33(5):495-499.

74. Lahat A, Lang A, Ben-Horin S. Impact of cannabis treatment on the quality of life, weight and clinical disease activity in inflammatory bowel disease patients: a pilot prospective study. *Digestion.* 2012;85(1):1-8.

75. Kafil TS, Nguyen TM, MacDonald JK, Chande N. Cannabis for the treatment of Crohn's disease and ulcerative colitis: evidence from Cochrane Reviews. *Inflamm Bowel Dis.* 2020;26(4):502-509.

76. Martínez V, Iriondo De-Hond A, Borrelli F, Capasso R, Del Castillo MD, Abalo R. Cannabidiol and other non-psychoactive cannabinoids for prevention and treatment of gastrointestinal disorders: useful nutraceuticals? *Int J Mol Sci.* 2020;21(9):3067. doi:10.3390/ijms21093067

77. Alammar N, Wang L, Saberi B, et al. The impact of peppermint oil on the irritable bowel syndrome: a meta-analysis of the pooled clinical data. *BMC Complement Altern Med.* 2019;19(1):21.

78. Black CJ, Yuan Y, Selinger CP, et al. Efficacy of soluble fibre, antispasmodic drugs, and gut-brain neuromodulators in irritable bowel syndrome: a systematic review and network meta-analysis. *Lancet Gastroenterol Hepatol.* 2020;5(2):117-131.

79. Black CJ, Moayyedi P, Quigley EMM, Ford AC. Peppermint oil in irritable bowel syndrome. *Gastroenterology.* 2020;159(1):395-396.

80. Madisch A, Holtmann G, Plein K, Hotz J. Treatment of irritable bowel syndrome with herbal preparations: results of a double-blind, randomized, placebo-controlled, multi-centre trial. *Aliment Pharmacol Ther.* 2004;19(3):271-279.

81. Rosch W, Liebregts T, Gundermann KJ, Vinson B, Holtmann G. Phytotherapy for functional dyspepsia: a review of the clinical evidence for the herbal preparation STW 5. *Phytomedicine.* 2006;13(suppl 5):114-121.

82. Lapina TL, Trukhmanov AS. Herbal preparation STW 5 for functional gastrointestinal disorders: clinical experience in everyday practice. *Dig Dis.* 2017;35(suppl 1):30-35.

83. Madisch A, Vinson BR, Abdel-Aziz H, et al. Modulation of gastrointestinal motility beyond metoclopramide and domperidone: pharmacological and clinical evidence for phytotherapy in functional gastrointestinal disorders. *Wien Med Wochenschr.* 2017;167(7-8):160-168.

84. Ruxton CH, Reed SC, Simpson MJ, Millington KJ. The health benefits of omega-3 polyunsaturated fatty acids: a review of the evidence. *J Hum Nutr Diet.* 2007;20(3):275-285.

85. Patenaude A, Rodriguez-Leyva D, Edel AL, et al. Bioavailability of α-linolenic acid from flaxseed diets as a function of the age of the subject. *Eur J Clin Nutr.* 2009;63(9):1123-1129.

86. Parian AM, Limketkai BN, Shah ND, Mullin GE. Nutraceutical supplements for inflammatory bowel disease. *Nutr Clin Pract.* 2015;30(4):551-558.

87. Wild GE, Drozdowski L, Tartaglia C, Clandinin MT, Thomson AB. Nutritional modulation of the inflammatory response in inflammatory bowel disease—from the molecular to the integrative to the clinical. *World J Gastroenterol.* 2007;13(1):1-7.

88. Serhan CN, Arita M, Hong S, Gotlinger K. Resolvins, docosatrienes, and neuroprotectins, novel omega-3-derived mediators, and their endogenous aspirin-triggered epimers. *Lipids.* 2004;39(11):1125-1132.

89. Abdolmaleki F, Kovanen PT, Mardani R, Gheibi-Hayat SM, Bo S, Sahebkar A. Resolvins: emerging players in autoimmune and inflammatory diseases. *Clin Rev Allergy Immunol.* 2020;58(1):82-91.

90. Bassaganya-Riera J, Hontecillas R. CLA and n-3 PUFA differentially modulate clinical activity and colonic PPAR-responsive gene expression in a pig model of experimental IBD. *Clin Nutr.* 2006;25(3):454-465.

91. Shoda R, Matsueda K, Yamato S, Umeda N. Therapeutic efficacy of n-3 polyunsaturated fatty acid in experimental Crohn's disease. *J Gastroenterol.* 1995;30(suppl 8):98-101.

92. Cleland LG, James MJ, Proudman SM. Fish oil: what the prescriber needs to know. *Arthritis Res Ther.* 2006;8(1):202.

93. Aslan A, Triadafilopoulos G. Fish oil fatty acid supplementation in active ulcerative colitis: a double-blind, placebo-controlled, crossover study. *Am J Gastroenterol.* 1992;87(4):432-437.

94. Stenson WF, Cort D, Rodgers J, et al. Dietary supplementation with fish oil in ulcerative colitis. *Ann Intern Med.* 1992;116(8):609-614.

95. Barbosa DS, Cecchini R, El Kadri MZ, Rodriguez MA, Burini RC, Dichi I. Decreased oxidative stress in patients with ulcerative colitis supplemented with fish oil omega-3 fatty acids. *Nutrition.* 2003;19(10):837-842.

96. Scaioli E, Sartini A, Bellanova M, et al. Eicosapentaenoic acid reduces fecal levels of calprotectin and prevents relapse in patients with ulcerative colitis. *Clin Gastroenterol Hepatol.* 2018;16(8):1268-1275 e1262.

97. Almallah YZ, Richardson S, O'Hanrahan T, et al. Distal procto-colitis, natural cytotoxicity, and essential fatty acids. *Am J Gastroenterol.* 1998;93(5):804-809.

98. Seidner DL, Lashner BA, Brzezinski A, et al. An oral supplement enriched with fish oil, soluble fiber, and antioxidants for corticosteroid sparing in ulcerative colitis: a randomized, controlled trial. *Clin Gastroenterol Hepatol.* 2005;3(4):358-369.

99. Lorenz R, Weber PC, Szimnau P, Heldwein W, Strasser T, Loeschke K. Supplementation with n-3 fatty acids from fish oil in chronic inflammatory bowel disease—a randomized, placebo-controlled, double-blind cross-over trial. *J Intern Med Suppl.* 1989;731:225-232.

100. Turner D, Zlotkin SH, Shah PS, Griffiths AM. Omega 3 fatty acids (fish oil) for maintenance of remission in Crohn's disease. *Cochrane Database Syst Rev.* 2009;(1):CD006320.

101. Turner D, Shah PS, Steinhart AH, Zlotkin S, Griffiths AM. Maintenance of remission in inflammatory bowel disease using omega-3 fatty acids (fish oil): a systematic review and meta-analyses. *Inflamm Bowel Dis.* 2011;17(1):336-345. doi:10.1002/ibd.21374

102. Lev-Tzion R, Griffiths AM, Leder O, Turner D. Omega 3 fatty acids (fish oil) for maintenance of remission in Crohn's disease. *Cochrane Database Syst Rev.* 2014;(2):CD006320.

103. Turner D, Zlotkin SH, Shah PS, Griffiths AM. Omega 3 fatty acids (fish oil) for maintenance of remission in Crohn's disease. *Cochrane Database Syst Rev.* 2007;(2):CD006320.

104. Lorenz-Meyer H, Bauer P, Nicolay C, et al. Omega-3 fatty acids and low carbohydrate diet for maintenance of remission in Crohn's disease: a randomized controlled multicenter trial. Study Group Members (German Crohn's Disease Study Group). *Scand J Gastroenterol.* 1996;31(8):778-785.

105. Romano C, Cucchiara S, Barabino A, Annese V, Sferlazzas C. Usefulness of omega-3 fatty acid supplementation in addition to mesalazine in maintaining remission in pediatric Crohn's disease: a double-blind, randomized, placebo-controlled study. *World J Gastroenterol.* 2005;11(45):7118-7121.

106. Belluzzi A, Brignola C, Campieri M, Pera A, Boschi S, Miglioli M. Effect of an enteric-coated fish-oil preparation on relapses in Crohn's disease. *N Engl J Med.* 1996;334(24):1557-1560.

107. Belluzzi A, Campieri M, Belloli C, Boschi S, Cottone M, Rizzello F. A new enteric coated preparation of omega-3 fatty acids for preventing post-surgical recurrence in Crohn's disease. *Gastroenterology.* 1997;112(4):A494.

108. Zdrenghea MT, Makrinioti H, Bagacean C, Bush A, Johnston SL, Stanciu LA. Vitamin D modulation of innate immune responses to respiratory viral infections. *Rev Med Virol.* 2017;27(1):e1909.

109. Martineau AR, Jolliffe DA, Hooper RL, et al. Vitamin D supplementation to prevent acute respiratory tract infections: systematic review and meta-analysis of individual participant data. *BMJ.* 2017;356:i6583.

110. Wu D, Yang XO. TH17 responses in cytokine storm of COVID-19: an emerging target of JAK2 inhibitor Fedratinib. *J Microbiol Immunol Infect.* 2020;53(3):368-370.

111. Miraglia del Giudice M, Indolfi C, Strisciuglio C. Vitamin D: immunomodulatory aspects. *J Clin Gastroenterol.* 2018;52(suppl 1):S86-S88.

112. Fawaz L, Mrad MF, Kazan JM, Sayegh S, Akika R, Khoury SJ. Comparative effect of 25(OH)D3 and 1,25(OH)$_2$D3 on Th17 cell differentiation. *Clin Immunol.* 2016;166-167:59-71.

113. Wang F, Hou H, Luo Y, et al. The laboratory tests and host immunity of COVID-19 patients with different severity of illness. *JCI Insight.* 2020;5(10):e137799.

114. Chen G, Wu D, Guo W, et al. Clinical and immunological features of severe and moderate coronavirus disease 2019. *J Clin Invest.* 2020;130(5):2620-2629.

115. Podolsky DK. Inflammatory bowel disease (2). *N Engl J Med.* 1991;325(14):1008-1016.

116. Podolsky DK. Inflammatory bowel disease (1). *N Engl J Med.* 1991;325(13):928-937.

117. Rode A, Fourlanos S, Nicoll A. Oral vitamin D replacement is effective in chronic liver disease. *Gastroenterol Clin Biol.* 2010;34(11):618-620. doi:10.1016/j.gcb.2010.07.009

118. Pappa HM, Gordon CM, Saslowsky TM, et al. Vitamin D status in children and young adults with inflammatory bowel disease. *Pediatrics.* 2006;118(5):1950-1961.

119. Ananthakrishnan AN, Khalili H, Higuchi LM, et al. Higher predicted vitamin D status is associated with reduced risk of Crohn's disease. *Gastroenterology.* 2012;142(3):482-489.

120. Ananthakrishnan AN, Cagan A, Gainer VS, et al. Normalization of plasma 25-hydroxy vitamin D is associated with reduced risk of surgery in Crohn's disease. *Inflamm Bowel Dis.* 2013;19(9):1921-1927.

121. Jorgensen SP, Agnholt J, Glerup H, et al. Clinical trial: vitamin D3 treatment in Crohn's disease—a randomized double-blind placebo-controlled study. *Aliment Pharmacol Ther.* 2010;32(3):377-383.

122. Narula N, Cooray M, Anglin R, Muqtadir Z, Narula A, Marshall JK. Impact of high-dose vitamin D3 supplementation in patients with Crohn's disease in remission: a pilot randomized double-blind controlled study. *Dig Dis Sci.* 2017;62(2):448-455.

123. Lichtenstein GR, Sands BE, Pazianas M. Prevention and treatment of osteoporosis in inflammatory bowel disease. *Inflamm Bowel Dis.* 2006;12(8):797-813.

124. Gammoh NZ, Rink L. Zinc in infection and inflammation. *Nutrients.* 2017;9(6):624.

125. Prasad AS. Zinc in human health: effect of zinc on immune cells. *Mol Med.* 2008;14(5-6):353-357. doi:10.2119/2008-00033

126. Ehrlich S, Mark AG, Rinawi F, Shamir R, Assa A. Micronutrient deficiencies in children with inflammatory bowel diseases. *Nutr Clin Pract.* 2020;35(2):315-322.

127. Lee IC, Huo TI, Huang YH. Gastrointestinal and liver manifestations in patients with COVID-19. *J Chin Med Assoc.* 2020;83(6):521-523. doi:10.1097/JCMA.000000000000031.

128. Lih-Brody L, Powell SR, Collier KP, et al. Increased oxidative stress and decreased antioxidant defenses in mucosa of inflammatory bowel disease. *Dig Dis Sci.* 1996;41(10):2078-2086.

129. Duan H, Lu S, Qin H, et al. Co-delivery of zinc and 5-aminosalicylic acid from alginate/N-succinyl-chitosan blend microspheres for synergistic therapy of colitis. *Int J Pharm.* 2017;516(1-2):214-224.

130. Siva S, Rubin DT, Gulotta G, Wroblewski K, Pekow J. Zinc deficiency is associated with poor clinical outcomes in patients with inflammatory bowel disease. *Inflamm Bowel Dis.* 2017;23(1):152-157.

131. Mezzaroba L, Alfieri DF, Colado Simao AN, Vissoci Reiche EM. The role of zinc, copper, manganese and iron in neurodegenerative diseases. *Neurotoxicology.* 2019;74:230-241.

132. Ueno PM, Oria RB, Maier EA, et al. Alanyl-glutamine promotes intestinal epithelial cell homeostasis in vitro and in a murine model of weanling undernutrition. *Am J Physiol Gastrointest Liver Physiol.* 2011;301(4):G612-G622.

133. Tremel H, Kienle B, Weilemann LS, Stehle P, Furst P. Glutamine dipeptide-supplemented parenteral nutrition maintains intestinal function in the critically ill. *Gastroenterology.* 1994;107(6):1595-1601.

134. Severo JS, da Silva Barros VJ, Alves da Silva AC, et al. Effects of glutamine supplementation on inflammatory bowel disease: a systematic review of clinical trials. *Clin Nutr ESPEN.* 2021;42:53-60.

135. Budai MM, Varga A, Milesz S, Tozser J, Benko S. *Aloe vera* downregulates LPS-induced inflammatory cytokine production and expression of NLRP3 inflammasome in human macrophages. *Mol Immunol.* 2013;56(4):471-479.

136. Langmead L, Feakins RM, Goldthorpe S, et al. Randomized, double-blind, placebo-controlled trial of oral *Aloe vera* gel for active ulcerative colitis. *Aliment Pharmacol Ther.* 2004;19(7):739-747.

137. Langhorst J, Wulfert H, Lauche R, et al. Systematic review of complementary and alternative medicine treatments in inflammatory bowel diseases. *J Crohns Colitis.* 2015;9(1):86-106.

138. Gao Z, Yu C, Liang H, et al. Andrographolide derivative CX-10 ameliorates dextran sulphate sodium-induced ulcerative colitis in mice: involvement of NF-κB and MAPK signalling pathways. *Int Immunopharmacol.* 2018;57:82-90.

139. Tang T, Targan SR, Li ZS, Xu C, Byers VS, Sandborn WJ. Randomised clinical trial: herbal extract HMPL-004 in active ulcerative colitis—a double-blind comparison with sustained release mesalazine. *Aliment Pharmacol Ther.* 2011;33(2):194-202.

140. Sandborn WJ, Targan SR, Byers VS, et al. *Andrographis paniculata* extract (HMPL-004) for active ulcerative colitis. *Am J Gastroenterol.* 2013;108(1):90-98.

141. Krebs S, Omer TN, Omer B. Wormwood (*Artemisia absinthium*) suppresses tumour necrosis factor alpha and accelerates healing in patients with Crohn's disease—a controlled clinical trial. *Phytomedicine.* 2010;17(5):305-309.

142. Ren J, Tao Q, Wang X, Wang Z, Li J. Efficacy of T2 in active Crohn's disease: a prospective study report. *Dig Dis Sci.* 2007;52(8):1790-7. doi:10.1007/s10620-007-9747-y

143. Kaliora AC, Stathopoulou MG, Triantafillidis JK, Dedoussis GV, Andrikopoulos NK. Chios mastic treatment of patients with active Crohn's disease. *World J Gastroenterol.* 2007;13(5):748-753. doi:10.3748/wjg.v13.i5.748

144. Holleran G, Scaldaferri F, Gasbarrini A, Curro D. Herbal medicinal products for inflammatory bowel disease: a focus on those assessed in double-blind randomised controlled trials. *Phytother Res.* 2020;34(1):77-93.

145. Ben-Arye E, Goldin E, Wengrower D, Stamper A, Kohn R, Berry E. Wheat grass juice in the treatment of active distal ulcerative colitis: a randomized double-blind placebo-controlled trial. *Scand J Gastroenterol.* 2002;37(4):444-449.

146. Ng SC, Lam YT, Tsoi KK, Chan FK, Sung JJ, Wu JC. Systematic review: the efficacy of herbal therapy in inflammatory bowel disease. *Aliment Pharmacol Ther.* 2013;38(8):854-863.

147. Pan Y, Ouyang Q. [Effects of Bawei Xilei San on mice with oxazolone-induced colitis and the mechanisms]. *Zhong Xi Yi Jie He Xue Bao.* 2010;8(6):568-574.

148. Fukunaga K, Hida N, Ohnishi K, et al. A suppository Chinese medicine (xilei-san) for refractory ulcerative proctitis: a pilot clinical trial. *Digestion.* 2007;75(2-3):146-147.

149. Zhang F, Li Y, Xu F, Chu Y, Zhao W. Comparison of Xilei-san, a Chinese herbal medicine, and dexamethasone in mild/moderate ulcerative proctitis: a double-blind randomized clinical trial. *J Altern Complement Med.* 2013;19(10):838-842.

150. Mizoguchi A, Yano A, Himuro H, Ezaki Y, Sadanaga T, Mizoguchi E. Clinical importance of IL-22 cascade in IBD. *J Gastroenterol.* 2018;53(4):465-474.

151. Xiao HT, Peng J, Wen B, et al. *Indigo naturalis* suppresses colonic oxidative stress and Th1/Th17 responses of DSS-induced colitis in mice. *Oxid Med Cell Longev.* 2019;2019:9480945.

152. Naganuma M, Sugimoto S, Fukuda T, et al. *Indigo naturalis* is effective even in treatment-refractory patients with ulcerative colitis: a post hoc analysis from the INDIGO study. *J Gastroenterol.* 2020;55(2):169-180.

153. Xu HH, Wang MX, Tan HL, et al. [Effect of clinical doses of Realgar-*Indigo Naturalis* formula and large-dose of realgar on CYP450s of rat liver]. *Zhongguo Zhong Yao Za Zhi.* 2017;42(3):593-599.

154. Nishio M, Hirooka K, Doi Y. Pulmonary arterial hypertension associated with the Chinese herb *Indigo naturalis* for ulcerative colitis: it may be reversible. *Gastroenterol.* 2018;155(2):577-578.

155. Naganuma M. Treatment with *Indigo naturalis* for inflammatory bowel disease and other immune diseases. *Immunol Med.* 2019;42(1):16-21.

156. Naganuma M, Sugimoto S, Suzuki H, et al. Adverse events in patients with ulcerative colitis treated with *Indigo naturalis*: a Japanese nationwide survey. *J Gastroenterol.* 2019;54(10):891-896.

25

Ethical and Legal Considerations in Gastrointestinal Nutrition Interventions

Denise Baird Schwartz, MS, RD, FADA, FAND, FASPEN
Albert Barrocas, MD, FACS, FASPEN

KEY POINTS

- Ethical and legal considerations are important factors in the decision making process regarding the use of gastrointestinal nutrition interventions.
- Many tools and resources are available to assist health care practitioners in weighing the ethical and legal considerations associated with such interventions.
- Practitioners should feel empowered to apply ethical and legal considerations and information in their practice.

Introduction

Gastrointestinal (GI) nutrition interventions can present ethical and legal issues for health care practitioners, patients, family members, and surrogate decision makers (SDMs). The artificial administration of nutrition and hydration—whether directly into the GI tract (enteral nutrition[EN]) or through intravenous lines (parenteral nutrition[PN])—is a medical therapy. Although the term *artificial nutrition and hydration* is often used, in this chapter the term *artificially administered nutrition and hydration* (AANH) is used to emphasize that it is the route of feeding through a tube or intravenous line that is artificial, not the nutrition or the hydration.

Decisions about the initiation, continued use, or discontinuation of AANH pose important ethical and legal questions, such as these:

- Who is empowered (legally and ethically) to make these decisions?
- On what basis should these decisions be made by the patient, the family, or the SDM? Should they be made on the basis of quality of life (QOL) or likely clinical outcomes? Should they be made on the basis of cultural values, religious beliefs, and ethnic background? Or should they be based on country of origin, regional identity, or geographical location?
- What types of institutional policies and procedures might help health care practitioners and the patients, family members, and SDMs reach timely and ethical decisions for care?

This chapter explores the ethical and legal questions related to the use of AANH in adults and offers guidance for health care practitioners navigating this challenging aspect of patient care. Readers unfamiliar with the terminology used when dealing with ethical and legal aspects of GI nutrition interventions will find a list of definitions in Box 25.1. Box 25.2 includes a list of useful resources for advance care planning.

BOX 25.1

Glossary of Terms for Ethical and Legal Issues in Nutrition Support

Artificially administered nutrition and hydration (AANH): Nutrition in any form other than taking food and fluid by mouth (orally). AANH comprises enteral nutrition (EN), which is nutrition delivered through various tubes into the gastrointestinal tract, and parenteral nutrition (PN), which is nutrition delivered through intravenous lines.

Bioethics committee: An interdisciplinary committee whose functions are to provide ethics consults, policy development and review, and ethics education within an institution. The composition and functions of committees vary among facilities and states.

- *Ethics consults:* Consults performed by a small group of bioethics committee members who are involved in conflict resolution. Ethics consults can occur during patient care between practitioners or between health care practitioners and the patient, family, or surrogate decision maker (SDM). The goal is to achieve a consensus that is patient-centered, meaning it represents the patient's wishes and is in the best interest of the patient, does no harm, and is fair in its provision of health care delivery.
- *Policy development and review:* Policy work that supports the standards of care that are aligned with the values and mission of the organization. Examples of clinical polices may include code status, treatment decisions at the end of life, organ donation, and determination of death by neurological criteria.
- *Composition:* Generally composed of physicians, nurses, social workers, registered dietitian nutritionists, risk managers, chaplains, administrators, community members, and others as needed.

Cue-based patient and family discussion: A discussion that uses key words or phrases to help patients, families, and SDMs understand their role in health care options and to empower them to provide information to the practitioner. For example, during discussion of EN initiation, a seated practitioner, speaking slowly and listening attentively, would state the following: 1) patient-centered care is based on the patient's wishes; 2) the family's or SDM's role is to express what the patient would want; 3) the family's or SDM's role is to represent the patient's wishes and not their own; 4) the patient, family, and SDM are the center of the health care team.

Decisional capacity: The ability of a person to make decisions. Adults are presumed capable unless declared incapable by the practitioners treating them or incompetent by a court of law or judge. Some states require two physicians to determine decisional capacity of a particular person. Decisional capacity is specific to a point in time and a specific decision.

Ethical principles: The key ethical principles guiding the use of gastrointestinal nutrition interventions are the following:

- *Autonomy:* the right and ability of a capable person to make their own health care decisions (self-determination is a legal right)
- *Beneficence:* providing beneficial care based on the patient's best interests and clinical status
- *Nonmaleficence:* not doing harm to individuals
- *Justice:* the right of all individuals to receive health care that is fair through an equitable process, and the appropriate distribution of health care resources

Evidence-based medicine: Medical practice that relies on research and clinical expertise to guide decisions about the health care of individual patients.

Forgoing life-sustaining treatment: Doing without a medical intervention. Forgoing includes withholding (noninitiation) and withdrawing (stopping).

Health care agent, proxy, or surrogate decision maker (SDM): A person appointed by a patient to make health care

Box continues

BOX 25.1 (CONTINUED)

decisions in the event that the patient becomes incapable of making decisions (no longer had decisional capacity). Decisions made by the agent, proxy, or SDM should be based on the patient's preferences and carry the same legal weight as patient-made decisions.

Health literacy: The ability of an individual to obtain, process, and understand the health information needed to make informed health decisions.

Interdisciplinary team: A multidisciplinary group of health care practitioners from diverse fields who work in a coordinated and collaborative fashion toward a common goal for a patient.

Life-sustaining treatments: Medical therapies including, but not limited to, cardiopulmonary resuscitation, mechanical ventilation, EN, and PN.

Palliative care: Care that aims to prevent and relieve suffering and to support the best possible quality of life for patients and their families, regardless of disease stage or the need for other therapies. Palliative care includes optimizing patient function and helping with decision-making. It can be delivered concurrently with life-prolonging care or be the main focus of care.

Preventive ethics: Activities performed within a health care organization to identify, prioritize, and address systemic ethical issues rather than addressing ethical dilemmas on a case-by-case basis. A preventive ethics approach proposes that ethical conflict is preventable if commonly occurring triggers are identified and proactively managed by interventions at the organizational, unit, and individual levels.

Shared decision-making: A patient-centered approach in which practitioners relinquish the traditional authoritative role and train to become more effective patient partners. In this approach, patients are educated about the essential role they play in decision-making and are given effective tools to help them understand their options and the consequences of their decisions, without censure from their health care practitioners.

Surrogate committee: A subcommittee of a bioethics committee that functions in an advisory role, at the request of a physician, for a patient identified as "unrepresented," incapacitated, and without an advance directive, clear preferences, or SDM. The committee employs diverse perspectives to weigh the benefits against the burdens and risks of medical decisions in the best interest of the patient. It collectively functions as an advisor, and the physician ultimately functions as the decision maker. Current state laws are supplemented by institutional policies, organizational recommendations, and standards regarding decisions about the limitation or continuation of life-sustaining treatments.

Teach-back method of education: The practice of asking a patient (or family member or SDM) to explain or demonstrate what they have been taught by a practitioner in order to confirm that they understand the information presented by the practitioner. If the response indicates a lack of comprehension, then the practitioner reteaches the information using a different method or wording. The patient (or family member or SDM) is asked again to explain or demonstrate what they have been taught to confirm comprehension.

Transdisciplinary function: The concept of working in a cross-functional fashion in which function supersedes form. The most capable and available member of the patient care team is selected to carry out the desired function, despite that individual's formal discipline. Each individual team member functions within the limits of their state or federal certification, registration, or license.

Triage committee: A group of health care practitioners, preferably led by a physician, that implements the established protocols for allocating limited medical resources, when necessary.

BOX 25.2

Advance Care Planning Resources for Health Care Professionals and the Public

Breathe: A True Story of Letting Go of My Parents Gracefully for I Will See Them Again, by Anne Bland (www.breathe-annebland.com): A health care professional tells her story, written under a pen name, to help individuals begin a dialogue with family about end-of-life health care decisions. The focus is on dealing with family relationships, religion, and values that affect health care decisions. The book is intended for health care professionals and the public.

The Conversation Project (https://theconversationproject.org): Developed in collaboration with Institute for Healthcare Improvement, this project aims to have every person's end-of-life preferences expressed and respected. The project provides a starter kit to help individuals gather their thoughts and then have conversations with loved ones about their wishes for end-of-life care.

Five Wishes (a program of Aging With Dignity) (https://fivewishes.org): This program provides individuals with a useful guide and documentation tool written in everyday language for communicating their health care wishes. It helps start and structure important conversations about care in times of serious illness.

National Healthcare Decisions Day (NHDD) (https://theconversationproject .org/nhdd): Held annually on April 16, NHDD is a collaborative effort of national, state, and community organizations in the United States with the goal of inspiring, educating, and empowering the public and providers about the importance of advance care planning. The website provides resources for activities to promote NHDD.

POLST (www.polst.org): POLST has different names in different states. At the national level, it is simply called POLST: Portable Medical Orders, or POLST for short. It is a program comprising a process, a conversation, and a medical form that is designed to improve the quality of care people receive at the end of life. Emphasis is on the effective communication of patient wishes.

The indications and contraindications for EN and PN in adults are addressed in Chapters 19 and 20, respectively. A careful understanding of this material is important to ethical decision-making. Additionally, those chapters discuss the potential complications of EN and PN, which need to be discussed with the patient, family, or SDM before initiating therapy. When it comes to the use of AANH, practitioners participate with patients, family members, or SDMs in a shared decision-making process that involves discussion of the benefits vs the burdens and risks of the particular nutrition therapy being considered.

The indications and contraindications for EN and PN in pediatric patients are addressed in Chapter 21, and an understanding of this material is useful for ethical decision-making. For further considerations of ethical aspects of AANH in infants and children, refer to the American Society for Parenteral and Enteral Nutrition (ASPEN) position paper on this topic.[1]

Ethical Principles Guiding the Use of Nutrition Interventions

Health care practitioners should apply the ethical principles of *autonomy, beneficence, nonmaleficence,* and *justice* when making decisions regarding the use of GI nutrition interventions, as follows[2]:

- Autonomy refers to the patient's right to self-determination. Practitioners must respect patient autonomy.
- Beneficence means doing good for patients and always acting in their best interest.

- Nonmaleficence means practitioners should do no harm; this can include not providing ineffective treatments.
- Justice requires that all patients be treated equally and fairly by health care practitioners, allowing for differences in their clinical requirements.

Legal Aspects of Gastrointestinal Nutrition Interventions in End-of-Life Decisions

The legal history related to the use and discontinuation of EN spans several decades. Box 25.3 summarizes three of the landmark court cases that have shaped current legal opinion.[2-5] A more in-depth discussion of this area of law is beyond the scope of this chapter. Legal positions on end-of-life care are continually evolving, and local and state laws and regulations can vary. Therefore, health care providers should seek appropriate legal counsel to guide their own practice.

BOX 25.3

Notable Adult Legal Cases Related to Ethics and Tube Feedings in the United States[2-5]

Karen Ann Quinlan (1954–1985)

In 1975 Quinlan had a brain injury that left her in a persistent vegetative state (PVS) and dependent on tube feeding and ventilator support. In 1976 the New Jersey Supreme Court ruled that the ventilator, a life-sustaining measure, could be removed if the prognosis was "no reasonable possibility of a patient returning to a cognitive, sapient state" and a hospital ethics committee could confirm such a conclusion.

Quinlan was removed from a ventilator and found not to be ventilator dependent, so tube feeding continued. The following are implications of this case for ethical decision-making:

- The case supported the "substitutional judgment" or "subjective test," which allows a proxy (surrogate) to decide what the individual would have wanted.
- The case provided for criminal and civil legal protection for all parties involved in the decision-making process.
- The case assisted in establishing hospital ethics committees and enacting "living will" legislation at the state level.

Nancy Beth Cruzan (1957–1990)

In 1983 Cruzan sustained injuries in a car accident that left her in a PVS. In 1990 the Missouri Supreme Court determined that her feeding tube could lawfully be removed only if there was "clear and convincing evidence" that removal was in accordance with her wishes.

In 1990 the US Supreme Court:

- acknowledged the constitutional right that grants a competent person the right to refuse life-saving hydration and nutrition, ruled that a surrogate may act for the patient in electing to withdraw treatment, and indicated that clear and convincing evidence of an incompetent person's wishes to withdraw treatment was an appropriate standard of proof;
- upheld the state of Missouri's heightened evidentiary requirements;
- rejected the contentions of Cruzan's coguardians that the state must accept the substituted judgment of close family members, and established artificially administered nutrition and hydration (AANH) as a life-sustaining medical treatment, no different from ventilators and hemodialysis; and
- recommended the use of durable power of attorney for health care (DPAHC) and living wills as valuable safeguards to a patient's interest in directing medical care.

Box continues

BOX 25.3 (CONTINUED)

Cruzan's tube feeding was stopped.

This case stimulated increased use of health care proxies or DPAHC, and it was the reason for the enactment of the Patient Self Determination Act of 1990,[5] which requires hospitals, skilled nursing facilities, home health agencies, hospice programs, and health maintenance organizations to:

- inform patients of their rights under state law to make decisions concerning their medical care;
- periodically inquire as to whether a patient executed an advance directive and document the patient's wishes regarding their medical care;
- not discriminate against persons who have executed an advance directive;
- ensure that legally valid advance directives and documented medical care wishes are implemented to the extent permitted by state law; and
- provide educational programs for staff, patients, and the community on ethical issues concerning patient self-determination and advance directives.

Theresa Marie (Terri) Schiavo (1963–2005)

In 1990 Schiavo went into cardiac arrest, which left her in a PVS. In 1998 her husband filed a Florida petition to have her feeding tube removed on the grounds that Schiavo would not wish to be maintained in a PVS. Her parents argued the opposite position. Their legal debate led to two feeding tube removals and reinsertions, four rejected appeals to the US Supreme Court, and intervention by the Florida legislature and governor, US Congress, and the president.

In 2005 the federal district court refused to order the reinsertion of the feeding tube, and Schiavo's tube feeding was permanently stopped.

The political reaction to this case resulted in refinement of living will legislation with regards to AANH in several states. Also, it addressed the requirement of a patient's clearly expressed wishes in an advance directive for forgoing of AANH in patients who are incapable of making their own health care decisions.

A 2016 review article identified answers to common legal questions concerning nutrition support.[6] Box 25.4 on page 458 presents some of those questions and answers, along with some updated answers; resources are provided.[6-16]

Recommendations from Professional Societies

In clinical practice, the inclusion of an interprofessional perspective is essential to achieving the best outcomes for the patient. For this reason, practitioners must understand the positions, recommendations, and suggestions of organizations and practitioners involved in health care, nutrition care (in the United States and internationally), and advance care planning.[1,13,17-24] Common themes in these recommendations include:

- respect for autonomy;
- patient-centered care that incorporates the patient's health care wishes, cultural values, religious beliefs, and ethnic background, as well as the national, regional, and geographical considerations of the patient and family;
- use of informed SDMs when patients are unable to speak for themselves;
- consideration of the benefits vs the burdens and risks associated with life-sustaining therapies, in accordance with the individual's QOL goals;
- recognition that EN is a medical therapy;

BOX 25.4

Some Common Legal Questions and Answers Concerning Nutrition and Ethics[6-16]

What are the legal obligations for early nutritional status evaluation, documentation, and intervention?

The Joint Commission is an independent, not-for-profit organization that accredits, certifies, and manages health care organizations in the United States.[7] The commission's standards and elements of performance include provision of care, treatment, and services that pertain to the function of registered dietitian nutritionists (RDNs).[8] Tort law requires a provider to deliver care and treatment that is consistent with the "standard of care," as defined by the local medical community, national societies, and regulatory agencies.[6] Not adhering to the standard of care exposes the provider and institution to potentially viable claims of medical malpractice.[6]

What are the legal obligations for "informed consent"?

It is critical that the language used in conversations and consent forms be easily understood by both the patient and the family.[6] The American Medical Association (AMA) offers ethics guidance, but that guidance is not intended to establish standards of clinical practice or rules of law. Informed consent to medical treatment is fundamental in both ethics and law. The process of informed consent occurs when communication between a patient and practitioner results in the patient's authorization to undergo a specific medical intervention.[9] The potential benefits vs burdens and risks discussed should include not only those immediately associated with the procedure but also the long-term expected outcomes and prognoses.[6]

A 2017 article discussed the considerable differences in legislation and case law among European countries regarding informed consent in the management of percutaneous endoscopic gastrostomy in patients who are incapable of making their own decisions.[10]

What is decisional capacity vs competence?

There is a fundamental distinction between *decisional capacity*, as a clinical term established by qualified practitioners, and *competency*, as a legal term.[6]

The AMA *Code of Medical Ethics* addresses patient decision-making capacity, mental competence, and surrogate decision-making for those who are unable, over the short term or the long term, to make their own health care decisions.[11,12]

The American Nurses Association indicates that a patient with decision-making capacity or a surrogate decision maker (SDM) who is aware of the patient's preference or has knowledge of the patient's values and beliefs will be supported in their decision-making about accepting or refusing clinically appropriate nutrition and hydration at the end of life.[13]

What is the process for managing patients who lack decisional capacity or competency?

Practitioners have an ethical responsibility to identify an appropriate surrogate when a patient lacks decision-making capacity. SDMs should base their decisions on the *substituted judgment* standard—meaning they should use their knowledge of the patient's preferences and values to determine what the patient would want. If the patient's preferences are not known, then the decision should be based on the best interests of the patient.[10,11]

Box continues

BOX 25.4 (CONTINUED)

What are the legal implications of portable medical orders (previously known as Physician Orders for Life-Sustaining Treatment, POLST)?

POLST is national, but it may have different names in different states.[14] A shared decision-making process involving a conversation between a patient and their practitioner about the patient's goals is at the core of the POLST paradigm. POLST also consists of a set of medical orders, including the order for nutrition by tube. Authorization to execute POLST forms must fit within state regulations and scope-of-practice rules. There may be state-specific variations in the form.[15]

What is the legal definition of death?

A 2020 report provides recommendations for the minimum clinical standards for determination of brain death/death by neurologic criteria, with clear guidance for various clinical circumstances.[16]

- recognition of the role of palliative care for serious illness, not just for end of life; and
- the importance of advance care planning for individuals aged 18 years and older.

For RDNs, the positions and recommendations of the Academy of Nutrition and Dietetics[17,24] and ASPEN[1,20] are of particular relevance, and these perspectives are presented here.

The Academy of Nutrition and Dietetics Perspective

In 2009, the Academy of Nutrition and Dietetics and its credentialing agency, the Committee on Dietetics Registration, developed and approved a code of ethics for the Nutrition and Dietetics Profession. Essential components of the code of ethics (updated in 2018 and consisting of four general principles and 32 specific standards) and a 2015 article on applying the code to ethical decisions for withholding or withdrawing medically assisted nutrition and hydration are presented in Box 25.5 on page 460.[17,24-32] These two publications provide insight into the Academy of Nutrition and Dietetics perspective on AANH. Box 25.6 on page 461 identifies the general code of ethics approach to ethical decision-making in patient care.[24]

BOX 25.5

Key Components of the Academy of Nutrition and Dietetics Code of Ethics in Its Application to Medically Assisted Nutrition and Hydration[17,24-32]

Code of ethics principle[24]	Key standards[24]	Key concepts and skills for person-centered, family-oriented care; and resources in clinical ethics[17]
1. Competence and professional development in practice (**nonmaleficence**)	Nutrition and dietetics practitioners shall: • act in a caring, respectful manner; • demonstrate in-depth scientific knowledge; • incorporate the patient's unique values and cultural and ethnic diversity; • practice within their scope and collaborate with an interprofessional team; • apply an evidence-based approach to decision-making.	Key concepts: • cue-based patient and family discussion • health literacy • preventive ethics • shared decision-making • teach-back method of education
2. Integrity in personal and organizational behaviors and practices (**autonomy**)	Nutrition and dietetics practitioners shall: • respect the patient's autonomy.	Key resources[a]: • Choosing Wisely (Feeding Tubes for People with Alzheimer's)[25] • Five Wishes (an Aging with Dignity program)[26] • National Healthcare Decisions Day[27] • Portable Medical Orders (previously known as Physician Orders for Life-Sustaining Treatment, POLST)[14] • The Conversation Project[28]
3. Professionalism (**beneficence**)	Nutrition and dietetics practitioners shall: • demonstrate respect, constructive dialogue, and professionalism in all communications; • participate in decisions that affect the patient; • respect the values, rights, knowledge, and skills of other professionals.	Key resources: • Dietitians in Nutrition Support dietetic practice group (www.dnsdpg.org) • Advanced Practice Residency in Adult Nutrition Support[29] • American Society for Parenteral and Enteral Nutrition (ASPEN) International Clinical Ethics section[30]
4. Social responsibility for local, regional, national, global nutrition and well-being (**justice**)	Nutrition and dietetics practitioners shall: • collaborate with others to reduce health disparities and protect human rights; • promote fairness and objectivity with fair and equitable treatment.	Key skills: • participation in bioethics committees, patient SDM committees, interdisciplinary rounds, and consultations with the palliative care team[31] • ability to articulate the role of triage committees and their impact on nutrition therapies in a pandemic[32]

[a] See the Appendix for additional information on these resources.

BOX 25.6

Academy of Nutrition and Dietetics Code of Ethics Approach to Ethical Decision-Making in Patient Care[24]

Step 1: State the ethical dilemma.

Identify the nature and components of the dilemma:

- Is it an ethical issue, or is it a communication problem, practitioner-patient issue, or legal matter?
- What are the facts of the situation?
- What, objectively, is the issue?
- Who are the key participants?
- What are your (the practitioner's) perceptions and values?
- What further information is needed?

Step 2: Connect ethical theory to the dilemma in practice.

Use the four key principles of ethical theory: autonomy, nonmaleficence, beneficence, and justice.

Step 3: Apply the code of ethics to the issue and decision-making.

Apply the four principles of the code:

- competence and professional development in practice
- integrity in personal and organizational behaviors and practices
- professionalism
- social responsibility for local, regional, national, and global nutrition and well-being

Step 4: Select the best alternative and justify the decision.

Identify the possible alternatives, having considered the following factors, and make a final decision:

- cultural influences affecting your decision-making process
- how the alternative solutions track with your values and your institution's values
- your ability to defend the ultimate decision
- how the decision might affect others and whether they will support it

Step 5: Develop strategies to successfully implement the decision.

Seek additional knowledge to clarify or contextualize the situation as needed and then implement the chosen resolution.

Step 6: Evaluate outcomes and how to prevent similar occurrences in the future.

Monitor outcomes, ensuring the intended outcome or outcomes are achieved, and determine strategies to prevent future similar issues.

Adapted from Academy of Nutrition and Dietetics; Commission on Dietetic Registration. Code of Ethics for the Nutrition and Dietetics Profession.[24]

The American Society for Parenteral and Enteral Nutrition Perspective on Ethical Decision-Making in Patient Care

In 2014, members of the International Clinical Ethics Section of ASPEN published a special report on gastrostomy tube (G-tube) placement in patients with advanced dementia or who are near the end of life.[20] Box 25.7 provides the executive summary from the paper.[20]

BOX 25.7

American Society for Parenteral and Enteral Nutrition Special Report: Gastrostomy Tube Placement in Patients with Advanced Dementia or Near End of Life[20]

Executive Summary

The following approach is recommended for patients with advanced dementia or other near end of life conditions who are being considered for [gastrostomy-tube (G-tube)] placement. Throughout this paper, the term G-tube refers to any long-term enteral access device:

1. The decision to withhold or withdraw tube feeding in end-stage illness is supported by current scientific evidence.
2. Advanced dementia should be seen by the health care team as a terminal illness, and health care team members should clearly communicate this perspective to the patient's family, significant others, caregivers, and/or [surrogate decision maker (SDMs)].
3. A thorough discussion should take place with the patient, family, significant others, caregivers, and/or SDMs. The conversation should cover the most updated evidence-based findings regarding short-term and long-term risks, burdens, and benefits.
4. Alternatives such as assisted oral feeding and other innovative oral interventions should be thoroughly explored and discussed with the patient, family, significant others, caregivers, and/or SDMs.
5. The autonomy of the patient or SDM should be respected. Emphasis should be placed on functional status and quality of life. An essential aspect of the process involves cultural, religious, social, and emotional sensitivity to the patient's value system. A time-limited trial of nasogastric feedings may be considered if a decision to proceed in the future with a G-tube is made.
6. The final informed decision should be reached via a patient-centered approach, including family, significant others, caregivers, and/or SDMs.
7. Clinicians in health care institutions, both hospitals and long-term care facilities, should develop a process that is interdisciplinary, collaborative, proactive, integrated, and systematic in order to facilitate decision making that engages the patient, family, significant others, caregivers, and/or SDMs. The process should promote advance directives that provide health care based on the patient's wishes and best interest.

Reprinted with permission from Schwartz DB, Barrocas A, Wesley JR, et al. Gastrostomy tube placement in patients with advanced dementia or near end of life. Nutr Clin Prac. 2014;29(6):829-840. doi:10.1177/0884533614546890[20]

Figure 25.1 describes the decision-making algorithm to be used prior to G-tube placement in patients with declining oral intake and possible aspiration.[20] For example, an alternative to G-tube placement is comfort feeding only, for individuals exhibiting feeding problems resulting in weight loss, which can be common in advanced stages of dementia.

Use of the phrase *comfort feeding only*, as a physician's order, provides clear language and specifies the patient's goals of care. Additionally, the order to discontinue any AANH might be misunderstood as an order that means do not feed; but "comfort feeding only" would involve attentive eating assistance. This order would provide an individualized feeding care plan, which would include careful hand feeding.[33,34]

FIGURE 25.1 Decision-making algorithm for use prior to gastrostomy tube placement in patients with declining oral intake and possible aspiration

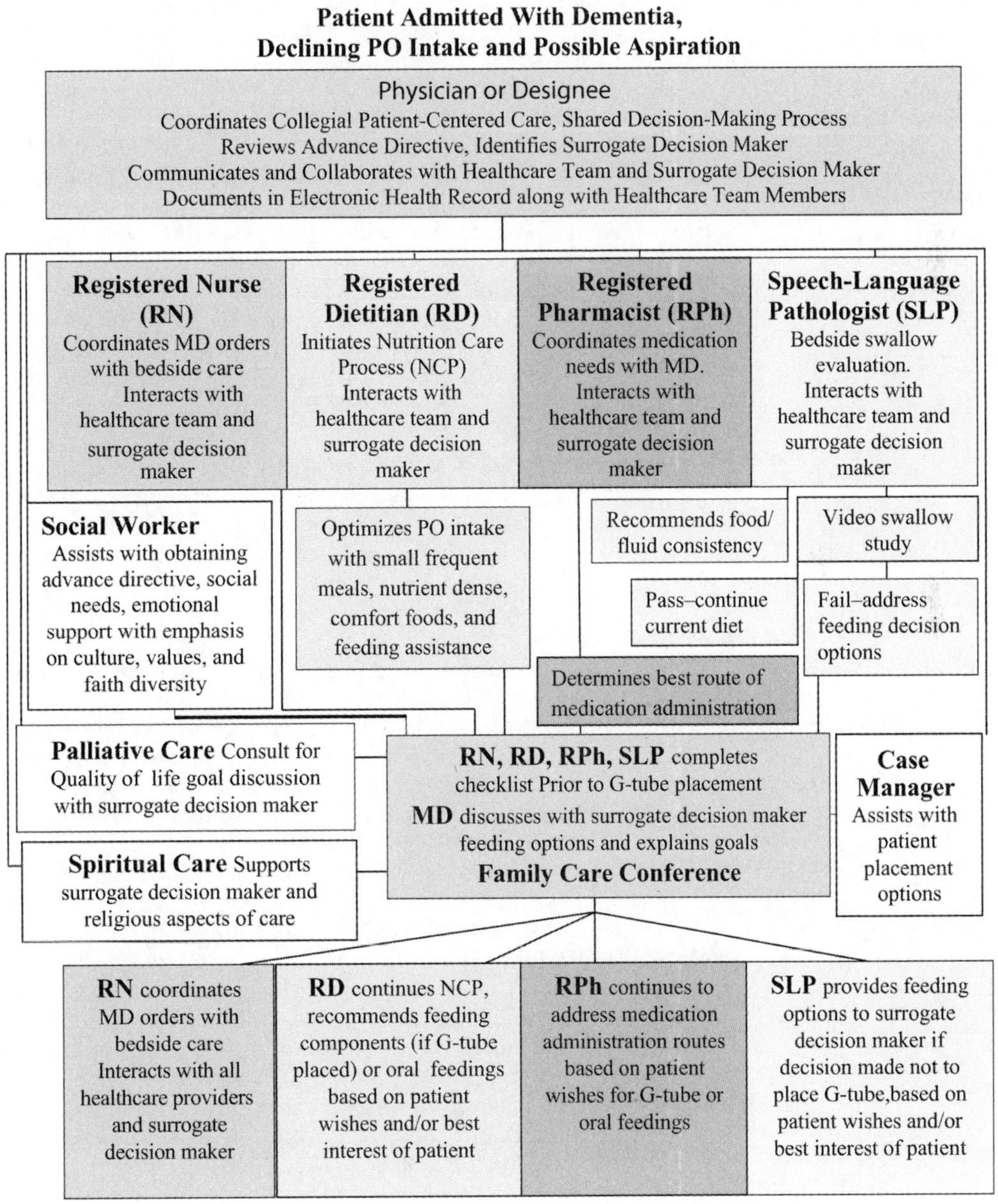

Abbreviations: G-tube = gastrostomy tube | MD = doctor of medicine | PO = by mouth (per os) | RDN = registered dietitian nutritionist | NCP = Nutrition Care Process | QOL = quality of life | RN = registered nurse | RPh = registered pharmacist | SLP = speech-language pathologist
Reproduced with permission from Schwartz DB, Barrocas A, Wesley JR, et al. Gastrostomy tube placement in patients with advanced dementia or near end of life. *Nutr Clin Prac.* 2014;29(6):829-840.[20]

A 2021 ASPEN position paper addresses the major ethical and legal issues related to AANH and offers guidance for practitioners confronted with these dilemmas.[1] The following specific patient conditions are included because of their potential for ethical issues: coma, decreased consciousness, and dementia; advanced dementia; cancer; eating disorders; and end-stage disease or terminal illness. The position paper covers the topic of ethical decisions during a pandemic and includes a legal summary of ethical issues. International authors address the similarities and differences within their own countries or regions and compare them with the US perspective. Box 25.8 provides key points listed in the position statements section of this paper.[1]

BOX 25.8

2021 American Society for Parenteral and Enteral Nutrition Position Statements on the Ethical Aspects of Artificially Administered Nutrition and Hydration[1]

1. Artificial nutrition and hydration is a medical treatment. The word *administered* in *artificially administered nutrition and hydration* (AANH) clarifies the route is artificial, not the nutrition or hydration.
2. The four ethical principles of autonomy, beneficence, nonmaleficence, and justice should be equally applied to patient care.
3. Advance care planning (ACP) with establishment of an advance directive, including designation of a surrogate decision maker (SDM), is recommended.
4. The cultural values, religious beliefs, and ethnic background of patients and families, as well as national, regional, and geographical considerations, need to be respected to the extent that they are consistent with the ethical principles and duties and legal requirements.
5. The use of interdisciplinary committees and teams and meetings with the patient and family or SDM is recommended for AANH discussions.
6. A surrogate committee should be created from bioethics committee members to perform an advisory role upon request for an *unrepresented* patient, without an advance directive or clear preferences or a designated SDM.
7. Limited-time trials are an acceptable alternative when the benefits of AANH are questionable and when the trial nature of AANH is communicated and agreed upon by the patient and family or SDM prior to its initiation.
8. Clinicians should not be ethically obligated to offer AANH if, in their clinical judgment, there is not adequate evidence for the therapy or if the burden or risk of the intervention far outweighs its benefit.
9. From a scientific, ethical, and legal perspective, there should be no difference between withholding and withdrawing of AANH; the term for both is *forgoing*.
10. If unable to resolve conflicts, despite an ethics consult, consultation with another provider and/or institution should be considered. Thereafter, if necessary, an orderly transfer of care is recommended to a qualified and willing clinician and/or institution, and care includes ensuring that these persons do not feel abandoned.
11. Scientific evidence related to the physiology of patients with brain death, in a coma, or in a . . . persistent vegetative state . . . indicates these patients do not experience thirst or hunger and, therefore, may not suffer.
12. AANH neither stops dementia disease progression nor prevents imminent death, and the decision to forgo [enteral nutrition (EN)] in end-stage illness is supported by current scientific evidence.
13. For individuals with cancer, use of a patient-centered communication style—if the patient, family, or SDM desires—incorporates a shared decision-making process. Conflicts between the clinician obligations and the patient's preferences involving AANH use should be acknowledged and evaluated on a case-by-case basis.
14. There is a delicate balance in treating eating disorders when AANH becomes a nonnegotiable aspect of an individual's treatment, and AANH may be required when nutrition rehabilitation involves reversing the effects of life-threatening malnutrition.

Box continues

15. For persons at the end of life (EOL), their preferences and quality of life (QOL) goals with acceptance or refusal of modified-consistency food and fluids provided orally or AANH must be respected.
16. Institutions should establish triage committees and develop protocols based on an ethical framework for the management of limited resources during pandemics in order to avoid perceptions or charges of inconsistent decision-making.
17. Forgoing AANH in infants and children at the EOL may be ethically acceptable when competent parents and the medical team concur that the intervention no longer confers a benefit to the child or creates a burden that cannot be justified.
18. The particular laws of state and national governments have to be considered when addressing whether or how to use AANH at the EOL and the role of informed consent.
19. States may apply a "clear and convincing" evidentiary standard in looking for evidence that the patient would want to forgo AANH, if the patient did not expressly give instructions on EOL preferences.
20. In the majority of cases, international ethical guidelines and practices are similar. The same is not true when considering legal mandates.

Reprinted with permission from Schwartz DB, Barrocas A, Annetta MG, et al. Ethical aspects of artificially administered nutrition and hydration: an ASPEN position paper. Nutr Clin Pract. 2021;36(2):254-267. doi:10.1002 /ncp.10633[1]

American Medical Association Ethical Guidance for Practitioners Caring for Patients at End of Life

The American Medical Association (AMA) *Code of Medical Ethics* includes a chapter on caring for patients at the end of life.[23] The opinions in the chapter are ethical guidance for practitioners; however, these opinions are not intended to establish standards of clinical practice or rules of law. Pertinent opinions from the AMA chapter are presented in Box 25.9 on page 466.[23]

Cultural, Religious, Ethnic, National, Regional, and Geographical Considerations

A patient's cultural values, religious beliefs, and ethnic background, as well as their national and regional identities and geographical considerations, can shape their views on end-of-life care and the use of life-sustaining therapies, such as EN. Box 25.8 identifies differences among religious perspectives on end-of-life decisions.[4,35-39] In general, among all three faiths included in Box 25.10 on page 467—Christianity, Islam, and Judaism—there is an emphasis on respect for the patient's autonomy and QOL, while striving for a peaceful experience at the end of life. Additional faith-based perspectives on ethics and AANH at the end of life are available in the literature.[2-4,36-38] The 2021 ASPEN position paper on ethics and AANH and the *ASPEN Adult Nutrition Support Core Curriculum* both provide information on ethical considerations for outside the United States and resources for additional information.[1,4] This information highlights the importance of learning about a patient's specific ethnic background as well as their country of origin, regional identity, and geographical considerations. It is important to acknowledge that each patient is unique and may follow a belief system based not only on religion but also on ethnicity and cultural values as well as and other factors when making decisions.[2,36-38]

BOX 25.9

American Medical Association Ethical Guidance for Practitioners Caring for Patients at End of Life[23]

Advance care planning and advance directives

Engage the patient in advance care planning by:

- incorporating the discussion into the medical record;
- periodically reviewing with the patient their goals, preferences, and choice of surrogate decision maker (SDM).

Prior to initiating or continuing medical treatments:

- assess the patient's decision-making capacity;
- determine whether the patient has an advance directive, whether it reflects the patient's current values and preferences, and whether the patient has designated an SDM.

Obtain assistance from an ethics committee or other appropriate institutional resource:

- if conflicts arise between the advance directive and the wishes of the patient's SDM;
- when a patient who lacks decision-making capacity has no advance directive and there is no SDM.

Withholding or withdrawing life-sustaining treatment

Review the patient's advance directive, values, goals for care, and treatment preferences.

Include the patient's SDM in the conversation.

Document all information in the medical record.

Discuss the option of initiating an intervention and evaluating its clinical effectiveness, noting that if the intervention does not achieve agreed-on goals, it can be withdrawn.

Explain that the SDM can make decisions to withhold or withdraw life-sustaining interventions when the patient lacks decision-making capacity.

Request a consultation with an ethics committee, palliative care team, or other appropriate resource.

Medically ineffective interventions

Obtain assistance from an ethics committee or other appropriate institutional resource if the patient or SDM continues to request care that you (the practitioner) deem not medically appropriate.

Respect the patient's right to appeal when the review does not support the patient's request.

Consider transferring care to another practitioner or institution that is willing to provide the desired care if the disagreement cannot be resolved through available mechanisms.

If a transfer is not possible, you (the practitioner) are under no ethical obligation to offer the intervention.

Develop an institutional policy that addresses these ethical issues.

BOX 25.10

Religious Perspectives on Health Care and End of Life[4,35-39]

Christianity

The various traditions and denominations making up the Christian faith have theological variations that may influence end-of-life decisions.[36]

Catholicism

Catholicism holds that there is a duty to preserve lives, although that duty is not absolute.[39] The following are key directives for Catholic health care services:

- Practitioners should help patients prepare for death; this includes providing necessary information for decision-making.
- A patient may forgo extraordinary or disproportionate means of preserving life; there is no moral obligation to use disproportionate or too-burdensome treatments.
- There is a general obligation to provide nutrition and hydration, including medically assisted, if the benefits outweigh the burdens.
- Practitioners should respect the informed judgment of a competent patient to accept or refuse life-sustaining treatment.

Regarding the distinction between ordinary and extraordinary treatments, *extraordinary care* means optional procedures that involve a grave burden for oneself (the patient) or another. Discontinuing medical procedures that are burdensome, dangerous, extraordinary, or disproportionate to the expected outcome can be legitimate; it is considered the refusal of overzealous treatment.[37]

In the United States, practitioners with a Roman Catholic connection are more likely to object to withdrawal of life support than are Protestants, Jews, and those with no religious designation, according to a systematic review of religious beliefs about end-of-life issues.[38] This conclusion is based on a study that analyzed data from a national survey of 1,144 physicians who objected to physician-assisted suicide, terminal sedation, and withdrawal of artificial life support, and examined associations between practitioner ethnicity, religious characteristics, and experience with patients at the end of life.[35]

Protestantism

Attitudes toward end-of-life questions differ widely among the many subgroups within the Protestant Church.[37]

When there is little hope for recovery, individuals generally understand and accept the withholding or withdrawing of a therapy.[4]

Decisions to forgo treatment are made by practitioners after informing and knowing the patient's wishes, when the practitioner deems recovery from illness impossible, or when the burden of treatment is not tolerated by the patient.[36]

Islam

In Islam, nutrition support is considered basic care and not medical treatment. If forgoing artificially administered nutrition and hydration (AANH) results in starvation, this is seen as being of greater harm than potential treatment complications. Starvation has to be avoided. However, the principle of avoiding or minimizing harm has to be followed and also applied to the delivery of AANH.[36]

Box continues

BOX 25.10 (CONTINUED)

The decision to forgo AANH in a terminally ill patient is made with informed consent, taking into account the clinical context of minimizing harm with input from the patient, family members, health care providers, and religious scholars.[36]

Premature death should be prevented, but treatments can be forgone in terminally ill individuals when practitioners are certain that death is inevitable and that treatment will not improve the patient's condition or quality of life.[4]

In a systematic review, the dignity of patients was found to be important to practitioners in their decision-making, along with religious and legal concerns.[38]

The responsibility for making the final decision regarding life-saving therapy should fall to the practitioners, who are well-informed about saving lives.[38]

Judaism

Jewish law is specific on end-of-life care; however, rabbinic interpretations may provide flexibility in approaches to end-of-life decisions.[36]

Fluids and food are considered to be basic needs and not treatment.[38]

Withdrawal of continuous life-sustaining therapy is not allowed, but withholding further treatment is allowed, as part of the dying process if the intervention is an intermittent life-sustaining treatment and if withholding treatment is a clear patient wish.[4]

Rabbinic involvement in medical decision-making may challenge conventional patient autonomy, particularly at the end of life. A careful explanation of the potential treatments and prognosis is vital to enabling the family to make decisions together with rabbis.[36]

When a patient is approaching the end of life, and if food and fluids may cause suffering or complications, it is permissible to withhold them if it is known that this is the patient's wish.[37]

Creating Institution-Specific Ethics Policies and Procedures

Despite the availability of legal precedents, position papers, and sociocultural information, a gap may still exist in clinical practice when it comes to the ethical decision-making process surrounding EN and PN as life-sustaining medical therapies. To optimize clinical practice, health care facilities should establish a proactive, integrated, systematic process and encourage increased communication of patients' health care wishes and advance care planning. A sample quality-improvement project for ethics in EN and PN is presented in Box 25.11. The purpose of such a project would be to determine whether EN and PN are being provided appropriately in the intensive care unit (ICU) based on patients' advance directive content or their preferences for health care as indicated by SDMs. Also, the project could reveal the need for more family care conferences, palliative care consults, and ethics consults. An institutional policy could be developed from this project by an interdisciplinary committee consisting of practitioners from nutrition, nursing, medical, and pharmacy services. Either nutrition or nursing services could be responsible for updating the policy and presenting the document at the meetings of various medical committees, including nutrition and metabolic, nursing, pharmacy and therapeutics, palliative care, and ICU committees, as well as any other committees that influence patient care.

Box 25.12 on page 470 offers an example of a communication policy and associated procedures for EN and PN–related health care decision-making in the ICU. Development of this type of policy and procedures would involve an interdisciplinary health care team.

1. Determine the number patients in the intensive care unit (ICU) receiving artificially administered nutrition and hydration (AANH) and the percentage of these patients who have an advance directive in their medical chart and who have had a family care conference, palliative care consult, and ethics consult.
2. Collect patient data for all individuals receiving AANH and analyze the data with an interprofessional health care team.
3. Compare the results of the analysis with current benchmarked data in the literature.
4. In collaboration with the health care team, develop an institutional policy and associated procedures for communication and ethical decision-making in patients receiving AANH; obtain approval of the policy and procedures through medical committees.
5. Educate the interdisciplinary health care team on the policy and procedures and implement them.
6. Recount the number of patients in the ICU receiving AANH to determine the effects of the change in practice and assess its sustainability.
7. Share best practices for ethics in the use of AANH among health care institutions and organizations.

The protocol would incorporate a review of the position papers, statements, and guidelines issued by relevant national organizations[13,16-24] and would be modified for the specific institution's patient population, as appropriate. Although the example focuses on the ICU patient, it can serve as a model for other units to develop a similar policy and set of procedures to be used with variation in other sections of the hospital, such as the emergency room and general medical-surgical units. Each facility would need to modify the policy and procedures based on its access to palliative care teams and the staff available for screening. Nursing services could be responsible for updating the policy and presenting the document at meetings of various medical committees, including nutrition and metabolic, nursing, pharmacy and therapeutics, palliative care, and ICU committees, as well as any other committees that influence patient care.

Health care facilities that develop a proactive, integrated, systematic process for ethical EN and PN decision-making may improve the communication process for patients, family members, SDMs, and health care practitioners. Written documentation in the medical record is important, and verbal communication between the patient, family, or SDM and the health care team about the patient's wishes for medical therapies, including EN and PN, is beneficial. For example, a discussion between the health care team and the patient, family, or SDM about the uses and potential benefits of EN and PN vs the burdens and risks may provide an opening for a broader conversation about the goals of care and use of other life-sustaining medical therapies. Ideally, the decision-making process should start early, before a patient is ill and hospitalized, with individuals engaging in and becoming empowered by advance care planning.

Ethical Considerations During a Pandemic

The COVID-19 pandemic has presented the US health care system with unprecedented ethical challenges. Beyond the ethical principles already discussed, there are some nuances that need to be considered during a pandemic.

First, special attention needs to be paid to the health care staff. The principles of beneficence and nonmaleficence are of particular importance when delivering care at the bedside, and it is imperative that routines for the monitoring and delivery of care, including nutrition interventions, be modified in order to provide the patient with the necessary care. Yet, there is an ethical obligation to also minimize the risks to the health care team and keep them safe

BOX 25.12

Sample Communication Policy and Procedures for Enteral and Parenteral Nutrition–Related Health Care Choices in the Intensive Care Unit

Policy: It is the policy of this institution to provide ethically and medically appropriate enteral nutrition (EN) and parenteral nutrition (PN) in the hospital instensive care unit (ICU) setting, based on evidence-based guidelines and recommendations of national organizations.

Purpose: The purpose is to promote health literacy and written documentation in the medical record concerning health care decisions about EN and PN. The intent is to promote early communication between health care practitioners, patients, family members, and surrogate decision makers (SDMs), with attention given to spiritual or faith needs and cultural diversity.

Important considerations: [Include here components from guidelines of the Academy of Nutrition and Dietetics, American Society for Parenteral and Entereal Nutrition (ASPEN), American Medical Association (AMA), and other organizations as appropriate for the institution population, culture, and religious affiliation.]

Procedures:

- Health care practitioners should participate in training sessions on communication, spiritual and cultural diversity, difficult topics, role playing, and the teach-back method of communication.
- Practitioners should complete an evaluation tool after a discussion with the patient, family, or SDM. This tool should incorporate both the health care practitioner's evaluation and the patient, family, or SDM evaluation. The results should be reviewed for revisions and reevaluated periodically.
- Information obtained about a patient's health care choices for EN and PN must be communicated both verbally with health care team and in writing in medical record.
- Patients in the ICU for 3 or more days should be screened for palliative care needs based on defined screening criteria, as developed by the palliative care team. Patients should be identified during ICU rounds as being at high risk for palliative care needs in order to facilitate health care choices to meet quality-of-life (QOL) goals, including EN and PN use.
- Family care conferences are recommended for patients expected to be in the ICU for 5 to 7 days or less. These conferences should incorporate a discussion of EN and PN, as appropriate. Conference outcomes and recommended plans should be documented in the progress notes.

References: [Add citations of relevance to the facility.]

Approval: [Signed and dated by the medical committee]

---

and healthy. An example of a modified routine might be the clustering of care to minimize the number of entries into a patient's room.

Second, it is essential to recognize the potential for an increased sense of isolation and depression in patients, for in most cases no visitors, or only a limited number of visitors, are allowed in the hospital during a pandemic. Ensuring that patients have frequent audio and visual communications with loved ones via current technology may reduce feelings of isolation and depression, as well as delirium, which is particularly seen in elderly patients and those with dementia. In addition, health care professionals can exercise beneficence and justice for patients by assuring that every patient is provided with optimal nutrition screening, assessment, and intervention in a timely manner, regardless of their circumstances.

Third, although it is unlikely that nutrition products and equipment would become scarce to the same degree that other interventions (eg, ventilators and personal protective equipment) would during a pandemic, health care institutions should have written protocols in place to deal with the appropriate and standardized allocation of limited resources.

Establishing a framework for developing such protocols is helpful. Suggested frameworks have been published.[32,40-48] When rationing resources, a deviation from the usual hierarchy of ethical principles is sometimes necessary. Whereas respect for individual autonomy is usually the most important of the four ethical principles, in the presence of resource scarcity, the interest of the state or community may supersede that of the individual. The principle of distributive justice may override individual autonomy in order to save the most lives or maximize improvements in individuals after treatment by providing medical therapies to the greatest number in order to decrease the total number of people harmed. Codifying an institutional or regional protocol that provides for a fair and consistent decision-making process in these situations can mitigate, to a larger extent, the potential for legal claims of unilateral and capricious actions.

Bioethics committees are available in institutions for individual conflict resolutions. These committees usually consist of administrators, health care professionals, community members, patient representatives, and other stakeholders. A bioethics committee should have a similar ethnic, religious, and cultural makeup to the institution's patient population, as cultural competency and the ability to form trusting bonds are essential to resolving conflicts. Additionally, committee members participate in protocol development. However, in times of limited resources, as during a pandemic, the execution of the protocols should be carried out by a separate group, often referred to as a triage committee, that does not include any of the treating team's members. Although these committees and the health care team are considered multidisciplinary and interdisciplinary in their administrative and organizational structures, they should work in a transdisciplinary, or cross-functional, manner such that the most capable and available individual carries out the required function, regardless of their discipline. However, each individual team member must still function within limits of their state or federal certification, registration, or license.

In sum, a pandemic such as COVID-19 presents health care practitioners with additional and at times divergent ethical considerations while at the same time recognizing that ethics and law are but two of the three challenges practitioners face in these situations. The third one is *technology*, which at times presents unforeseen difficulties, further complicating the other two. The conundrum resulting from what can be done technologically, what should be done ethically, and what must be done legally has been dubbed "the troubling trichotomy."[49]

Summary

Ethical and legal issues related to the use and discontinuation of EN have been addressed for decades. Several national health care organizations, including the Academy of Nutrition and Dietetics and ASPEN, have provided recommendations on this topic. Common themes in these recommendations are patient autonomy, use of informed SDMs when individuals are unable to speak for themselves, the need for an interdisciplinary approach, consideration of the benefits vs the burdens and risks associated with life-sustaining therapies based on the individual's QOL goals, and the importance of advance care planning.

An individual's views on end-of-life care and use of life-sustaining therapies, such as EN, may be shaped by their religious convictions and ethnic and cultural background. Health care providers need to respect the values and uniqueness of every individual in their care. To this end, health care facilities should consider developing institutional policies and procedures to assist health care practitioners in ethical and legal areas and empower patients in their own advance care planning. Additional policies and procedures incorporating ethical considerations should be developed to deal with providing health care during a pandemic or other crisis situation when resources are limited.

References

1. Schwartz DB, Barrocas A, Annetta MG, et al. Ethical aspects of artificially administered nutrition and hydration: an ASPEN position paper. *Nutr Clinc Prac.* 2021;36(2):254-267. doi:10.1002/ncp.10633

2. Schwartz DB. Ethical considerations in the critically ill patient. In: Cresci G, ed. *Nutritional Therapy for the Critically Ill Patient: A Guide to Practice.* 2nd ed. Taylor and Francis; 2015:635-652.

3. Barrocas A, Schwartz DB. Ethical considerations in nutrition support in critical care. In: Seres DS, Van Way III CW, eds. *Nutrition Support for the Critically Ill.* Springer International Publishing; 2016:195-227.

4. Schwartz DB, Barrocas A. Ethics and law. In: Mueller C, Lord LM, Marian M, McClave SA, and Miller S, eds. *The ASPEN Adult Nutrition Support Core Curriculum.* 3rd ed. American Society for Parenteral and Enteral Nutrition; 2017:785-804.

5. Patient Self Determination Act of 1990, HR 4449, 101st Cong (1989-1990). Accessed January 26, 2021. www.congress.gov/bill/101st-congress/house-bill/4449

6. Barrocas A, Cohen ML. Have the answers to common legal questions concerning nutrition support changed over the past decade? 10 questions for 10 years. *Nutr Clin Prac.* 2016;31(3):285-293.

7. The Joint Commission. Accessed January 26, 2021. www.jointcommission.org

8. Academy Nutrition and Dietetics. The Joint Commission. Accessed January 26, 2021. www.eatrightpro.org/practice/quality-management/national-quality-accreditation-and-regulations/the-joint-commission

9. American Medical Association. Informed consent. In: *Code of Medical Ethics.* American Medical Association. 2016:chap 2, opinion 2.1.1. Accessed January 26, 2021. www.ama-assn.org/sites/default/files/media-browser/code-of-medical-ethics-chapter-2.pdf

10. Sukkar S, Barranco R, Ventura F, Molinelli A. Informed consent and percutaneous endoscopic gastrostomy (PEG): the difficulties of a single European viewpoint. *Prog Nutr.* 2017;19(4):359-368. doi:10.23751/pn.v19i4.5939

11. Chaet DH. AMA *Code of Medical Ethics'* opinions on patient decision-making capacity and competence and surrogate decision making. *AMA J Ethics.* 2017;19(7):675-677. doi:10.1001/journalofethics.2017.19.7.coet1-1707

12. Reddy R, Chaet DH. AMA *Code of Medical Ethics'* opinions related to end-of-life care. *AMA J Ethics.* 2018;20(8):E738-742. doi:10.1001/amajethics.2018.738

13. ANA Center for Ethics and Human Rights. Position statement: nutrition and hydration at the end of life. Effective 2017. Accessed January 16, 2021. www.nursingworld.org/~4af0ed/globalassets/docs/ana/ethics/ps_nutrition-and-hydration-at-the-end-of-life_2017june7.pdf

14. National POLST. Honoring the wishes of those with serious illness and frailty. Accessed January 26, 2021. https://polst.org

15. *National POLST Legislative Guide.* 2020. Accessed January 26, 2021. https://polst.org/wp-content/uploads/2020/11/2020-POLST-Legislative-Guide.pdf

16. Greer DM, Shemie SD, Lewis A, et al. Determination of brain death/death by neurologic criteria: the World Brain Death Project. *JAMA.* 2020;324(11):1078-1097. doi:10.1001/jama.2020.11586

17. Schwartz DB. Ethical decisions for withholding/withdrawing medically assisted nutrition and hydration. *J Acad Nutr Diet.* 2015(3);115:440-443. doi:10.1016/j.jand.2015.01.002

18. Hospice and Palliative Nurses Association. HPNA position statement: medically administered nutrition and hydration. January 2020. Accessed August 18, 2020. https://advancingexpertcare.org/position-statements

19. Alzheimer's Association. Feeding issues in advanced dementia. 2015. Accessed January 26, 2021. www.alz.org/media/Documents/feeding-issues-statement.pdf

20. Schwartz DB, Barrocas A, Wesley JR, et al. Gastrostomy tube placement in patients with advanced dementia or near end of life. *Nutr Clinc Prac.* 2014;29(6):829-840. doi:10.1177/0884533614546890

21. American Academy of Hospice and Palliative Medicine: five things physicians and patients should question. Choosing Wisely website. Revised January 14, 2021. Accessed January 26, 2021. www.choosingwisely.org/societies/american-academy-of-hospice-and-palliative-medicine

22. American Geriatrics Society Ethics Committee and Clinical Practice and Models of Care Committee. American Geriatrics Society feeding tubes in advanced dementia position statement. *J Am Geriatr Soc.* 2014;62(8):1590-1593. doi:10.1111/jgs.12924

23. American Medical Association. Opinions on caring for patients at the end of life. In: *Code of Medical Ethics.* American Medical Association; 2016:chap 5. Accessed January 7, 2021. www.ama-assn.org/sites/default /files/media-browser/code-of-medical-ethics-chapter -5.pdf

24. Academy of Nutrition and Dietetics; Commission on Dietetic Registration. Code of Ethics for the Nutrition and Dietetics Profession. Accessed January 26, 2021. www.eatrightpro.org/-/media/eatrightpro-files/career /code-of-ethics/codeofethicshandout.pdf

25. Feeding tubes for people with Alzheimer's: when you need them—and when you don't. Choosing Wisely website. May 2013. Accessed January 23, 2021. www .choosingwisely.org/patient-resources/feeding-tubes -for-people-with-alzheimers

26. Five Wishes. Accessed January 26, 2021. https:/ /fivewishes.org/Home

27. National Healthcare Decisions Day—April 16. The Conversation Project website. Accessed March 2, 2022. https://theconversationproject.org/nhdd

28. The Conversation Project. Accessed January 26, 2021. https://theconversationproject.org

29. Cleveland Clinic Center for Human Nutrition, Dietitians in Nutrition Support Dietetic Practice Group. Advanced practice residency in adult nutrition support. Accessed March 10, 2022. https://my.clevelandclinic .org/departments/digestive/medical-professionals /education/adult-nutrition-advanced-practice -residency

30. ASPEN. ASPEN's international clinical ethics section. Accessed March 10, 2022. www.nutritioncare.org /about_aspen/membership/sections/international _clinical_ethics_section/international_clinical _ethics_section

31. Schwartz DB, Pavic-Zabinski K, Tull K. Role of a nutrition support clinician on a hospital bioethics committee. *Nutr Clinc Prac.* 2019;34(6):869-880.

32. Barrocas A, Schwartz DB, Seres DS, Hasse JM, Mueller CM. Ethical framework for nutrition support resource allocation during shortages: lessons from COVID-19. *Nutr Clinc Prac.* 2020;35(4):599-605.

33. Palacek EJ, Teno JM, Cassaret DJ, et al. Comfort feeding only: a proposal to bring clarity to decision-making regarding difficulty with eating for persons with advanced dementia. *J Am Geriatrics Soc.* 2010;58(3):580-584.

34. Cardenas D. Ethical issues and dilemmas in artificial nutrition and hydration. *Clin Nutr ESPEN.* 2021;41:23-29. doi:10.1016/j.clnesp.2020.12.010

35. Curlin FA, Nwodim C, Vance JL, et al. To die, to sleep: US physicians' religious and other objections to physician-assisted suicide, terminal sedation, and withdrawal of life support. *Am J Hosp Palliat Care.* 2008;25(2):112-120. doi:10.1177/1049909107310141

36. Choudry M, Latif A, Warburton KG. An overview of the spiritual importances of end-of-life care among the five major faiths of the United Kingdom. *Clin Med (Lond).* 2018;18(1):23-31. doi:10.7861/clinmedicine.18 -1-23

37. Druml C, Ballmer PE, Druml W, et al. ESPEN guideline on ethical aspects of artificial nutrition and hydration. *Clin Nutr.* 2016;35(3):545-556.

38. Chakraborty R, El-Jawahri AR, Litzow MR, Syrjala KL, Parnes AD, Hashmi SK. A systematic review of religious beliefs about major end-of-life issues in the five major world religions. *Palliat Support Care.* 2017;15(5):609-622. doi:10.1017/S1478951516001061

39. United States Conference of Catholic Bishops. *Ethical and Religious Directives for Catholic Health Care Services.* 6th ed. United States Conference of Catholic Bishops; 2018. Accessed March 4, 2022. www.usccb .org/about/doctrine/ethical-and-religious-directives /upload/ethical-religious-directives-catholic-health -service-sixth-edition-2016-06.pdf

40. Gostin LO, Friedman EA, Wetter SA. Responding to COVID-19: how to navigate a public health emergency legally and ethically. *Hastings Cent Rep.* 2020;50(2): 8-12.

41. Emanuel EJ, Persad G, Upshur R, et al. Fair allocation of scarce medical resources in the time of Covid-19. *N Engl J Med.* 2020;382:2049-2055.

42. White DB, Lo B. A framework for rationing ventilators and critical care beds during the COVID-19 pandemic. *JAMA.* 2020;323(18):1773-1774.

43. Cohen IG, Crespo AM, White DB. Potential legal liability for withdrawing or withholding ventilators during COVID-19: assessing the risks and identifying needed reforms. *JAMA.* 2020;323(19):1901-1902.

44. Berlinger N, Wynia M, Powell T, et al. Ethical framework for health care institutions and guidelines for institutional ethics services responding to the coronavirus pandemic. The Hastings Center. March 16, 2020. Accessed January 26, 2021. www .thehastingscenter.org/ethicalframeworkcovid19

45. Kramer JB, Brown DE, Kopar PK. Ethics in the time of coronavirus: recommendations in the COVID-19-pandemic. *J Am Coll Surg.* 2020;230(6):1114-1118.

46. Prachand VN, Milner R, Angelos P, et al. Medically necessary, time-sensitive procedures: scoring system to ethically and efficiently manage resource scarcity and provider risk during the COVID-19 pandemic. *J Am Coll Surg.* 2020;231(2):281-288.

47. Angelos P. Surgeons, ethics and COVID-19: early lessons learned. *J Am Coll Surg.* 2020;230(6):1119-1120.

48. Binkley CE, Kemp DS. Ethical rationing of personal protective equipment to minimize moral residue during the COVID-19 pandemic. *J Am Coll Surg.* 2020;230(6):1111-1113.

49. Barrocas A. The troubling trichotomy 10 years later: where are we now? *Nutr Clin Pract.* 2016;31(3):295-304.

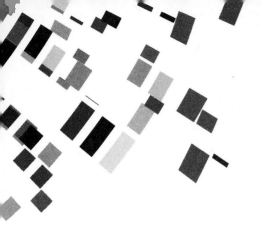

Continuing Professional Education

The second edition of the *Health Professional's Guide to Gastronintestinal Nutrition* offers readers 12 hours of Continuing Professional Education (CPE) credit from the Comission on Dietetic Registration. Readers may earn credit by completing the interactive quiz at:

https://publications.webauthor.com/HPG_to_GI_2nd

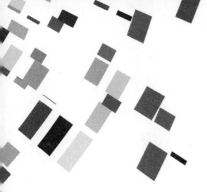

Index

Letters *b*, *f* and *t* after page number indicate box, figure, and table, respectively.

A

AAAs. *See* aromatic amino acids
AAD. *See* antibiotic-associated diarrhea
AANH. *See* artificially administered nutrition and hydration
abundance, of intestinal microbiome, 225*b*
Academy of Nutrition and Dietetics
    on cancer nutrition screening, 158
    Code of Ethics of, 459, 460*b*–461*b*
    on malnutrition documentation, 19
    on nutrition screening, 3
    on obesity diets, 179
acid-base balance, 7
AcipHex. *See* rabeprazole
ACP. *See* advance care planning
Actigall. *See* ursodeoxycholic acid
acute-phase proteins, 18
Acute Physiology and Chronic Health Evaluation II (APACHE II), 4, 5*b*
acute renal insufficiency, 195
adalimumab, 28*b*
Addison disease, 94*b*
adjustable gastric banding (AGB), 306, 308, 309, 310*f*, 311–314, 322*t*
α2-adrenergic receptor antagonist, 67*b*
advance care planning (ACP), 452, 455*b*, 457, 465*b*
aflatoxins, 149*t*
AGB. *See* adjustable gastric banding
alanine aminotransferase (ALT), 415*b*
albumin
    as acute-phase protein, 18
    HPEN and, 415*b*
alcohol
    after bariatric surgery, 320
    cancer and, 149*t*
    esophageal cancer and, 163
    liver disease from, 109
    osteoporosis and, 123
    pancreatitis and, 127
alkaline phosphatase (ALP), 415*b*
Alli. *See* orlistat
allytic sulfides, 150*b*
aloe vera, 434–435

for IBD, 443*b*
    for IBS, 83*t*, 84
alopecia areata, 94*b*
ALP. *See* alkaline phosphatase
alpha-gal syndrome, 209
ALT. *See* alanine aminotransferase
AMA. *See* American Medical Association
amenorrhea, 199*b*
American Medical Association (AMA)
    on EOL, 465, 466*b*
    on informed consent, 458*b*
American Society for Parenteral and Enteral Nutrition (ASPEN)
    on AANH, 455, 464, 464*b*–465*b*
    on cancer nutrition screening, 158
    on critically ill patients, 16–17
    on gastrostomy, 462–463, 462*b*, 463*f*
    on HPEN shortages, 417*b*
    on malnutrition documentation, 19
    on nutrition screening, 3
    on protein requirements, 18
    on Tralement, 416, 416*t*
amino acids. *See also* branched-chain amino acid
    AAAs, 121–122
    pancreas and, 126
    in pediatric PN, 386*t*
    in PN, 366, 366*t*
amoxicillin and clavulanic acid (Augmentin)
    for pediatric dysmotility, 144
    for SBS, 67*b*
amylase-trypsin inhibitors (ATIs), 80
AN. *See* anorexia nervosa
anal fissures
    flexible sigmoidoscopy for, 30
    pediatric constipation and, 145
anaphylaxis, 208–209, 209*b*
Andrographis paniculata (HMPL-004), 443b
anemia
    eating disorders and, 192*b*, 199*b*
    gastric surgery and, 295, 297*b*
    with IBD, 46–47
    iron deficiency, 94*b*
anorectal motility study, 35–36
anorexia, 186
    from antineoplastic therapy, 156*b*
    esophageal cancer and, 163
anorexia nervosa (AN), 185
    diagnostic criteria for, 187*b*

Human Milk Banking Association of North America (HMBA-NA), 379
β-hydroxy-beta-methylbutyrate (HMB), 155
hyperaldosteronemia, 196, 199*b*
hyperammonemia, 390
hyperamylasemia, 198*b*
hypereosinophilic syndrome, 139
hyperglycemia
    with EN, 356*b*
    with HPEN, 413*b*
    with liver disease, 123
    with pediatric PN and, 390–391
    with PN, 372*b*
hyperlipidemia
    eating disorders and, 198*b*
    obesity and, 307*t*
    waist circumference and, 12
hypermagnesemia, 193, 195–196
hypernatremia
    with EN, 356*b*
    with licorice root, 436
hyperphosphatemia, 357*b*
hypertension. *See also* portal hypertension
    alcohol-related liver disease and, 109
    CF and, 137
    obesity and, 305*b*, 307*t*
    waist circumference and, 12
hypertriglyceridemia
    with pediatric PN, 392, 392*t*
    with PN, 372*b*
hypochloremia, 198*b*
hypoglycemia
    eating disorders and, 198*b*
    with EN, 356*b*
    with HPEN, 413*b*
    MSUD and, 141
    with PN, 372*b*
hypokalemia
    eating disorders and, 199*b*
    with HPEN, 414*b*
    with licorice root, 436
hypomagnesemia
    eating disorders and, 193
    with HPEN, 414*b*
hyponatremia
    cirrhosis and, 111, 112
    eating disorders and, 193
hypophosphatemia
    eating disorders and, 193, 198*b*
    with HPEN, 414*b*
hypothyroidism
    constipation and, 145
    obesity and, 175
hypoventilation syndrome, 305*b*
hypovolemia, 193

I

IBD. *See* inflammatory bowel disease
IBD-AID. *See* anti-inflammatory diet for IBD
Iberogast. *See* STW 5
IBS. *See* irritable bowel syndrome
IBS-D. *See* diarrhea-predominant IBS
ibuprofen, 137
ideal body weight (IBW), 10
    protein and, 18
idiopathic dilated cardiomyopathy, 94*b*
IgA. *See* immunoglobulin A
IgE. *See* immunoglobulin E
IgG. *See* immunoglobulin G
IL-6. *See* interleukin-6
ILE. *See* intravenous lipid emulsion
ileostomy, 298, 299*b*
immune system
    intestinal microbiome and, 228, 228*b*
    prebiotics and, 258*b*, 259
    probiotics and, 268–269
immunoglobulin A (IgA), 94*b*, 96–97, 96*t*
immunoglobulin E (IgE)
    food allergies and, 208–213, 210*b*–211*b*
    IBS and, 76
immunoglobulin G (IgG)
    celiac disease and, 97
    for food allergies, 211*b*
immunomodulating diets, 129
immunotherapy, 156*b*
Imodium. *See* loperamide
inborn errors of metabolism, 140–141
    EN infant formulas for, 382
Indigo naturalis (Qing-Dai), 445*b*
indoles, cancer prevention from, 152*b*
infant formulas, 379–383, 380*b*, 381*b*, 383*b*
infertility
    eating disorders and, 199*b*
    obesity and, 305*b*
inflammatory bowel disease (IBD), 42–55. *See also* Crohn's disease; ulcerative colitis
    anemia with, 46–47
    bone health and, 46
    clinical presentation of, 44
    colonoscopy for, 30
    diets for, 49–54, 50*b*–53*bb*
    EN for, 48–49
    flexible sigmoidoscopy for, 30
    IBS and, 74
    intestinal microbiome and, 228, 230
    malabsorption and, 45
    malnutrition and, 44–46
    marijuana for, 439
    nutraceutical supplements for, 433, 442, 443*b*–445*b*
    nutrition management of, 44–48, 46*t*

K

ketogenic diet, 241b, 243
keystone species, of intestinal microbiome, 225b
Korsakoff syndrome, 199b

L

lactic acidosis, 61
lactose intolerance
    IBS and, 76–77
    with RYGB, 317
    SBS and, 60
lactulose, 121
lansoprazole (Prevacid), 66b
lanugo, 199b
late dumping syndrome, 316
laxatives. See also specific types
    AN and, 186
    for colonoscopy, 30
    drug-nutrient interactions with, 424, 425b
    eating disorders and, 193, 195–196
LC-MC/MC. See liquid-chromatography with tandem mass spectrometry
LDL-C. See low-density lipoprotein-cholesterol
legal issues
    of AANH, 452–471, 453b–462b, 463f, 464b–470b
    common questions on, 458b–459b
    of EOL, 456–457, 456b–457b
    with QOL, 452
legumes, 238b, 239–240
leukopenia, 192b, 199b
Levaquin. See levofloxacin
levetiracetam, 142
levofloxacin (Levaquin), 67b
licorice root (Glycyrrhiza glabra), 436
life-sustaining treatment, 454b
lignans, 152b
lignin, 152b
α-linoleic acid, 150b
lipase, 192b
lipid-regulating drugs, 429–430, 430b
lipids. See also dyslipidemia; hyperlipidemia
    intestinal microbiome and, 228b
    pancreatitis and, 130
    in pediatric PN, 386t
    in PN, 367, 368t
    profile, 7
liquid-chromatography with tandem mass spectrometry (LC-MS/MS), 28b
liraglutide (Saxenda), 181t, 329
lisdexamfetamine, 201
liver cancer, 149b
    cirrhosis and, 111

liver disease, 109–123. See also cirrhosis; hepatitis
    CF and, 135, 137
    clinical presentation and diagnosis of, 110–112, 111f, 112b
    complications of, 121–123, 122f
    eating disorders and, 196–197
    ERCP for, 34
    with HPEN, 414b
    intestinal microbiome and, 228b
    malnutrition and, 109, 113–121, 115b–117b, 118b–120b
    nutraceutical supplements for, 433
    pathogenesis of, 109–110
    tests for, 28b
liver transplantation
    for CF, 137
    for cirrhosis, 113
Lomotil. See diphenoxylate with atropine
Look AHEAD, 179
loperamide (Imodium)
    drug-nutrient interactions of, 423
    for SBS, 66b
low-density lipoprotein-cholesterol (LDL-C), 259–260
low-residue diet, 53b
lumacaftor, 137
luteinizing hormone, 192b
lycopene, 152b
lysosomal acid lipase, 28b

M

macronutrient-based diet, 177–178
macronutrients. See also carbohydrate; fat; protein
    after bariatric surgery, 319–320
    eating disorders and, 192–193
magnesium. See also hypermagnesemia; hypomagnesemia
    in antacids, 423b
    antidiarrheals and, 423
    eating disorders and, 195–196
    gastric surgery and, 295
    HPEN and, 415b
    liver disease and, 120b
    pediatric neurologic impairments and, 142
    in PN, 363t, 367, 368t
magnesium gluconate, 64t
magnesium lactate, 64t
malabsorption, 7
    with celiac disease, 101
    CF and, 135
    with EN, 352, 355b
    gastric surgery and, 295
    HPEN and, 410b
    IBD and, 45
    inborn errors of metabolism and, 140
    pancreatic cancer and, 165–166
    PEI and, 130–131

personality disorders, 190

PERT. *See* pancreatic enzyme replacement therapy

Pertzye, 426

PG-SGA. *See* Patient-Generated Subjective Global Assessment

phenobarbital, 142

phenolic acid, 153*b*

phentermine HCl, 181*t,* 329

phenytoin, 142

phosphate
> in antacids, 423*b*
> in EN infant formulas, 382

phosphorus
> celiac disease and, 102*b*
> gastric surgery and, 295
> HPEN and, 415*b*
> liver disease and, 120*b*
> PN and, 363*t,* 367, 368*t*
> for SBS, 64*t*

PN. *See* parenteral nutrition

PNAC. *See* parenteral nutrition-associated cholestasis

PN-associated liver disease (PNALD), 68

pneumothorax, 372*b*

policy development and review, 453*b*

pollen-food allergy syndrome (oral allergy syndrome), 210

POLST. *See* portable medical orders

polyacetylene, 153*b*

polycystic ovary syndrome, 305*b*

polyethylene glycol
> for AN, 195
> for CF, 137
> for colonoscopy, 30
> for constipation, 137, 145, 195

polymerase chain reaction (PCR), 28*b*

polyphenolic acids, 151*b*

polyphenols, 437

polyunsaturated fatty acids (PUFAs)
> in fish oils, 440
> IBD and, 43
> intestinal microbiome and, 230, 245*b*

portable medical orders (POLST), 455*b,* 459*b*

portal hypertension
> CF and, 137
> cirrhosis and, 111

potassium. *See also* hypokalemia
> antidiarrheals and, 423
> eating disorders and, 195
> HPEN and, 415*b*
> IBD and, 47*t*
> in PN, 363*t,* 367, 368*t*

potassium chloride, 64*t*

PPIs. *See* proton pump inhibitors

prealbumin, 18

prebiotics, 233–234, 254–260
> benefits of, 257–260, 257*b*–258*b*
> in diet, 256–257
> in EN infant formulas, 383*b*

vs. fiber, 255–256, 255*f*
> for hepatic encephalopathy, 122
> for IBS, 81–82
> polyphenols as, 437
> recommended intake of, 260

PREDIMED. *See* Prevención con Dieta Mediterránea

pregnancy
> after bariatric surgery, 328–329
> celiac disease and, 96

Prevacid. *See* lansoprazole

Prevención con Dieta Mediterránea (PREDIMED), 179

preventive ethics, 454*b*

Prilosec. *See* omeprazole

probiotics, 233–234, 265–279
> benefits of, 268–269, 269*f*
> for CDI, 271–272
> for Crohn's disease, 267, 273–274
> for diarrhea, 270–273
> efficacy of, 267–268
> in EN, 345*b*
> in EN infant formulas, 383*b*
> for Helicobacter pylori, 273
> for hepatic encephalopathy, 122
> for IBD, 273–275
> for IBS, 81–82, 275–278, 276*b*–277*b*
> nomenclature for, 268*b*
> for pancreatitis, 129
> safety of, 278–279
> taxonomy of, 267, 267*b*
> for ulcerative colitis, 267, 274–275

prochlorperazine, 426*b*

prokinetic agents
> drug-nutrient interactions of, 428–429, 428*b*
> peppermint oil as, 439

protectants, 426–428, 427*b*

protein
> after bariatric surgery, 319
> for cancer, 159–160
> in EN, 341*b*–345*b,* 346
> in EN infant formulas, 380–381, 380*b*
> intestinal microbiome and, 245*b*
> liver disease and, 118*b*
> nitrogen balance and, 18, 18*b*
> obesity diet and, 177–178
> pancreas and, 126
> pancreatitis and, 129*b,* 130
> for pediatric dysmotility, 144
> in pediatric PN, 387
> profile, 7
> refeeding syndrome and, 201
> requirements for, 17–18
> surgery and, 286

prothrombin time (PT), 415*b*

Protonix. *See* pantoprazole

proton pump inhibitors (PPIs)
> for AAD, 270

V